ROSS & WILSON
PATHOPHYSIOLOGY

ROSS & WILSON PATHOPHYSIOLOGY

Allison Grant BSc, PhD, FHEA
Lecturer, School of Health and Life Sciences
Glasgow Caledonian University
Glasgow
UK

ELSEVIER

Notices

Practitioners and researchers must always rely on their own experience and knowledge in evaluating and using any information, methods, compounds or experiments described herein. Because of rapid advances in the medical sciences, in particular, independent verification of diagnoses and drug dosages should be made. To the fullest extent of the law, no responsibility is assumed by Elsevier, authors, editors or contributors for any injury and/or damage to persons or property as a matter of products liability, negligence or otherwise, or from any use or operation of any methods, products, instructions, or ideas contained in the material herein.

ISBN: 978-0-7020-7771-5

Content Strategist: Andrae Akeh
Content Project Manager: Fariha Nadeem
Design: Margaret Reid
Illustration Manager: Muthukumaran Thangaraj
Marketing Manager: Deborah Watkins

Printed in India

Last digit is the print number: 9 8 7 6 5 4 3 2 1

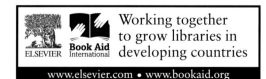

Contents

Preface   vi

Acknowledgements   vii

1   Introduction to Pathophysiological Processes   1

2   Genetics and Disease   24

3   Neoplasia   61

4   Disorders of Immunity   88

5   Disorders of Blood   110

6   Disorders of Cardiovascular Function   132

7   Disorders of Respiratory Function   168

8   Disorders of Neurological Function   197

9   Disorders of the Special Senses   238

10   Disorders of Endocrine Function   251

11   Disorders of Gastrointestinal Function   272

12   Disorders of Renal Function   300

13   Disorders of Musculoskeletal Function   322

14   Disorders of Reproductive Function   348

15   Skin   375

Index   391

Preface

The human body is a wonderful machine: complex, sophisticated, truly beautiful, and—if looked after—generally pretty reliable. From ancient times, early medical practitioners have studied anatomy (the structure of the body), physiology (the mechanisms by which the body functions), and therapeutics (remedies used to cure illness or to alleviate its signs and symptoms). Pathology is the study of disease, and pathophysiology is the study of disordered function of body systems and processes that follow disease, ageing, or injury, as well as the causes and consequences of this disordered function. It is a relatively young branch of medical science; it draws on the disciplines of anatomy, physiology, pathology, microbiology, genetics, biochemistry, molecular biology, and cell biology. Increased life expectancy and medical advances that allow people to survive diseases that carried significant mortality even a few decades ago have led to rising numbers of people living with chronic disorders. A sound knowledge of pathophysiology is an essential part of any healthcare professional's toolkit: understanding the underlying disease processes identifies risk factors, explains associated signs and symptoms, informs on prognosis and anticipated consequences, and is fundamental to choosing optimal treatments.

This textbook explains the pathophysiology of a comprehensive range of important diseases and disorders. It goes beyond simple descriptions and explains the underlying processes, without getting bogged down in excessive detail. To put the pathophysiology in context, each chapter begins with a brief summary of key anatomy and physiology relevant to the content of the chapter. Because this book is primarily aimed at students and practitioners in the medical and healthcare professions, each section includes a short summary of the main treatments most likely to be currently offered (although the field of therapeutics moves rapidly!).

I hope that this book is a useful addition to the current library of medical literature. It offers a middle ground between the many excellent, advanced, and highly detailed pathophysiology resources available and the body of simplified texts, which offer an accessible introduction but which may lack adequate background and explanation to meet the needs of some readers.

This project has been long in the making, and the timing happened to encompass the lockdowns, restrictions, and turbulent living and working patterns that the SARS-CoV-2 (COVID) pandemic brought as it swept across the world. I suppose at least it meant that with all concerts, shows, socialising, and other entertainments cancelled and nothing better to do, I probably had more time to get on with the book. I am very proud of it, but I welcome suggestions, corrections, and comments from students and colleagues. Academic resources are always improved by collaboration, discussion, and co-operation!

Allison Grant
April 2023

Acknowledgements

The preparation of an academic textbook of this scope and magnitude is a major undertaking. There were times when I wondered why I had ever embarked on this task, and I am so very pleased and proud to see it come to fruition. I have said 'my book', but there has been an army of people with me all the way through without whom not one word would have seen the light of day.

The team at Elsevier encouraged, supported, and advised me. Thank you in particular to Fariha Nadeem, who has been a constant, practical, and calm presence. Thanks are due also to Robert Edwards, Poppy Garraway, and Marie Dean, who patiently and skilfully translated my rough drawings into clear and detailed illustrations. There is also a team of professionals at Elsevier with whom I never have direct contact but who actually converted my submitted manuscript into the final product: thank you all.

Thanks to Pauline Graham, formerly of Elsevier, who suggested the project in the first place. Thank you too to Anne Waugh, my co-author on Ross and Wilson Anatomy and Physiology in Health and Illness, who reviewed some of the content and made helpful and constructive suggestions. My debt of thanks owed to Anne goes much further back than this project: as an experienced academic author taking a rookie under her wing many years ago, she has always been a patient teacher, a reliable guide and advisor, the most eagle-eyed proof-reader I have ever met, and a good friend.

I also want to thank my departmental friends and colleagues in the Department of Biological and Biomedical Sciences at Glasgow Caledonian University. They didn't actually help me write any of this (so cannot be blamed for any errors), but I greatly value the collegiate and supportive environment to be found in our workplace.

I have taught many students over the years, and every one of them has shaped my professional career and practice. The 'lightbulb moment' when a student's face changes because they suddenly 'get' it never fails to make me smile. Students' interest and curiosity, and watching and guiding their development as they move along their learning path from first years to postgraduates, are such an important part of academic job satisfaction. Thank you to you all: keep asking questions; don't expect me to have all the answers; be prepared to go out and find the answers for yourselves; and if I have helped you to do that, I'll be happy.

I am very grateful for the love and support of my friends and family. They listened patiently when I was stressed and tired. Not once did anyone tell me to put a sock in it and just get on with the job. Finally, I have very special thanks for my two gorgeous kids, Seona and Struan. COVID wasn't an easy time for anyone, but you made it so much more bearable. Thanks for the cups of coffee, for the tolerant ear listening to how anxious/frustrated/hacked off I became at regular intervals along the way, for the support and love, and the bottle of champagne when the manuscript was finally submitted. You're both magic.

Allison Grant
April 2023

For my beloved grandmother: Margaret (Peggy) McCrindle (15/2/1914–18/9/2014), who always told me I'd write a book one day.

Introduction to Pathophysiological Processes

1

CHAPTER OUTLINE

KEY CONCEPTS AND DEFINITIONS OF DISEASE
THE IMPORTANCE OF EPIDEMIOLOGY
THE CELLULAR BASIS OF DISEASE
Cells and tissues
Cell structure
   Intracellular organelles
   Cell–cell and cell–matrix adhesion
CELLULAR AND TISSUE RESPONSE TO INJURY
AND INFECTION

The inflammatory response
   The main events of the acute inflammatory
response
   Chronic inflammation
   Indications of systemic inflammation
Pathogenicity and infection
   Pathogenic groups
   Sepsis

Disease is an unavoidable consequence of being alive. Creatures that inhabited the Earth long before humans evolved have left evidence of their pathologies in the fossil record. Many of the disorders and malformations that affected both them and our earliest human ancestors are familiar to modern medicine, indicating that the underlying mechanisms and processes causing disease are fundamental to living cells and tissues. The disease burden that humans carry today can be evaluated in different ways. The human cost—in terms of pain, suffering, disability, and grief—is immeasurable. The economic price—in terms of lost workdays, premature deaths, ageing populations, and the vast and expanding costs of healthcare systems—represents a huge proportion of the economic turnover of countries worldwide.

Disease is not the opposite of health, but it is an important factor in determining the degree of an individual's health status. The World Health Organisation (WHO) definition of health, dating from 1946 when the WHO's constitution was adopted, states that health is a state of complete physical, mental, and social well-being, and not merely the absence of disease or infirmity. Disease can be considered a condition affecting all or part of the body that impairs function beyond what is considered normal for an individual. The concepts of physiological 'normal' and interindividual variation are important in human biology, emphasising that function changes or is naturally different among individuals (e.g., between males and females; among those at different stages of development, such as fetal development, childhood, adolescence, maturity, and older age).

KEY CONCEPTS AND DEFINITIONS OF DISEASE

A wide range of diseases are discussed in this textbook, but even so this is nowhere near a comprehensive collection of all or even most human disorders, of which there are an enormous number. In addition, with advancing technology, it is increasingly possible to identify subcategories in diseases previously considered to be one condition. This produces detailed classification and subclassification systems that may be confusing to all but specialists working in the area; nevertheless, these classifications are increasingly important for identifying treatment options and allowing healthcare teams to offer therapies that target the underlying disease mechanisms as closely as possible. For example, there are several subtypes of breast cancer, each of which has a different molecular profile that may respond better to particular drugs. However, there are several key definitions and concepts that apply across the board in the study of disease.

Pathology, pathophysiology, and pathogenesis: what's the difference?

In its broadest sense, **pathology** is the study of disease. It is often used to mean study of the diseased tissues themselves, a study that improves understanding of the underlying disease processes and helps in diagnosis. For example, to identify which form of arthritis is present, a tissue biopsy from a painful knee joint can be studied under the microscope to identify abnormalities, and the tissue could be tested for the presence of abnormal immune cells or proteins; this would allow the pathologist to make a diagnosis of, for example,

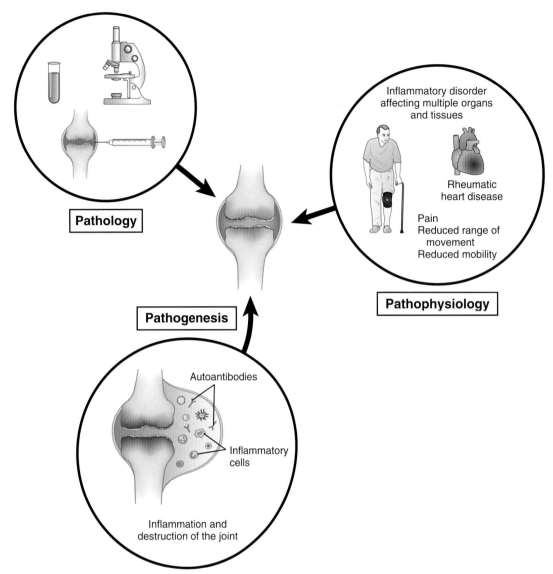

Fig. 1.1   Pathology, pathophysiology, and pathogenesis in rheumatoid disease.

rheumatoid arthritis. **Pathophysiology** is the study of altered function in an organ or tissue as the result of a disease process. Considering the arthritis example: an arthritic joint functions differently from a healthy joint. Its range of movement may be limited, it is likely to be painful, and it may be unable to bear the normal loading associated with walking and other weightbearing activities. In addition, rheumatoid disease damages organs other than the joints, for example, the heart, so functional changes are seen here, too. **Pathogenesis** refers to the cellular and molecular mechanisms that generate the disease; the main changes in the rheumatoid joint are mediated by an excessive inflammatory and immune response (Fig. 1.1).

Aetiology
Aetiology is the study of the cause of disease, and there is a very wide range of possible causes. Tissues can be injured by physical force or trauma, by extremes of temperature, or by chemical damage (e.g., extremes of pH). Genetic mutation, described in more detail in Chapter 2, causes a wide range of diseases—some inherited and some acquired—and the family of diseases we call cancer. Pathogenic organisms invading and establishing themselves in body tissues cause disease by a variety of processes. The body's defence mechanisms are powerfully cytotoxic and can lead to significant tissue injury if activated inappropriately or if not adequately controlled. Autoimmunity, in which body tissues are damaged by an inappropriate immune response, is discussed on page 103, and the inflammatory response is described in this chapter. Radiation—including ultraviolet radiation in sunlight, background environmental radiation, and radiation used in therapeutic and diagnostic medicine—damages living tissue.

The aetiology of a disease is frequently multifactorial, with more than one factor playing a part in increasing an individual's risk of developing the disease. Sometimes the aetiology is not known (idiopathic disease). Some disorders increase the risk of developing others; for example, there is a known association between ulcerative colitis and colon cancer.

Signs and symptoms: what's the difference?

A **sign** is an indication of disease that may be measured and/or assessed objectively by people other than the patient. Examples include high blood pressure or abnormal blood glucose levels. A **symptom** is experienced by the patient and is usually fairly subjective, for example, someone complaining of headache, fatigue, or flashing lights in the field of vision is reporting symptoms. Sometimes an indication of disease can be both sign and symptom because it is evident to both patient and others: a skin rash, a cough, or hair loss are examples.

Morbidity and mortality: What's the difference?

Mortality is death associated with a disease. **Morbidity** is incapacitation, illness, or disability resulting from disease.

Prognosis

Prognosis is the anticipated outcome of disease. It predicts features of the disease including the length of illness, the nature and duration of signs and symptoms, and the timeline of recovery (or, indeed, whether recovery is unlikely). Prognosis can also suggest the likelihood of any long-term consequences of the disease and whether quality of life is expected to be fully normal or reduced in some way after recovery. It is often notoriously difficult for healthcare providers to give accurate prognoses because of individual differences and unforeseen complications, but it is usually an aspect of their disease that patients are intensely concerned about.

Complications

A **complication** is an unwanted consequence of disease that develops as a result of the main disease process. For example, bacterial pneumonia may develop after a viral upper respiratory tract infection, because the virus suppresses normal immune defences and increases the risk of further infections.

Remission and relapse

Some chronic diseases are characterised by fluctuating health status, with periods of worsening, more active disease (**relapse**) alternating with periods of better, even normal, health (**remission**). Multiple sclerosis and ulcerative colitis are examples.

Congenital and acquired diseases

Congenital disease is present at birth. It may be the result of genetic abnormality in either the sperm or the ovum, or a mutation occurring after conception in the early stages of embryonic development. It may also be caused by an injury to the developing fetus; for example, placental insufficiency can cause intrauterine hypoxia and brain damage. **Acquired disease** is the result of exogenous factors after birth, and the list of possible agents is long: some important ones are listed under the Aetiology section.

Iatrogenic and idiopathic disease: What's the difference?

Iatrogenic disease is caused, however unintentionally, by medical interference, procedures, or hospitalisation. **Idiopathic** illness has no known cause (aetiology) and arises apparently spontaneously. Clearly, idiopathic disease must be caused by one or more factors, but by definition they have not yet been discovered.

Syndromes

A syndrome is a collection of signs and symptoms with a common underlying pathology but one that may be associated with more than one disease. For example, Cushing syndrome encompasses the wide range of signs and symptoms associated with excessively high glucocorticoid levels (p. 269), which can be caused by a range of causes, for example, steroid treatment, or an adrenal tumour secreting these hormones.

THE IMPORTANCE OF EPIDEMIOLOGY

Epidemiology is the study of the factors that determine the distribution of health and disease in populations, and quantifying and applying this knowledge to predict, control, and treat disease. Some key epidemiological definitions are given in Box 1.1. Epidemiological analysis can be done on a local, national, or international scale. It informs healthcare providers about changing burdens of disease, allows evaluation of healthcare systems, initiatives and policies, and can be used to predict future trends in health and disease. The largest global epidemiological project to date is the Global Burden of Disease (GBD) study. Begun in 1990 as an

---

Box 1.1 Some key epidemiological definitions

Term	Definition
Incidence	The number of new events occurring in a defined population during a specified time period (e.g., the number of males aged 30–50 who had a heart attack in Scotland in 2008 is a measure of incidence). It may be expressed as events per number of the population (e.g., 3.8 per 100,000) or as a percentage (e.g., 0.0038%).
Prevalence	The proportion or percentage of a named event in a defined population at a specific point in time or during a specified time period (e.g., the prevalence of the common cold in the general population in Alaska in December 2020 was 37%, meaning that 37% of the population had a cold sometime in December 2020).
Risk	Risk is the probability that an event will occur in a defined population at some point (e.g., lifetime risk). Risk factors are events or conditions that increase the likelihood of that event occurring. In health statistics, relative risk is often used, meaning that risk of an event occurring in certain populations is expressed compared with the risk in other populations; e.g., the risk of developing certain skin cancers in fair-skinned people may be three times higher than in dark-skinned people.

international collaboration now involving more than 145 countries, it examines risk factors, mortality, and morbidity in a range of important diseases and injury in populations across the world. Analysis of this data allows researchers to quantify health loss, including death rates, in people across countries, time, socioeconomic status, ethnicity, age, and sex, which in turn should allow policymakers to make better decisions regarding allocation of resources and how best to meet the needs of the people for whom they are responsible.

THE CELLULAR BASIS OF DISEASE

Although disease is often considered at the whole-organism level ('I have a cold'), or at the organ/system level ('He had a heart attack'), the mechanisms of disease occur at the cellular level and involve a huge array of biochemical processes operating and controlling every aspect of normal cell function. Cells do not operate independently; each of the approximately 50 trillion cells making up the human body lives in a controlled environment, and every cell contributes its own specialised activity to ensure that the whole organism remains healthy–that is, the sum of their total activities maintains homoeostasis.

CELLS AND TISSUES

A **tissue** is a collection of cells of the same type. There are four types of tissue in the human body: epithelial tissue, connective tissue, nervous tissue, and muscle tissue. Each is associated with its own function and architecture, and contains the specialised tissue cells embedded in varying amounts of a gelatinous supporting meshwork called extracellular matrix (ECM) or ground substance. Fig. 1.2A illustrates a fibroblast, the main cell type responsible for synthesising ECM substances, embedded within its ECM.

The extracellular matrix
The ECM provides scaffolding to which the cells attach themselves. It holds a large amount of water, allowing nutrients and wastes to diffuse between the tissue and its blood supply, and it absorbs and distributes the mechanical stressors applied to body tissues, protecting the living cells within it. It is also a biologically active component of tissues, and directs cell division and migration, cell healing, and embryonic development. ECM composition varies from tissue to tissue, but two main structural components are described in this chapter.

The collagens. Collagen is the fundamental structural protein of tissues and represents about 30% of the total protein content of the body. The fibrillar collagens (types I, II, III, V, and XI) form strong, inelastic, flexible fibres providing the internal structure of most connective tissue. Type I collagen is the commonest protein in the body. This is the collagen laid down in osteoid to which calcium and phosphate crystals are bound, forming mature bone tissue. Collagen gives bone great tensile strength (i.e., it cannot be stretched), and the calcium phosphate content gives it rigidity. The combination is a shatter-resistant tissue stronger than steel-reinforced concrete and capable of bearing large loads. Tightly packed type I collagen fibres form the tendons that anchor skeletal muscle to bone (Fig. 1.2B). The fibrillar collagens are abundant in blood vessel walls, joints, the cornea of the eye, the wall of the gastrointestinal tract, and other tis-

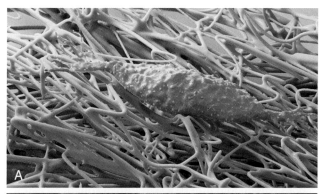
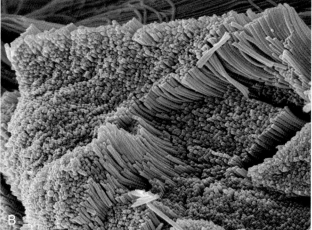

Fig. 1.2   The extracellular matrix (ECM). (A) A fibroblast embedded in its ECM. (B) Collagen fibres in a tendon. (Sources: (A) Nanoclustering/ Science Photo Library; (B) Steve Gschmeissner/Science Photo Library.)

sues. Connective tissue disorders caused by the production of faulty fibrillar collagens (e.g., Ehlers-Danlos syndrome) are characterised by reduced mechanical strength of body structures.

Some collagens form sheets rather than fibres. Type IV collagen, along with a protein called *laminin*, forms the basement membrane on which epithelial cells sit. Because epithelial cells form the membranes covering and lining body organs and cavities, faulty type IV collagen leads to a loss of epithelial integrity. Goodpasture syndrome (p. 307) is caused by dysfunctional type IV collagen, affecting the glomerular membrane of the kidney and the alveolar membrane of the lung.

Other collagens are used as linking materials to secure structures to each other. For example, type VII collagen forms extended fibrils called *anchoring fibrils* that attach the basement membrane of epithelial layers, including the skin, to the connective tissue below. In one form of epidermolysis bullosa, a collection of skin blistering disorders, autoantibodies to type VII collagen destroy these anchoring fibrils and the epidermis sloughs away from the dermis beneath.

Glycosaminoglycans (GAGs). These very large sugar molecules form a substantial proportion of the matrix of many connective tissues, including cartilage, elastic tissue, and loose connective tissues. They are frequently found bound to proteins, forming even larger molecules called *proteoglycans*.

GAGs contribute key properties to the biology of the ECM. They trap water and therefore contribute to the shock-absorbing properties of connective tissues, particularly important in the musculoskeletal system. A fully hydrated single molecule of hyaluronan, the largest GAG, is enormous in molecular terms–over 200 nm in diameter. Their ability to absorb water makes them ideal space fillers and gives elasticity to body structures. Their huge size restricts the movement of water, macromolecules, and microorganisms through connective tissues, keeping tissues well hydrated and resisting changes in the local environment, including limiting the spread of infection. They act as adhesion molecules for growth factors, concentrating them in tissues during embryonic development, growth, and healing. They prevent the deposition of minerals in soft tissues and act as adhesion molecules for inflammatory cells, allowing, for example, lymphocytes to gather in areas where immune protection is needed. When present in fluid, they thicken it, making it viscous and slippery; for example, they are present in synovial fluid, which lubricates and nourishes synovial joints.

Changes in GAG content of tissues, either through ageing or in disease (the mucopolysaccharidoses; p. 342), affect their physical and chemical properties and contribute to age-related deterioration in connective tissue, for example, stiffening and reduced ability to heal.

Epithelial tissue

Epithelial cells grow in layers, forming the membranes that cover, line, and protect body organs and internal cavities and passageways. They regulate what can pass from one side of the membrane to the other, and so they have a barrier function, controlling movement of cells and substances between body spaces. They do this using specialised cell-cell junctions, which have varying degrees of permeability (see below) and also with an array of pumps, carriers, and channels in the cell membranes of each cell. Because they are frequently exposed to mechanical stress, they regenerate rapidly and usually contain considerable numbers of stem cells, from which new cells are continuously being produced. This is a factor in the high rate of cancers originating in epithelial tissues. If the epithelial layer is only one cell thick, it is a simple epithelium; if there are multiple layers, it is called *stratified*. The basal epithelial cells produce a thin layer of a collagen-rich substance to which they attach firmly; this is called the *basement membrane*. Epithelial cells may be thin and flat (squamous), cube-shaped (cuboidal), or tall and thin (columnar), depending on the function of the membrane they form (Table 1.1). The cells are packed tightly together, and there is very little ECM within the tissue.

Connective tissue

This represents a diverse range of tissues (Fig. 1.3), but most contain significant quantities of ECM, and the cells within are dispersed and not necessarily in direct contact with one another. Some connective tissues have specialised functions (e.g., blood, bone, and cartilage), but others are found widely in all parts of the body, supporting, connecting, and protecting body structures. Connective tissue cells include **adipocytes**, which store fat in the form of triglycerides; **chondrocytes**, which build and maintain

---

Table 1.1 Characteristics and function of epithelial cells

Cell shape	Characteristics	Example	Function
Squamous			
Simple squamous	Forms a thin membrane, usually to allow rapid exchange of substances	Lining the alveoli of the lungs	Rapid gas diffusion
Stratified squamous	Constantly renewing from basal layer; the upper layers can be shed because they are continually replaced from below. May be keratinised for extra protection (e.g., skin) or non-keratinised (e.g., mucous membranes)	Skin	Protection
Cuboidal			
Simple or stratified cuboidal	The increased cell volume compared with squamous epithelial cells accommodates cell organelles for manufacture and secretion of substances and being thin enough to allow materials to cross	Lining glands	Produce and secrete (e.g., hormones)
Columnar			
Simple columnar	Tall cells protect the underlying tissues. There may be additional specialised features (e.g., microvilli on the upper (free) surface for absorption, as in the small intestine)		
Pseudostratified ciliated columnar	All cells are attached to the basement membrane, but they are so squashed in and tightly packed that under the microscope it appears that some are not. Cilia are motile structures that beat in synchrony and generate movement in the fluids above the cells	Lining most of the upper respiratory tract	Cilia move the mucus blanket, along with trapped particles, away from the lungs to protect against infection

cartilage; and **osteocytes**, which maintain bone. Other important connective tissue cells include **fibroblasts**, which produce collagen; **mast cells**, which store and release histamine as an important part of the inflammatory response; and white blood cells, including **macrophages** and **lymphocytes**, whose function is defensive. Some macrophages live in connective tissue, providing permanent populations of defensive cells to protect local tissues (e.g., dust cells in the alveoli of the lung). Others are constantly on the move, patrolling body tissues and prepared to activate inflammatory and immune defence mechanisms if they detect damage or infection.

Adipose tissue (Fig. 1.3A). Adipose (fat) tissue consists of **adipocytes** packed closely together with relatively little ECM in between. The adipocytes are swollen with fat, and the tissue has little blood supply. Adipose tissue is an important energy store, and subcutaneous fat insulates the body. In addition, it packs round organs (e.g., the heart and the eye in its bony orbit), padding and cushioning them.

Cartilage (Fig. 1.3B). Cartilage is mainly a collagen and proteoglycan matrix with its cells (chondrocytes) scattered through the tissue, either singly, in pairs, or in very small clusters. The cells live in little pockets called *lacunae*, and they maintain the matrix of the tissue. There are no blood vessels in cartilage. It is tough and slightly pliable but not elastic; it is a very good shock absorber and resists compression. Its mechanical strength is important in **fibrocartilage** (which contains a high proportion of tough collagen fibres), which forms intervertebral discs of the spinal column. **Hyaline cartilage** coats the end of bone ends at joints, preventing bone-bone contact and cushioning the loading forces applied to joints when doing load-bearing work. **Elastic cartilage** has extra elastic fibres and so is very deformable and found, for example, in the outer ear and in the larynx.

Blood (Fig. 1.3C). This is a fluid connective tissue, in which the blood cells (**erythrocytes, leukocytes,** and **platelets**) are suspended in plasma, the equivalent of the tissue matrix. The functions of the different components of blood are discussed in Chapter 5.

Bone (Fig. 1.3D). The matrix in bone tissue is about two-thirds calcium and phosphate salts laid down on a collagen matrix. This combination gives great mechanical strength (from the calcium and phosphate content) and the capacity to absorb shock and resist shattering (from the tough and resilient collagen fibres). The cells (**osteocytes**) live in lacunae and lay the bone down in layers called *lamellae* around a central (Haversian) canal. The cells are widely dispersed in the tissue but communicate with each other through tiny channels in the bone called *canaliculi*. Bone is described in more detail on p. 324.

Loose connective (areolar) tissue (Fig. 1.3E). This tissue is found throughout the body as a key component connecting and supporting all body structures; it contains a range of connective tissue cells, including **adipocytes**, **fibroblasts**, **lymphocytes**, **mast cells**, and **macrophages**. The matrix is made up of collagen, which gives it tensile strength (that is, it resists being pulled apart), along with elastic fibres, so it recoils after being stretched. The underlying ground substance is mainly proteoglycans, but there are other ECM substances present as well, including laminin, fibronectin, and hyaluronic acid.

Nervous tissue

This includes nerve cells (**neurones**), which generate and conduct electrical impulses, and their support cells (**glial cells**). Nervous tissue is discussed in more detail in Chapter 8.

Muscle tissue

The body possesses three functionally distinct types of muscle: skeletal, cardiac, and smooth. Key characteristics of these three muscle types are described in Table 1.2.

CELL STRUCTURE

Human cells are classified as eukaryotes, meaning that their genetic material (i.e., DNA) is enclosed within its own nuclear membrane (compare with bacteria, whose DNA is distributed throughout their cytosol and are called *prokaryotes*; see below). Each cell is enclosed in a specialised cell (plasma) membrane. Collectively, the contents of the cell membrane are called the **cytoplasm**. Cytoplasm is a water-based substance called **cytosol** in which a variable number of specialised structures called *organelles* are suspended. A representative human cell is shown in Fig. 1.4.

INTRACELLULAR ORGANELLES

Although human cells come in a wide range of shapes and sizes (a liver cell looks very different to a nerve cell), most possess a range of essential structures called organelles to perform key functions essential for their own survival and the health of the body. Each organelle has its own specialised role, whether in energy production, protein synthesis, or the packaging of cellular wastes.

The cell nucleus

This is usually the largest organelle and is generally located centrally within the cell. It contains the cell's DNA, organised into sausage-like structures called *chromosomes*. DNA is the body's largest molecule and contains the coded information that the cell needs to synthesise all essential proteins. The role of the nucleus and DNA in protein synthesis is described in Chapter 2.

Mitochondria

Mitochondria (singular: mitochondrion) produce adenosine triphosphate (ATP), the cell's energy currency. The number of mitochondria per cell varies, but metabolically active cells like liver and skeletal muscle may contain thousands. Mitochondria are packed with multiple folded membranes equipped with enzyme pathways to produce ATP from nutrients they import from the cell cytosol. The ATP they manufacture is exported from the mitochondria into the cell cytosol to fuel the activities of other cell organelles. Mitochondrial disorders therefore disrupt the cell's ability to generate energy. Mitochondria also contain a small quantity of DNA, which contains genes that mainly code for proteins involved in energy metabolism.

The cell membrane

The main constituent of the cell membrane is phospholipid, along with cholesterol and other lipids. Phospholipid molecules are formed from a glycerol molecule attached to two long-chain fatty acids. These molecules align themselves in a double layer, with the fatty acid 'tails' orientated inwards (because they are repelled by the watery cytosol

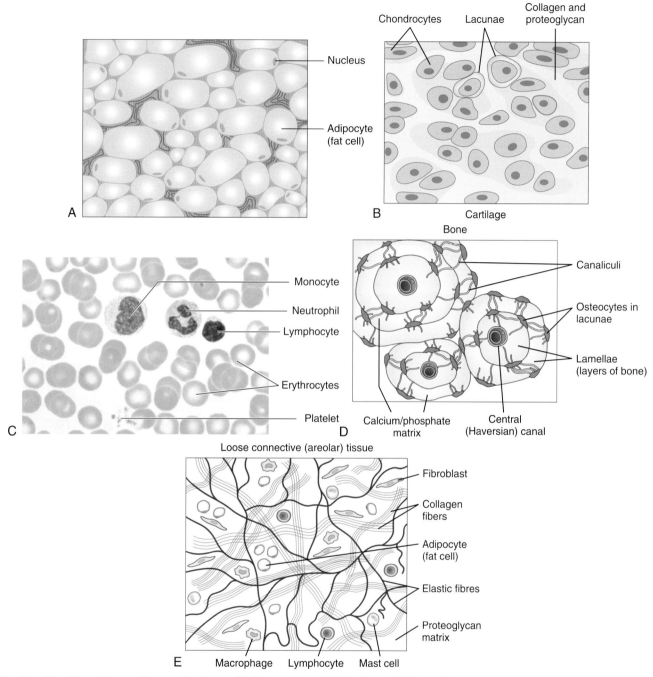

Fig. 1.3 The different types of connective tissue. (A) Adipose tissue. (B) Cartilage. (C) Blood. (D) Bone. (E) Loose connective (areolar) tissue. (Modified from (A) Waugh A and Grant A (2018) *Ross & Wilson anatomy and physiology in health and illness,* 13th ed, Fig. 3.20A. Oxford: Elsevier Ltd; (B) Waugh A and Grant A (2018) *Ross & Wilson anatomy and physiology in health and illness,* 13th ed, Fig. 3.23A. Oxford: Elsevier Ltd; (C) Biophoto Associates/Science Photo Library. Reproduced with permission; (D) Waugh A and Grant A (2018) *Ross & Wilson anatomy and physiology in health and illness,* 13th ed, Fig. 4.2. Oxford: Elsevier Ltd; (E) Waugh A and Grant A (2018) *Ross & Wilson anatomy and physiology in health and illness,* 13th ed, Fig. 3.19. Oxford: Elsevier Ltd.)

within the cell and the watery extracellular fluids outside the cell) and the glycerol 'heads' pointing outwards. This molecular arrangement gives a characteristic 'sandwich' appearance under the electron microscope. Functionally, the cell membrane is far more than a simple wrapping holding the cell contents together. It is studded with a wide range of proteins and glycoproteins performing a variety of functions (Fig. 1.5). Some form pores, channels, and specialised pumps that permit the cell to import and export substances and regulate its internal composition. Some act as receptors for hormones, cytokines, growth factors, and other chemical messengers, allowing the cell to communicate with other body cells and to respond to signals in its local environment. The cell membrane expresses adhesion molecules to anchor itself in position to its local matrix, but also in some cases to allow other cells to attach; for example, damage to the endothelial cells lining a blood vessel stimulates them to produce adhesion molecules for white blood cells, allowing

Table 1.2   The three types of muscle tissue

Muscle cell type	Control	Location	Structural features	Image
Smooth	Involuntary	In the walls of blood vessels and the respiratory, gastrointestinal, and genitourinary tracts; the iris of the eye	Spindle-shaped cell with single nucleus; not striated	Nucleus
Skeletal	Voluntary	Mostly associated with the skeleton; the diaphragm	Long cylindrically shaped with multiple nuclei; striated	Nuclei
Cardiac	Involuntary	In the heart	Branching striated cell with single nucleus	Branching cell / Nucleus / Intercalated disc

Source: Figures adapted from Waugh A, Grant A (2023) *Ross & Wilson anatomy and physiology in health and illness,* 14th ed, Figs. 3.24A, 3.25A and 3.26. Oxford: Elsevier Ltd.

them to attach and migrate into the damaged tissue for protection and repair. Additionally, specialised structures that fasten cells to their neighbours (e.g., desmosomes and gap junctions, see below) are integrated into the cell membrane. Some proteins are completely enclosed within the membrane (intrinsic proteins), some are associated with but not part of the membrane (extrinsic proteins), and others span the thickness of the membrane (transmembrane proteins). Nerve and muscle cell membranes are electrically excitable, capable of generating, and transmitting action potentials.

The endoplasmic reticulum (ER)

This is an extensive network of flattened bags and tubules of membranes within the cell. Much of the membrane surface of a cell's ER is coated in tiny granules called *ribosomes* (this is called **rough ER**), which produce and process proteins. ER without ribosomes, called **smooth ER**, detoxifies drugs and produces lipids, including steroid hormones. Smooth ER also stores calcium, particularly important in muscle cells, which need a constant supply of calcium for contraction.

Golgi apparatus

The Golgi apparatus is formed of stacks of membranous bags. Its main function is to store, package, and modify the proteins and lipids produced in the ER for distribution both for the cell's own use but also so that they can be exported (e.g., an endocrine cell producing a hormone needs to be able to store it and secrete it when required).

Lysosomes

These are membranous bags in which the cell digests unwanted substances and packages waste products, and they are packed with proteolytic and other degradative enzymes for this purpose. Because of this, the interior of the lysosome is highly toxic and would cause significant cell damage if released into the cytosol. To excrete the waste, the lysosomal membrane fuses with the cell membrane, releasing its contents into the extracellular fluids (exocytosis). Lysosomal disorders lead to accumulation of toxic materials within the cell and may cause cell death.

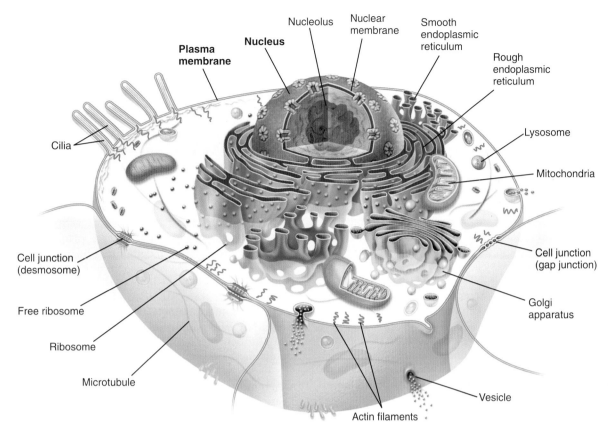

Fig. 1.4 A representative human cell. (Modified from Craft JA, Gordon CJ, Huether SE, McCance KL, Brashers VL, and Rote NS (2019) *Understanding pathophysiology*, 3rd ed. Sydney: Elsevier.)

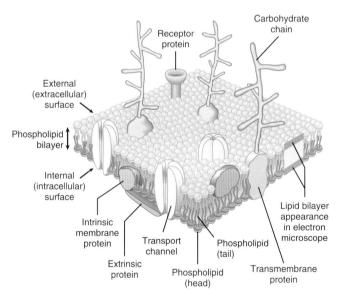

Fig. 1.5 Structure of the cell membrane. (Modified from Standring S (2021) *Gray's anatomy*, 42nd ed, Fig. 1.3. Oxford: Elsevier Ltd.)

Cytoskeleton

The cell needs mechanisms to direct internal movement of materials, and also sometimes to permit the whole cell to migrate from one place to another. This is provided by an intracellular network of three main types of fibrous protein: microtubules, actin, and intermediate filaments.

Microtubules

In cell division, the cell's DNA is copied, and each copy distributes to opposite ends of the nucleus, requiring the equivalent of tramlines to guide the travelling chromosomes. Microtubules assemble into a framework that guides the chromosomes as they separate in preparation for cell division (p. 54). Transport of materials along nerve axons (axonal transport) and the movement of organelles around within the cell are also guided by microtubules.

Actin

Networks of actin proteins, anchored to the internal surface of the cell membrane, give the cell internal support and shape. Cilia, whose beating action moves the mucus blanket lining the airways, are anchored in the cell membrane by actin proteins. Cell motility—for example, white blood cells travelling through tissues or cell migration during wound healing—results from assembly of actin networks, forming cell pseudopodia, and allowing amoeboid motion.

Intermediate filaments

Intermediate filaments are anchored at the cell membrane in structures called *desmosomes* (see below) and reinforce the membrane at points where the cell membrane is attached to adjacent cells or to the ECM.

CELL–CELL AND CELL–MATRIX ADHESION

Tissues are highly organised structures. Cells must be able to interact with one another, to maintain their place in the overall architecture of the tissue via cell-cell adhesion mechanisms, and to anchor themselves to their ECM for stability and to maintain tissue strength and integrity. Cell membranes possess specialised adhesion structures for this purpose (Fig. 1.6). Cell–cell and cell–matrix adhesion abnormalities, in which cells cannot adhere appropriately to each other or to their ECM, are associated with significant diseases, including cancer and blistering disorders of the skin.

Cell–cell junctions

The main types of cell–cell junctions are shown in Fig. 1.6.

Tight junctions

As the name suggests, in this form of junction between adjacent cells, the plasma membranes are held very tightly together, making it very difficult or impossible for substances to pass between the cells. Specialist proteins called **claudins** are tightly woven through both membranes, stitching them firmly together. When epithelial cells are linked with tight junctions, they form a relatively impermeable barrier that separates one compartment from another. An example is the endothelial layer lining capillaries supplying much of the brain. Normally, capillaries are fairly leaky vessels because the single layer of endothelial cells forming their walls are loosely attached to one another. This formation is essential to allow nutrients, gases, and wastes to exchange between the blood and the tissues. However, in the brain, greater selectivity is needed to protect the delicate brain tissues, and the endothelial cells of brain capillaries are joined with tight junctions, greatly reducing transfer of materials between the blood and the brain (the blood–brain barrier, p. 207). Tight junctions also allow cells to generate concentration gradients because, by preventing passive diffusion of small particles, for example ions, they can then use pumps to keep the concentration of a particular substance on one side of the membrane much higher than on the other side. This is important, for example, in the kidney, which relies on maintaining ionic gradients to control reabsorption, and impaired claudin/tight junction function in the kidney can lead to kidney disease. In the stomach, *Helicobacter pylori* releases a toxin that disrupts the tight junctions between the gastric epithelial cells, allowing the acidic stomach juices to penetrate to deeper layers, contributing to peptic ulcer formation.

Gap junctions

These are areas in the plasma membranes of adjacent cells that form communicating channels between their interiors, meaning that cells can directly and rapidly exchange ions, nutrients, and other substances with one another. This is the commonest type of cell-cell junction, and many body cells communicate with each another this way; for example, respiratory epithelial cells use gap junctions to co-ordinate the synchronised beating of their cilia, and cardiac muscle cells use them to ensure rapid and co-ordinated spread of the cardiac action potential through adjacent cardiac myocytes. Some nerve cells also use gap junctions for rapid transmission of signals and for myelin production. The proteins essential to gap junction structure are the **connexins**. Inherited disorders of connexins can cause deafness and other neurological disorders.

Desmosomes

Desmosomes are formed from dense plaques of proteins packed into the plasma membrane, which attach firmly to similar structures in the plasma membrane of adjacent cells. They anchor intermediate filaments to the cell membrane, as discussed above. In pemphigus vulgaris (p. 385), antibodies to the key protein **desmoglein** in the desmosomes of keratinocytes destroy desmosome structure, leading to loss of cell-cell adhesion between the layers of the epidermis and mucous membranes.

Adherens junctions

These junctions use actin filaments to attach cells to one another. They are the earliest form of cell-cell adhesion to appear in embryonic development and allow migrating cells to adhere to one another in developing tissues.

Cell-ECM adhesion

Cells attach themselves to adjacent ECM molecules using a range of specialised proteins called **integrins**. One important mechanism is the **hemidesmosome**, so called because, unlike desmosomes, the dense attachment plaque is only found on the plasma membrane of one cell. Epithelial cells use hemidesmosomes to anchor themselves to their basement membrane by attaching either to laminin or to collagen. In the blistering disorder bullous pemphigoid, antibodies to components of the hemidesmosome structure disrupt it, reducing cell-cell

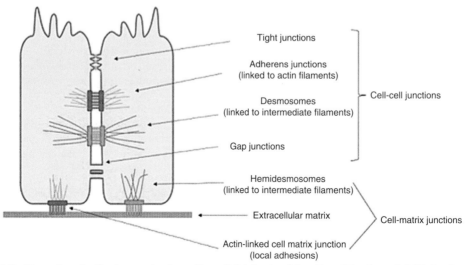

Fig. 1.6 The main cell adhesion mechanisms. (From Cell Adhesion, https://en.wikipedia.org/wiki/Cell_adhesion.)

adhesion and allowing the epidermis to separate from the dermis. Epithelial cells can also use actin filaments to anchor themselves to the ECM.

CELLULAR AND TISSUE RESPONSE TO INJURY AND INFECTION

Human cells live in the body's protected environment, whose complex homeostatic mechanisms operate constantly to maintain this environment at optimal conditions. Infection, trauma, radiation injury, chemical injury, drugs and other toxins, extremes of temperature, biochemical or metabolic disturbances, and genetic damage are all capable of significantly disrupting cellular function, and therefore disrupting tissue and organ function (Fig. 1.7). Any factor that tends to alter or disrupt normal cellular operation at any level is called a *stressor*. Stressors need not necessarily cause damage; for example, regular weightbearing exercise is a stressor, but used appropriately it stimulates bone growth and increases bone density, improving skeletal health. Excessive weightbearing exercise will, however, cause microfractures, weaken the bone, and, with increasing stress, eventually fracture. Sustained exposure to stressors can lead to adaptive changes in tissue morphology, especially in epithelial tissues, as explored in Chapter 3.

THE INFLAMMATORY RESPONSE

The inflammatory response is a collection of cellular and biochemical events that follow tissue injury, however trivial. It does not imply infection, although infection is much likelier in injured tissue than in healthy tissue. It is usually a local response, restricted to the damaged area, but if the injury is major, the products of tissue damage circulating in the bloodstream and the powerful response of the defence and immune systems may cause systemic consequences (the systemic inflammatory response). A range of inflammatory mediators, released by damaged tissues and inflammatory cells, regulate the inflammatory response.

Ultimately, the inflammatory response is protective: it attracts protective white blood cells and stimulates other body defences; it limits tissue damage, activates the clotting cascade, prevents or limits infection, and promotes healing. However, it is also the case that, through the release of powerful inflammatory mediators and the activation of aggressive inflammatory cells, the inflammatory response can significantly damage healthy tissues.

THE MAIN EVENTS OF THE ACUTE INFLAMMATORY RESPONSE

The cardinal signs of tissue inflammation are redness, heat, pain and swelling. The inflammatory response can be studied according to the main cells and events involved, although it must be emphasised that this description is for convenience and that during the inflammatory response, these processes develop with considerable overlap. Fig. 1.8 summarises the main events of the inflammatory response.

Blood vessel response in inflammation

Within seconds of tissue injury, blood flow through the affected area increases as the tiny arterioles feeding blood into the capillaries dilate. The increased blood flow brings additional white blood cells and antibodies into the tissues for defence. In addition, local capillaries become more permeable because the single layer of endothelial cells that form their walls pull apart from each other, producing gaps through which plasma fluid and white blood cells can escape into the tissues. The fluid carries antibodies and other proteins, including the clotting

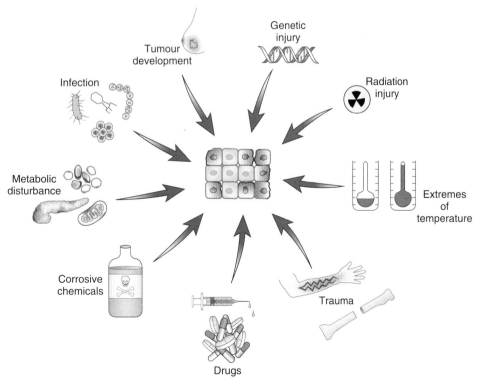

Fig. 1.7 Potential causes of tissue injury.

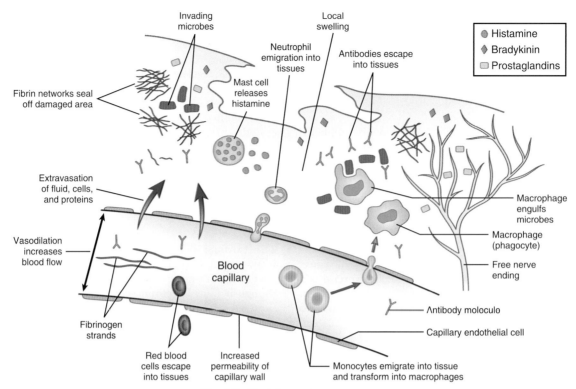

Fig. 1.8 The inflammatory response.

protein fibrinogen. In the tissues, fibrinogen is converted to fibrin, producing a sticky network of fibres that helps to limit the movement of any invading bacteria. The additional heat brought with the higher blood flow has two main benefits. First, it helps to reduce the risk of infection. Bacteria that may have entered a wound from the exterior prefer a cooler temperature, ideally no more than normal body temperature, and they grow less well in the heat of an inflamed tissue. Second, the phagocytic activity of the white blood cells being attracted in large numbers to the injury is enhanced by the additional heat. The swelling that develops as the tissue spaces become engorged with fluid cushions the damaged area and causes pain by compressing nerve endings. The pain is a constant reminder of the injury and tends to lead to behaviours that protect the area and limit its use, both of which will favour healing.

White blood cell arrival and activity

Within a few minutes, phagocytic neutrophils and other leukocytes begin to congregate in the injured tissue in increasing numbers. This is not random chance but is driven by **chemotaxis**, in which chemicals released by damaged tissues and any invading organisms attract inflammatory cells into the area. Chemotactic substances (**chemotaxins**) include bacterial proteins, lipids, and a range of inflammatory mediators and cytokines such as complement proteins, leukotrienes, and interleukins.

Leukocyte emigration

Fluid leaking through the permeable capillary walls makes the blood more viscous and slower flowing than usual, making it easier for white blood cells to make contact with the endothelium (margination). Neutrophils are the first leukocytes to migrate into damaged tissue. Having made contact with the endothelium, they roll along it and then adhere to it. This happens because the endothelium lining the microcirculation in inflamed tissues begins to produce specialised adhesion molecules to which neutrophils attach. Once attached, the neutrophil crawls through the blood vessel wall by amoeboid motion and enters the tissues (emigration) (Fig. 1.9). Neutrophils are active phagocytes and act as scavengers in inflamed tissues, consuming and destroying bacteria, other microbes, and dead and dying body cells. Phagocytic macrophages are slower to arrive at the site of injury, taking 24 to 48 hours for their numbers to rise to significant levels, but they are larger and longer lived than neutrophils, and they are an important link cell responsible for activating the immune response (p. 90). The release of damaging enzymes and toxins when leukocytes are activated is an essential part of their antimicrobial activity but can cause significant injury to host tissues.

Important inflammatory mediators

A wide range of chemicals is synthesised or activated in response to tissue injury, responsible for initiating, co-ordinating, and controlling the complex interaction of events of the inflammatory response. Collectively, these substances are called inflammatory mediators. They include a number of **cytokines**. Cytokines are small proteins released by a range of body cells, mainly lymphocytes and other white blood cells, but also activated blood vessel endothelium, epithelial cells, and connective tissue cells. They regulate immune and inflammatory responses, and the main stimuli for their release are infection and tissue injury. Increasingly, cytokine inhibitors (so-called *biologics*) are used therapeutically in the treatment of inflammatory and immunological disorders.

The most important inflammatory mediators are discussed below but represent only a small number of the overall total.

Arachidonic acid products

Arachidonic acid is an essential component of cell membranes. After cell injury, arachidonic acid is released from damaged

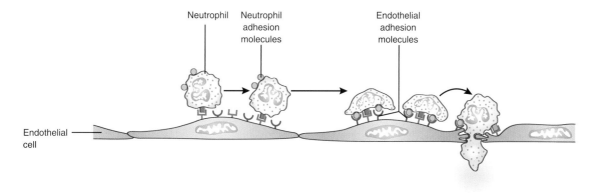

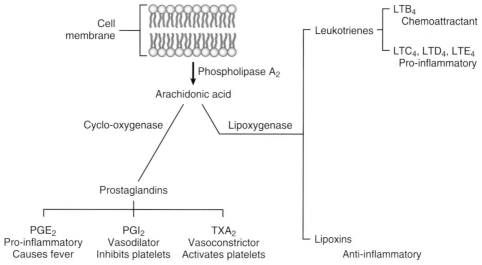

Fig. 1.9 Neutrophil rolling, adhesion, and emigration. (Modified from Zimmerman J and Rotta AT (2023) *Fuhrman and Zimmerman's pediatric critical care*, 6th ed, Fig. 110.2. St. Louis: Elsevier Inc.)

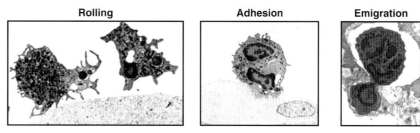

Fig. 1.10 The metabolic fates of arachidonic acid.

membranes by the enzyme phospholipase A_2 and may then be acted on by two main enzymes: cyclo-oxygenase, which ultimately generates **prostaglandins**; and lipoxygenase, which ultimately generates **leukotrienes** and **lipoxins** (Fig. 1.10).

Prostaglandins. Prostaglandins (PGs) are so named because they were originally isolated from the prostate gland, although in fact they are produced by nearly all body cells. They are a family of very short-lived inflammatory mediators responsible for a range of inflammatory events including vasodilation, increased vascular permeability and pain. The main family members are PGE_2, PGI_2, and thromboxane $(TX)A_2$. PGE_2 additionally has a role in fever (see below). TXA_2 is a potent platelet activator and a powerful vasoconstrictor, helping to slow blood flow through injured tissue, which facilitates leukocyte emigration and triggers clotting, which also reduces blood flow and minimises blood loss. Although this section discusses only their pro-inflammatory

functions, it is worth noting that PGs have a number of additional roles including gastric mucosal protection and regulation of blood flow through key body organs including the kidneys.

Leukotrienes and lipoxins. Leukotrienes (LTs) are mainly synthesised by inflammatory cells, including mast cells and white blood cells. LTB_4 is a very important chemoattractant for leukocytes, attracting them into damaged tissues in large numbers. LTC_4, LTD_4, and LTE_4 all increase vascular permeability, cause intense vasoconstriction, and are potent bronchoconstrictors. Lipoxins act as brakes on the inflammatory response and inhibit the adhesion of leukocytes to the endothelium and chemotaxis.

Histamine

This important inflammatory mediator is synthesised from the amino acid tryptophan by mast cells and stored in granules bound to the anticoagulant heparin. Mast cells (Fig. 1.11) are abundant in most connective tissues, especially in the skin and gastrointestinal and respiratory tracts, all key areas for defence because they are constantly exposed to the external environment and are particularly vulnerable to damage from infection or trauma. They degranulate and release their contents in response

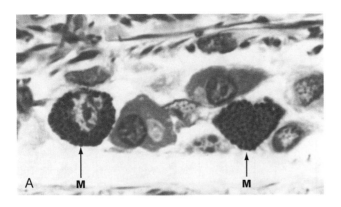

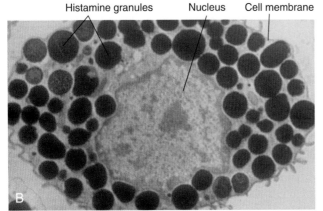

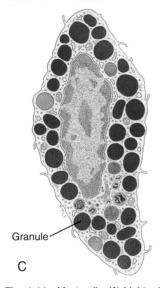

Fig. 1.11 Mast cells. (A) Light micrograph of mast cells (labelled M), showing their dense staining. (B) False-coloured electron micrograph of a mast cell. The histamine granules are coloured deep red. (C) Artist's representation of a mast cell. (Modified from (A) Young B, Lowe J, Stevens A et al (2006) *Wheater's functional histology*, 5th ed, Fig. 4.18. Edinburgh: Elsevier Ltd; (B) Patton KT, Bell FB, Thompson T et al (2022) *Anatomy and physiology*, 11th ed, Fig. 32.4. St. Louis: Elsevier Inc. and; (C) Lentz T, Yale Medical School, New Haven, CT in book Cell Fine Structure.)

to a range of stimuli, including activated complement proteins, physical injury to the tissue in which they are living, and a range of allergens (this is strongly associated with type I hypersensitivity, p. 99). Histamine is a potent vasodilator, increases vascular permeability, and causes itch.

Serotonin
Serotonin, also called 5-hydroxytryptophan (5-HT), is found in large quantities in platelets, some nervous tissue, and the gastrointestinal tract. It causes vasoconstriction and is essential for normal clotting.

The interleukins (ILs)
The interleukins are a group of cytokines initially thought to be produced only by leukocytes (hence the name) but have since been shown to be released by other body cells. They are mainly involved in regulation of the inflammatory and immune responses, and also promote and control the development, differentiation, and function of inflammatory and immune cells. IL release is stimulated by tissue injury or by the presence of microbes or microbial products in body tissues. There are over 60 identified to date, but only three—IL-1, IL-2, and IL-8—are briefly described in the following sections.

Interleukin-1. IL-1 is released by macrophages, B cells, and fibroblasts, among others. It activates T cells, B cells, macrophages, and other inflammatory and immune cells. IL-1 has a wide range of pro-inflammatory effects, including increased leukocyte adhesion to blood vessel endothelium and increased blood cell synthesis. It stimulates the acute phase response (see below) in the systemic response to injury or infection and induces fever (IL-1 was originally called *endogenous pyrogenic factor* when first discovered in the 1940s). It is thought to be involved in a number of autoimmune and inflammatory disorders, including inflammatory bowel disease, rheumatoid arthritis, and psoriasis, and IL-1 antagonists are becoming increasingly important in the treatment of such disorders.

Interleukin-2. IL-2 is released mainly by T cells and accelerates proliferation of inflammatory and immune cells. It is likely to be particularly important in autoimmune and inflammatory disorders that involve abnormalities in T-cell function (e.g., type IV hypersensitivity; p. 101).

Interleukin-8. This interleukin is released by a wide range of inflammatory and immune cells, keratinocytes, hepatocytes, and connective tissue cells like chondrocytes and fibroblasts. Its most significant function is as a chemoattractant for white blood cells, but it also stimulates bone marrow to increase blood cell production. IL-8 levels are elevated in infection and in many inflammatory and autoimmune disorders.

The kinins
The main kinin is **bradykinin**, a small peptide of only nine amino acids released by injured tissues from a larger protein called *kininogen*. Bradykinin increases vascular permeability, causes vasodilation, and stimulates intense pain by irritating local free nerve endings. It is rapidly broken down but has been implicated in some disorders (e.g., hereditary angioneurotic oedema; p. 93), in which its continual production causes rapid and sustained swelling.

Tumour necrosis factor alpha (TNFα)

This important, multifunctional cytokine is produced mainly by macrophages and promotes inflammation and the activation of white blood cells.

Complement

This collection of defensive proteins, found in blood and throughout body tissues, is a key component of the body's defences and is described in detail on p. 89.

Consequences of acute inflammation

Generally, acute inflammation can be expected to resolve, accompanied with the elimination of any infecting organism and tissue healing. Depending on the degree of damage, healing may not involve complete replacement of the original tissue and can involve varying degrees of scar formation. Tissues with a high cell turnover (e.g., skin, gastrointestinal lining) or the capacity for significant regeneration (e.g., the liver) generally heal the most completely. If full healing cannot take place e.g., in continuous or repeated injury, because of infection or in immunosuppression, a chronic inflammatory response may develop.

Two main mechanisms are involved in tissue healing: repair and fibrous (scar) tissue formation. Many injuries heal with a combination of the two.

Repair

Repair is the replacement of damaged tissues with newly formed tissue of the same type. Division and proliferation of healthy cells adjacent to the site of injury, sometimes with the contribution of recruited stem cells (p. 61), restore the integrity of the tissue with the same structure as it had before the injury. This is most likely to be complete if the injury is minor and there is no infection.

Scar formation

Deposition of fibrous connective (scar) tissue at the site of injury by fibroblasts supplements healing when complete repair is not possible, perhaps because the damage was extensive or if the tissue is subject to sustained irritation or injury. The inflammatory response at the site is followed by the appearance of granulation tissue, a loose connective tissue rich in active fibroblasts and characterised by developing networks of newly sprouting blood vessels. Injured tissue is progressively cleared from the site by macrophages and is replaced by granulation tissue. With time, a network of connective tissue fibres is steadily laid down throughout the granulation tissue, strengthening and stabilising it, and eventually evolving into the scar (Fig. 1.12) This is called *organisation of the granulation tissue*. Scar tissue helps to seal the wound, join wound edges together, and provide mechanical

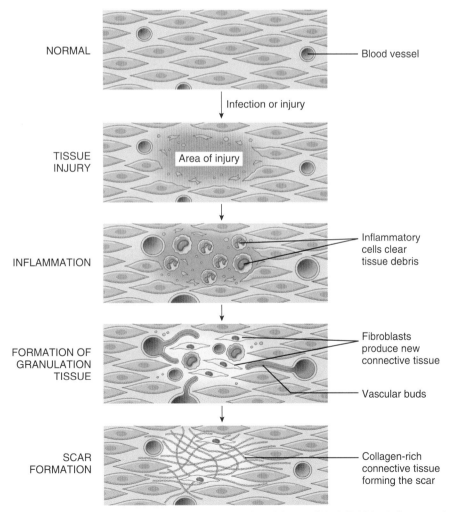

Fig. 1.12 The development of scar tissue. (Modified from Kumar V, Abbas A and Aster J (2017) *Robbins & Cotran pathologic basis of disease: general pathology, vol 1: First Bangladesh edition*, Fig. 3.26. New Delhi: RELX India Pvt. Ltd.)

strength, although typically, a mature scar only achieves about 70% of the strength of the original tissue. However, because it does not have the functional capacity of the original tissue, the organ involved may be seriously compromised if the fibrous tissue is extensive; for example, scar tissue in the heart after a myocardial infarction can seriously interfere with its pumping action, and fibrous tissue in the lung cannot participate in gas exchange.

Keloid scars. A keloid is a mass of excessive scar tissue raised above the skin surface and extending beyond the margins of the original wound. Keloids are benign tumours produced by abnormal healing and usually occur on areas of the skin that are subject to most stretching forces (e.g., across the chest and shoulder, on the flexor surfaces of the limbs). Although they never become malignant, they can have considerable cosmetic impact when they occur on exposed areas of skin, and they can cause significant deformity (Fig. 1.13). Collagen synthesis in keloids is up to 20 times higher than in normally healing scars, and the collagen fibres are not adequately cross-linked, which reduces the strength of the repair. Keloids are more common after deep injuries and in people with highly pigmented skin.

CHRONIC INFLAMMATION

This is an extended and sustained response, with no evidence of healing or resolution. The inflammatory cell population is different compared with acutely inflamed tissues, in which neutrophils and macrophages predominate. Chronically inflamed tissues are populated mainly with lymphocytes, plasma cells, which make antibodies (p. 92) and macrophages. Most cases of chronic inflammation follow an acute inflammatory response that fails to resolve but may occasionally develop spontaneously in otherwise apparently healthy tissues. Factors that increase the risk of an acute inflammatory condition becoming chronic include the following.

Suppurative infection and abscess formation. Suppuration means pus formation and is almost always associated with infection. Pus contains dead and dying leukocytes and tissue cells, and microbes and microbial products. If the infection is close to the body surface or an internal body cavity or passageway, the pus can often drain away and does not collect in significant quantities within the tissues. However, deeper

in the tissues where there is no easy drainage route available, pus accumulates, and pressure from the expanding body of pus triggers a fibrotic response from local fibroblasts, which manufacture a wall of fibrous tissue (the abscess capsule) to enclose it. This forms an abscess, producing a reservoir of infection not easily accessed by defence cells or antimicrobial substances, including antibiotics (Fig. 1.14) A chronic inflammatory response can follow.

The presence of indigestible or persistent inflammatory agents. Asbestos fibres in the alveoli, bone fragments at the site of fracture or foreign bodies (e.g., undissolved sutures, fragments from external materials, or surgical materials left by mistake after an operation) cannot be removed and digested by the body's phagocytes. Their efforts to destroy the unwanted materials cause persistent and sustained chronic inflammation at the site.

Chronic exposure to an irritant. In general, avoiding a known irritant substance leads to resolution (e.g., avoiding cosmetics or laundry products that irritate the skin), but continued application or exposure cause a sustained and chronic response (e.g., the respiratory epithelium in cigarette smoking).

Consequences of chronic inflammation

The main healing mechanism in chronic inflammation involves deposition of granulation tissue and production of fibrous scar tissue. Tissues become thickened, less flexible, and sometimes lose function, depending on the degree of fibrosis. A persistent inflammatory environment, which favours cellular proliferation and is rich in growth factors, is directly linked to the pathogenesis of neoplastic disease (p. 79).

Granuloma formation

A granuloma is a mass of chronically inflamed tissue that has been walled off by fibroblasts to protect adjacent tissues (Fig. 1.15). Granuloma formation is associated with infections caused by microbes resistant to body defences (e.g., tuberculosis and syphilis), some parasitical worm infections, some chemicals that cannot be adequately cleared (e.g., beryllium), and certain rare phagocyte deficiencies (e.g., chronic granulomatous disease). Granulomas can block passageways and compress and damage adjacent structures.

INDICATIONS OF SYSTEMIC INFLAMMATION

Circulating inflammatory mediators and microbial products can affect multiple body organs (a systemic response). Triggers of a systemic inflammatory response include infection, physical exhaustion, burns, cancer, pancreatitis, and myocardial infarction. Signs and symptoms include weight loss, fatigue, general malaise, loss of appetite, and nausea. The systemic inflammatory response in conjunction with infection (sepsis) is considered below.

Acute phase reactants

Blood levels of certain proteins are increased in the systemic inflammatory response, a useful clinical sign. Termed *acute phase reactants*, their role is defensive; they activate protective mechanisms, including complement, and help limit infection. **C-reactive protein** (CRP) is produced mainly in the liver and has a number of protective roles in inflammation and infection, including activating complement and binding to

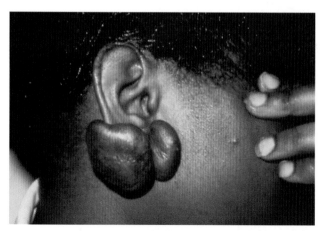

Fig. 1.13 Keloid. Excessive collagen production during healing generates a raised, bulky scar (keloid). (From Townsend C (2022) *Sabiston textbook of surgery*, 21st ed, Fig. 6.6. Philadelphia: Elsevier Inc.)

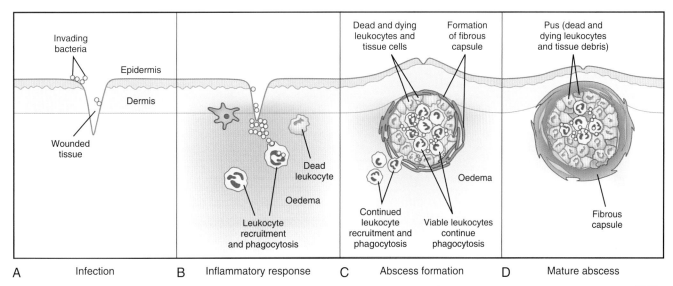

Fig. 1.14 Abscess formation. (A) Tissue injury and infection. (B) Recruitment and activation of leukocytes, which phagocytose microbes. (C) The developing abscess contains a mixture of dead and dying leukocytes and tissue debris. (D) The mature abscess, contained in a fibrous capsule.

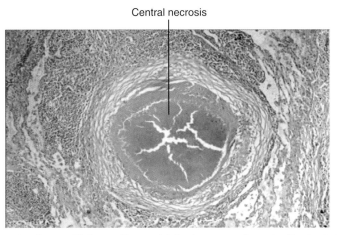

Fig. 1.15 Tuberculosis granuloma, a focal area of inflammation containing immune cells and active bacteria. The central area is hypoxic and necrotic. Reprinted with permission from Elsevier (Lawn SD, Zumla AL (2011) Tuberculosis, *Lancet* 378(9785):57–72).

microbes, increasing their destruction by phagocytes. Its levels usually begin to rise within 6 to 8 hours of the initial insult.

A raised **erythrocyte sedimentation rate** (ESR) is also a non-specific marker of systemic inflammation. Erythrocytes in a blood sample treated with an anticoagulant sink to the bottom of the test tube. In inflammatory or infective conditions, they tend to clump together and therefore sink faster than normal. Other non-specific acute-phase reactants include **fibrinogen** (its levels tend to fall because clotting is activated in systemic inflammation and infection). **Procalcitonin**, the precursor of calcitonin, is elevated in bacterial infections, sepsis, some malignancies, and serious illness (e.g., burns, major surgery, and severe trauma).

Fever (pyrexia)

The hypothalamus in the brain hosts a number of important regulatory centres, including the body's temperature control centre. The hypothalamic thermostat keeps the body's core temperature at about 36.8°C (98.2°F). In infection, circulating microbial products—in particular **lipopolysaccharide** (LPS), a component of some bacterial cell walls—stimulate cytokine release (e.g., IL-1, IL-6, and TNFα) from inflammatory cells. These cytokines reset the hypothalamic thermostat to a value higher than normal (Fig. 1.16), and the hypothalamus initiates mechanisms to generate and conserve heat to bring body temperature up to the new set point. Products of tissue damage and other inflammatory mediators have the same effect on the hypothalamus. Substances that increase body temperature above normal are called **pyrogens**. To achieve the new elevated body temperature, metabolic rate increases to generate more heat, shivering is initiated, there is widespread vasoconstriction in the skin, and the individual may put on extra clothes or wrap up to conserve heat. As with the localised rise in temperature of inflamed tissue, fever reduces the ability of pathogenic bacteria to establish themselves in the body and enhances the activity of defensive phagocytes.

PATHOGENICITY AND INFECTION

It has been estimated that there are a trillion species of microbes on Earth. Microbes, or microscopic organisms, take

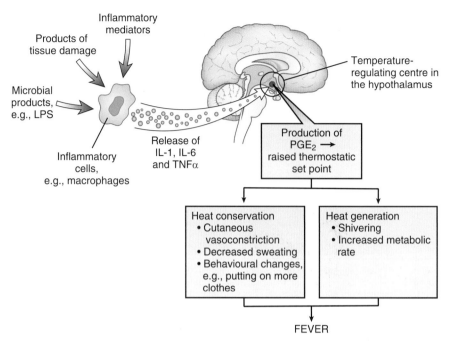

Fig. 1.16 The generation of fever. *IL-1,* Interleukin 1; *IL-6,* interleukin 6; *TNFα,* tumour necrosis factor alpha; *LPS,* lipopolysaccharide; *PGE₂,* prostaglandin E₂. (Modified from Brown D, Edwards H, Buckley T, et al. (2020) *Lewis's medical-surgical nursing,* 5th ed, Fig. 10.3. Sydney: Elsevier Australia.)

many forms, including bacteria, viruses, fungi, and protozoa. Only a very small proportion of these are pathogenic in humans (i.e., cause human disease), and many microbial species inhabit body spaces and surfaces in a peaceful and sometimes beneficial coexistence. Such microbes are called *commensals.* The microbial population (microbiome) living in the human gastrointestinal tract has significant effects, both positive and negative, on health.

Microbes inhabited Earth long before humans, who were therefore obliged to evolve sophisticated and effective defence mechanisms to survive infection. Some of these are described previously (inflammation, fever) and in Chapter 4, and reduced effectiveness of defence and immunity greatly increases the risk and severity for infection.

In the modern era of medicine, when the principles of microbial transmission and the importance of basic hygiene are well understood and antimicrobial drugs are globally available, it might seem at first glance that humans should have conquered the threat of infection. In many countries, the incidence and mortality associated with infections that were once very common, such as maternal infection after childbirth, typhoid fever, and many sexually transmitted diseases, have fallen dramatically. The development of vaccines against many common and potentially lethal infections and the implementation of vaccination programmes have contributed significantly to reducing the burden of infection on human health. However, infection is still very common and is the most frequent adverse outcome associated with healthcare settings (also called **nosocomial infection**). Overuse of antibiotics and other antimicrobial agents has led to the emergence of multiple strains of microbes that no longer respond to drug treatment, so-called *resistant strains.* The regular emergence of infections that reach pandemic proportions (i.e., spread rapidly from country to country, infecting people worldwide) is in

part the result of cheap and easy travel, and the widespread transport of goods and materials around the world. The Spanish flu pandemic of 1918 to 1919 infected a third of the world's population and killed over 50 million people. Human immunodeficiency virus (HIV) probably emerged from chimpanzees in the 1920s, spread to humans, and is estimated to have caused over 25 million deaths since the 1980s. The virus SARS-CoV-2, thought to have originated in bats in China, emerged in 2019, spreading rapidly from its region of origin to cause the COVID-19 pandemic. The human and economic toll of infection is, unsurprisingly, significantly greater in under-resourced and financially poorer countries.

Infections specific to particular body systems are described in relevant chapters. The following sections consider the principal characteristics of the main groups of pathogenic microbes and some of the systemic consequences of infection.

PATHOGENIC GROUPS

From a clinical point of view, identifying the specific organism responsible for a particular infection is essential in identifying the pathophysiological changes likely to occur and to choose appropriate treatments. The ability of a microbe to cause disease depends on a range of factors; the infecting organism must have an effective route of transmission, be able to survive and reproduce in one or more of the environments within the body, and be able to avoid or resist host defences. The stages of infection are shown in Fig. 1.17. The capacity of a pathogen to harm its host is called *virulence;* the more virulent the organism, the more damage it can do. Microbes enter the body through a variety of routes, including skin wounds or via the respiratory, genitourinary, or gastrointestinal tracts. It must also be remembered that for many infections, especially when chronic, the body's defensive and immune response contribute significantly to the tissue damage associated with the infection.

Naming microorganisms

Conventionally, microbes (except viruses) are identified with two names, both of which should be italicised. The first name is the **genus** (pl. genera) to which it belongs. Each genus contains numerous subgroups called **species**, and the second part of the microbe's name identifies its species. Hence, *Staphylococcus aureus* and *Staphylococcus epidermidis* are two species of bacteria within the genus *Staphylococcus*. The genus portion is often shortened according to a conventional list of abbreviations: hence, *Streptococcus pyogenes*

is *S. pyogenes*, *Helicobacter pylori* is *H. pylori*, and *Staphylococcus aureus* is *Staph. aureus*.

Bacteria

The main parts of a bacterial cell are shown in Fig. 1.18. There is no nucleus, and bacterial DNA is usually formed of an extended single DNA molecule present in the cytoplasm. Cells with no nucleus are termed **prokaryotes**. Because bacteria require protection from their external environment, most have a rigid, protective outer cell wall, below which lies their plasma membrane, a phospholipid bilayer like the plasma membrane of mammalian cells. There may also be an outer protective capsule. Like mammalian cells, bacteria produce proteins on their ribosomes, but there is no endoplasmic reticulum, and ribosomes are scattered free in the cytoplasm. The cytoplasm may contain inclusions of stored nutrients, and many bacteria have flagellae: long, spiral, thread-like extensions used for propulsion through the external medium. Short, threadlike filaments called *fimbriae* or *pili* (singular: fimbria and pilus) extend from the cell wall and allow the bacterium to adhere to adjacent structures, including other bacteria and to human cells.

Some bacteria, notably *Clostridium* and *Bacillus* species, form **spores** when exposed to unfavourable environmental conditions. Spores are dormant, meaning they have no metabolic activity and are incapable of reproduction, but they are very robust and allow the bacterium to survive for extended periods, sometimes hundreds of years, in adverse conditions. When conditions become more favourable, the spore germinates and reverts to the normal bacterial form. Food contaminated with *Clostridium* and *Bacillus* spores can therefore cause food poisoning, even after cooking or preservation procedures.

Mechanisms of bacterial pathogenicity

After entry into the body, bacteria adhere to target cells via their fimbriae and attach to specific receptors present on the plasma membrane. They grow and divide and establish themselves on or within a body tissue e.g., in food poisoning, when the epithelium of the gastrointestinal tract is colonised. From here, they may invade deeper tissues and spread to distant sites via the lymphatics or bloodstream. Some bacteria enter body cells and survive and proliferate within them. These bacteria are called **intracellular pathogens** and include *Mycobacteria* and *Chlamydia* species. Hidden within body cells, they are protected from the body's

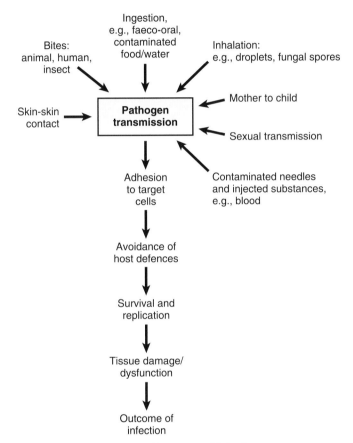

Fig. 1.17   The stages of infection.

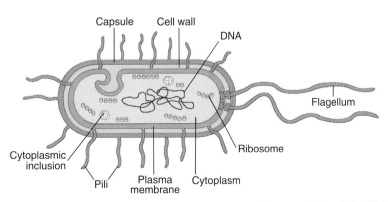

Fig. 1.18   The main features of a bacterial cell. (Modified from Goering R, Dockrell H, Zuckerman M, et al. (2018) *Mims medical microbiology*, 6th ed. Philadelphia: Elsevier.)

Table 1.3   The pathogenic effects of some bacterial toxins

Organism	Effects of toxin
Clostridium botulinum (food poisoning)	Blocks transmission at the neuromuscular junction
Vibrio cholerae (cholera)	Triggers water and electrolyte secretion in the gastrointestinal tract
Clostridium tetani (tetanus)	Triggers painful, sustained skeletal muscle contraction
Staphylococcus aureus (multiple infections and secretes a range of toxins)	Haemolysis (caused by toxins called *lysins*)
	Fever (pyrogenic toxins)
	Vomiting (enterotoxins)
	Dermo-epidermal separation (epidermolytic toxin)
Shigella species (bacterial dysentery)	Profuse and watery diarrhoea
Bacillus pertussis (whooping cough)	Inhibits ciliary action and suppresses immune function

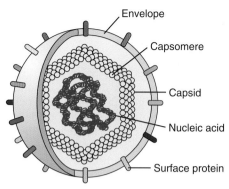

Fig. 1.19   General structure of a virus. (Modified from VanMeter K and Hubert R (2022) *Microbiology for the healthcare professional*, 3rd ed, Fig. 5.2. St Louis: Mosby.)

immune system. Bacterial proliferation kills the host cell, releasing more bacteria into the local environment and spreading the infection.

Many bacteria release toxins that directly damage body tissues (e.g., enterotoxins from *Escherichia coli*), and other organisms responsible for food poisoning damage gastrointestinal epithelial cells. Bacterial toxins reaching the bloodstream can cause widespread organ damage not restricted to the focus of infection. Other toxins damage cell membranes, activate a damaging inflammatory response, or suppress host immune responses. Table 1.3 lists some important bacterial toxins and their effects.

Some organisms release enzymes that damage or break down tissue constituents (e.g., elastases that destroy elastin and phospholipases that damage cell membranes). *Helicobacter pylori*, which infects the stomach mucosa, produces urease, an enzyme that produces ammonia and raises gastric pH, an important factor in the pathology of *H. pylori* infection (p. 288).

Some medically important pathogenic bacteria

A wide range of microbes cause disease, most of which are considered in the relevant sections of this textbook, but two of the most important genera of pathogenic bacteria, streptococci and staphylococci, are described here.

Streptococcus. Streptococci are berry-shaped bacteria that tend to grow in pairs or in chains and usually prefer anaerobic (the absence of oxygen) conditions. Some species growing in the mouth and throat are useful commensal organisms and secrete microbicidal substances that prevent other microbes from establishing themselves on these membranes. However, others cause significant infections. *S. pyogenes* (group A streptococcus) causes pharyngitis ('strep sore throat'), scarlet fever, and skin infections, including erysipelas and cellulitis. These infections can trigger an abnormal immune response responsible for rheumatic fever and post-streptococcal glomerulonephritis. *S. pneumoniae* (pneumococcus) is found in the respiratory tracts of up to

70% of otherwise healthy people but can cause a range of serious infections including pneumonia, meningitis, and endocarditis.

Staphylococcus. Staphylococcal species are berry-shaped bacteria that grow in clusters. They are anaerobic organisms and can be isolated from the skin and upper respiratory tract of many healthy people. They are adaptable and diverse, they rapidly develop resistance to a range of antibiotics, and they cause a wide variety of human infections. *Staphylococcus aureus*, which grows as golden colonies on nutrient agar (hence the name: aureus means *gold* in Latin), is responsible for many of these, including skin infections (e.g., boils, impetigo, and scalded skin syndrome), wound infections (including post-surgical infection), food poisoning, osteomyelitis, pneumonia, endocarditis, and blood-borne infection. Many strains of *S. aureus* produce heat-stable toxins, which are responsible for some of their pathogenicity (e.g., food poisoning and scalded skin syndrome). Methicillin-resistant *S. aureus* (MRSA) was first isolated in 1961 in the UK and rapidly spread to become a global problem. It continues to cause serious infections that present considerable treatment challenges, and despite extensive study of this microbe, medical science has not yet found a way to control its spread or pathogenicity.

Viruses

Viruses are not living cells, in the sense that they are not capable of independent life and must infect a host cell before they can reproduce. The simplest viral particles consist of a short section of nucleic acid and a few essential viral enzymes wrapped in an external symmetrical capsid made of proteins called capsomeres (Fig. 1.19). Some viruses carry their genetic material in the form of DNA, whereas others possess the simpler, single-stranded form RNA. The surface of the virus displays a range of proteins, including enzymes to help the viral particle move through host tissues and receptors that allow them to attach to host cell membranes, an essential step in infection. Some may also possess a lipid-rich envelope, acquired from the host cell when pushing through the cell's membrane when leaving it.

The viral life cycle is shown in Fig. 1.20. Viruses bind to body cells via cell-surface receptors and are absorbed through the cell membrane. Once within the host cell, the virus uncoats; that is, it opens its capsid to release the enzymes and viral nucleic acid within. The host cell then reads

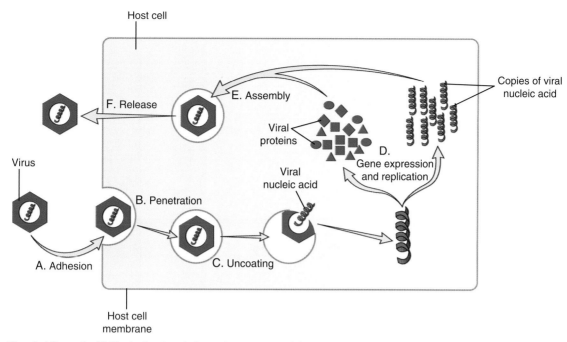

Fig. 1.20 The viral life cycle. (A) Viral adhesion via its surface proteins. (B) Virus enters host cell. (C) Virus uncoats. (D) Virus uses host cell machinery to synthesise new viral nucleic acids and proteins. (E) Assembly. New viral particles are produced. (F) Release. Viruses may now carry an envelope of lipids from host cell membrane. (Modified from Ryu WS (2017) *Molecular virology of human pathogenic viruses*, Fig. 3.1. Boston: Academy Press.)

the viral nucleic acid to produce new viral proteins and also makes multiple copies of the viral nucleic acid. If its nucleic acid is in the form of DNA, this can be inserted directly into the host cell's DNA and used to produce viral proteins. If the viral nucleic acid is single-stranded RNA, the process is a little more complicated: these viruses, called **retroviruses**, also carry an enzyme called *reverse transcriptase*, which generates double-stranded DNA from the RNA. This DNA is then used by the host cell to produce viral proteins. Finally, new viral particles are assembled and released, which may happen in one of two ways. Some viruses simply reproduce continually in the host cell until the host cell lyses (bursts), releasing new viruses suddenly and in great numbers into local tissues to infect adjacent cells. Alternatively, the new viral particles may be released in a slower stream through the host cell membrane so that the infected cell remains alive and capable of generating virus over an extended period of time. Such viruses often cause chronic infection.

Mechanisms of viral pathogenicity

Viruses can kill cells via lysis as described previously. Other mechanisms of virally induced tissue damage include the production of enzymes and toxins that damage or destroy essential cell components, including the cell membrane, disabling or killing the host cell. Because viruses interfere with the host cell DNA and the cell cycle machinery, some viral infections are associated with an increased risk of cancer. Notable examples include the human papilloma virus (HPV) and cervical cancer, and Epstein-Barr virus (EBV) and Burkitt's lymphoma.

Some medically important pathogenic viruses

Most viral infections are short-lived and self-limiting, but viruses have caused some of the most devastating epidemics in human history. Important viruses include the human immunodeficiency virus, influenza virus, and hepatitis viruses.

Herpesviruses. There are at least 100 different viruses in this family, of which eight infect humans. They include herpes zoster virus (HZV), herpes simplex virus (HSV, p. 382), EBV, and cytomegalovirus (CMV). They are all associated with **latency**, which means that the virus may remain dormant within tissues for long periods of time; during this time, the virus is not replicating, and there is no evidence of infection. However, the virus may be reactivated, often more than once, so that initial infection is followed by variable periods of remission and episodes of active disease. The herpesvirus family cause a range of common infections (Table 1.4).

Fungi

Fungal cells are more highly evolved than bacterial cells or viral particles, with complex membrane systems similar to those of human cells. Their outer boundary, like bacteria, is a rigid and protective cell wall, below which lies the fungal cell membrane. They may grow as branched cords (hyphae) formed from individual fungal cells joined end-to-end forming a dense intertwined network called a *mycelium*. Mycelia can grow to phenomenal sizes: the largest living thing on Earth, growing in the soil in an Oregon forest, is an enormous honey fungus thought to be at least 3.8 km wide. Fungi that form mycelia are called **moulds**. **Yeasts** are fungi that usually exist as individual, ovoid cells that reproduce by budding, a process by which the cell grows an extension of itself that eventually separates as a new cell. Although there are more than 100,000 species of fungi, fewer than 1% cause disease in animals or humans. Fungal infection in humans is usually associated with immunocompromise, or where tissues are unusually

Table 1.4   The main herpesviruses

Virus name	Comments
Herpes simplex 1 (HSV1) and herpes simplex 2 (HSV2)	Cause oral, genital, and skin infections and meningitis
Varicella zoster virus (VZV)	Causes chickenpox and shingles
Epstein-Barr virus (EBV)	Causes glandular fever
Cytomegalovirus (CMV)	Causes a range of infections in immunocompromised people; congenital CMV infection can impair intrauterine development; respiratory infection in children
Kaposi's sarcoma-associated herpes virus (KSHV)	Strongly associated with Kaposi's sarcoma, usually only seen in immunocompromised patients (e.g., in AIDS)

Box 1.2   Risk factors for sepsis

Those under 1 year	Neonates, especially prematurity
	Maternal infection or fever
	Maternal group B streptococcal infection, either in this pregnancy or in a previous pregnancy
Pregnancy	Within 6 weeks of giving birth, having a termination, miscarriage, or stillbirth.
	Extended period between rupture of membranes and delivery
	Post-delivery vaginal infection
	Medical intervention (e.g., caesarean section, forceps delivery)
	Gestational diabetes, diabetes, or other coexisting medical conditions
	Contact with group A streptococcal infection
Older age	Over 75 years
	Frailty
Immunocompromise	Steroid or other immunosuppressant treatment
	Recent surgery or other invasive procedures
	Indwelling urinary catheters or lines
	Chemotherapy
	Intravenous drug users
	Splenectomy
	Skin wounds, infections, burns, or blistering disorders
Chronic illness	Diabetes
	Liver cirrhosis
	Kidney disease
	HIV infection
	Autoimmune disease
	Cancer
	Chronic obstructive airways disease
Hospitalised people/ those in healthcare institutions	

warm, moist, and infrequently washed (e.g., between the toes in particularly sweaty feet, or between skin folds in people with obesity).

Mechanisms of fungal pathogenicity

Fungi are among the normal flora of body membranes and are usually kept in check by other microbial populations present. However, they can flourish if the individual is immunocompromised or if other resident flora are destroyed by antibiotic treatment. Thrush, a fungal infection caused by *Candida albicans*, is a good example of this; oral thrush is sometimes seen after treatment with a broad-spectrum antibiotic. This is an example of an opportunistic infection. Some fungi colonise passageways and obstruct them; for example, inhaled *Aspergillus* spores can establish themselves in airways and produce dense masses of fungal tissue that block them completely. Organisms that use keratin as an energy source (dermatophytes) can establish themselves in the skin, hair, and nails, causing inflammation and tissue damage. Sometimes, fungal pathogenicity is associated with a specific fungal toxin, as in eating poisonous mushrooms. Additionally, allergic responses to fungal proteins may cause respiratory problems.

Protozoa

The protozoa are a diverse group of unicellular organisms responsible for a range of infections. They spend part of their life cycle in another living creature, and so the distribution of the disease caused by each is restricted to the habitat of the alternative host. They include the sporozoa (e.g., the malaria plasmodium), amoebae, some of which cause gastrointestinal infections (e.g., *Entamoeba histolytica*) and flagellated organisms. These include trichomonas (e.g., *Trichomonas vaginalis*) and trypanosomes (e.g., sleeping sickness).

Sleeping sickness (African trypanosomiasis)

The trypanosome causing this condition is *Trypanosoma brucei* and is endemic to sub-Saharan Africa. Its alternative host is the tsetse fly. The bite of an infected fly injects trypanosomes into the bloodstream, where they divide. They then infect multiple body tissues including the central nervous system, where they cause encephalitis, which is fatal if untreated.

SEPSIS

Sepsis is a continuum of progressive damage to body organs because of an excessive and overwhelming body response to an insult, usually bacterial infection. Severe sepsis is characterised by developing shock (p. 161) and life-threatening organ failure. It is important to realise that the initiating infection may not in itself be serious, and the risk of sepsis developing is significantly increased in vulnerable people. Risk factors for sepsis are given in Box 1.2. If sepsis causes circulatory failure or metabolic or cellular abnormalities that significantly increase mortality, it is considered to have progressed to septic shock. The WHO estimates that sepsis causes up to 6 million deaths annually, and low- and middle-income countries bear most of this mortality burden. It is a major cause of child and maternal deaths.

Pathophysiology

The initial infection activates the body's immune defences and an inflammatory response, with the production and release of cytokines and pro-inflammatory mediators. Leukocytes, particularly neutrophils, are activated, and they

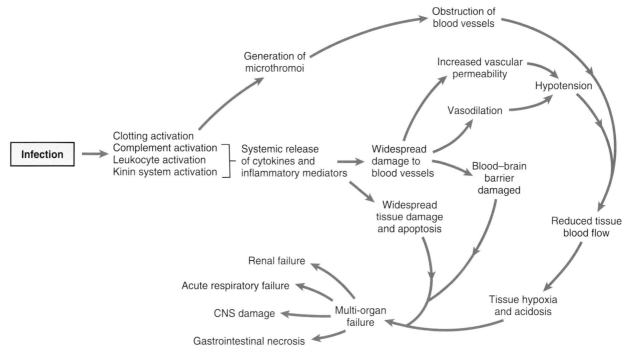

Fig. 1.21 The pathogenesis of sepsis. *CNS,* Central nervous system.

converge on the area of infection and release their own mediators. Normally, the inflammatory response is restricted to the area of infection, but in sepsis, it becomes systemic, causing widespread inflammation and tissue damage in multiple organs. This hyper-inflammatory phase is associated with activation of complement and the release of powerful inflammatory cytokines including TNFα and interleukins. These agents injure blood vessels, particularly the microvasculature, rendering them unable to control blood flow, impairing blood supply to organs and causing tissue ischaemia. Hypotension develops because damaged blood vessels dilate, and circulating inflammatory mediators and bacterial toxins increase the permeability of blood vessel walls, resulting in the loss of fluid into the tissues. The clotting cascade is activated, and microthrombi block small vessels, impairing blood flow even more and accelerating cell death and organ failure. The cytokines also trigger apoptosis (programmed cell death) in key immune cells, depleting them and reducing the body's ability to fight the infection. Microvascular damage in the central nervous system reduces the effectiveness of the blood–brain barrier, allowing aggressive immune cells and toxic inflammatory mediators to cross into the brain, leading to neurological dysfunction. Microvascular damage in the lungs causes pulmonary oedema and progressive lung dysfunction. Acute kidney injury is very common in sepsis and is associated with a poor outcome. Damage in the gastrointestinal tract disrupts the barrier function of the tract wall, which normally prevents bacteria crossing from the lumen into local blood vessels, and injury to gastrointestinal organs can cause release of digestive enzymes that degrade and destroy tissue. Fig. 1.21 summarises the key events in developing sepsis.

Signs and symptoms

The patient is tachycardic, with an elevated respiratory rate and low blood pressure. The patient may be unable to maintain adequate blood oxygen levels without oxygen treatment. Urine output is low, and the skin is blue or blue/grey and may be mottled. There may be indications of frank infection, for example, pyrexia, an infected surgical wound, or a urinary tract infection. Rising blood lactate levels cause metabolic acidosis, which correlates with a poorer outcome.

Management and prognosis

The Sepsis Trust recently implemented the Sepsis Six bundle, a package of six interventions that has been shown to significantly reduce mortality. Of the six interventions, three are to be given (oxygen, antibiotics, and fluids) and three are to be taken (bloods for arterial blood gases, glucose levels, lactate levels, and other standard tests; cultures to identify the infection; and regular readings of urine output to monitor renal function). Early identification is enormously important because rapid intervention interrupts the spiral of deteriorating function that accompanies developing sepsis, reduces mortality, and minimises long-term organ damage.

BIBLIOGRAPHY AND REFERENCES

Arkis, M., Burgler, S., Crameri, R., et al. (2011). Interleukins, from 1 to 37, and interferon-gamma: Receptors, functions, and roles in disease. *The Journal of Allergy and Clinical Immunology, 127*(3), 701–721.
Arwyn-Jones, J., & Sepis, B. A. (2019). Sepis. *Surgery, 37*(1), 1–8.
Vetter, T. R., & Jesser, C. A. (2017). Fundamental epidemiology terminology and measures: It really is all in the name. *Anesthesia & Analgesia, 125*(6), 2146–2151.

Useful websites

Global Burden of Disease home page: http://www.healthdata.org/gbd.
The Sepsis Trust: https://sepsistrust.org
WHO constitution: https://www.who.int/about/who-we-are/constitution
WHO factsheet on sepsis: https://www.who.int/news-room/factsheets/detail/sepsis

2 Genetics and Disease

CHAPTER OUTLINE

DNA, GENES, AND CHROMOSOMES
From DNA to proteins
  DNA and chromosomes
  The functional unit of DNA: the gene
  From gene to protein
Epigenetics
Mitochondrial DNA
PATTERNS OF INHERITANCE
  Autosomal inheritance
  Sex-linked inheritance
GENE DISORDERS
The principal monogenic disorders
  Cystic fibrosis (CF)
  Duchenne muscular dystrophy
  Fabry disease
  Fragile X syndrome
  Haemophilia
  Homocystinuria
  Huntington disease
  Leigh syndrome

Marfan syndrome
Neurofibromatosis
Osteogenesis imperfecta
Phenylketonuria (PKU)
Polycystic kidney disease (PKD)
Retinoblastoma
Sickle cell anaemia
Tay Sachs disease
Thalassaemias
Polygenic disorders
  Polygenic inheritance
CHROMOSOMES AND THEIR ABNORMALITIES
Mitosis, meiosis and the production of gametes
The main autosomal abnormalities
  Cri-du-chat syndrome
  Down syndrome
The principal sex chromosome disorders
  Klinefelter syndrome
  Turner syndrome

DNA, GENES, AND CHROMOSOMES

Genetics is the study of heredity and the variation of inherited characteristics between generations. Ancient civilisations recognised that characteristics of their plants and livestock were passed from generation to generation, and they knew to sow seed from the hardiest crops and breed from the strongest animals, but our understanding of the basis of heredity dates only from the end of the 19th century. The word *genetics* is a recent entry into the scientific dictionary and was coined by the English biologist William Bateson in 1906. Bateson was interested in evolution and in how characteristics of living creatures appeared, disappeared, and reappeared throughout generations. His work was strongly influenced by a paper that appeared in 1867, which would be fundamental to the emergence of the study of heredity as a rational and mathematical science. The author was a monk living in Moravia; his name was Gregor Mendel, and although his chosen vocation was a religious one, he had sound scientific training and a systematic approach to his investigations. Mendel (Fig. 2.1) performed experiments on generations of sweet pea plants, examining the inheritance of specific traits such as seed colour and plant height, and concluded that these characteristics were passed from parent to offspring in stable, transmissible units. He suggested that offspring inherited two of these units, one from each parent. This discovery was fundamental to the explosion of research in heredity dating from the early 20th century, and the rapid development of the science now called *genetics*. We call Mendel's transmissible units *genes*, and each nucleated cell (except gametes) contains around 20,000 genes, packaged into much larger structures called *chromosomes*. In 1956, human cells were shown to contain 46 chromosomes, arranged in 23 pairs and found in the cell nucleus. Chromosomes are built of the longest molecule in the human body: deoxyribonucleic acid (DNA). DNA contains the genetic code, written in the genes found along the length of the molecule, which determines the characteristics of every living organism on Earth.

The **genome** refers to all the genetic material belonging to an organism. The **genotype** refers to the genes belonging to an individual, and the result of that gene activity in the individual is called the **phenotype**; e.g., the genes

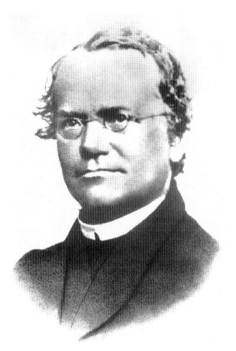

Fig. 2.1 Gregor Mendel (From Mendel's Principles of Heredity, by W. Bateson, 1909).

for eye colour are part of an individual's genotype and the colour of their eyes is the expression of those genes: their phenotype.

This chapter will explore the molecular structure of DNA, genes, and chromosomes; discuss the science of heredity; describe the main categories of genetic disorders; and consider advances in genetic medicine.

FROM DNA TO PROTEINS

Nearly all genes code for the production of proteins, although a few code for production of essential non-protein molecules, such as ribonucleic acid, whose function will be discussed later.

DNA AND CHROMOSOMES

DNA was discovered in the mid-19th century and was confirmed as the cell's genetic material in the mid-1940s by a group of researchers at New York's Rockefeller Institute. The problem of how the vast amount of information needed by the cell could be contained within such a simple molecule as DNA was solved when, in 1953, the British scientists Roger Watson and James Crick demonstrated its elegant double helix structure. Each nucleated cell contains DNA that would measure several metres in total length if pulled straight and measured end to end. The key to fitting such a huge quantity of DNA into the tiny cell nucleus, which is only about 6 μm in diameter, lies in the coiling and super coiling of lengths of DNA, producing dense, compact structures visible down the microscope as 46 individual chromosomes.

Chemically, DNA is very simple: it is composed of four bases—namely, adenine (A), cytosine (C), guanine (G) and thymine (T)—a sugar (deoxyribose), and phosphate groups. If the twisted, double-stranded structure

of DNA is compared with a twisted ladder, the ladder uprights are made of alternating sugar and phosphate groups, and the ladder rungs are made of base pairs. Base pairing is not random: if the base on one strand is cytosine, the matching base is always guanine; similarly, adenine is always paired with thymine. There are 3 billion base pairs in a cell's DNA, and the sequence of base pairs is the code in which the cell stores the information for producing all body proteins. A base (A, T, C, or G) plus its associated sugar and phosphate group is called a **nucleotide** (Fig. 2.2).

DNA is tightly coiled round small, positively charged proteins called **histones**, which facilitate DNA folding. Because DNA is negatively charged, DNA-histone ionic bonds stabilise the structure. In terms of mass, there is normally about the same volume of histone protein as DNA in the nucleus, but the histones allow such efficient folding and packaging of the DNA that the resultant 46 chromosomes fit within the tiny volume of the cell nucleus (Fig. 2.2) The term used for DNA and its associated proteins is **chromatin**.

Although chromosomes are sometimes described as thread or sausage-shaped, each chromosome is narrowed at a point called the *centromere*, giving it a 'waist' and dividing it into a short arm and a long arm. The short arm is called the *p arm* and the long arm is the *q arm*. Stained and viewed under the microscope, each chromosome displays a series of light and dark bands and sub-bands, which are useful when describing a specific location on the chromosome. At each end of the DNA strand packed into the chromosome is a repeating sequence called a **telomere**, which is responsible for limiting the number of times the cell can replicate (see also p. 64). Fig. 2.3 shows the general features of a chromosome pair.

In nucleated body cells, chromosomes are visible only at certain times of the cell cycle (p. 63), just before replication. The rest of the time, the chromatin is more diffuse and less organised. When visible, the 46 chromosomes are paired, and these pairs are numbered 1 to 23. Pairs 1 to 22 are called **autosomes**, and pair 23 comprises the **sex chromosomes**, which identify the individual as male or female. A male has an X chromosome and a Y chromosome (XY), and a female has two X chromosomes (XX). A cell's chromosomes can be extracted, paired, identified, and photographed: this is called **karyotyping**. An individual's karyotype represents the genetic inheritance from the parents, and of each pair of chromosomes, one came from the mother (in the ovum) and the other from the father (in the spermatozoon) (Fig. 2.4). A male child inherits his Y chromosome from his father and an X from his mother; a female child inherits her father's X chromosome and one of her mother's X chromosomes.

THE FUNCTIONAL UNIT OF DNA: THE GENE

Less than 2% of the cell's DNA actually codes for protein. The sections of DNA that do code for proteins are called *genes* and are found at specific places on specific chromosomes. The Human Genome Project, whose objectives were to identify the specific sequence of base pairs on all DNA in the human cell, to identify all its genes, and to precisely map their locations, completed its work in 2003. This massively important international collaboration provided mankind with the blueprint for making a human cell and opened

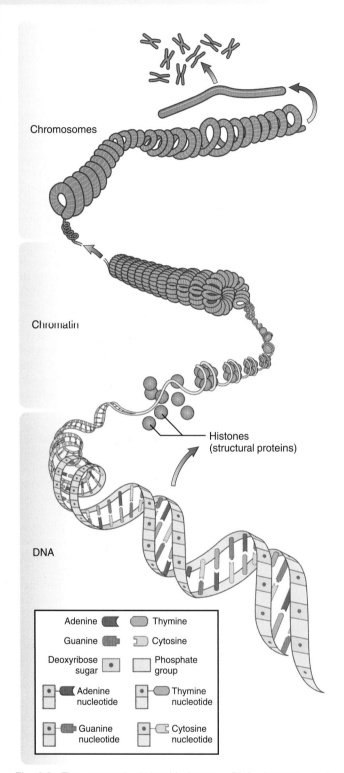

Chromosomes

Chromatin

DNA

Histones
(structural proteins)

Adenine	Thymine
Guanine	Cytosine
Deoxyribose sugar	Phosphate group
Adenine nucleotide	Thymine nucleotide
Guanine nucleotide	Cytosine nucleotide

Fig. 2.2 The structural relationship between DNA, chromatin, and chromosomes. (Modified from Waugh A and Grant A (2018) *Ross & Wilson anatomy and physiology in health and illness*, 13th ed, Fig 17.4. Oxford: Elsevier Ltd.)

countless opportunities for the prevention and treatment of disease.

Gene mapping

Every gene now has a molecular 'address', which pinpoints its precise size and chromosomal location, and which uses

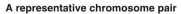

A representative chromosome pair

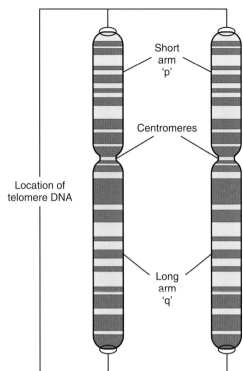

Short arm 'p'

Centromeres

Location of telomere DNA

Long arm 'q'

Fig. 2.3 A representative chromosome pair.

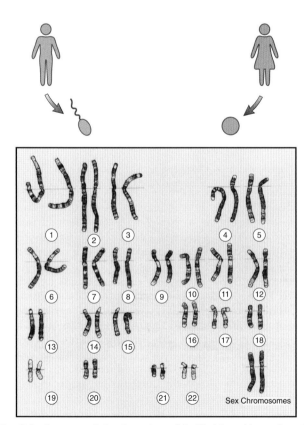

1 2 3 4 5
6 7 8 9 10 11 12
13 14 15 16 17 18
19 20 21 22 Sex Chromosomes

Fig. 2.4 A representative karyotype. (Modified from Hagen-Ansert S (2018) *Textbook of diagnostic sonography*, 8th ed, Fig. 55.3. St Louis: Elsevier Inc.)

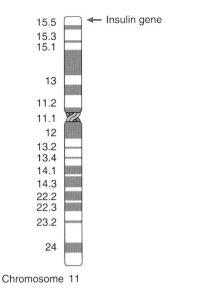

← Insulin gene

Chromosome 11

Fig. 2.5 Chromosome 11 showing the location of the insulin gene. (Modified from McPherson R (2022) *Henry's clinical diagnosis and management by laboratory methods,* 24th ed, South Asia Edition, Fig. 71.24. New Delhi: Elsevier India.)

a specific nomenclature understood by the international genetics community. For example, the gene that codes for the production of insulin is found on the short arm of chromosome 11 at position 15.5 (band 15, sub-band 5), and its address is given as 11p15.5 (Fig. 2.5). Knowing the exact location of a specific gene and which other genes are nearby is significant because genes that are close to one another can affect one another's function and therefore may be more likely to stay together during the meiotic divisions that mix up genetic material in the production of gametes (ova and sperm) and so be inherited together. Fig. 2.6 shows a karyotype demonstrating the locations of some key genes whose mutation is associated with important genetic disorders.

Gene pairs: alleles

The ovum and spermatozoon that fuse at conception each carries one copy of chromosomes 1 to 23 so that the resulting zygote now has two of each chromosome, matched up to give the familiar 23 chromosome pairs forming the genome of the new individual. The genes found along these chromosomes are located at the same place on each chromosome of each pair, whether the chromosome came from the

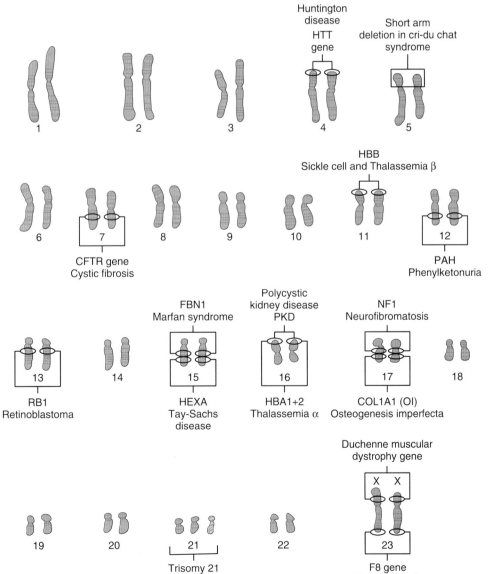

Fig. 2.6 Karyotype showing the location of gene mutations and chromosomal abnormalities associated with some important genetic disorders.

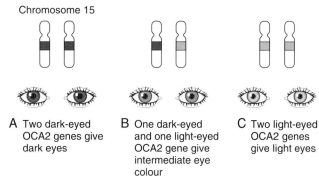

Fig. 2.7 The effect of polymorphism of the *OCA2* gene on eye colour. The *OCA2* locus on chromosome 15 is shown. (A) Two dark-eyed *OCA2* genes give dark eyes. (B) One dark-eyed gene and one light-eyed gene give intermediate eye colour. (C) Two light-eyed *OCA2* genes give light eyes.

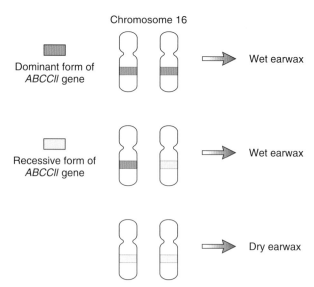

Fig. 2.8 Expression of dominant and recessive genes.

mother or the father. For example, as described previously, the gene that codes for insulin is found at 11p15.5 on the maternal chromosome and at exactly the same place (**locus**, plural loci) on the paternal chromosome. The zygote therefore has two copies of the insulin gene. These paired genes are called **alleles**. Although they sit on corresponding loci on the paired chromosomes 11, the two genes may not be identical. In most individuals, both genes will be normal and both code for insulin. However, sometimes the gene from one parent is mutated or abnormal in some way. In that case, the individual relies on the other gene from the other parent being fully functional for normal insulin production.

Another example is the genes that code for eye colour. Unlike the insulin gene, which is the only gene in the entire genome that codes for insulin, eye colour is determined by multiple genes, resulting in a wide variety of human eye colourings. This is determined by the type of the pigment melanin in the iris. At least 15 genes are thought to be involved in determining eye colour, but the main one is found on chromosome 15. This gene is called *OCA2* and it makes a protein called P protein, which increases melanin production in the iris. Some forms of the *OCA2* gene make a great deal of P protein, which means melanin levels in the iris are high and the eyes are dark, and other forms of the gene produce less, leading to lighter eyes. If an individual inherits two light-eyed forms of the gene, they are more likely to have lighter eyes that someone who inherits a light-eyed and a dark-eyed gene. Different forms of the same gene are called **polymorphisms** (Fig. 2.7) If both alleles for a given gene are identical, the individual is said to be **homozygous** for that gene. If the two genes are not identical, the individual is **heterozygous** for that gene.

Gene polymorphism is not the only factor affecting an individual's phenotype. Alleles are not always equally strongly expressed. When an individual is heterozygous for a gene (i.e., possesses two different forms of that gene), one is often responsible for determining the phenotype; this is called **dominance**. The other gene, whose effects may be completely masked by the dominant allele, is called **recessive**. Very few traits are coded for by a single gene. Many of those once thought to be single-gene traits, such as tongue rolling and hairline shape, are now known to be the product of more than one gene. However, earwax consistency is determined by a single gene, the *ABCC11* gene, which regulates the

secretory activity of an ion channel that controls how wet or dry the earwax is. The normal allele for wet earwax (commonest in European and African populations) is dominant over the mutant allele for dry earwax. This means that an individual with two dominant wet earwax alleles will have wet earwax, an individual with one wet earwax allele and one dry earwax allele will also have wet earwax, and an individual with two dry earwax alleles will have dry earwax. Only one copy of a dominant gene is required for its trait to be expressed (Fig. 2.8). The mutant, recessive form for dry earwax is different from the dominant allele by only a single base pair in the gene sequence.

FROM GENE TO PROTEIN

The DNA base pair sequence along the length of a gene determines the precise order of amino acids that will be assembled into a new protein. Each gene is marked at one end with a start sequence of bases, indicating the beginning of the coding sequence, and a stop sequence at the other end. Within the gene, however, the base sequence does not all code for protein. On average, a gene contains nine **exons**, which are base sequences that carry the code for the protein, interspersed with **introns**, which are not code. Fig. 2.9A shows a hypothetical gene, with its stop and start sequences. This gene has four coding sequences (exons 1–4) and three sections of non-coding introns in between. How the intron sections are dealt with in production of the final protein is described below.

Junk DNA and satellites

The genes on a chromosome are found at intervals along the chromosomal length, separated by long stretches of apparently useless, 'junk' DNA. The 98% of DNA that does not code for protein is made up of repeated base sequences in groups of two, three, four, five, or more bases. If it is not coding for protein, what is its function? Is it redundant, and why is it present? We know that our genetic material is evolving and changing, and some of this apparently non-functional DNA may once have coded for genes that are no longer used. Although much of the remaining, repetitive DNA has no known role, some of it is essential to normal gene

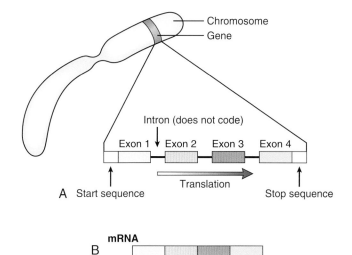

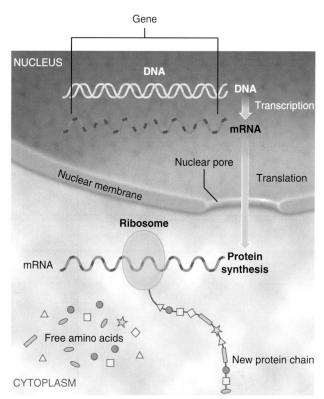

Fig. 2.10   The relationship between DNA, RNA, and protein synthesis. (Modified from Waugh A and Grant A (2018) *Ross & Wilson anatomy and physiology in health and illness*, 13th ed, Fig. 17.5. Oxford: Elsevier Ltd.)

Fig. 2.9   Gene structure. (A) Showing introns, exons, and stop and start regions. (B) The RNA produced from this gene, with the introns edited out. (Modified from Cross S (2019) *Underwood's pathology: a clinical approach*, 7th ed, Fig. 3.3. Oxford: Elsevier Ltd.)

function, and errors in its structure, especially in the vicinity of a gene, are associated with some inherited diseases.

Satellite DNA

About 10% to 15% of the non-coding DNA is made up of short sequences of base pairs, repeated many times and forming large blocks within the non-coding DNA. This is called **satellite DNA**, and although it does not code for protein, some of it has key functions in the cell. For example, the telomeres that protect the ends of chromosomes are satellite DNA and have a well-understood role in DNA replication and cell senescence (p. 64). Some sections of satellite DNA are unique to each individual and are used for DNA fingerprinting, now a common tool in paternity testing and in forensic science.

Gene expression

Gene expression is the production of a protein from the instructions written in a gene. The first part of this process is called **gene transcription**, during which a copy of the genetic code is produced in the form of a molecule of messenger RNA (mRNA). In the second stage, **translation**, the messenger RNA leaves the nucleus and travels to ribosomes in the cell cytosol so that the new protein can be made from free amino acids (Fig. 2.10).

Transcription (Fig. 2.11)

The DNA along the length of the gene is split down the centre of the ladder, separating the base pairs and exposing the individual bases. Only one strand of the DNA, called the **template strand**, is used to transcribe a molecule of mRNA because RNA is single stranded, not double stranded. The structure of RNA is similar to DNA in that it contains phosphate groups, a sugar (ribose, not deoxyribose), and bases; however, its four bases are adenine, cytosine, guanine, and uracil instead of thymine. The new molecule of RNA is built by the enzyme RNA polymerase. After the transcription of a gene, enzymes rapidly recoil the DNA, restoring it to its original double helical structure. mRNA, carrying the coded message for

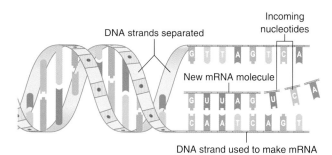

Fig. 2.11   Transcription. (Modified from Waugh A and Grant A (2018) *Ross & Wilson anatomy and physiology in health and illness*, 13th ed, Fig. 17.6. Oxford: Elsevier Ltd.)

synthesis of the protein, leaves the nucleus and attaches to a ribosome in the cytoplasm, where the protein is assembled.

As mentioned previously, genes contain coding sequences (exons) essential for producing the correct protein, but also introns, sequences of base pairs not represented in the final protein. Once the mRNA is transcribed from the gene, these intron sequences must be very accurately snipped out and the exon sequences carefully joined up before the mRNA is allowed to leave the nucleus (Fig. 2.9B). Precision here is critical because even a single nucleotide error alters the mRNA coding sequence and may completely change the final protein product. The process of intron mRNA removal and joining up of the exon sequences is called **splicing**, and splicing errors are responsible for some important genetic disorders (e.g., thalassaemia).

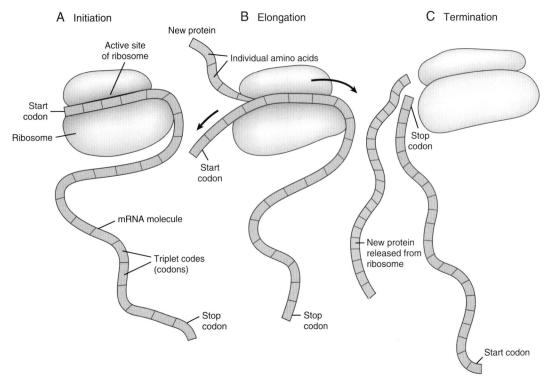

A Initiation

New protein

Active site
of ribosome

Individual amino acids

Start
codon

Ribosome

Start
codon

mRNA molecule

Triplet codes
(codons)

Stop
codon

B Elongation

Start
codon

Stop
codon

C Termination

Stop
codon

New protein
released from
ribosome

Start codon

Fig. 2.12   The three steps of translation. (A) Initiation. (B) Elongation. (C) Termination.

mRNA translation and protein assembly (Fig. 2.12**)**
Converting the code in mRNA to a final protein molecule
is called translation and takes place on ribosomes. The code
in mRNA is written in four bases: A, G, C, and U, and there
are 20 amino acids used in human protein synthesis. The
code can therefore not be one base, one amino acid; or two
bases, one amino acid; there are not enough combinations.
The bases on mRNA are therefore read in triplets called
codons, giving 64 possible combinations. Of these possible
triplets, 61 code for amino acids. For instance, UUU codes
for phenylalanine, AAA codes for lysine, and CCC codes for
proline. There is significant duplication because there are
64 possible triplet codes and only 20 amino acids; therefore,
for example, there are four codons for serine: UCU, UCC,
UCA, and UCG. AUG codes for methionine and is also an
important start signal. The three codons that do not code
for start or an amino acid—UAA, UAG, and UGA—are stop
signals and indicate that the protein is now complete and
should be released from the ribosome. The three stages of
translation are described below (Fig. 2.12).

Initiation (Fig. 2.12A). The first step in translation is attachment of the mRNA to a ribosome at a special active site.
The code written in the mRNA is read three bases at a time
(i.e., in the triplet codes). The start signal is usually an AUG
codon. The ribosome scans along the mRNA molecule looking for this start codon, and it will usually begin protein synthesis at the first one it finds.

Elongation (Fig. 2.12B). Once the mRNA is correctly bound
to the ribosome and the start signal is identified, protein assembly begins. The first amino acid added is usually methionine because the main start codon AUG codes for methionine. Amino acids are then added to the growing protein
chain according to the triplet code and joined together with
peptide bonds. As each codon is read and the appropriate

amino acid is added, it moves out of the active site to make
room for the next incoming amino acid.

It is critical that the ribosome starts in the right place and
that there are no errors in the base sequence because this
would throw the sequence out. Such mistakes are called
frameshift errors because they shift the reading frame
used by the ribosome. Adding in bases (insertions) or deletion of bases shifts the reading frame either to the right
or to the left, respectively, changes the code, and leads to
the production of a non-functional protein. For example,
take the hypothetical codon sequence AUG CCA UGU
GAA UAG (Fig. 2.13). This codes for methionine-proline-
cysteine-glutamate-STOP. AUG (methionine) is the start
codon. If any bases are missing or additional bases are inserted in the start codon, then the start signal is lost, and
protein synthesis will not begin in the right place. Likewise,
if any of the bases in UAG are missing or there is another
base inserted, the stop signal is missed and protein synthesis
will proceed. For example, if the first C is missing, the sequence now becomes AUG CAU GUG AAU AG..., coding
for methionine-histidine-STOP. If there is an additional C
inserted after the first C, the base sequence becomes AUG
CCC AUG UGA AAU G...–and the amino acid order becomes methionine-proline-methionine-STOP.

Termination (Fig. 2.12C). Protein synthesis stops when a
stop codon on the mRNA arrives at the ribosome's active
site. This triggers the release of the new protein from the
ribosome.

EPIGENETICS

Epigenetics is the study of factors that influence gene expression but are not caused by changes in the nucleotide
sequence in the gene. Increasingly, the important role of

these influences is recognised in inherited diseases and can make prediction of risk and disease occurrence quite challenging, even if the inheritance pattern of a particular hereditable disease is well understood. Epigenetic factors can suppress or activate gene expression and are themselves hereditable: that is, they are permanent features of DNA and are passed from parent to child.

Epigenetic control is essential for normal development and differentiation, and it is responsible for suppressing gene activity in cells and tissues for which the gene product is not required. For example, every nucleated body cell has a gene for insulin production, but only pancreatic β-cells actually use it, because these are the cells responsible for insulin synthesis. In all other body cells, the gene is silenced. This is a good example of how cells with identical genomes do not demonstrate identical function.

Another example of epigenetic gene modulation is the silencing of one X chromosome in females. Females, with two X-chromosomes, would produce twice as much X-related protein than males. To even this up between the sexes, one of their X-chromosomes is silenced. This is called **lyonisation**.

Epigenetic modifications of genes may relate to the influence of environmental and lifestyle factors in inherited disease, explain why genetically identical twins can have different phenotypes, and help explain why maternal behaviours have consequences for the health of their children throughout the children's lives. Because epigenetic factors are so important in determining gene behaviour, they are an active area of research in the treatment of genetic disease.

Three important mechanisms of epigenetic modulation are through DNA methylation, through histone modifications, or by interfering with RNA.

DNA methylation

Addition of methyl groups to DNA at cytosine residues usually leads to gene suppression. Cancer was the first disorder in which DNA methylation was implicated when it was discovered that methylation of tumour suppressor genes (p. 75) inactivates them and disengages normal cell growth control mechanisms. Conversely, undermethylation of tumour promotor genes (p. 76) leads to growth stimulation. Inherited

diseases attributable to faults in normal DNA methylation include Prader-Willi syndrome.

Histone modification

Histones are more than just supporting material; they influence the expression of their associated genes. If the DNA is tightly wound around the histones and the packaging is compact, then the gene is inaccessible and likely to be silenced. However, if the histone-DNA arrangement is looser and less compact, it is more available to the factors that trigger transcription and it is more likely to be expressed.

In addition, changes in histone structure alter the overall structure of the chromatin and can inhibit or increase the expression of genes. These modifications can also act as markers for enzymes controlling transcription, either to indicate that genes are to be transcribed or to indicate that the gene is inactive and should not be transcribed. Inherited disorders associated with abnormal histone modification include X-linked mental retardation.

RNA interference

The process of gene expression can also be interrupted at the mRNA level. Remember that mRNA is produced by reading the triplet code on an active gene. This mRNA is then translated on the ribosome, and the corresponding protein is produced (see Fig. 2.10). One standard mechanism used by the cell to regulate gene activity is by producing fragments of double-stranded mRNA, which bind to the protein-coding mRNA from the nucleus and render it useless, meaning that, although the gene has been read and mRNA synthesised, its protein is not made. Using this approach to prevent the production of abnormal proteins by mutated genes has been an active area of research in the hunt for drugs to treat genetic disease. The first gene-silencing drug that works in this way, **patisiran**, was approved in 2018 for the treatment of a rare disorder called hereditary transthyretin amyloidosis. In this disorder, a mutated gene in liver cells produces amyloid protein that deposits in neurological tissue, causing polyneuropathy and progressive neurological dysfunction. The active agent in patisiran is RNA specifically designed to bind to the mRNA produced by the mutated liver gene, and prevents it being translated into the damaging amyloid protein (Fig. 2.14).

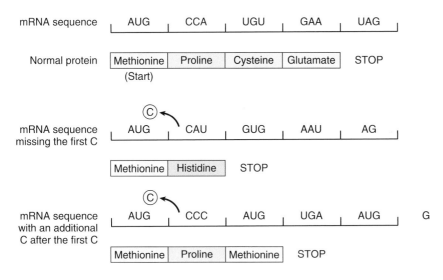

Fig. 2.13 Frameshift mutation.

MITOCHONDRIAL DNA

Although most DNA is found in the cell nucleus, 37 genes are located on a circular chromosome in mitochondria. These genes code mainly for proteins needed for the energy-producing pathways in mitochondria. Inherited mitochondrial disorders therefore involve failure of energy transfer processes in the cell and are inherited through the mother because spermatozoa do not carry mitochondria. Mitochondrial DNA (mtDNA) produces a larger number of spontaneous mutations than nuclear DNA, often without any clinical signs or symptoms, although they accumulate as the individual ages. Mitochondrial activity also decreases with age, and the associated decline in the efficiency of energy pathways probably contributes to features of ageing such as cell senescence and the diminishing ability of stem cells to regenerate tissues. It is noteworthy that the decline in mitochondrial numbers and efficiency with age is not unavoidable. Regular physical exercise stimulates the production of new mitochondria in various tissues including brain and muscle.

Every cell has thousands of copies of mtDNA, which explains why cells can tolerate a fairly large proportion of mutations. Provided there are enough normally functioning mitochondrial chromosomes in the cell, there will be enough protein produced to supply the cell's needs. If every mitochondrial chromosome in the cell is identical, the cell is said to show **homoplasmy**. However, as mutations arise, the chromosomes begin to show variability, and this is called **heteroplasmy**. The wide range of mutations, along with the different proportions of mutated DNA from cell to cell, gives rise to a wide range of clinical presentations in inherited mitochondrial disorders. Generally, they feature myopathy (including the heart) and neurological disturbances because muscle and nervous tissue are particularly dependent on aerobic respiration for their high energy requirements. Primary mitochondrial disorders include Leigh syndrome (p. 44).

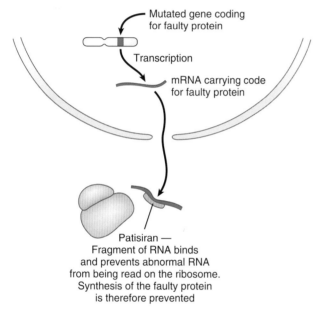

Fig. 2.14 The action of patisiran in gene silencing.

PATTERNS OF INHERITANCE

An individual inherits 50% of his or her chromosomes from the mother and 50% from the father, so the child's genetic makeup is therefore a combination of genes from both parents. Siblings who resemble one parent more than the other have inherited specific genes from that parent (e.g., genes that determine the shape of the face, the size and shape of the nose) that are dominant over the genes inherited from the other parent (Fig. 2.15). However, heredity is immensely complex. Most traits are the product of multiple gene interactions; as our knowledge of genetics expands, it is becoming more and more evident that characteristics and traits once believed to be single-gene activity are in fact the product of several genes. Even if a gene is dominant, it may

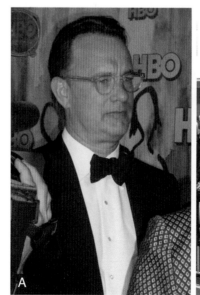
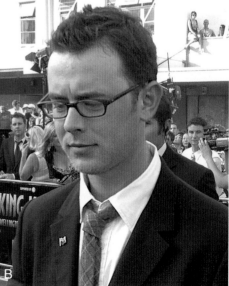

Fig. 2.15 Family resemblance (From (A) Tom Hanks (kristin.eonline.com - HBO Post-Emmys Party, Pacific Design Center, Sept. 21, 2008) and (B) Colin Hanks (jonzerthemighty - edit of https://www.flickr.com/photos/jonzer/242223176).

not be fully expressed because of epigenetic influences and environmental and lifestyle factors.

Additionally, as seen in the example of eye colour mentioned previously, multiple genes frequently have a part to play in what we perceive as a simple physical characteristic. It is important, therefore, that the difference between inheritance of a gene, which is often predictable and can be tracked through generations of a family, and its expression in an individual is clearly understood. Having a gene that predisposes an individual to cancer does not necessarily mean that the individual will develop the disease: the activity of that gene will be affected by other genes, epigenetics, the environment, lifestyle factors, and other variables. Even identical twins, both carrying such a gene, may have different outcomes, with one developing cancer and the other remaining disease-free. Despite this complexity, tracing the transmission of a gene through a family tree is a very useful tool in identifying at-risk individuals and studying patterns of gene expression.

Inheritance patterns depend on whether the gene is located on an autosome or a sex chromosome and whether it is dominant or recessive. Here we will consider some well-understood patterns of inheritance that allow family genetic histories to be mapped and the prediction of emergence of characteristics or disease through generations.

Consanguinity

Inherited disorders are more common in children whose parents are related (e.g., first or second cousins) because they are descendants from the same gene pool and therefore more likely to have inherited the same gene mutations from both parents. In cultures where interfamily marriages are traditional, the incidence of congenital disorders is much higher than in cultures where it is forbidden or not common practice. The preference for intermarriage within the related royal families of Europe, for example, led to an unusually high incidence of a rare form of haemophilia in the descendants of Queen Victoria. She probably developed the causative mutation spontaneously and then passed it, through two of her five daughters and their European royal marriages, to her descendants. Once the haemophilia gene appeared in the royal gene pool, intermarriage between distantly related family members greatly increased the likelihood that children from these marriages would inherit the gene and therefore suffer from haemophilia.

AUTOSOMAL INHERITANCE

Genes located on the autosomes show no sex difference in affected individuals, and the expression of that gene in an individual depends mainly on whether it is dominant or recessive. However, it is important to remember that having a dominant gene does not guarantee expression of that gene because of the influence of other genes or environmental factors. **Penetrance** and **variable expressivity** are two factors that influence gene expression and make it difficult, if not impossible, to accurately assess and predict the risk of developing an inherited disease in members of an affected family.

Penetrance

Penetrance is the degree to which an autosomal dominant gene known to be present in an individual is actually expressed through their descendants. It might be assumed, from the explanation previously given, that all children inheriting a dominant form of a gene from one parent should express that gene because dominant genes by definition are expressed. When this is the case, penetrance is said to be 100% (complete). However, this does not always happen because gene expression is modified by epigenetic, environmental, and other factors, and so not all children inheriting the gene express the trait or disease. This is called **incomplete penetrance**. An example is Huntington disease, which is caused by an abnormal number of CAG repeats in an exon belonging to the *Huntingtin (HTT)* gene on chromosome 4. The normal gene has up to 35 repeats. This was first mapped in 1993, and later work showed that the number of extra repeats affected the likelihood that the disease would appear at all, and strongly correlated with the age of onset. The more CAG repeats there are, the higher the penetrance (i.e., the greater the chance that the individual will develop Huntington disease, and the younger they are likely to be when symptoms first appear). People with 36 to 39 repeats may not develop the disease at all (incomplete penetrance). Over 40 repeats give 100% penetrance; that is, everyone will develop Huntington disease if they live long enough. Over 60 repeats cause the onset of disease in childhood (Fig. 2.16).

Expressivity

Expressivity is the range of phenotypes seen in individuals with the same genes. Gene expression can vary significantly, even in closely related individuals, so that family members who have inherited a particular disease gene do not all present with identical clinical pictures. For example, four siblings may all inherit the gene for polydactyly (more than five digits on a hand or a foot). This trait displays incomplete penetrance because not all these siblings may have extra digits, despite having the faulty allele. However, of those who do, the extra digits may not be identical, and not on the same hand or foot. The gene is therefore expressing itself in different ways in different siblings. This is expressivity.

Autosomal dominant inheritance

A dominant allele is usually expressed in all family members who possess it, whether they are homozygous (two dominant alleles) or heterozygous (one dominant, one recessive

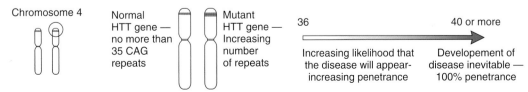

Fig. 2.16 The relationship between additional CAG repeats in the *HTT* gene and the penetrance of Huntington disease.

allele). Transmission of the gene usually follows a predictable pattern. If a parent is heterozygous for the gene, that parent has a 50% chance of passing either form to a child; and if that parent is homozygous, then every child will inherit it and probably express it in their phenotypes. This can be demonstrated in a Punnett square (Fig. 2.17), showing all possible combinations of any given gene in a couple's children. Conventionally, a dominant gene is indicated with

a capital letter, and a recessive gene with a lowercase letter. This example demonstrates that if both parents are heterozygous for gene A, meaning that each parent has one copy of the dominant gene (A) and one copy of the recessive gene (a), it is possible for them to produce children who are homozygous dominant (AA), homozygous recessive (aa), and heterozygous (Aa). An individual who carries a mutant gene but does not express it is called a **carrier**. Although the carrier is not affected by the faulty gene, he or she can pass it on to children.

Most disease-related genes are recessive, and there are few examples of autosomal dominant inheritance of disease. One example, however is Huntington disease. In this case, the affected gene, the *Huntingtin* gene, is dominant and much less common in the general population than the normal recessive form.

If a couple (Generation A), of whom the father is heterozygous for the *Huntingtin* gene (i.e., carries one normal gene and one mutant gene) and the mother is homozygous recessive (i.e., has two copies of the normal gene), have four children, statistically 50% of the pregnancies will result in a fetus carrying the mutant dominant *Huntingtin* gene (Fig. 2.18A). There is no sex difference because the gene is carried on an autosome, so male and female children are equally likely to be affected and, although in this example

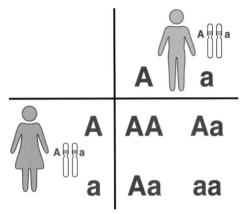

Fig. 2.17 Representative Punnett square showing the possible combinations of gene A in children of two heterozygous parents.

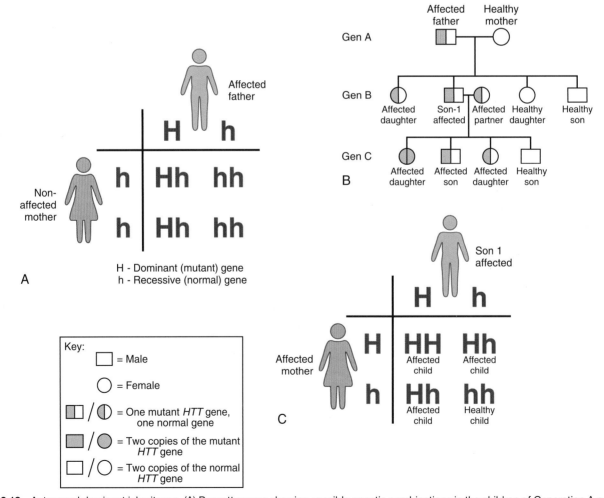

Fig. 2.18 Autosomal dominant inheritance. (A) Punnett square showing possible genetic combinations in the children of Generation A parents. (B) Inheritance tree. (C) Punnett square showing possible genetic combinations in the children of son 1 and a heterozygous partner.

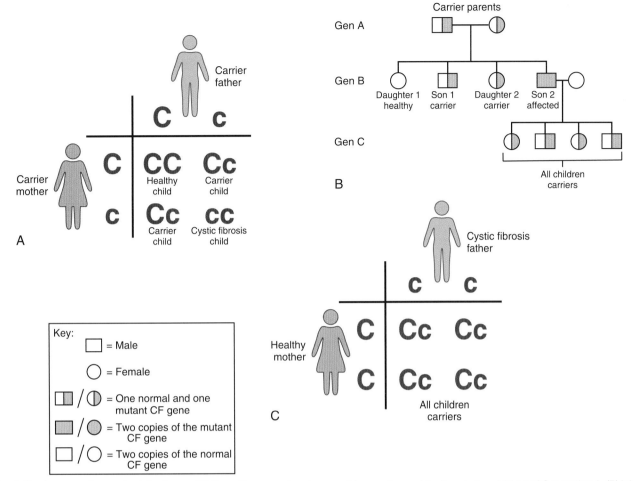

Key:

☐ = Male

◯ = Female

◫ / ◐ = One normal and one mutant CF gene

▦ / ⬤ = Two copies of the mutant CF gene

☐ / ◯ = Two copies of the normal CF gene

Fig. 2.19 Autosomal recessive inheritance. (A) Punnett square showing possible genetic combinations in the children of Generation A. (B) Inheritance tree. (C) Punnett square showing possible genetic combinations in the children of son 2 and a homozygous dominant partner.

only the father can pass it to this couple's children, clinically it does not matter which parent carries the gene. Fig. 2.18B shows an inheritance tree illustrating the possible transmission routes for the Generation A father's faulty gene in his children and grandchildren. The statistical likelihood is that half of his children (Generation B) will inherit the faulty dominant gene and may themselves develop the disease. Son 1, an affected child, has produced four children (Generation C) with a partner who also carries the *Huntingtin* gene, and the statistical likelihood is that only one of their children will inherit two copies of the normal gene and be free of the disease (Fig. 2.18C). Note, from the discussion above, that presence of an affected gene does not guarantee that Huntington disease will develop, and note too that this discussion presents the statistical likelihood of these inheritance patterns occurring, not a predictable set of events for an individual family.

Autosomal recessive inheritance

If an individual is autosomal recessive for an allele, its inheritance pattern is the same as for autosomal dominant (i.e., a homozygous recessive parent, with two copies of the recessive gene, will pass a recessive gene to all their children because that is the only form that the parent has). If they are heterozygous, with a recessive allele and a dominant allele, the chance of passing the recessive gene to a child is 50:50.

However, the pattern of expression is different. Unless both parents pass a recessive allele to the child, the gene will not be expressed.

One example of a disease inherited as an autosomal recessive trait is cystic fibrosis. In Fig. 2.19, two carrier parents, Generation A, both heterozygous for the trait, have four children (Generation B). The Punnett square in Fig. 2.19A shows the possible gene combinations in children of Generation A parents. Statistically, one in four children will inherit two recessive copies of the gene, one from each parent and therefore will have cystic fibrosis: in this example, son 2. Two in four will inherit one recessive gene from one parent and a dominant gene from the other and be carriers of cystic fibrosis, like their parents. In this example, these children are son 1 and daughter 2. One in four will inherit two dominant, healthy genes from their parents and therefore have no recessive alleles at all: here, daughter 1 (Fig. 2.19B). In this example, only son 1 has produced children (Generation C). Even though his partner is homozygous dominant (i.e., has two normal genes), all their children will carry the recessive, faulty CF gene (Fig. 2.19C) because that is the only gene he has to give them.

SEX-LINKED INHERITANCE

Sex-linked inheritance means that the gene is located on the sex chromosomes, X and Y. Females, with two X

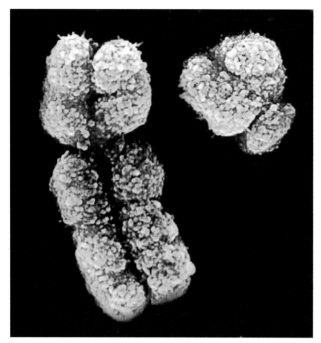

Fig. 2.20 The sex chromosomes. (From Fitzgerald-Hayes M and Reichsman F (2010) *DNA and biotechnology*, 3rd ed, Fig. 6.15. San Diego: Academic Press.)

chromosomes, must pass an X chromosome to all their children. All female ova therefore carry one X chromosome. Males, however, with an XY pairing in their sex chromosomes, can pass either. Spermatozoa therefore carry either an X or a Y chromosome, and this determines the sex of the baby. If the ovum is fertilised with a spermatozoon carrying an X chromosome, the baby will be a girl; if it carries a Y, the baby will be a boy. Unlike autosomal pairs 1 to 22, the X and Y chromosomes are not matched in size: the Y chromosome is much smaller than the X and carries only a few dozen genes, whereas the X-chromosome bears about 800. This means that females, with two matching X-chromosomes, have two copies of every X-linked gene. Males, however, have one X and one Y. Both the p and q arms of the Y chromosome are much shorter than on the X, so that most of the genes carried on the man's X chromosome do not have a corresponding allele on his Y (Fig. 2.20).

The Y chromosome genes are mainly related to expression of male-related proteins and functions. For example, the *SRY* gene on the short arm of the Y chromosome produces a protein that triggers testicular development in the fetus and inhibits development of female reproductive organs, and there is no corresponding *SRY* gene on the X chromosome. However, the X-chromosome, being much bigger than the Y chromosome, carries hundreds of genes not found on the Y chromosome and which are unrelated to sex determination, including some related to colour vision and blood and muscle physiology. Because a male has only one copy of these genes, on the X chromosome inherited from his mother, that gene will be expressed, whether it is recessive or dominant, faulty or normal. An inherited trait or disorder carried on an X-linked gene but not matched on the Y results in expression of the trait or disease in males and is called a **sex-linked (X-linked) disorder**. An example

of an X-linked trait is colour blindness, and important X-linked diseases include haemophilia and Duchenne muscular dystrophy.

Transmission patterns in X-linked inheritance

Transmission of an X-linked characteristic is through the maternal line, and usually (although not exclusively) expressed in males. The pathophysiology of haemophilia A is discussed on p. 42, and its inheritance pattern discussed here. The gene for clotting factor VIII is located on the long arm of the X chromosome, and the Y chromosome lacks this gene. When this gene is mutated and abnormal, it causes the clotting disorder haemophilia A. The Punnett square in Fig. 2.21A shows the possible genetic combinations in the children of a couple, of whom the father is haemophiliac and the mother is normal. Punnett squares showing inheritance of sex-linked characteristics must also include the sex chromosomes because the sex of the children is important when considering inheritance patterns. The father has only one copy of the gene to pass to his children, on his X chromosome, and it is the recessive, faulty gene. He cannot transmit it to his sons because he passes them his Y chromosome. However, all his daughters will receive his X chromosome with the haemophilia A gene. The mother has two normal alleles on her two X-chromosomes. The four possible genetic combinations in their children are shown in generation B: two girls and two boys. Both boys inherit their father's healthy Y chromosome and a normal X from their mother and are healthy. Both girls must inherit the haemophilia gene from their father, and a normal gene from their mother. As the normal gene is dominant, the girls are healthy, but they are carriers and may pass the faulty gene to their own children. In generation C, the possible genetic combinations of children of daughter 1 (a carrier) and a normal man are shown as a Punnett square (Fig. 2.21.C). Here, statistically, half of their daughters will be carriers and half will be healthy. Half of their sons will be healthy, but half will have haemophilia.

If daughter 1 from Generation B has children with a haemophiliac partner, the inheritance pattern is very different, because both parents have a haemophilia gene and may pass it to their children. In this scenario, 50% of their sons will be haemophiliac and 50% healthy; 50% of their daughters will be carriers and 50% will be normal (Fig. 2.22) It is therefore possible for women to express X-linked traits, and correspondingly X-linked disease, but it is much less common than in males.

GENE DISORDERS

Mutations in the base sequence of a gene produce incorrect sequences in the corresponding mRNA molecule in transcription, and so the amino acid sequence in the newly synthesised protein is also wrong. This can lead to reduced or lost function in that protein; for example, an enzyme may lose its activity, or a structural protein may no longer be the correct shape or fit to be assembled into body tissues. Although this may seem trivial, even minor errors in gene sequences can lead to life-threatening or life-changing genetic disorders. DNA mutations are common; most occur spontaneously, but some are the consequence of exposure to mutagenic factors such as ionising radiation (see Chapter 3). Mutations in gene sequences can occur in several ways.

Substitution

Substitution is the replacement of one nucleotide with a different one. This can either eliminate or introduce stop or start codons, leading to incorrect sections of the gene being transcribed and the production of non-functional proteins. It may change the codon from one amino acid to another, leading to insertion of an incorrect amino acid, which may mean that the new protein is non-functional. If the incorrect nucleotide is close to a splice site, the removal of introns from a transcribed mRNA molecule could be inaccurate, again leading to sequence mistakes in amino acid addition to the new protein. Substitution errors are the commonest form of mutation (Fig. 2.23), and genetic disorders caused by this form of mutation include sickle cell anaemia. Here, a single substitution of the normal adenine base in the sixth triplet of the gene sequence with a thymine base changes the amino acid sequence in the final β-globin protein, replacing the correct amino acid glutamate with incorrect valine. This seems like such a trivial error, but it produces seriously abnormal haemoglobin and the devastating condition of sickle cell anaemia.

Deletion

If sections of the gene are lost, the mutation is called a *deletion*. If the deleted sequence removes complete nucleotide triplets, then the amino acids those triplets represent will be missing from the final protein; however, if the deletion removes only one or two of the three bases from the base triplet, then the reading sequence is disrupted: this is a frameshift mutation (see Fig. 2.13), and the amino acid sequence in the final protein is likely to be completely wrong beyond the mutation point. The larger the chunk missing from the gene, the more abnormal the final protein is, and the more likely it is to be non-functional. In cystic fibrosis, there is a mutation in the *CFTR* gene. The commonest mutation is deletion of an entire codon in the gene. Without this codon, a phenylalanine amino acid is missing from the final protein, leading to impaired production of chloride channels, the underlying cause of cystic fibrosis.

Insertion

Even a single base inserted in error disrupts the gene code and leads to errors in the final protein. One or two extra bases cause a frameshift mutation (see Fig. 2.13). Extra bases may create inappropriate start or stop codons, disrupt existing ones, or lead to additional amino acids being inserted in the protein. The larger the insertion, the more

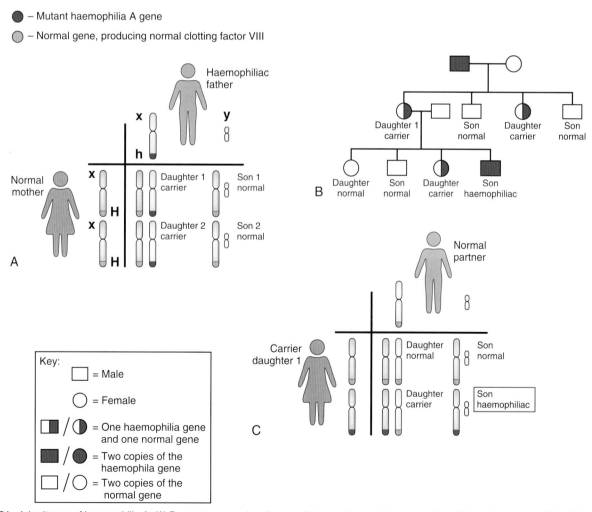

Fig. 2.21 Inheritance of haemophilia A. (A) Punnett square showing possible genetic combinations in the children of a haemophiliac father and a normal mother. (B) Inheritance tree. (C) Punnett square showing the possible genetic combinations in the children of daughter 1 and a normal father.

abnormal the protein is likely to be. Some insertions take the form of increased numbers of trinucleotide repeats, either in the intron or exon portions of genes (e.g., Huntington disease).

THE PRINCIPAL MONOGENIC DISORDERS

Monogenic disorders, in which the genetic error lies with a single identified gene, include some of the most common inherited disorders. Although these disorders involve only one gene, there are usually a number of different mutations possible, producing a spectrum of signs and symptoms in individuals presenting with the disease. For example, there are over 1000 possible defects in the gene responsible for cystic fibrosis, partly accounting for the variability in disease severity and the pattern of signs and symptoms.

Sometimes gene mutations are inherited from a parent; however, a large proportion of single gene disorders result from a spontaneous mutation in either the spermatozoon or the ovum, which then appears in the genotype of the new baby. In this case, there is no family history, although the mutation can be passed on to the new individual's children. Although individual monogenic diseases are each relatively rare, there are at least 10,000 identified, and their overall prevalence is estimated at between 1% and 2% of the population, with significant morbidity and mortality.

Inborn errors of metabolism

The biochemistry of life depends on a huge array of essential metabolic pathways, including those producing energy, directing the use of key substances such as vitamins and trace elements, and regulating the production and use of proteins, carbohydrates, lipids, and nucleic acids. The enzymes that drive these key processes are coded for by single genes. If an enzyme-coding gene mutates, and the production of the enzyme is reduced or stopped, metabolism can be severely disrupted. Inherited disorders involving mutations in these genes are called *inborn errors of metabolism* (IEMs). Although there is often enough residual enzyme activity in affected people to allow adequate function, when enzyme deficiency is severe, the consequences can be serious. These disorders include phenylketonuria, cystinuria, familial hypercholesterolaemia, and albinism. Other IEMs are listed in Table 2.1.

CYSTIC FIBROSIS (CF)

CF is the commonest autosomal recessive disorder in populations of white European descent, occurring on average between 1/2000 and 1/3000 live births. It is much rarer in

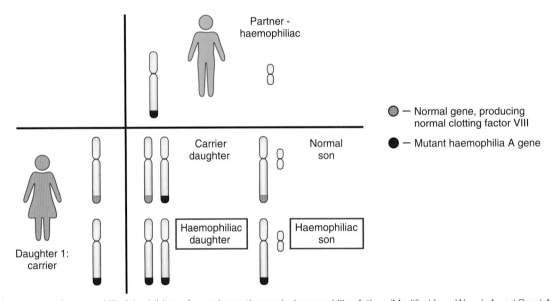

Fig. 2.22   Inheritance of haemophilia A in children of a carrier mother and a haemophiliac father. (Modified from Waugh A and Grant A (2018) *Ross & Wilson anatomy and physiology in health and illness*, 13th ed, Fig. 17.11. Oxford: Elsevier Ltd.)

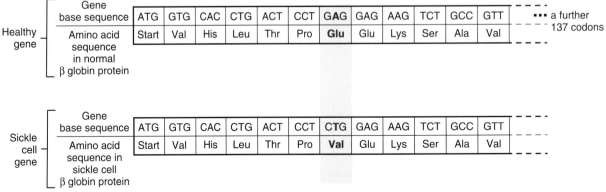

Fig. 2.23   Substitution error in the gene for the β-globin chain of haemoglobin in sickle cell anaemia.

Table 2.1   Some inborn errors of metabolism

Type of disorder	Examples of disorders	Some key facts
Lysosomal storage disorders Lysosomes normally break down cellular metabolites, which accumulate in these disorders, causing progressive disability in affected children	Hurler syndrome, Hunter syndrome	Associated with accumulation of intracellular polysaccharides, causing progressive multisystem problems and cognitive deterioration; death usually occurs in the midteens.
	Tay-Sachs disease (p. 49) Gaucher disease Fabry disease (p. 41) Niemann-Pick disease	Associated with accumulation of sphingolipid, a key component of cell membranes, disrupting cognitive development and other aspects of brain, liver, and spleen function; death usually occurs in childhood.
Protein metabolism disorders	Phenylketonuria (p. 47) Albinism	Melanin production is disrupted, causing unpigmented hair, iris, hair, and retina; visual problems include nystagmus, low visual acuity, photophobia, strabismus, and poor depth perception; there is significantly higher risk of skin cancers, including squamous cell carcinoma and malignant melanoma, which may reduce life span.
	Maple syrup urine disease	The metabolism of the amino acids leucine, valine, and isoleucine is blocked, leading to their accumulation to toxic levels especially in the central nervous system; death occurs within a few weeks of birth unless the dietary intake of these amino acids is restricted.
	Homocystinuria (p. 43)	
Glycogen storage disorders (GSDs) Glycogen is the storage form of glucose, and in these disorders, glycogen accumulates within cells, but the ability of the cell to release glucose from glycogen for energy is impaired	Pompe disease Von Gierke disease Cori disease	There are around 30 GSDs; there is usually hypoglycaemia, and muscle function, including in the heart, is impaired because of this; there is often abnormal liver function because the liver is so important in glucose processing.
Metal/trace element metabolic disorders	Wilson disease	The affected gene codes for an enzyme essential to copper excretion. Accumulation of copper damages the liver, the nervous system, and muscle. D-penicillamine is a chelating agent, given orally, which binds to and removes copper from tissues, increasing its excretion in the urine and reduces total body copper levels.
	Haemochromatosis	Any one of several genes that produce enzymes important in the absorption, transport, and storage of iron may be responsible, so clinical presentations are variable. Widespread iron accumulation impairs the function of many organs, including the liver, muscle, heart, joints, and pancreas (diabetes is likely).
Porphyrias In these disorders, haem production is deficient and the precursor molecules accumulate.	A range of conditions, depending on which enzyme in the pathway is affected	The build-up of haem precursor molecules is toxic to tissues. Haem is essential to the function of all body organs, so symptoms are widespread. Skin involvement is common, with photosensitivity, blistering and skin fragility. The nervous system, the liver and other internal organs are also frequently affected.

individuals of African or Asian descent. The diagnosis is usually confirmed before the age of 2 years. Although life expectancy in CF has improved, this disease significantly shortens life. Only about 50% of sufferers reach 40 years of age.

Genetics

The CF gene is located on the long arm of chromosome 7; its locus was identified in 1985. It was named the *CFTR* (cystic fibrosis transmembrane conductance regulator) gene, and the normal, dominant form produces the protein that forms chloride channels in the cell membranes of secretory epithelial cells. The chloride channels allow the cell to export chloride and bicarbonate ions into airway, gastrointestinal, and reproductive secretions. This draws water with it and keeps the cell secretions well hydrated. When the channel is faulty, it becomes much less

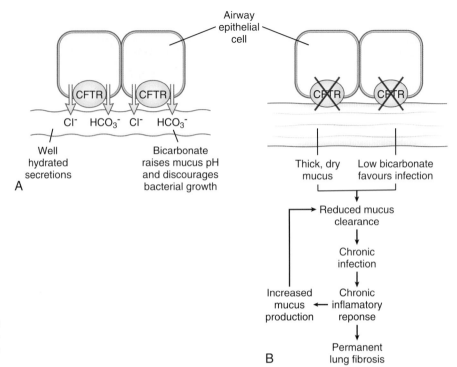

Fig. 2.24 Cystic fibrosis in the airways. (A) Normal chloride channel function. (B) Impaired chloride channel function in cystic fibrosis.

permeable to chloride, chloride export fails, and the ionic and water content of cellular secretions is reduced. This gives viscous, sticky secretions that resist normal clearance mechanisms, block body passageways, and act as a reservoir for infection.

Pathophysiology

The principal signs and symptoms usually relate to respiratory function (Fig. 2.24). Because the mucus produced is dry, thick, and sticky, the mucociliary escalator cannot clear it normally, and over time chronic and repeated infections lead to airway narrowing, inflammation, increased mucus production, airway obstruction by mucus, and progressive pulmonary fibrosis. The deficiency in bicarbonate secretion increases the risk of infection because bicarbonate is antibacterial. *Staphylococcus aureus* colonises the airways at an early stage, followed by less common organisms, including *Pseudomonas aeruginosa*, which frequently develop antibiotic resistant strains because of repeated antibiotic treatment. Pulmonary fibrosis restricts blood flow into the lungs from the pulmonary veins, increasing pulmonary blood pressure and the workload of the left side of the heart, possibly leading to heart failure. Children cough, wheeze, and fail to thrive, and their skin tastes salty, a sign to doctors as far back as mediaeval times that the child did not have long to live. Salty skin is also related to the faulty chloride channel; in normal sweat production, chloride, and, indirectly, sodium, and water are reabsorbed from the sweat duct before the sweat is excreted onto the skin, but this does not happen in CF.

Thick gastrointestinal secretions partly or completely obstruct the gastrointestinal tract. Viscous meconium (the bowel contents in newborn babies) can completely obstruct the intestine. Most individuals with CF have some pancreatic impairment, although this is very variable. This reduces or completely inhibits the production and release of pancreatic digestive juices into the duodenum. Up to 50% of people with CF develop diabetes because the affected pancreas cannot produce insulin. Cholelithiasis (p. 297) is also common. Male infertility is almost universal because the vas deferens fails to develop correctly.

Management and prognosis

Newborns are routinely screened for blood levels of immunoreactive trypsin, an indirect marker for CF. This is one of the tests performed at about 5 days old on the blood taken from a heel prick. It is not 100% accurate, but an uncertain diagnosis can be confirmed by genetic testing. There is no cure for CF, and treatment includes regular chest physiotherapy to loosen and clear secretions, aggressive antibiotic treatment of infections, oral replacement of pancreatic enzymes, and monitoring and management of CF-related diabetes. Because a single gene is affected in CF, the condition is a highly attractive candidate for the use of gene therapy, in which the *CFTR* gene is introduced into the body with the aim of its being taken up into body cells and used to produce normal chloride channels. This research has concentrated on the lungs because the pulmonary consequences of this disease are the most debilitating. The first study to show modest, but significant, stabilisation of lung function using *CTFR* DNA was published in 2015 by the UK Cystic Fibrosis Gene Therapy Consortium. This group inserted normal *CTFR* gene into tiny fat droplets called liposomes and delivered them into the lungs of 62 CF patients by inhalation. Their work has extended into further clinical trials. Other approaches include gene repair, where the incorrect gene sequence is enzymatically removed and the correct gene sequence inserted in its place. This has the advantage over gene therapy in that it is a permanent repair. Newer agents—ivacaftor and lumacaftor—enhance CFTR function in patients with certain specific mutations.

DUCHENNE MUSCULAR DYSTROPHY

Duchenne muscular dystrophy was named for Guillaume Duchenne, a French doctor who described a case in 1861. The incidence is 1 in 3500 male children, and it is rare in females because it is transmitted as a sex-linked condition. It is the commonest inherited muscle wasting condition.

Genetics

The affected gene, *DMD*, normally codes for a protein called **dystrophin**, which anchors actin, one of the proteins responsible for contraction, to the inside of the muscle cell membrane. Dystrophin therefore provides mechanical strength to the muscle cell and prevents damage when the cell is contracting. *DMD* is located on the short arm of the X chromosome, so the mother passes the disorder to her children. Because affected boys often do not survive to her children, and so do not pass on their defective *DMD* gene, the high incidence of the disease reflects a high spontaneous mutation rate: probably about a third of cases are new mutations.

DMD is a huge gene, possessing 79 exons, which probably accounts in part for the high spontaneous mutation rate. The commonest mutations in Duchenne's are deletions and frameshift mutations, leading to a complete loss of dystrophin production, but a wide range of mutations has been reported. Some mutations code for the production of abnormal but still partially functional dystrophin, giving a related, but generally milder, form of muscular dystrophy called Becker muscular dystrophy.

Pathophysiology

Muscular dystrophy causes progressive damage and loss of function in skeletal and cardiac muscle cells, which worsen with time because of the cells' poor internal mechanical support. Although affected children generally reach their developmental milestones in the first few months, once they begin learning to walk, progress typically slows, and problems with gait, balance, co-ordination, muscle strength, and rapid fatigability become apparent. Calf muscles can be larger than normal (pseudohypertrophy), but this does not mean increased muscle bulk: the increased size is caused by deposition of fat and fibrotic scar tissue. The disease is usually rapidly progressive, and many children need a wheelchair for all or part of the time before their teens. Upper body weakness may restrict use of the arms and lifting the hands above the head may become impossible. Weakness in the diaphragm and other respiratory muscles, and in cardiac muscle, leads to breathing and cardiovascular complications, including respiratory infections and life-threatening heart failure. Cognitive impairment is often seen. Although this disorder is almost never seen in women, some carriers can experience mild symptoms, such as muscle weakness and cramps, because of the effects of X-chromosome inactivation. If the normal X-chromosome is suppressed (lyonisation, p. 31), the effect of the abnormal gene can be magnified.

Management and prognosis

Diagnosis may be based on family history, if there is one, but if not, a careful history and monitoring of the physical signs and symptoms gives a reliable picture. Muscle cell death increases serum creatinine kinase levels in the early years, which fall as muscle mass reduces. Genetic testing confirms a dystrophin mutation. There is no cure. Life expectancy is drastically shortened, and treatment is supportive. Good management of respiratory infections and cardiac function can extend life. Boys are living longer because of better care, and some live into their 30s and beyond, although most do not survive beyond the late teens or early 20s.

FABRY DISEASE

This X-linked IEM, one of the lysosomal storage disorders, affects approximately 1 in 50,000 males and all main racial groups.

Genetics

The faulty gene in Fabry disease is the *GLA* gene, which produces the enzyme alpha-galactosidase. This enzyme is responsible for breaking down the lipid **globotriaosylceramide** in lysosomes. In this disorder, not enough enzyme is produced, and the lipid accumulates inside cells, with widespread consequences.

Pathophysiology

Skin symptoms include reduced sweat production. Globotriaosylceramide deposition in the cornea causes corneal cloudiness, and the auditory apparatus in the ear is progressively damaged, with hearing loss. Progressive kidney damage leads eventually to renal failure and damage to blood vessels causes tissue ischaemia and fibrosis and increases the risk of early cerebrovascular disease. The disorder is associated with episodes of severe pain, especially in the hands and feet, because of impaired circulation.

Management and prognosis

Diagnosis is usually made in childhood or early adolescence, although in milder cases, it may be later. Symptom management (e.g., pain control, treating hypertension, and other cardiovascular manifestations) and maintaining good general health is key. New treatments, available in some countries, include enzyme replacement. However, even with appropriate support, affected males usually die before reaching their forties.

FRAGILE X SYNDROME

Fragile X syndrome is one of the commonest inherited causes of learning disability, autism, and cognitive impairment, affecting about 1 in 4000 male births and 1 in 8000 females. Affected children can show significant developmental delay, and diagnosis is usually made between the ages of 3 and 4 years.

Genetics

The specific defect lies with the *FMR1* gene on the X chromosome. This gene produces a protein called FMRP (fragile X mental retardation protein), which is essential to the development of normal synaptic function, and therefore communication between nerves in the central nervous system. In the normal gene, the first exon contains between 5 and 40 lengths of a repeat sequence of CGG triplets. In fragile X syndrome, this repeat sequence expands to over 200 copies, resulting in silencing of the gene. The absence of this protein disrupts normal neurological development, including the loss of normal synaptic plasticity essential for learning and memory. The *FMR1* gene is located very close to the

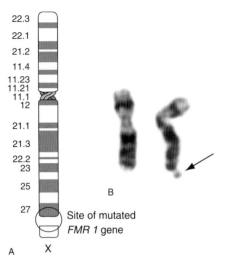

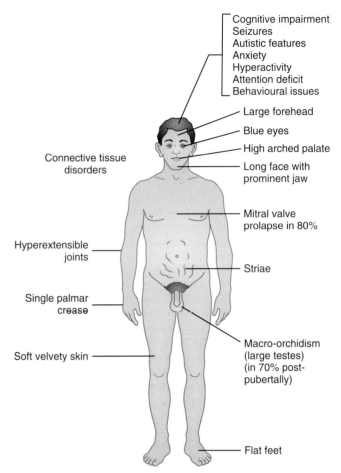

Fig. 2.25 Fragile X. (A) Drawing of chromosome showing the location of the breakage point. (B) Photograph of affected chromosome, with the breakage point indicated (arrow). (Modified from McPherson R and Pincus M (2022) *Henry's clinical diagnosis and management by laboratory methods*, 24th ed, Fig. 71.26. Philadelphia: Elsevier Inc.)

Fig. 2.26 Typical features in Fragile X syndrome. (Modified from Puri BK, Laking PJ, and Treasaden IH, 2002, *Textbook of psychiatry*. Edinburgh: Churchill Livingstone.)

end of the long (q) arm of the X chromosome, and the multiple repeats lead to a fragile site on the chromosome, an area where the chromosome is likely to break, and clearly visible with appropriate staining under the microscope, giving the disease its name (Fig. 2.25).

The gene is inherited in an X-linked dominant pattern, and so the disease is primarily expressed in males; in addition, men are usually more seriously affected than women. Individuals (males or females) with between 50 and 200 repeats are said to have a premutation, and most have normal intellectual development, although some display mild signs and symptoms. Permutations, however, are unstable and can expand into the full mutation during meiotic divisions in the production of ova in an affected female, meaning that her sons could inherit the full mutation and display the condition.

Pathophysiology

Affected children show varying degrees of developmental delay, including difficulties with speech, social interaction, and intellectual and cognitive functions. Intellectual ability tends to decline with age, especially in males. Other key features of the condition are shown in Fig. 2.26. About a quarter of affected individuals suffer from epilepsy.

Management and prognosis

Diagnosis is 99% accurate with genetic testing. There is no cure, and treatment aims to maximise the individual's potential, using appropriate interventions such as speech therapy and educational support. Problems such as anxiety and attention deficit disorder may be treated with appropriate medications.

HAEMOPHILIA

Although the aetiology of haemophilia has only recently been firmly understood after the discovery of clotting factors in the 1940s and 1950s, it is an ancient disease, referred to in Biblical and second-century Jewish writings. Haemophilia is usually inherited, although spontaneous mutations

account for about one third of cases. There are two forms, haemophilia A and haemophilia B, of which haemophilia A is the more common, occurring in 1 in 5000 live male births compared with 1 in 30,000 for haemophilia B. Haemophilia B is sometimes called *Christmas disease*, after the first patient diagnosed with this disorder in 1952. In both forms, clotting is impaired, leading to spontaneous bleeding, usually into muscles or joints, and failure to clot after injury. The incidence is equal across all racial and ethnic groups, although males are more commonly affected than females because the abnormal gene is X-linked.

Acquired haemophilia is not inherited and is caused by the production of autoantibodies to factor VIII. It may develop in pregnancy, cancer, or other conditions, but the cause is often never identified.

Genetics

The production of two clotting factors (factor VIII in haemophilia A and factor IX in haemophilia B) is either reduced or absent because the genes that code for their production are abnormal. The clotting factor VIII gene, called *F8*, and the clotting factor IX gene, *F9*, lie close to one another on the long arm of the X chromosome and are inherited in an X-linked recessive pattern. The factor VIII gene contains 26 exons, and multiple mutations have been identified, including deletions, insertions, and frameshift mutations. The factor IX gene, with only 8 exons, is much smaller but over 800 different mutations have been reported.

Pathophysiology

Both forms are characterised by excessive bleeding, either spontaneous or after even minor trauma. There is significant variation in FVIII and FIX levels between affected people; in some, the clotting factor may be completely absent, and others have higher clotting factor production and almost normal clotting times. Normal plasma levels of FVIII are between 50 and 150 IU/dL, and values over 5 IU/dL are associated with mild disease. Less than 1 IU/dL causes severe disease, with spontaneous and regular bleeding. Values in between give intermediate symptoms. Bleeding into joints and muscles is common because of the physical stress to which the musculoskeletal system is subjected. Bleeding into the joints is painful, limits mobility, and can cause permanent deformity. Bleeding after surgery or dental work may be difficult to control, and haematoma formation may occur after even non-traumatic tissue compression (e.g., lifting a child under the arms, or a tumble in a child learning to walk). Although the disease almost always affects males, carrier females may have reduced levels of either clotting factor. This is because even though they have a normal copy of the *F8* or *F9* gene, one of their X chromosomes is silenced (lyonisation, p. 31), which may be the chromosome with the normal gene.

Management and prognosis

Mild haemophilia may not be diagnosed until a traumatic event in adult life leads to unexpectedly slow clotting, but more serious disease is generally picked up in early childhood, often when the child starts to become independently mobile. Diagnosis can be made in utero if there is a family history. Molecular analysis of chorionic villus samples, taken between weeks 10 and 13 of pregnancy, confirms the mutation. Measurement of clotting factor levels identifies the type of haemophilia. The standard treatment is clotting factor replacement, preferably with genetically engineered products rather than factors extracted from plasma, to reduce the risk of transmitting a blood borne infection. With adequate management, life expectancy should be normal. However, a significant (up to 30%) number of haemophiliac people treated with replacement clotting factors begin to develop IgG antibodies to them, neutralising the factors in the blood. The use of immunosuppressants in these patients usually effectively suppresses antibody production but brings additional complications such as increased susceptibility to infection.

HOMOCYSTINURIA

This IEM is not evenly globally distributed, with much higher-than-average incidence in some populations: 1 in 1800 in Qatar, 1 in 6400 in Norway, 1 in 17,800 in Germany, and 1 in 65,000 in Ireland, compared with a global average between 1 in 50,000 and 200,000.

Genetics

The disease is caused by an inability to metabolise the amino acids methionine and homocysteine. Any one of several genes may be affected, so there are different forms of the disorder, all inherited as autosomal recessive traits. The commonest form is caused by a mutation in the *CBS* gene, which produces cystathionine β-synthase. This enzyme normally converts homocysteine to cysteine for excretion. In its absence, homocysteine and the closely related amino acid methionine accumulate in the blood and in body tissues.

Pathophysiology

Accumulation of homocysteine causes short sightedness and an increased incidence of lens dislocation. Nervous system involvement includes impaired intellectual development and seizures. Involvement of the bone marrow may include megaloblastic anaemia. Physically, the affected individual may resemble someone with Marfan syndrome, with characteristic long limbs, fingers, toes, and other skeletal features. The risk of stroke and other cardiovascular events is significantly higher than average, and they are common causes of death.

Management and prognosis

Many cases are picked up by newborn screening with a routine heel prick test measuring plasma homocysteine levels. Older children presenting with myopia and lens dislocation should have blood homocysteine levels measured. Starting treatment early may slow the development of the disorder. Administration of pyridoxine (vitamin B_6) decreases homocysteine levels by increasing its conversion to cysteine, which is excreted; however, only about 50% of patients respond to this. Low protein diets restrict methionine intake and therefore reduce circulating methionine blood levels.

HUNTINGTON DISEASE

Worldwide, the prevalence of this neurological disorder is about 5 in 100,000, although it is most common in populations of European descent. It generally manifests itself in young or middle-aged adults, but there is a juvenile form. Most cases of Huntington disease are found in families known to carry the abnormal gene, but spontaneous mutations do occur, leading to the appearance of the disease in people with no family history. Up to 14% of cases may be caused by new mutations.

Genetics

The gene affected in Huntington disease is the *Huntingtin* (*HTT*) gene, located on chromosome 4 and which produces the Huntingtin protein. The normal gene is recessive and produces normal Huntingtin protein, which is found throughout body tissues, but its highest concentrations are found in the brain.

As described earlier, the mutation is an insertion (p. 37). The normal gene contains fewer than 35 CAG triplet repeats. Increasing number of repeats not only increases the risk of developing the disease and its severity, but also decreases the stability of the gene. In other words, the more CAG repeats there are in a parent's gene, the more likely it is that the gene will expand even further during meiosis in the production of their spermatozoa or oocytes, and explains why the disease can become significantly more severe through generations. This phenomenon is called **anticipation**. Over 40 repeats guarantees the development of the disease, assuming the individual lives long enough.

Pathophysiology

Despite ongoing research, the exact function of the normal Huntingtin protein is still not certain, although it seems to facilitate the movement of proteins and other substances within cells and may have a role in activating or deactivating gene transcription. The dominant, mutated gene produces an abnormal Huntingtin protein, which appears to fold incorrectly and disrupts normal nerve function. It is not understood why neurons are selectively targeted, when the protein has been found in all body tissues, but its accumulation leads to nerve cell death, particularly in the basal ganglia, which are essential for controlled, integrated voluntary muscle movement. Postmortem examination of the brain of an individual affected with Huntington disease shows atrophy of the basal ganglia, particularly of the caudate nucleus.

Symptoms usually begin between the ages of 30 and 50, except in the childhood form. The clinical course shows progressive neurological deterioration, steady loss of motor function, and a gradual decline in cognitive and intellectual ability. The first movement changes may include twitching, restlessness, fidgeting, clumsiness, or changes in gait and balance. Failing memory, impaired concentration, an inability to plan and organise normal daily activities, and reduced ability to cope with changes in routine or unexpected events are common. Behavioural and emotional changes include irritability, impulsiveness, irrationality, and anxiety. The signs and symptoms are usually initially quite subtle but become more marked as the disorder progresses. Late-stage disease is associated with physical incapacitation, loss of speech, impaired swallowing, potentially violent jerking of the head and limbs, and dementia. Death usually occurs within 15 to 25 years of diagnosis.

Management and prognosis

Antenatal testing is possible, but it is usually performed only if termination of the pregnancy is being considered. Children of an affected parent have a 50:50 chance of inheriting the gene (see Fig. 2.18), and counselling and support is essential for people opting for genetic testing to identify whether they have inherited their parent's mutation. This has been available only since 1993 and can be performed in symptomatic people to confirm a diagnosis, or in asymptomatic people to predict (from the number of CAG repeats in their gene) the likelihood of their developing the disease. The test is 98% to 99% accurate and is particularly useful in symptomatic individuals with no family history.

There is no cure for Huntington disease. Anti-depressants, muscle relaxants/anti-spasmodics, speech therapy, psychiatric support, and other interventions can relieve symptoms and maximise quality of life.

LEIGH SYNDROME

This disorder of energy production is very uncommon in most populations worldwide (average global incidence 1:40,000), but the affected gene is concentrated in certain populations, leading to clustering of cases; for example, the incidence in the Faroe Islands is 1:1700.

Genetics

Leigh syndrome can be caused by mutations either in mitochondrial DNA (mtDNA) or in nuclear DNA. Mutations in at least 70 different genes have been associated with this disorder, but all lead to faulty cellular energy production and an inability to produce ATP. Because it can be caused by mtDNA or nuclear DNA mutations, its inheritance pattern is not consistent. About 20% of cases are caused by mtDNA mutation, inherited through the mother (p. 000) because a newly formed zygote's mitochondria come from the oocyte, not the spermatocyte. A very small number of cases are X-linked, but most inherited cases of Leigh syndrome follow an autosomal recessive inheritance pattern.

Pathophysiology

The presentation of this disorder varies greatly between affected individuals because of the wide range of genetic abnormalities that can cause it. In most cases, abnormal function mainly involves the nervous system. Leigh syndrome is characterised by damage to particular parts of the brain: the basal ganglia and corpus striatum, which are involved in the co-ordination of voluntary movement; the cerebellum, also involved in control of movement and balance; and the brainstem, which regulates key life support activities including respiration and cardiovascular control. Generally, symptoms show early in life, with loss of motor function and movement disorders, and nervous system symptoms such as deafness, dysphagia, nystagmus, and paralysis of the muscles that control eye movement.

Management and prognosis

Diagnosis is made by evaluation of the symptoms, including motor and intellectual developmental delay with associated brainstem and/or basal ganglia deficiency. Molecular genetic testing confirms the diagnosis and also identifies the faulty gene and its location, either on mtDNA or nuclear DNA. Because there is no cure, treatment is symptomatic and supportive, and it manages individuals according to their specific needs.

MARFAN SYNDROME

This connective tissue disorder is relatively common, affecting 1 in 5000 to 10,000 people. Of all cases, 75% are inherited, with the remaining quarter caused by spontaneous mutation. There is no gender difference, and it is found in all races and ethnic groups.

Genetics

Marfan syndrome is inherited in an autosomal dominant fashion. The gene almost always responsible, *FBN1,* is found on the long arm of chromosome 15 and is a large gene with 65 exons. The healthy gene codes for a protein called **fibrillin**, an important component of elastic connective tissue. More than 600 different mutations have been reported in *FBN1,* most of which produce faulty fibrillin that does not polymerise correctly within the elastic fibres. This huge number of mutations gives rise to a wide range of phenotypic variations in individuals with the disorder and can make diagnosis a challenge. Less commonly, a gene called *FBN2,* on the long arm of chromosome 5, can be mutated, which also produces faulty fibrillin.

Pathophysiology

Elastic connective tissue is an important structural constituent of extracellular matrix in multiple body tissues, including ligaments, the aorta, and the supporting fibrils

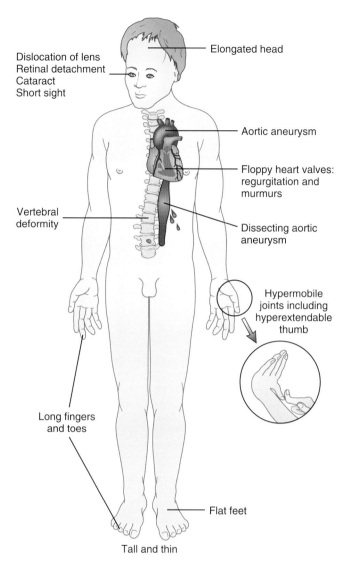

Dislocation of lens
Retinal detachment
Cataract
Short sight

Elongated head

Aortic aneurysm

Floppy heart valves:
regurgitation and
murmurs

Vertebral
deformity

Dissecting aortic
aneurysm

Hypermobile
joints including
hyperextendable
thumb

Long fingers
and toes

Flat feet

Tall and thin

Fig. 2.27 The main features of Marfan syndrome. (Modified from Damjanov I (2017) *Pathology for the health professions*, 5th ed, Fig. 5.12. St Louis: Elsevier Inc.)

of the lens of the eye. Abnormal fibrillin changes the mechanical properties of these supporting connective tissues and affected tissues are weaker than normal. Individuals with Marfan syndrome (Fig. 2.27) are tall and thin, with hypermobile joints because of lax ligaments, and long fingers and toes. Almost diagnostic of the syndrome is a hyperextendable thumb, which can be bent right back against the wrist. The upper body is disproportionately shorter than the lower body and there are often spinal deformities such as kyphosis and scoliosis. The chest wall is often deformed and asymmetrical. Aortic dilation can lead to aortic dissection, with blood forcing its way between the layers of the aortic wall, significantly weakening it and predisposing to rupture. This is clearly life-threatening and needs to be monitored. Mitral valve regurgitation is also a feature of this syndrome because the cardiac valves are floppy and poorly supported, and the chordae tendineae that normally prevent the valve flaps from prolapsing back up into the atria during ventricular contraction are too long. Cardiovascular manifestations are the greatest risk to life in this illness. Ocular symptoms can vary significantly from patient to patient, but

most commonly involve dislocation of the lens of the eye, either into the anterior or posterior cavity of the eyeball. The lens can be so seriously displaced that it lies directly against the retina. Lens dislocation is called *ectopia lentis* and is very rare in the otherwise healthy eye.

Management and prognosis

The variable clinical picture, and the large number of possible genetic abnormalities underlying this condition, can make accurate diagnosis very difficult. It is important to get the diagnosis correct, however, to monitor and manage the most life-threatening consequences. Careful physical examination and the use of a detailed set of diagnostic criteria, called the *Ghent criteria*, in which points are allocated to a range of possible signs and symptoms, are key tools in accurate diagnosis. Marfan syndrome is a significantly life-shortening disorder, with the average survival time being only 32 years, and the commonest cause of death is aortic rupture. Cardiac workload can be reduced with beta-blockers, which also reduce the stress on the aorta, and surgery is indicated if aortic root expansion reaches a diameter of over 5 cm.

NEUROFIBROMATOSIS

This relatively common (1 in 3000) disorder comes in two main forms: neurofibromatosis types 1 and 2 (NF1 and NF2). NF1, also called *von Recklinghausen's disease* after the German pathologist who coined the term *neurofibroma*, is the commoner form and carries the better prognosis and is the only form discussed here.

Genetics

NF1 is inherited as an autosomal dominant trait and the gene, *NF1*, is found on the long arm of chromosome 17. Normal *NF1* codes for a protein called **neurofibromin**. About half of cases are inherited, and the other half result from spontaneous mutations. This is an extremely high spontaneous mutation rate, and it is not known why this gene is so susceptible, although its large size (61 exons) probably contributes. Multiple mutations, including insertions and deletions, have been reported in the gene, most of which lead to the production of such abnormal neurofibromin that it is completely non-functional.

The gene is most likely to mutate in males, so inheritance is more often associated with the sperm than the oocyte, and the incidence increases with increasing paternal age. A child born to an affected parent has a 50% chance of inheriting the gene, and penetrance is 100%, so all children inheriting the faulty gene will express the disease, with signs and symptoms usually showing before the age of 5. Expressivity is however very variable from individual to individual, even within families, although identical twins usually manifest very similar clinical presentations. The disease distributes evenly across ethnic and racial groups.

Pathophysiology

Neurofibromin is widely produced in body tissues, including the nervous system. It is one of a family of tumour suppressor proteins that inhibits the activity of ras protein, a tumour promoter (p. 76). When mutated, the neurofibromin protein is non-functional or poorly functional, and ras protein becomes overactive, triggering inappropriate cell proliferation and

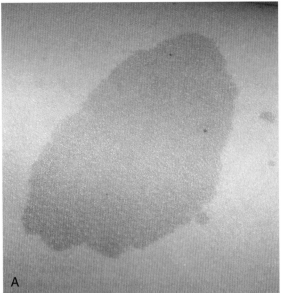

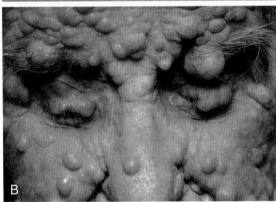

Fig. 2.28 Neurofibromatosis. (A) Café au lait spot: well-demarcated brown macule on the back. (B) Neurofibromata. (Courtesy, Julie V. Schaffer, MD. Bolognia J, Schaffer J, Duncan K et al (2022) *Dermatology essentials*, 2nd ed, eFig. 92.3. Oxford: Elsevier Inc. and (B) Paul Parker/ Science Photo Library.)

leading to the skin and nervous system tumours associated with this disease. Sufferers develop flat, irregularly shaped, pigmented patches called *café au lait spots* on the skin, and neurofibromata, benign, fleshy skin growths either developing under the skin or growing out on pedicles (Fig. 2.28).

Neurofibromata of the skin often become larger and more numerous with age, and although they do not become cancerous, they present significant cosmetic problems. They may also develop along nerves, including the optic nerve (optic glioma), where they may transform and become malignant. In the brain, they can cause epilepsy and other neurological complications, and they are associated with slow or abnormal neurological development in children, including delayed speech, attention deficit and learning disability. Large neurofibromas, called *plexiform neurofibromas*, can grow around nerves anywhere in the body, including the spinal cord, and may cause neurological deficit, significant deformity, and disfigurement. Individuals with NF1 also have an increased risk of non-NF1 cancers.

Management and prognosis

There is no cure, so symptoms are monitored and managed if and when they become troublesome. Skin or nerve tumours may be surgically removed if they are disfiguring or causing symptoms. Extra educational support, speech therapy, and family counselling are used to bring affected children to their greatest potential. Physiotherapy, pain management, and psychological support are important.

OSTEOGENESIS IMPERFECTA

Also called *brittle bone disease*, this disorder was named in 1835 by a German/French surgeon called Jean Lobstein (it is sometimes referred to as *Lobstein's disease*), but it dates back at least to ancient Egypt. There are at least eight forms of the disease, each caused by a defect in one of the genes responsible for type I collagen synthesis, and a spectrum of clinical presentations, although all are characterised by bone fragility and increased risk of fracture. The prevalence of osteogenesis imperfecta (OI) is about 1 in 20,000 births. The commonest type, type 1 OI, is the mildest form, and type II OI is the most severe form. The other types have clinical courses that fall somewhere in between these two extremes.

Genetics

The most commonly involved genes, *COL1A1* and *COL1A2*, cause more than 90% of all OI cases. Type 1 OI is usually caused by *COL1A1* gene mutations. *COL1A1* is inherited as an autosomal dominant trait, is located on the long arm of chromosome 17, and produces one of the proteins essential to the structure of the final collagen molecule. *COL1A2* is inherited in an autosomal recessive fashion, is located on the long arm of chromosome 7, and produces another of the protein chains found in healthy collagen. Over 800 different mutations in these genes have been reported.

Pathophysiology

The abnormal collagen produced in OI cannot be used in the helical structure of mature collagen. Collagen (p. 4) is an essential component of the body's connective tissue framework. Healthy bone is about one-third collagen by mass, and collagen is the fundamental structural protein in tendons, the sclera of the eye, cartilage of the musculoskeletal system, ligaments, teeth, and skin. OI is therefore characterised by fragile bones and repeated fractures, loose joints, small stature, and osteoporosis. The most severe form can lead to in utero fractures, gross skeletal deformity, underdeveloped ribcage and lungs, and perinatal death.

Management and prognosis

Diagnosis can often be made accurately on the clinical signs and symptoms and confirmed with genetic testing and collagen biopsy. There is no cure for OI. Management focuses on maximising musculoskeletal health (through exercise, weight management and physiotherapy) and other supportive interventions aimed at improving quality of life. Bones can be splinted to reduce fracture incidence, and some studies have shown some benefit using bisphosphonates, which, like natural phosphate, are deposited in bone tissue, strengthening it. The affected individual's lifespan depends on the form of disease present. The most severe forms are drastically life-limiting, with respiratory failure the commonest cause of death in affected children because the chest is small and the ribcage may be deformed, leading to respiratory insufficiency.

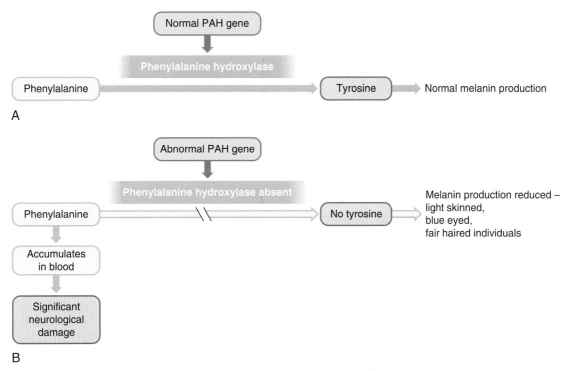

Fig. 2.29 The metabolic pathway in phenylketonuria. (From Waugh A and Grant A (2018) *Ross & Wilson anatomy and physiology in health and illness*, 13th ed, Fig. 17.12. Oxford: Elsevier Ltd.)

PHENYLKETONURIA (PKU)

PKU is the commonest IEM, first identified in 1953. Its global incidence varies significantly between populations; in American Caucasians, it is 1:10,000 to 1:15,000 newborns, but in the African American population it is only 1:50,000. In Japan, the incidence is only 1:125,000, whereas in China it is 1:17,000. The UK figure is 1:14,300.

Genetics

The mutated gene, *PAH*, codes for the enzyme phenylalanine hydroxylase, which normally metabolises the amino acid phenylalanine. In its absence, phenylalanine levels in the blood and tissues rise significantly. *PAH* is located on the long arm of chromosome 12, and hundreds of different mutations in this gene have been identified. PKU is inherited as an autosomal recessive trait.

Pathophysiology

If treatment is not rapidly initiated in an affected newborn, accumulating phenylalanine, highly toxic in nervous tissue because it damages the myelin sheath of nerve fibres, blocks intellectual development, and can cause seizures. The amino acid tyrosine is normally produced from phenylalanine, and tyrosine in turn is converted to melanin (Fig. 2.29). In the absence of phenylalanine hydroxylase, melanin production is reduced, and affected individuals are often light skinned, fair haired, and blue eyed. Children of mothers with PKU, even when well controlled, are more likely to have learning impairments, possibly because there is an inadequate supply of tyrosine to the developing baby.

Management and prognosis

Neonatal screening programmes reliably pick up affected babies, and treatment, based on restriction of dietary phenylalanine, is lifelong. This means a low protein diet, but phenylalanine is also present in other foodstuffs, for example those sweetened with aspartame, which is manufactured from phenylalanine. The best-case scenario with effective treatment is complete absence of any learning disability, but there is a slightly increased incidence of intellectual impairment in PKU-affected people.

POLYCYSTIC KIDNEY DISEASE (PKD)

This common disorder affects organs in addition to the kidney, including liver and blood vessels. There are two forms: one inherited as a dominant allele, and one inherited as a recessive form. The dominant form is far more common than the recessive form and affects 1 in every 500 to 1000 people globally. This disease is distributed equally between genders, races, and ethnicities.

Genetics

Most cases are inherited, but about 10% occur as spontaneous mutation with no family history. The genes involved in the autosomal dominant form are *PKD1* (found on the short arm of chromosome 16) and *PKD2* (found on the long arm of chromosome 4), which code for proteins called **polycystin-1** and **polycystin-2**, respectively. Together, these proteins co-operate in development of normal renal nephron epithelium and the function of cilia in the nephron. Disruption of normal polycystin function triggers cell proliferation and the formation of multiple, large cysts within the kidney tubules. *PKD1* mutation causes 85% of cases. A wide range of different mutations in these genes has been reported, leading to a range of clinical presentations in affected people.

The gene responsible for the autosomal recessive disease, *PKHD1*, is found on the short arm of chromosome 6.

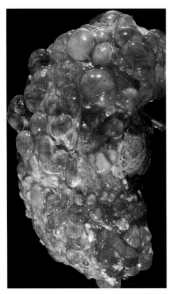

Fig. 2.30 Polycystic kidney. (From Kumar V, Abbas A, and Aster J (2021) *Robbins & Cotran pathologic basis of disease*, Fig. 20.43. Philadelphia: Elsevier Inc.)

Although this form of the disease is much rarer than the autosomal dominant type, it is significantly more serious, manifesting itself in infancy and usually lethal in early childhood.

Pathophysiology

The kidneys are enlarged and swollen, and the multiple dilated cysts, 3 to 4 cm in diameter, are very obvious (Fig. 2.30). The kidneys can expand enormously, compressing adjacent structures and causing loin pain and a sense of weight or dragging in the back. There may be haematuria, recurrent infections, renal colic from blood clots, and proteinuria. Hypertension is common, and, as kidney tissue is progressively destroyed, renal failure develops, affecting half of all sufferers by the age of 60. Cysts appear in the liver in 40% of cases and are usually asymptomatic, although large cysts cause compression and pain. Cardiac valvular abnormalities are common, but again often asymptomatic; however, aneurysms in the cerebral circulation can cause stroke and account for 4% to 10% of deaths in individuals with PKD.

Management and prognosis

For individuals with a family history, diagnosis is usually straightforward once symptoms appear. Ultrasound, computed tomography (CT), and magnetic resonance imaging (MRI) scans confirm renal enlargement and the presence of cysts. Genetic testing identifies the mutation. There is no cure for PKD. Pain management, controlling infections, and treating hypertension, which accelerates kidney failure, are all important.

RETINOBLASTOMA

This highly malignant eye tumour is the commonest malignant eye disease in children, affecting both sexes equally, although there is global variation in incidence. The average worldwide incidence is 1 in 16,000 to 18,000 live births, but higher rates are found in children of African, Indian, and Native American origin. The rate is also higher in lower socioeconomic groups and in children whose mothers have low educational attainment, suggesting a significant environmental influence.

Genetics

The affected gene, *RB1*, is a tumour suppressor gene (p. 75) essential to controlling the cell cycle. It is located on the long arm of chromosome 13, and its normal protein product, pRB, helps control cell division by acting as a brake on growth, and also functions in cell differentiation and apoptosis. Loss of this gene through mutation releases the affected cell from normal growth controls, and tumour formation results. *RB* mutations are found in many different types of cancer, but in retinoblastoma the cell suffering the *RB* mutation is a retinal neuronal stem cell.

About one third of affected children inherit one mutation from one parent. Provided that the other allele from the other parent is normal, the individual is higher risk (about 10,000 times greater than normal) but otherwise healthy. However, a spontaneous mutation in this normal allele leads invariably to malignant change. In the heritable form, the trait is inherited in an autosomal dominant fashion. The remaining two thirds of cases arise from spontaneous mutation in both alleles, a case of seriously bad luck. This form is not hereditable, and the affected child cannot pass the disease to his or her children because the mutation is present only in the eye cells and not in the gametes.

Pathophysiology

Retinoblastoma, especially inherited retinoblastoma, usually presents in the first few years of life. Two thirds (usually the spontaneous form) present with only one eye affected, but in one third, generally those with the inherited form, the disease is bilateral. The child may present with a squint (strabismus), a red or inflamed eye, or leucocoria (the pupil appears cloudy rather than black because of the pale tumour in the posterior cavity; Fig. 2.31A). The cell of origin is thought to be a retinoblast, a precursor cell in the lineage that produces the different types of specialised retinal nerve cells.

Management and prognosis

The tumour is often clearly visible through the pupil and can occupy a significant proportion of the posterior eye cavity (Fig. 2.31B). Ultrasound and CT scan of the orbit confirm its presence. Removal of the eye is curative, assuming that the tumour has not spread to nearby structures. Loss of the eye is obviously a major event for the patient, and if both eyes are removed, the child is left blind, a devastating event, so clinical decision making needs to balance the priorities of saving the child's life and preserving vision. Chemotherapy, radiotherapy, cryotherapy, and laser therapy are used to eradicate the tumour in cases where the eye can be saved and can often preserve useful vision in the treated eye. When adequately treated, survival rates are over 90%.

SICKLE CELL ANAEMIA

Individuals originating from sub-Saharan Africa, Saudi Arabia, India, and Mediterranean countries have significantly higher risk than other populations. In some badly affected areas, 1 child in 50 is born with the disorder. Because possessing one copy of the affected gene confers resistance to malaria, the sickle cell gene is widespread in regions where

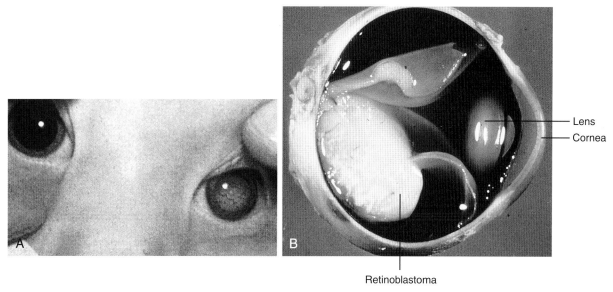

Lens
Cornea

Retinoblastoma

Fig. 2.31   Retinoblastoma. (A) The pupil is white rather than black (leukocoria) because of the tumour in the eye. (B) Section of an eye showing retinoblastoma in situ. (From (A) Abramson D (2022) Retinoblastoma, *CA Cancer J Clin* 1982(32): 130–140; and (B) Turnpenny P, Ellard S, and Cleaver R (2020) *Emery's elements of medical genetics and genomics*, 16th ed, Fig. 14.6. Philadelphia: Elsevier Inc.)

malaria is endemic. Sickle cell disease is the commonest inherited haemoglobin disorder.

Genetics

The affected gene, called *HBB*, is found on the short arm of chromosome 11 and is inherited as an autosomal recessive trait. The healthy gene codes for β-globin, one of the four chains of haemoglobin (Hb), the oxygen-transporting protein in erythrocytes. Multiple mutations of this gene have been reported, producing different forms of abnormal Hb. Hb containing chains of sickle cell β-globin is called *haemoglobin S* (HbS). The mutation involves replacement of a particular T nucleotide for an A in a single triplet in the gene, leading to insertion of a glutamate amino acid instead of a valine in the β-globin chain. This single substitution changes the conformation of the final protein, leading to polymerisation (i.e., the molecules clump together) of the Hb molecules under low oxygen conditions, and the characteristic 'sickling' of the red blood cells (Fig. 2.32A and B).

Survival and proliferation of the gene within the populations mentioned previously are evolutionarily favoured because carriers with one *HBB* mutation (i.e., heterozygous for the sickle cell trait but whose Hb is clinically normal) are resistant to malaria. However, homozygous individuals (i.e., those with two copies of the recessive sickle cell gene) do not benefit from this protection. The number of carriers in these populations is very high, which in turn keeps the birth rate of homozygous children high. Carriers are usually asymptomatic unless exposed to extremes of cold, severe hypoxia, or other significant circumstances. Other precipitating factors include infection, inflammation, and dehydration.

Pathophysiology (Fig. 2.32C)

There is a wide range of presentations in terms of severity; some patients are significantly more affected than others. HbS polymerisation causes the characteristic sickling of the red blood cells, which is initially reversible but eventually leads to permanent deformity of the erythrocyte. Once sickling becomes permanent, the red blood cells lose their streamlined shape, their ability to flex and fold to pass through narrow capillariesm, and their ability to stack in the bloodstream for smooth laminar flow. Instead, they clump and block the tiny blood vessels of the microcirculation, causing ischaemia and necrosis of the tissues. Vaso-occlusive crises, in which the blood supply to tissues is obstructed, particularly affect the hands and feet and lead to severe pain and hospitalisation events. Red cell membranes become fragile, and the cells rupture in the bloodstream and are targets for haemolysis in the spleen and liver, leading to varying degrees of anaemia. The lysing red blood cells trigger microthrombi formation in the circulation, contributing to poor tissue perfusion. Pulmonary complications are common because blood flow through the lungs is compromised. Infections are common, particularly in tissues whose blood supply is significantly compromised by obstruction. Impaired blood flow to the central nervous system may cause convulsions, transient ischaemic attacks, stroke, and bleeding into brain tissue. The bones are a common site for vaso-occlusive crises, impairing bone development in childhood and increasing risk of osteomyelitis (i.e., bone infection; p. 334).

Management and prognosis

Specific tests reliably detect HbS in blood samples, and an examination of blood smears clearly shows the distinctive, abnormal sickled shape of affected erythrocytes. Avoiding precipitating factors is a key element of management. Treatment of acute attacks includes analgesia, oxygen therapy to reverse hypoxia, intravenous fluid administration to improve blood flow, and antibiotic treatment of infection.

TAY-SACHS DISEASE

This IEM affects mainly individuals of Eastern and Central European Jewish descent. In some affected populations, it

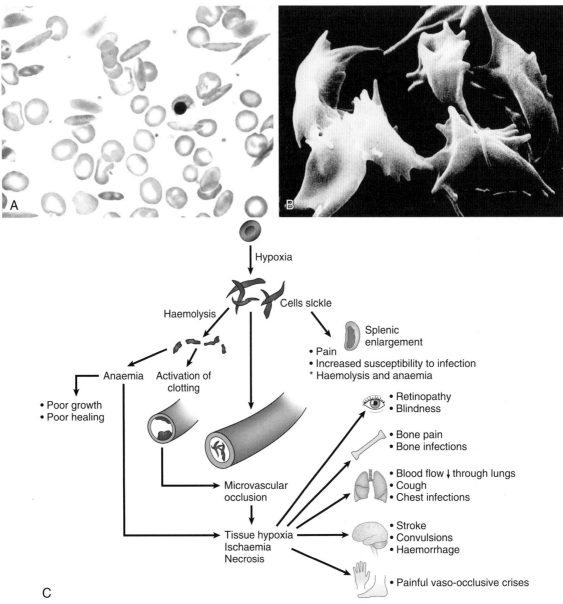

Fig. 2.32 Sickle cell disease. (A) Blood smear showing normal and sickled erythrocytes. (B) Scanning electron micrograph of deoxygenated sickled cells. (C) Pathophysiology of sickle cell anaemia. (From (A) Hudnall S (2024) *Hematology: a pathophysiologic approach*, 2nd ed, Fig. 5.1. Philadelphia: Elsevier Inc., (B) from Young NS, et al. (eds) (2006) *Clinical hematology*, p. 39. Philadelphia: Mosby.)

has been calculated that one in 25 people is a carrier. In the general population, the disease is very rare.

Genetics

The disease is transmitted as an autosomal recessive trait. The gene, called *HEXA*, was identified in 1985 and is located on the long arm of chromosome 15. The healthy form of the gene codes for part of an enzyme called β-hexosaminidase, which breaks down substances called **gangliosides**. Mutated *HEXA* produces a non-functional enzyme, and gangliosides accumulate inside cells, causing the devastating clinical course described in the next section (Fig. 2.33). More than 100 different mutations in *HEXA* have been reported.

Pathophysiology

Gangliosides are important constituents of cell membranes and participate in normal cell-cell interactions, especially in the brain. However, if they are allowed to accumulate, they cause massive damage in the central nervous system and other tissues, including the heart and liver. In the absence of β-hexosaminidase, ganglioside levels increase steadily, causing progressive neurodegeneration and motor impairment.

The disease course is relentless and always fatal. The baby seems normal at birth, but developmental regression and other symptoms such as loss of muscle tone usually appear by about 6 months. Blindness, deafness, confusion, paralysis, and profound cognitive impairment are typical. By the age of 2 years, the child is generally in a persistent vegetative state, and survival beyond 3 years old is rare. There are rarer forms, in which the disease does not manifest until later in childhood or young adulthood, but similar neurological and motor impairment develops, and the lifespan is short.

Management and prognosis

Screening for carrier status is by genetic analysis, and β-hexosaminidase levels can be measured in the blood. Prenatal testing can be done about 11 weeks of pregnancy by chorionic villus sampling, or at about 16 weeks by amniocentesis. There is no cure, and treatment is symptomatic and supportive. Current research is examining the possibility of an approach called *chaperone therapy*, in which the activity of the mutated enzyme is increased, enhancing ganglioside breakdown, but this work is still in its very early stages.

THALASSAEMIAS

These haemoglobinopathies were first described in a cohort of Italian children in 1925, although historical evidence

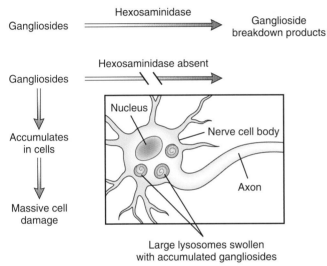

Fig. 2.33 The biochemical fault in Tay-Sachs disease. (A) Normal. (B) Hexosaminidase deficiency.

shows that they are ancient diseases. Thalassaemia affects males and females equally, and global distribution shows increased incidence in the Mediterranean region, Africa, the Middle East, India, and Southeast Asia, probably because carrier status confers resistance to malaria (as with sickle cell disease). The two main types are alpha-thalassaemia (sometimes called *thalassaemia A*) and beta-thalassaemia (sometimes called *thalassaemia B*). The genetic mutations in the two forms are different, although the clinical presentations are very similar because both forms are associated with production of abnormal haemoglobin, the oxygen-carrying pigment in red blood cells.

Genetics

Alpha-thalassaemia

Alpha-thalassaemia is caused by a mutation in one or more of four alleles that code for the production of **α-globin**, an essential sub-unit of haemoglobin. These genes, called *HBA1* and *HBA2*, sit close to each other on the short arm of chromosome 16. Healthy people have four copies of the allele (two alleles associated with each gene), and the different types of alpha-thalassaemia result from the loss of one or more of these alleles (Fig. 2.34). The more mutated alleles present, the lower the production of normal α-globin and the more severe the disease. Loss of one allele yields a silent carrier, an individual with no symptoms and normal haemoglobin levels. Loss of two alleles is also generally asymptomatic, although the chance of passing the mutant alleles to children is increased. Three lost alleles yield symptomatic disease, and four mutations, with complete failure of α-globin production, was inevitably fatal before birth until the development of intrauterine blood transfusion. A wide range of mutations has been reported in these genes, including deletions and splice mutations (see above).

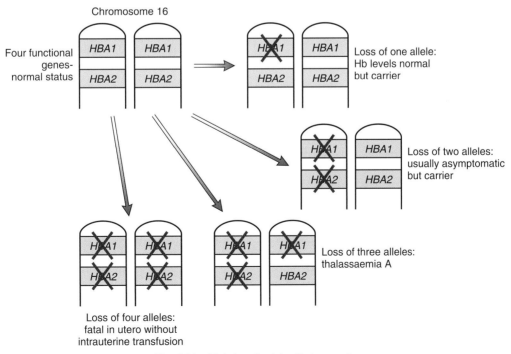

Fig. 2.34 Allele loss in alpha-thalassaemia.

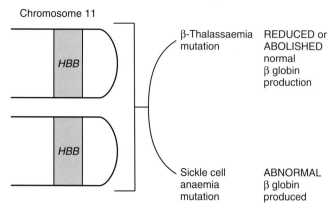

Fig. 2.35 *HBB* mutations in beta-thalassaemia and sickle cell disease.

Beta-thalassaemia

Mutations in the *HBB* gene cause beta-thalassaemia, which is inherited in an autosomal recessive fashion. As discussed earlier, *HBB* codes for the **β-globin** chain of haemoglobin and is also the gene responsible for sickle cell anaemia. In sickle cell anaemia, the mutation produces a faulty β-globin, whereas in beta-thalassaemia, the mutation either reduces or abolishes β-globin production (Fig. 2.35). In the most severe form of beta-thalassaemia, thalassaemia major, there is complete failure of β-globin production, and the commonest mutation is a splicing error, when introns are being cut out of the transcribed mRNA molecule before it relocates to the ribosome for translation. Thalassaemia major is usually associated with the homozygous recessive genotype (i.e., the individual has two copies of faulty recessive *HBB*). In the less severe form, thalassaemia minor, β-globin production is reduced but some is still produced; individuals are usually heterozygous, with one normal allele and one faulty allele.

Pathophysiology

In thalassaemia, production of either α or β globin chains is inadequate, although some people have reduced production of both. This leads to an imbalance between the levels of the α and β chains, which are insoluble unless they are matched up in the correct proportions. The normal haemoglobin molecule contains two of each, and if either globin is in short supply, the relative excess of the other precipitates out during red cell synthesis, interfering with erythrocyte production and causing varying degrees of anaemia. The severest form of alpha-thalassaemia, with all four α-globin alleles non-functional, causes severe anaemia in utero, which in turn causes heart failure and oedema in the fetus (hydrops fetalis). Less severe forms of both α and β thalassaemia are associated with reduced erythropoiesis, anaemia, and bone changes as red bone marrow, normally found only within spongy bone, expands into compact bone to increase erythrocyte production. Children's growth can be stunted, and the risk of infection is increased. Blood smears show a microcytic and hypochromic anaemia. Hepatomegaly (an enlarged liver) occurs because regular transfusions, the standard treatment, increase the body's iron load, and the liver collects and stores this excess iron. An enlarged spleen (splenomegaly) is also common, mainly because the abnormal erythrocytes are cleared rapidly by the monocyte-macrophage system here. In inadequately treated individuals, there may be heart failure caused by chronic anaemia.

Management and prognosis

Family history is important for identifying at-risk pregnancies. Prenatal testing of amniotic fluid identifies any genetic abnormality, important in thalassaemia major, which requires prenatal treatment. The mainstay of management is regular blood transfusion, although this brings additional complications including iron overload, which can be treated with iron chelation therapy. Removal of the spleen reduces the rate at which erythrocytes are eliminated and can reduce the number of transfusions needed. Cure is sometimes possible, especially in younger patients, with bone marrow transplant.

POLYGENIC DISORDERS

In contrast to monogenic disorders, in which the deficiency is linked to a fault in a single gene, polygenic disorders are associated with multiple gene mutations. They are associated with a family history and clustering of the disease within groups of blood relatives, but the pattern of disease expression is more random, infrequent, and unpredictable than in monogenic inheritance. In polygenic inheritance, multiple genes each play a small, additive part in the expression of the disorder. Environmental factors generally play a major part in determining whether a polygenic disorder will be expressed, and if so, how severe it will be. Many common disorders are associated with polygenic inheritance, including cardiovascular disease, asthma, type 2 diabetes, Alzheimers disease, multiple sclerosis, and schizophrenia (to name but a few).

POLYGENIC INHERITANCE

It is harder to prove that a disease has a genetic component if there is no clear inheritance pattern, and, even though some families are clearly more susceptible to the disorder, its expression seems sporadic and irregular. Such family clustering could be, for example, caused by the fact that families may share multiple behavioural and environmental preferences that could account for higher disease rates. Evidence to support a genetic input comes from family and twin studies, migrant studies, and the association of particular traits with particular forms of certain genes.

Family and twin studies

It is easier to identify a disease with an inherited component when it is relatively rare in the general population but occurs more regularly in certain families, but even then it is hard to determine whether the increased family incidence relates to a genetic influence or shared environmental factors. Identical twin studies, especially if the twins are separated and brought up by different families, can give clear direction here. If a disorder appears in identical twins separated at birth, a genetic link is much likelier than not. Another piece of supporting evidence for a hereditable component is the appearance of more severe defects in a susceptible family compared with the general population. For example, cleft lip and cleft palate have an inherited component, and families with higher-than-average incidence of these defects are often more likely to have more extreme forms of the defect, and to have both cleft lip and cleft palate appear together, than the general population, suggesting abnormal gene concentration in these families. Other family studies have shown that in cluster families with defects that affect one sex more than the other, such as pyloric stenosis (mainly male children), the rate of occurrence in female babies is also higher than in the general population. This suggests that the genes responsible are present in higher-than-average proportions in the family gene pool, increasing the chance that female babies will also be affected.

Disease in migrant populations

The incidence of certain diseases is not evenly distributed across populations within countries, or even regions within those countries. How can it be decided if this variation is caused by the local environment or behavioural factors, or if it is caused by a shared genetic ancestry? If a population group migrates to a different country where the incidence of a particular disease is either significantly lower or higher, and the migrant group incidence remains the same as when the group was in its home country, it suggests that genetic factors within that group are at play. However, if the incidence changes to match the local population, environmental factors such as diet, climate, or other influences are probably responsible, and are likely to be more important than any genetic contribution (e.g., in multiple sclerosis).

The association between traits and gene polymorphisms

Certain genes are present in populations in a wide range of variations, giving rise to a range of phenotypes. For example, the genes that code for eye colour come in a variety of different forms, generating the spectrum of colours and patterns seen in the human iris. Such variations are called **polymorphisms**. Other examples include the genes that code for 'self' antigens on the surfaces of all nucleated body cells. These genes, called **HLA genes**, are found on chromosome 6 and there are over 200 of them clustered in the same area on the chromosome. Some of these genes have hundreds of different forms (alleles). There is a very strong association between certain alleles of HLA genes and some diseases, suggesting a genetic link in the aetiology of such diseases. For example, the inflammatory joint disease ankylosing spondylitis is strongly associated with one form of one of the HLA genes, HLA-B27. Identifying the specific subtype of this gene in an individual suspected of having ankylosing spondylitis is a very useful diagnostic tool. Other disorders strongly associated with certain subtypes of some HLA genes include type 1 diabetes, rheumatoid arthritis, and Graves disease. Inheriting particular subtypes of these HLA genes from a parent therefore increases the risk of developing these disorders.

CHROMOSOMES AND THEIR ABNORMALITIES

Chromosomal abnormalities occurring in gamete formation are more likely to lead to spontaneous pregnancy loss than single gene defects and are commonly responsible for first trimester miscarriages. Many chromosomal defects can be clearly seen under the light microscope: extra or absent chromosomes are easily identified, and the damage in chromosomes with extra or missing sections is also often obvious. Smaller defects, involving only small sections of one or more chromosomes, require more sophisticated molecular techniques for identification.

The number of chromosomes may be incorrect. Normal gametes have 23 (**haploid**), and normal body cells have 46 (**diploid**). Cells with 69 (3x23) are **triploid**, and those with 92 (4x23) are tetraploid. Triploidy and tetraploidy do not usually lead to a live birth, and when they do, the baby dies shortly afterwards.

Aneuploidy is the state of an abnormal number of chromosomes but not in a multiple of 23. Sometimes a cell can inherit an extra copy of a chromosome pair (**trisomy**) or only one of the pair instead of two (**monosomy**). Autosomal monosomy is lethal: a developing fetus that does not contain two copies of any one of the autosomes will not survive to term. However, trisomy of some of the chromosome pairs may be compatible with life, although with varying degrees of deficiency. As for the sex chromosomes, no cell can survive without at least one copy of the X chromosome, but relatively large variations in numbers of X and/or Y can be tolerated.

Chromosomal breakages are common and are usually rapidly repaired, retaining their original structure and with no loss of genetic material. However, errors in repair mechanisms, or faulty cell division, may lead to loss of sections of a chromosome (**deletions**), addition of genetic material to a chromosome (**insertions**), exchange of material between chromosomes belonging to different pairs (**translocations**), or broken sections reinserted the wrong way round (**inversions**). In these chromosomal abnormalities, the total chromosomal number is often normal, but one or more of the chromosomes contains structural faults (Fig. 2.36)

Key to the outcome of chromosomal abnormalities for the affected individual is whether the karyotype remains balanced. If all the genetic material from all 46 chromosomes is retained, even if genes are in the wrong place or on the wrong chromosome, the situation is described as **balanced** and generally gives rise to no problems for the affected individual (but children inheriting the abnormal chromosome will be affected). However, if there is extra genetic material present, or (usually more problematically) material missing, this is described as **unbalanced** and gives rise to clinically significant consequences in the affected individual.

Deletions

In a deletion, a chromosome breaks in two places, the middle section is lost, and repairing enzymes join the free ends of the two end pieces. This means that the resulting chromosome may lack some of its genes, and the cell therefore has only one copy of these genes instead of two (Fig. 2.36A). The larger the missing section, the more likely it is that the consequences in an affected zygote will be severe. One example of an inherited condition caused by deletion of genes is cri-du-chat syndrome.

Insertions

In simple insertions, a section of a chromosome broken away from its original site is inserted into another chromosome (Fig. 2.36B). Simple insertions result in a balanced

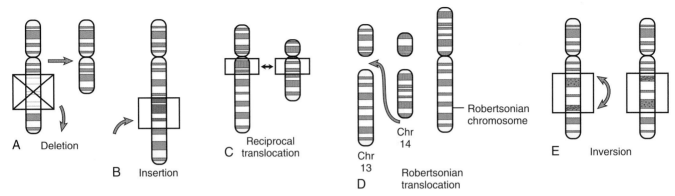

Fig. 2.36 Chromosomal abnormalities. (A) Chromosomal deletion. (B) Chromosomal insertion. (C) Reciprocal translocation. (D) Robertsonian translocation. (E). Inversion.

karyotype in the affected individual even though the resulting chromosomes are either shorter or longer than normal, but passing the abnormal chromosomes to the next generation in gametes leads to imbalances in the karyotypes of the children. However, other insertions can add material into a chromosome, leading to an unbalanced karyotype. Repeated sections of a gene cause significant mutations in, for example, Huntington disease and myotonic dystrophy, and significantly change the functionality of the gene.

Translocations

In translocations, chromosomal material is exchanged between non-homologous chromosomes (i.e., chromosomes from different chromosome pairs). If this does not result in any genes being lost, the individual is likely to be clinically normal because, although their genes are out of order and in the wrong place, the overall gene complement is present. However, if a faulty chromosome is then incorporated into one of the individual's gametes and passed to a zygote, its genetic complement will not be balanced, leading either to loss in pregnancy or inherited disease in a live born child.

There are two types of translocation: **reciprocal translocation** and **Robertsonian translocation**. Reciprocal translocation (Fig. 2.36C) is breakage of two chromosome pairs into two sections, and a straightforward swap between the pairs, leading to the formation of two new pairs of chromosomes but with the overall genetic content remaining the same. This results in a balanced rearrangement for the affected individual, although passing the abnormally structured chromosomes to children leads to unbalanced arrangements. Reciprocal translocations are fairly common and seen in 1 in 500 individuals. The **Philadelphia chromosome**, commonly seen in chronic myeloid leukaemia, is an example of a reciprocal translocation that causes disease (p. 115). In Robertsonian translocations, chromosomes break apart at the centromeres, and the long arms of two different chromosomes unite, forming a large, new chromosome. This is seen only in chromosomes 13, 14, 15, 21, and 22. The short arms are lost, so the individual now has only 45 chromosomes. The commonest form of this abnormality is fusion of the long arms of chromosomes 13 and 14 (Fig. 2.36D).

For the individual, this is a balanced arrangement because, fortunately, the absent short arms contain no important genes, and so it does not matter that there is only one copy, and they still have two copies of all other genes. When

gametes are formed from cells that contain the Robertsonian chromosome, which is essentially two chromosomes in one, some will contain two copies of one of the chromosomes: the large, translocated chromosome plus a normal chromosome. If that gamete then fuses with a normal gamete at conception, it produces a zygote whose cells contain three copies of that chromosome (trisomy). Translocation involving chromosome 21 is one cause (about 4%) of Down syndrome, in which affected individuals inherit two copies of chromosome 21, two inherited from a translocation abnormality in the mother, and one from the father.

Inversions

When a chromosome breaks in two places, it can happen that the section is reinserted, but the wrong way round, so the sequence in the broken fragment is reversed (Fig. 2.36E). These rearrangements are balanced and do not cause problems unless the break point cuts through an important gene. However, the mutation causes problems in children because the reversed section of the chromosome in one gamete will not match the sequence in the normal chromosome in the other gamete. Inversions are important mutations in human disease, including haemophilia A. In this disorder, an inversion in the gene for factor VIII is found in 43% of cases.

MITOSIS, MEIOSIS AND THE PRODUCTION OF GAMETES

Gametes (the female ova and the male sperm) are produced in the gonads, the female ovary and the male testis. Gametes are haploid, containing only 23 chromosomes, one of each autosomal pair 1 to 22 and a sex chromosome, either X or Y. This means that at fertilisation the chromosome pairs match up, one from each parent (see Fig. 2.4), and the new cell produced by this fusion possesses a total of 23 pairs of chromosomes; it is diploid.

The division of somatic cells (any cell that is not a gamete) in growth, healing, and repair takes place by **mitosis**, which occurs in a sequence of steps called prophase, metaphase, anaphase, and telophase. The aim of mitosis is to produce two daughter cells identical in every respect to the parent cell. Therefore, before the onset of mitosis, every chromosome is carefully duplicated. The cell now has four chromosomes for each chromosome pair instead of just two. The copied chromosomes are called **chromatids**. In prophase, two centrioles appear and migrate to opposite ends of the

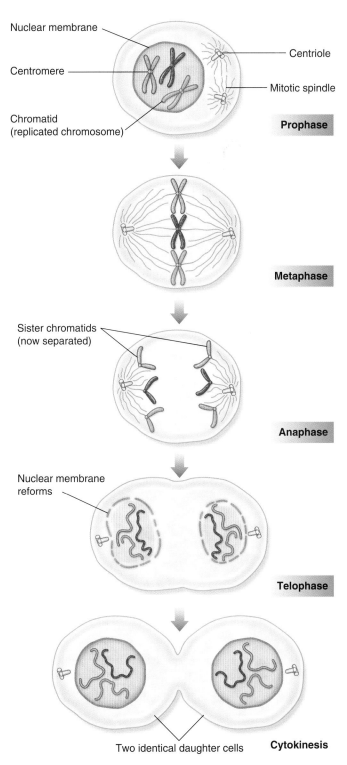

Nuclear membrane

Centriole

Centromere

Mitotic spindle

Chromatid
(replicated chromosome)

Prophase

Metaphase

Sister chromatids
(now separated)

Anaphase

Nuclear membrane
reforms

Telophase

Two identical daughter cells   **Cytokinesis**

Fig. 2.37 Mitosis. (From Waugh A and Grant A (2018) *Ross & Wilson anatomy and physiology in health and illness*, 13th ed, Fig. 3.11. Oxford: Elsevier Ltd.)

cell. Centrioles, and a network of microtubules called the *mitotic spindle* that links them, are the guidance system that directs chromatid separation. In metaphase, the chromatids align along the centre of the mitotic spindle. In anaphase, chromatids separate from each other and travel to opposite ends of the cell. In telophase, new nuclear membranes form around the chromatids, followed by cytoplasmic division, producing two new daughter cells identical to the parent cell (Fig. 2.37).

The process that generates gametes (ova and spermatozoa) is called **meiosis**. Meiosis is different to mitosis in three key respects: it involves two divisions, not just one; it produces four haploid cells instead of two diploid cells; and the daughter cells are all genetically different to each other and to the parent cell. The two cell divisions are called *meiosis I* and *meiosis II*, and during meiosis I, genes exchange between chromosomes of the same pair so that the gametes are all genetically different from one another. Errors in meiosis,

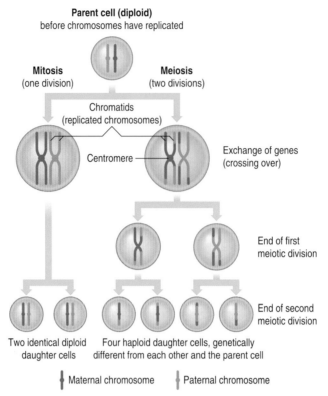

Fig. 2.38 Meiosis. (From Waugh A and Grant A (2018) *Ross & Wilson anatomy and physiology in health and illness*, 13th ed, Fig. 17.8. Oxford: Elsevier Ltd.)

leading to abnormal gamete production, are very common and these gametes are usually non-viable, leading to failure of fertilisation or early miscarriage of pregnancy.

Meiosis (Fig. 2.38)

As in mitosis, the first step is for the chromosomes to copy themselves, so there are now four chromatids for each chromosome pair. Remember that one chromosome has been inherited from the mother and the other from the father, and although the gene loci match for each chromosomal pair, there are likely to be significant differences between maternal and paternal alleles. For example, remember that there are multiple versions of the genes coding for eye colour. The maternal chromatids line up against the paternal chromatids and exchange genes. This means that the four new chromatids of a chromosome pair are all different from each other, each containing segments of both maternal and paternal DNA. This is called **crossing over** or **recombination**. When the cell divides at the end of meiosis I, the duplicated chromosomes are randomly allocated to one or other of the two daughter cells. The daughter cells from meiosis I are therefore haploid, with 23 chromosomes (each consisting of two chromatids) and are genetically different from each other and from the parent cell.

In the second meiotic division, the chromatids separate and one goes into one daughter cell, and the other goes into the other daughter cell.

Meiosis and gamete formation

The meiotic formation of sperm, driven by testosterone, is ongoing throughout the lifespan of the male, from puberty onwards, and often into an impressive old age. On the other hand, a female's population of ova is laid down in her ovary during embryonic development, and she produces no more after birth. The ova of a newborn baby girl have been paused in their meiotic development early in meiosis I, are still diploid, and are called **primary oocytes**. At puberty, under the influence of oestrogen and progesterone, one or more primary oocytes is released on a roughly monthly cycle at ovulation. At that point, meiosis is reactivated, the first meiotic division completed, and the ovum released as a haploid **secondary oocyte**. This only undergoes the second meiotic division if fertilised by a spermatozoon, producing a diploid zygote.

Nondisjunction

Nondisjunction occurs when a chromosome pair does not separate in meiosis I (Fig. 2.39B), or chromatids of a chromatid pair do not separate in meiosis II (Fig. 2.39C). Some gametes therefore receive twice as many chromosomes as they should, and some receive none. It is far more common for nondisjunction to occur in the ovum than the sperm, and it is believed that this is because of the detrimental effect of increasing maternal age on the oocyte. It seems likely that when the arrested meiotic division of the primary oocyte is reactivated at ovulation, the internal structures within older ova that are supposed to direct chromosome or chromatid movement fail to work effectively. This leads to errors in separating and guiding chromosomes or chromatids to the correct ends of the cell. Nondisjunction is the usual cause of conditions such as Down syndrome and Klinefelter syndrome, in which the fertilised ovum receives at least one extra copy of a chromosome.

Chromosomal mosaicism. If nondisjunction occurs during gamete production and a gamete with one or more extra chromosomes fuses with a normal gamete at fertilisation,

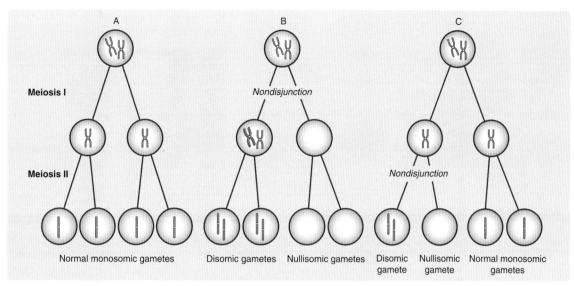

Fig. 2.39   Nondisjunction. (A) Normal meiosis. (B) Nondisjunction in meiosis I. (C) Nondisjunction in meiosis II. (From Newport M, Horton-Szar D, and Evans J (2008) *Crash course: cell biology and genetics*, Fig. 8.26. Edinburgh: Mosby Ltd.)

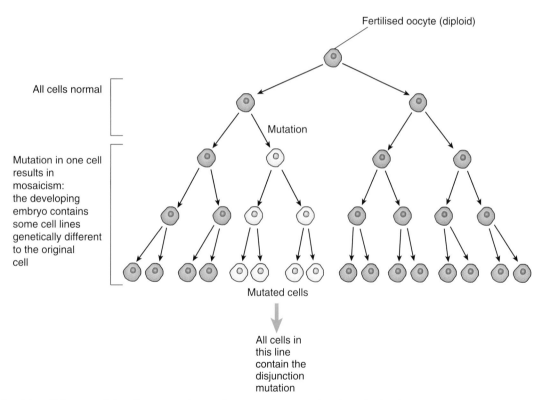

Fig. 2.40   Mosaicism. When nondisjunction occurs in a cell at an early stage of embryonic development, all cells descending from that cell inherit the mutation. (Modified from Nussbaum R, McInnes R, and Willard H (2018) *Thompson & Thompson genetics in medicine*, Fig. 7.17. Philadelphia: Elsevier Inc.)

all the cells in the new individual will inherit the additional material. However, sometimes the two gametes are normal at conception, but nondisjunction occurs at an early stage in embryonic development, leading to more than one genetically similar but different cell lines being established in the developing embryo. This is called **mosaicism** (Fig. 2.40). This is the origin of the trisomy 21 in 2% to 4% of people with Down syndrome. When only some body cells contain

the genetic abnormality, the resulting condition is often milder than when the mutation is found in all body cells.

THE MAIN AUTOSOMAL ABNORMALITIES

Chromosomal abnormalities are very common in both male and female gametes; at least 10% of sperm and up to 25% of oocytes are affected, but they are usually lethal. First

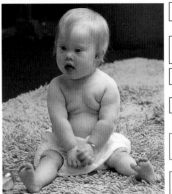

Intellectual impairment
Increased risk of Alzheimer disease

Upward sloping palpebral fissures

Pronounced epicanthic fold

Increased risk of leukaemia

Poor muscle tone

Growth retardation

Small ears

Flattened nose and face

Large tongue

Heart defects

Single palmar crease

Space between first and second toes

Fig. 2.41 Common features of Down syndrome. (Modified from Lissauer T and Clayden G (2007) *Illustrated textbook of paediatrics*, Fig. 8.2a. Edinburgh: Mosby.)

trimester loss occurs in up to one fifth of pregnancies because of a non-viable fetus, and an unknown further number of zygotes are lost so early after conception that the woman does not realise she has ever been pregnant.

CRI-DU-CHAT SYNDROME

The incidence of cri-du-chat (literally: cat's cry, because of the characteristic high-pitched wailing made by affected babies caused by an underdeveloped larynx) is rare, seen in only 1 in 50,000 live births. The disorder is found in all races, and females are affected more frequently than males in the ratio of 1:0.7.

Genetics

The condition is caused by a range of deletions on the short arm of chromosome 5, usually inherited from the father. The signs and symptoms can vary depending on the extent of the deletion. In the most extreme case, the entire short arm is missing and the disorder manifests in its most severe form.

Pathophysiology

Affected children show significant developmental delay, failure to thrive, microcephaly (small head), behavioural issues, cognitive impairment, hypersensitivity to sound, and characteristic facial features, including a flat nasal bridge, underdeveloped chin, plump cheeks, low-set ears, and a downturned mouth. They may also have low muscle tone and cardiac and musculoskeletal abnormalities.

Management and prognosis

The characteristic cry of the newborn is a significant pointer to diagnosis. Genetic studies confirm the loss of chromosome 5 material. A normal lifespan is possible if appropriate support is available. Respiratory or cardiac failure is usually the cause of death.

DOWN SYNDROME

This is the commonest inherited chromosomal abnormality and affects up to 1 in 800 births. It occurs across all races. The risk increases sharply with maternal age. Women aged 20 at conception have a risk of 1 in 1500 of conceiving a child with Down syndrome; this risk rises to 1 in 400 by the age of 35, and at 45 the risk is 1 in 30. The direct relationship between maternal age and risk is thought to relate to the age of the ovum, which is as old as the mother herself.

Genetics

Down syndrome is caused by the presence of three copies of chromosome 21 (trisomy 21; see Fig. 2.6), almost always derived from the ovum. The vast majority of cases arise because of nondisjunction of chromosomes during gamete formation. In Down syndrome, nondisjunction of chromosome 21 leads to the production of a primary oocyte with two copies of this chromosome, and when this gamete combines with a normal sperm cell, the zygote has three copies. A high proportion of trisomy 21 fetuses do not go to term but are lost through miscarriage or stillbirth. A small number (2%) of people with Down syndrome are identified as mosaics (p. 56) and the condition usually manifests itself more mildly.

Pathophysiology

The spectrum of clinical signs and symptoms in Down syndrome is wide (Fig. 2.41). High-functioning individuals may have only minimal cognitive and physical limitations, but in others the disorder manifests more severely. There is cognitive impairment, congenital cardiac abnormalities including patent ductus arteriosus and atrial and ventricular septal defects, growth retardation, and typical facial features including protruding tongue, small ears, pronounced epicanthic fold (of the upper eyelid), and upwardly sloping palpebral fissures, giving the appearance of upwardly sloping eyes. There is increased risk of leukaemia and Alzheimers disease.

Management and prognosis

The characteristic facial features can make diagnosis straightforward shortly after birth, and genetic testing confirms the presence of a third chromosome 21. Cardiac complications, an increased predisposition to respiratory infections and the higher-than-average risk of leukaemia can shorten life, but the average lifespan is now over 60 years. The development of Alzheimer disease is very common after the age of 40.

THE PRINCIPAL SEX CHROMOSOME DISORDERS

A cell without at least one copy of an X chromosome will not survive. However, significant variation in X and Y

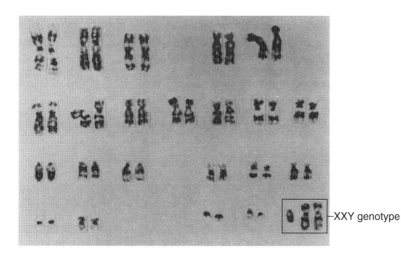

—XXY genotype

Fig. 2.42   Karyotype in Klinefelter syndrome. (Modified from Fitzsimmons JS (1980) *A handbook of clinical genetics*, Fig. 5.30. Butterworth-Heinemann.)

chromosomal complement in a zygote may be tolerated and the pregnancy result in a live birth.

KLINEFELTER SYNDROME

The occurrence of Klinefelter syndrome is somewhere around 1 in 650 male live births, although it is believed to be underdiagnosed because there is significant variability in signs and symptoms. There is equal spread between races.

Genetics

It was shown in 1959 that the condition is caused by one or more extra X chromosomes in a male karyotype. The commonest form is trisomy XXY, with a total chromosome count of 47 (Fig. 2.42). It is usually caused by nondisjunction of chromosomes during meiosis in gamete formation, frequently but not always the ovum. When the ovum is responsible, there is a positive correlation with maternal age. The degree of cognitive impairment and physical signs increases with the number of additional X chromosomes present. Some individuals show mosaicism, and these males may have less pronounced features of the disorder.

Pathophysiology

There is a range of clinical presentations, and not all individuals with Klinefelter syndrome demonstrate all of these features. Testicular underdevelopment leads to reduced testosterone levels, causing poor development of muscle mass, female-pattern distribution of body fat, low libido, small penis and testes, gynaecomastia, and infertility. Oestrogen levels may be higher than normal, and men with Klinefelter syndrome are at increased risk of breast cancer, osteoporosis, and autoimmune disorders such as rheumatoid arthritis and systemic lupus erythematosus. There is usually cognitive impairment.

Diagnosis and management

Diagnosis may be made on the clinical features and confirmed on karyotype analysis. Testosterone treatment can promote the development and maintenance of secondary sexual characteristics.

TURNER SYNDROME

This condition, first described by Henry Turner in 1938, affects only females and is found in all races. It is seen in about 1 in 2500 live births, although it is seen much more frequently in miscarriage or stillbirths. It is also likely to be underdiagnosed, as mild cases may not be picked up.

Genetics

Turner syndrome is caused by loss of all or part of the second X chromosome, usually because the paternal chromosome is absent or shortened.

Pathophysiology

Many women with Turner syndrome are of normal intelligence, although there may be reduced IQ, other cognitive impairment, and psychological issues. Physical signs include widely spaced nipples, low-set ears, and neck webbing (a thick fold of skin running from behind the ears to the shoulders). Affected women have shorter-than-average height and failure of ovarian development, leading to infertility and sexual immaturity. There is increased risk of type 2 diabetes, aortic coarctation, and inflammatory bowel disease.

Management and prognosis

Routine ultrasounds in pregnancy can detect babies with Turner syndrome: there may be generalised swelling or oedema around the neck. Although short stature is often the first indication of the condition and can lead to diagnosis in early childhood, Turner syndrome may not be diagnosed until adolescence or even later. Examination of the karyotype shows the missing or shortened second X chromosome. Growth hormone treatment and oestrogen replacement therapy minimise growth retardation and stimulate and maintain sexual maturity.

BIBLIOGRAPHY AND REFERENCES

Adams, D., Gonzales-Duarte, A., O'Riordan, W. D., et al. (2018). Patisiran, an RNAi therapeutic, for hereditary transthyretin amyloidosis. *New England Journal of Medicine, 379*(1), 11–21.

Alton, W. F. W., Armstrong, D. K., et al. (2015). Repeated nebulisation of non-viral CFTR gene therapy in patients with cystic fibrosis: A randomised, double-blind, placebo-controlled, phase 2b trial. *Lancet Respiratory Medicine, 3*(9), 684–691. https://doi.org/10.1016/S2213-2600(15)00245-3

Fijnvandraat, K., Cnossen, M. H., et al. (2012). Diagnosis and management of haemophilia. *BMJ, 344*(7855), 36–39.

Hamers, L. (2018). The first gene-silencing drug wins FDA approval. *Science News, 194*(5), 6.

Hemminki, K., Bermejo, L., & Forsti, A. (2006). The balance between heritable and environmental aetiology of human disease. *Nature Reviews Genetics, 7*, 958–965.

Pyeritz, R. E., Korf, B. R., & Grody, W. W. (Eds.). (2019). *Emery and Rimoin's principles and practice of medical genetics and genomics* (7th ed.) Elsevier.

Shawky, R. M. (2014). Reduced penetrance in human inherited disease. *Egypt J Med Hum Genet, 15*, 103–111.

Simmons, D. (2008). Epigenetic influences and disease. *Nature Education, 1*(1), 6.

Sirrs, S., Hollak, C., Merkel, M., et al. (2016). The frequencies of different inborn errors of metabolism in adult metabolic centres: Report from the SSIEM adult metabolic physicians group. *Journal of Inherited Metabolic Disease Reports, 27*, 85–91.

Sun, N., Youle, R. J., & Finkel, T. (2016). The mitochondrial basis of aging. *Molecular Cell, 61*(5), 654–666.

Turnpenny, P., & Ellard, S. (2017). *Emery's elements of medical genetics* (15th ed.). Elsevier.

Wastnedge, E., Waters, D., & Patel, S. (2018). The global burden of sickle cell disease in children under five years of age: A systematic review and meta-analysis. *Journal of Global Health, 8*(2). https://doi.org/10.7189/jogh.08.021103

Useful Websites

GeneReviews: A wide range of genetic conditions reviewed and explained. https://www.ncbi.nlm.nih.gov/books/NBK1116/.

Genetics Home Reference: Fantastic repository of information on genetics and genetic diseases. https://ghr.nlm.nih.gov.

National Organisation for Rare Diseases: Useful information on a range of inherited disorders. https://rarediseases.org.

University of Kansas Medical Centre: A wide range of materials and activities in genetics. http://www.kumc.edu/gec/.

Neoplasia

3

CHAPTER OUTLINE

INTRODUCTION
CANCER EPIDEMIOLOGY
Global trends in cancer incidence and survival
CELL DIVISION AND TISSUE GROWTH
The cell cycle and its control
  The M phase
  The G_1 phase
  The S phase
  The G_2 phase
Senescence and apoptosis
  Senescence
  Apoptosis
Adaptive adjustments in tissue growth patterns
CHARACTERISTICS OF NEOPLASMS
  Tumour nomenclature
  Tumour structure
Properties and behaviours of neoplastic cells
Differences between malignant and benign
  neoplasms
  Metastatic spread
CARCINOGENESIS: THE DEVELOPMENT OF
CANCER
  The genetics of cancer

Tumour suppressor and tumour promoter genes
The process of carcinogenesis: initiation and
  promotion
Risk factors for cancer
ASSESSMENT AND TREATMENT OF CANCER
The tumour burden and effects on the body
Assessment of cancer
Major treatment approaches
THE MAJOR CANCERS
Lung cancer
  Types of lung cancer
  Manifestations of lung cancer
  Management and prognosis
BREAST CANCER
  Types of breast cancer
  Manifestations of breast cancer
  Management and prognosis
COLORECTAL CANCER
  Types of colorectal cancer
  Manifestations of colorectal cancer
  Management and prognosis

INTRODUCTION

The average adult human body contains around 50 trillion cells, an impressive journey from the fusion of just two cells—a spermatozoon and an ovum—at conception. During embryonic and fetal development, the rate of cell division is significantly accelerated compared with adult tissues; on average, the newborn baby contains 5 trillion cells, which have differentiated (specialised) into over 200 different types and formed the body's organs. During infancy and childhood, cell division continues rapidly, and the child grows through youth to maturity, at which point cell proliferation slows and becomes largely restricted to replenishing and replacing old or injured tissues. This incredible feat of biology is tightly controlled by a complex system of growth regulators, which activate or inhibit cell replication at key points, permitting cell division when required and inhibiting it when not. Activating cell suicide pathways in old

or diseased cells, and regulating their replacement by managed cell proliferation, carefully maintain cell numbers.

Most cells in a tissue are **terminally differentiated**, meaning they have a specialised function and have lost the ability to divide. Most tissues, however, also contain a population of **stem cells**, self-renewing cells that are constantly dividing and which can differentiate into a number of different cell types as needed (Fig. 3.1). Stem cell division is very tightly controlled to prevent inappropriate or excessive tissue growth. Older cells grow and divide more slowly than younger cells, and most body cells have a built-in limit of about 60 divisions in total. Each time a cell divides, it must copy its DNA first, and errors (mutations) in DNA copying are quite common. If a mutated cell is not repaired or destroyed, its mutations are passed to daughter cells and accumulate in later generations of the cell so that older cells may have significant numbers of genetic mutations (Fig. 3.2). These errors may allow the cell to escape the body's normal growth control mechanisms, and

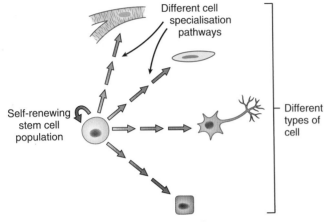

Fig. 3.1   Stem cells.

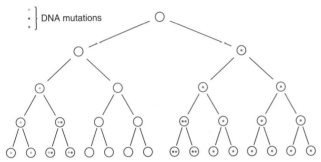

Fig. 3.2   Accumulation of mutation through successive cell generations.

acquire the ability to divide independently; this can lead to tumour development. Tumour formation is called **neoplasia** (neo = new, plasia = growth). Neoplastic growths may be benign or malignant; malignant growths cause cancer.

This chapter will explore some of the mechanisms and processes that contribute to tumour growth and development and will discuss some of the more common cancers.

CANCER EPIDEMIOLOGY

Cancer is second only to cardiovascular disease as the cause of death in developed countries. It may seem like a scourge of 21st-century life, because the rates of various forms of the disease are steadily increasing, but cancer is an ancient disease, suffered by people throughout human history. There is clear evidence in the fossil record of cancerous growths in early humans dating from over 1.5 million years ago, and skeletons from ancient Egypt bear damage indicating the presence of primary and secondary bone cancers. Although the disease was probably less common in those times than nowadays because the average lifespan was much shorter, and lifestyle choices like smoking and high saturated fat intake did not contribute, the capacity for malignant growth is clearly inbuilt within our cells.

GLOBAL TRENDS IN CANCER INCIDENCE AND SURVIVAL

International Agency for Research on Cancer (IARC) figures showed there were an estimated 19,292,789 new

cases of cancer globally in 2020. The three commonest cancers were breast, lung, and colorectal (Fig. 3.3), although death rates were highest in lung, colorectal, and liver cancers (IARC, 2020). The worldwide distribution of cancers varies hugely. For example, the highest burden of infection-related cancers (e.g., liver cancers related to hepatitis) is seen in the least wealthy countries, which have limited infection control measures and poor public health education programmes. The incidence of colorectal cancer, which is related to saturated fat intake, is lowest in the least wealthy countries such as sub-Saharan Africa and rising in developing and middle- to high-income countries, including the UK and Canada. It is actually falling in some high-income, highly developed countries, including the United States and Japan, where screening and early detection of pre-malignant lesions—and increasing awareness of lifestyle factors—may be driving these positive changes.

Survival rates also vary enormously worldwide. In the developed, middle- to high-income world, survival rates are usually better than in poorer countries. Wealthier countries generally have more sophisticated healthcare systems, superior diagnostic facilities, screening programmes, and effective public health education policies. For example, 5-year survival rates from breast cancer diagnosed in women between 2010 and 2014 were 90.2% in the United States but only 66.1 in India. Survival rates from gastrointestinal cancers are highest in southeast Asia, but in these same countries, survival rates from melanoma are among the worst in the world. Collection of population data on cancer incidence and survival is an important tool in decision-making in cancer control and management policy, especially in lower income countries.

CELL DIVISION AND TISSUE GROWTH

In a mature organism, cell numbers are carefully controlled by a complex set of mechanisms, governed by enzymes and regulatory proteins that are activated and deactivated at key points in the cell's life cycle. The **cell cycle** is a circular sequence of specific events that governs cell division and the rate at which new cells are produced. The more cells in a tissue participating in the cell cycle, the faster the tissue is likely to proliferate. The epithelial lining of the gastrointestinal tract, for instance, renews itself every 2 to 6 days or so, whereas brain neurones differentiated at birth probably never divide in an individual's lifetime and may therefore have to survive and function for a century or more.

As cells age, their function tends to deteriorate, and after multiple cell divisions, their DNA contains increasing numbers of mutations. To prevent old, abnormal, or dysfunctional cells from replicating and passing their damaged DNA to further generations, older cells are programmed to enter a senescence pathway or to activate a suicide pathway (**apoptosis**). Total cell numbers in a tissue therefore represent a balance between the numbers of new cells produced and the numbers destroyed. Malfunctions of both or either of these (i.e., either overproduction or under-destruction) are the fundamental platform for nearly all cancers.

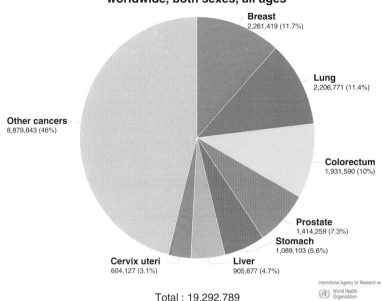

Estimated number of new cases in 2020, worldwide, both sexes, all ages

Breast
2,261,419 (11.7%)

Lung
2,206,771 (11.4%)

Other cancers
8,879,843 (46%)

Colorectum
1,931,590 (10%)

Prostate
1,414,259 (7.3%)

Stomach
1,089,103 (5.6%)

Cervix uteri
604,127 (3.1%)

Liver
905,677 (4.7%)

International Agency for Research on Cancer
World Health Organization

Total : 19,292,789

Fig. 3.3 Estimated number of new cases of the main cancers in 2020. (Reprinted from IARC, 2020.)

THE CELL CYCLE AND ITS CONTROL

The cell cycle (Fig. 3.4) represents the different stages in the life of the cell, including growth phases G_1 and G_2, the stage of DNA replication (the S phase) and cell division: mitosis (M phase). The enzymes controlling the cell cycle are in turn controlled by proteins called **cyclins**.

Some cell types, such as muscle and nerve cells, rarely divide and so spend most of their time in G_0. Other cell types, for instance epithelial cells, move in and out of the cell cycle much more frequently, increasing the rate of cell proliferation and allowing rapid tissue regeneration. Cells that spend a large proportion of their time in the cycle are more likely to acquire and retain genetic errors because their DNA is copied more frequently, increasing the likelihood of precancerous and cancerous mutations. In addition, the time taken for a cell to move through the cell cycle varies considerably; in epithelial tissues, the generation time can be as little as 8 hours, but slow-growing cells may take days to complete one cycle.

THE M PHASE

Cells going into the M phase have copied their DNA in the previous S phase and so have 92 chromosomes instead of 46. The first part of the M phase is mitosis (see Fig. 2.37), in which the duplicated chromosomes separate and collect at opposite ends of the cell. Cytokinesis, the second part, is division of the cytoplasm. It results in two daughter cells—each with 46 chromosomes—which are genetically identical to each other, assuming all has gone well during this stage. They are smaller than the parent cell and may either enter the first growth phase, G_1, or go directly into G_0.

THE G_1 PHASE

Cells can spend a variable length of time in the G_1 phase, during which they grow back towards the size of their parent cell, although at this stage they do not copy their DNA. Cell growth slows down if growth conditions are unfavourable

(e.g., if the nutrient supply is inadequate or if the tissue is exposed to other stressors). In addition, before leaving G_1, the cell's DNA is carefully checked for any damage. This checkpoint, sometimes called the **restriction point**, normally prevents cells from proceeding through the cycle if they are damaged or if the local conditions are not good enough to support expanding cell numbers. Restriction point malfunctions are associated with nearly all cancers and allow abnormal cells to continue dividing. If no further cell division is required at this time, cells exit the cell cycle during G_1 and enter G_0.

The G_0 phase

Most body cells live their lives in G_0, entering this stage as soon as they are produced. In G_0, the cell cycle is disabled, and the cell cannot reproduce. However, the cell is not dormant; it is fully differentiated and fully functional. Within most tissues and organs, most body cells have been diverted out of the cell cycle into G_0 and are carrying out the essential roles of their cell type, for example as liver, muscle, or epithelial cells. Under certain closely controlled circumstances, differentiated cells can re-enter the cell cycle, but most cell division takes place in stem cell populations.

THE S PHASE

During this stage, the cell copies its DNA so that it now has 92 chromosomes instead of 46.

THE G_2 PHASE

Once the S phase is complete, the cell usually moves swiftly through the G_2 stage, during which the enzymes required for mitosis are activated. There is a further checkpoint here, and the replicated chromosomes are examined for damage. Abnormal cells are usually blocked from entering mitosis and, if their DNA cannot be repaired, may have their apoptosis genes activated and undergo self-destruction. Normal cells rapidly enter the M phase and undergo mitosis.

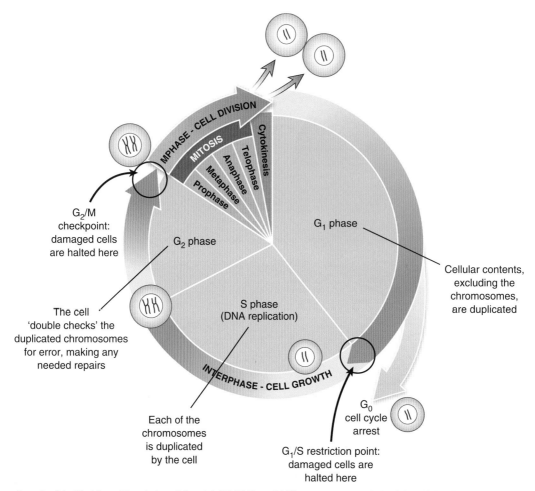

Fig. 3.4   The cell cycle. (Modified from Waugh A and Grant A (2018) *Ross & Wilson anatomy and physiology in health and illness*, 13th ed, Fig. 3.10. Oxford: Elsevier Ltd.)

SENESCENCE AND APOPTOSIS

Old, damaged, or abnormal cells can be shunted permanently out of the cell cycle and into a state of **senescence**, during which the cell may continue functioning but can never again divide. Senescence probably evolved to prevent mutated cells from transmitting their damaged DNA to future generations of cells and therefore to suppress the development of cancer. The alternative fate for old, damaged, or abnormal cells is **apoptosis**. Both processes are key to maintaining a controlled and healthy cell population.

SENESCENCE

Most body cells can divide between 50 and 60 times before entering senescence, although old age is not the only trigger. Other causes of senescence include DNA damage and strong mitogenic signals. Strong mitogenic signals can result from overactivity of **oncogenes**, which stimulate tissue growth. In the face of excessive or chronic activation of cell division, cells escape down the senescence pathway rather than keep rapidly dividing, which is a strong argument in favour of senescence being an anti-cancer mechanism.

As tissues age, they accumulate increasing numbers of senescent cells. Evidence suggests that although senescence in younger tissues provides an escape route for cells that are

being driven to divide faster than normal, in older tissues senescent cells provide an environment rich in inflammatory mediators that actually favours neoplastic growth. This relates strongly to the well-established observation that the incidence of cancer increases with age: most cancers occur in people over 55 years old. It is also well recognised that inflammation predisposes to cancer.

Telomerase and senescence

Telomeres are extended sequences of satellite DNA (p. 29) that 'cap' the ends of chromosomes. The enzymes of the cell cycle are programmed to join free DNA ends together as part of their repair function, which could lead them to mistakenly attach the end of one chromosome to the end of another. To prevent this, telomeres mark the ends of each chromosome and repair enzymes recognise that this is a terminal sequence; they do not join it to adjacent chromosomes. However, each time a cell copies its DNA for cell division, the telomeres capping the chromosomal ends get shorter. Eventually, they become critically short, and the DNA cannot be fully copied, which triggers cessation of cell division and the onset of senescence (Fig. 3.5) A few normal human tissues—for example, fetal cells and some adult stem cells—possess an enzyme called **telomerase**, which repairs the telomeres after cell

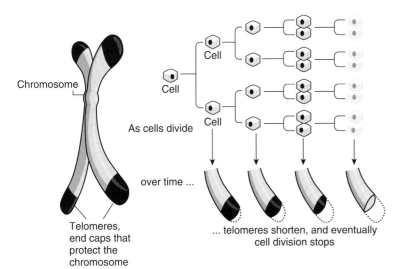

Chromosome

Telomeres, end caps that protect the chromosome

Cell

As cells divide

Cell

Cell

over time ...

... telomeres shorten, and eventually cell division stops

Fig. 3.5 Telomere shortening with successive DNA replications. (Adpated from Madiha F, Mehran R, Naseer A et al (2018) A systematic review of aging and its causes. *International journal of development research*, 8(11) 23904-23908.)

division. Most adult body cells are telomerase negative, do not express this enzyme, and so are limited to a set number of divisions. Cancer cells are usually telomerase positive, conferring immortality and producing a cell line that can replicate indefinitely.

Because telomerase is not expressed in most adult cells, there is a great deal of research interest in it as a potential target for anti-cancer therapy. Some anti-telomerase vaccines have shown promise in clinical trials, and telomerase inhibitors are also currently under investigation.

APOPTOSIS

Apoptosis is programmed cell death. All nucleated body cells contain genes that trigger apoptosis, and failure of apoptotic mechanisms is a significant contributor to the pathology of cancer. In healthy tissues, apoptosis ensures controlled destruction of defective, virally infected, excess or abnormal cells. The doomed cell shrinks and begins to lose its attachments to adjacent cells and to its basement membrane. Internally, its organelles disintegrate, and the cell substance breaks up into a collection of small 'blebs', membrane-bound cell fragments that are rapidly phagocytosed by defence cells, thus preventing an inflammatory response (Fig. 3.6). Apoptosis can be completed within an hour and is driven by a set of death-inducing enzymes called **caspases**, which are activated when the cell is first identified for termination.

Failure of apoptosis is a common contributor to the development of cancer. For example, in some B-cell lymphomas, a family of proteins called Bcl-2 proteins that protect abnormal cells from apoptosis are produced in elevated quantities and are thought to underpin the development of the disease. TP53 protein (p. 75), a very important growth inhibitor produced by the *p53* gene, normally blocks the cell cycle at the checkpoint between the G_1 and S phases and induces apoptosis in abnormal cells. It is released in large quantities in cells whose DNA has been damaged by, for example, ionising radiation. This blocks their ability to divide, ensuring that damaged cells do not progress in the cell cycle. If the *p53* gene is faulty, as it is in many cancers, TP53 protein

production is reduced, inhibiting the apoptotic destruction of these abnormal cells, which may survive and divide.

ADAPTIVE ADJUSTMENTS IN TISSUE GROWTH PATTERNS

Tissues exposed to unusual or excessive stresses undergo adaptive growth patterns as coping strategies (Fig. 3.7). Some of these may be precursors to malignant change.

Hyperplasia (Fig. 3.7A)

In hyperplastic tissues, cell numbers increase, increasing tissue mass. Hyperplasia is an adaptive response to, for example, constant wear and tear. The skin on the soles of the feet is much thicker than the skin on the calf of the leg because of the pressure and friction of walking and running. This is a normal and appropriate response, although it may be triggered by a viral infection (e.g., the common verruca). It may also be a forerunner of malignancy: for example, endometrial thickening can occasionally be a sign of future endometrial carcinoma. In hyperplasia, the cells look and behave as normal.

Hypertrophy (Fig. 3.7B)

In hypertrophy, tissue mass increases because cells enlarge. As in hyperplasia, this is a standard adaptive response in tissues subjected to additional stresses or increased workload. For example, skeletal muscle cells enlarge when regularly exercised, which increases the muscle mass.

Metaplasia (Fig. 3.7C and E)

In response to chronic irritation or injury, one tissue type can convert to another. Usually seen in epithelial tissues, this response is reversible if the stimulus is withdrawn, allowing the original tissue type to re-establish itself. For example, the upper respiratory passageways are lined with pseudostratified ciliated columnar epithelium. The cilia beat to propel mucus and trapped particles away from the lungs. In response to the chronic irritation and inflammation caused by cigarette smoking, this epithelium may replace itself with a thickened, stratified squamous epithelium, which better

Apoptosis

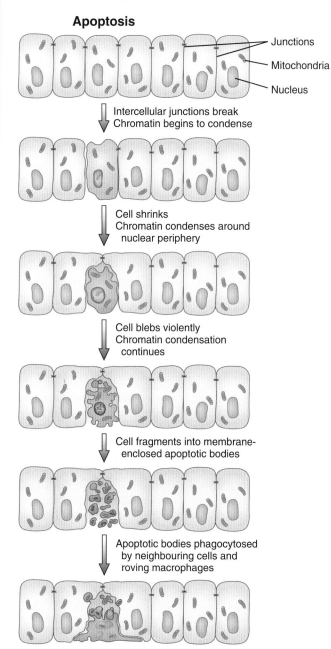

Junctions

Mitochondria

Nucleus

Intercellular junctions break
Chromatin begins to condense

Cell shrinks
Chromatin condenses around
nuclear periphery

Cell blebs violently
Chromatin condensation
continues

Cell fragments into membrane-
enclosed apoptotic bodies

Apoptotic bodies phagocytosed
by neighbouring cells and
roving macrophages

Fig. 3.6 Apoptosis. (From Pollard T, Earnshaw W, Lippincott-Schwartz J, et al. (2017) *Cell biology,* 3rd ed, Fig. 46.2. Philadelphia: Elsevier Inc.)

protects the underlying tissues but does not possess the cleaning cilia and so is less effective at protecting the deeper airways from inhaled contaminants. This change is potentially pre-cancerous and may be accompanied by the appearance of molecular markers of cancer. The cells, however, are of the correct shape and size for stratified squamous epithelium and are arranged in the orderly structure characteristic of the new tissue type.

Dysplasia (Fig. 3.7D and E)

This is irreversible change, often pre-cancerous, and, like metaplasia, usually associated with epithelial tissues. The architecture of the tissue is disorderly and abnormal, and the cells appear abnormal under the microscope. The nuclei can be bizarre and irregular in shape and size, and their chromosomal material unusually obvious, indicating that the cells are actively dividing. A dysplastic tissue that has not breached its underlying basement membrane is called carcinoma in situ and can usually be completely cured by surgery, provided that care is taken to remove all the abnormal cells.

CHARACTERISTICS OF NEOPLASMS

It is important to distinguish between a benign and a malignant neoplasm because, although they share certain features and behaviours, a malignant tumour is much more likely to lead to a poorer outcome. Identifying a growth as benign or malignant is therefore a critically important pathological distinction that will determine the clinical choices made regarding treatment and the prognosis for the patient.

TUMOUR NOMENCLATURE

It is not always possible to tell whether a tumour is benign or malignant from its name. Generally, for benign neoplasms of connective tissues, the first part of the name indicates its tissue of origin and ends in '-oma'. For example, a lipoma is a benign tumour of fat tissue. The nomenclature of benign epithelial tumours is not so consistent and may refer to the type of epithelial cell from which the neoplasm originates, regardless of the organ it is growing in, or to the architecture of the neoplasm itself. For example, an adenoma is a benign tumour of glandular epithelium, which could be growing in the kidney, in the pituitary gland, or in the skin. There are important exceptions: a melanoma, more properly called a *malignant melanoma*, originates in melanocytes, but it is definitely not benign; the inconsistent terminology has established itself despite not conforming to the general pattern.

Malignant tumours are classified according to the tissue type of origin. Solid connective tissue malignancies are called **sarcomas**: a liposarcoma is a malignant tumour of fat, and an osteosarcoma is a malignant tumour of bone. Blood is also a connective tissue, but a fluid, so the nomenclature is different: the terms leukaemia and lymphoma apply to malignancies of white blood cells. Epithelial cell–derived solid tumours are called **carcinomas**. An adenocarcinoma is therefore a malignant tumour of glandular origin.

Blastomas are malignancies developed from precursor cells (blasts) in embryonic tissue (e.g., retinoblastoma [p. 48]). These cancers usually affect children and can be highly aggressive. Some terms relating to tumour biology are given in Table 3.1.

TUMOUR STRUCTURE

Whether benign or malignant, a tumour is made up not only of neoplastic cells (the **parenchyma**) but also a meshwork of supporting connective tissue containing blood vessels and a variable proportion of host cells including fibroblasts, T cells, and macrophages, recruited and directed by the tumour cells to provide a tailored environment favourable to tumour growth (Fig. 3.8). This meshwork, called the **stroma**, is produced by the host cells under the direction of the tumour cells and is similar to the environment found in normally healing tissues (i.e., it favours cell division, the growth and proliferation of blood vessels, and expansion and remodelling

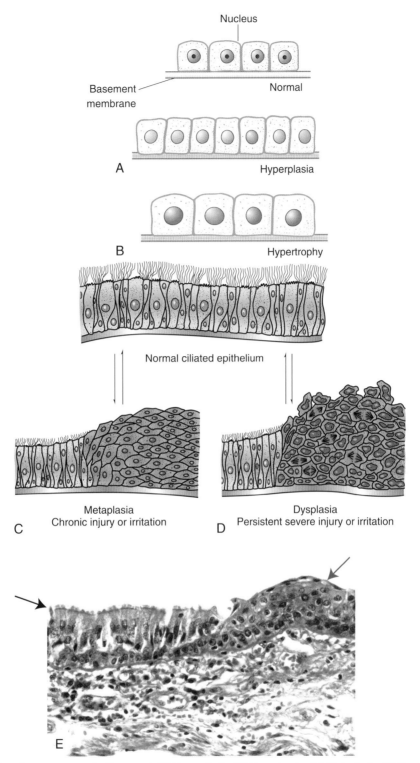

Fig. 3.7 Adaptive growth patterns compared with normal. (A) Hyperplasia. (B) Hypertrophy. (C) Metaplasia. (D) Dysplasia. (E) Section of bronchial epithelium, showing normal ciliated epithelium (black arrow) and metaplastic change to stratified epithelium (red arrow). (Modified from (A and B) Craft J, Gordon C, Huether S, et al. (2019) *Understanding pathophysiology ANZ*, 3rd ed, Fig. 4.7. Sydney: Elsevier Australia; (C and D) McCance K, and Huether S (2015) *Pathophysiology*, 7th ed, Fig. 2.6. St Louis: Mosby; (E) Kumar V, Abbas A and Fausto N (2007) *Robbins & Cotran pathologic basis of disease*, 8th ed. Philadelphia: Saunders.)

of the extracellular matrix, the network of proteins, and other substances that supports tissue cells). In damaged but otherwise healthy tissue, these processes are inhibited when healing is complete, but because tumour cells have been released from normal growth regulation,

inhibition does not occur and the tumour cells continue to proliferate.

Stromal consistency differs widely between tumours. The more connective tissue it contains, the firmer it is. **Scirrhous** tumours are rock-hard (skiros-hard [Greek]), because of

Table 3.1   Some terms related to tumour biology

Term	Definition
Extracellular matrix	The network of connective tissue proteins (e.g., collagen and elastin) in which cells live
Neoplasm	New growth (neo = new, plasm = growth)
Benign	A neoplasm whose cells retain close similarity to its parent tissue and that will almost certainly remain in its primary location
Malignant	A neoplasm whose cells are significantly different in appearance and behaviour to its parent tissue and that will almost certainly spread to distant sites
Stroma	The meshwork of supporting proteins, structures, and non-neoplastic cells (e.g., collagens, blood vessels, fibroblasts, and inflammatory cells) in which the neoplastic cells are growing
Parenchyma	The neoplastic cells of the tumour
Carcinoma	A malignant tumour of epithelial cell origin
Sarcoma	A malignant tumour of solid connective tissue origin
Blastoma	A malignant tumour arising from precursor cells (blasts)

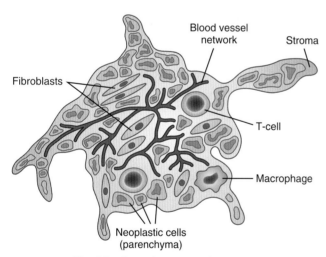

Fig. 3.8   General structure of a tumour.

the high connective tissue content, a characteristic of some breast cancers. Other tumours are soft and fleshy.

PROPERTIES AND BEHAVIOURS OF NEOPLASTIC CELLS

When a cell mutates and escapes the normal growth controls described previously, it may start to divide and form a tumour if it is in a solid tissue, or develop into a blood disorder if the abnormal cell is a blood cell precursor in the bone marrow. Whatever the specific mutations underlying an individual neoplasm, they confer a common set of properties

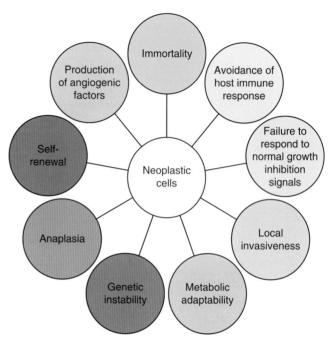

Fig. 3.9   Key properties of neoplastic cells.

on the transformed cell, each of which gives it a proliferative advantage over normal tissues (Fig. 3.9).

Immortality

Neoplastic cells have a limitless capacity to divide, avoiding senescence and apoptosis. Most cancer cells express telomerase (p. 64), a major factor in immortality. The oldest cell line known to science was isolated in 1951 from a 30-year-old American tobacco farmer called Henrietta Lacks, who suffered from a particularly aggressive cervical cancer. Named HeLa cells from the first two letters of her first name and her surname, her cells have been used worldwide in a multitude of applications, including development of polio vaccine, in vitro fertilisation, and cell cloning, and were the first human cells in space. Nearly 70 years later, this cell line is still globally important in science. HeLa cells are telomerase positive and show no signs of slowing their growth rate: in common with cancer cells in general, they have become immortal and seem to be capable of multiplying themselves indefinitely.

Failure to respond to normal growth inhibition signals

Healthy cells grown in the laboratory spread and divide on their growth medium until they contact adjacent cells, at which point cell division stops. A similar behaviour is observed in healing tissues. This is called **contact inhibition**. It was recognised many decades ago that cancer cells behave very differently and grow unrestrainedly over the top of each other, producing multiple disorganised layers of continuously dividing cells; in the body, such growth patterns produce an expanding tumour. Neoplastic cells also lose their ability to respond to the normal chemical signals that would shunt them out of the cell cycle into G_0 and prevent further cell division. Growth rates in neoplastic tissues are often faster than normal tissues, although this varies widely. For example, the rate of normal epithelial cell division in the healthy gastrointestinal tract is much faster than some slow-growing malignancies.

Self-renewal

Neoplastic cells divide repeatedly even without normal growth stimulation signals. As with their loss of responsiveness to growth inhibition signals, this escape from regulation leads to tumour expansion.

Metabolic adaptability

A growing tumour has high nutritional and energy demands, and neoplastic cells also have to compete with stromal cells and adjacent, healthy tissues for resources. Cancer cells can adjust their metabolic pathways to rapidly produce additional ATP and macromolecules required for their growth and survival, giving them a growth advantage.

Local invasion

Carcinoma in situ refers to dysplastic cells that have remained localised and are observing the natural boundaries of their basement membranes. An important step for a developing malignancy is the expression of enzymes that break down membranes and extracellular matrix components, allowing tumour cells to invade locally and cross barriers such as blood and lymphatic vessel walls to travel away from their tissue of origin. In addition, an invading tumour displays abnormal adhesion factors on its cell membranes. Adhesion molecules, such as **cadherins**, stabilise normal cells in the three-dimensional structure of their tissue, restricting their mobility, but are lost in cancer cells, freeing them to invade, migrate, and metastasise. **Metastasis**, a feature of malignant neoplasms, is a complex and difficult process, described later (p. 72), in which travelling fragments from the primary tumour establish secondary growths at distant sites. Metastasis is a significant clinical problem, a poor prognostic indicator, and often the cause of death.

Production of angiogenic factors

The growing tumour needs to develop its own blood supply. The production of a new network of blood vessels in a tissue is called **angiogenesis**. When a solid tumour is very small, its growth needs are supplied by diffusion of nutrients and oxygen from its surrounding environment. However, once past a diameter of half a millimetre, diffusion is inadequate to reach the core of the enlarging tumour, and the cells in the middle become hypoxic. Hypoxia is an important stimulator of angiogenesis and triggers the release of chemicals called angiogenic factors such as vascular endothelial growth factor (VEGF), which stimulate the development of capillary buds and a vascular network within the tumour. This new blood supply allows the tumour to continue growing.

The transition between early-stage tumours, which have not yet penetrated their basement membranes or begun to invade neighbouring tissues, is marked by a so-called angiogenic switch, characterised by the appearance of actively growing and aggressively invasive blood vessels. As with other components of the tumour stroma, the host cells produce the angiogenic chemicals responsible for stimulating angiogenesis, but they do this under instruction by the tumour cells. The blood vessels are often abnormal and defective and are clearly different from blood vessels in normal organs. The centres of solid tumours may be so hypoxic and

inhospitable that they become necrotic. However imperfect it may be, the blood supply feeds the expanding tumour and permits growth.

Avoidance of the host immune response

The interaction between the tumour cells and the host's immune cells is complex. The immune system has a range of protective measures in place to detect and destroy abnormal body cells, and these measures are generally very effective. Directed T cells are actively engaged in patrolling body tissues, hunting for and eliminating abnormal body cells, including cancer cells. Very abnormal cancer cells are obvious and easy targets, but cancer cells are also by definition genetically unstable, and as they divide will produce variants, some of which by chance will be less immunogenic (i.e., are more likely to be ignored by the T cells). These cells have a much higher chance of survival because they have evaded T-cell destruction. This subpopulation of cancer cells will survive and proliferate, unchecked by immune cells, until the tumour burden becomes great enough that signs and symptoms start to appear.

Immune function-related factors, such as incomplete resolution of acute inflammation and the development of a chronic inflammatory response, are strongly associated with malignancy: a range of cancers, including hepatocellular carcinoma and colonic cancer, are linked to chronic inflammation. Inflamed tissues show increased rates of cell division, migration and survival, and enhanced angiogenesis, providing a microenvironment suitable for neoplastic growth. Additionally, tumour cells are very good at suppressing the immune response: they recruit a subset of T cells called *regulatory T cells* (T-regs; p. 92) into the tumour stroma. T-regs are the 'brakes' of the immune system; their immunosuppressive action is thought to be important—for example, in pregnancy—and prevents the mother's T cells from attacking her genetically different fetus. A stromal environment rich in T-regs suppresses the immune response and protects the tumour cells. Tumour cells may also produce immunosuppressant factors like tumour growth factor alpha (TGFα) and a wide range of other chemicals that actively suppress the host's defences.

Anaplasia-loss of differentiation

De-differentiation, the loss of the cell's specialised features, is characteristic of neoplasia. The more malignant the tumour, the faster its cells lose their specialised features and the less they resemble the parent cell. As they de-differentiate, the tumour cells not only lose their own specialised markers and stop producing their own specialised proteins but increasingly display markers characteristic of undifferentiated fetal or stem cells (Fig. 3.10) Stable differentiated body cells, which are normally unable to divide, can revert to a stem-cell-like state if they are damaged by a procarcinogenic event, and re-enter the cell cycle and begin to produce tumour cells. The de-differentiation of tumour cells is such a fundamental property in cancer that pathological assessment of a tumour biopsy is graded according to how far along the de-differentiation pathway the cells are. The more de-differentiation they display, the higher the grade and the poorer the prognosis (Fig. 3.11). Identification of the parent tissue is important when the cancer presents as secondary disease: for example, a woman with breast cancer may initially go to the doctor because of back pain, which turns out to be caused by secondary

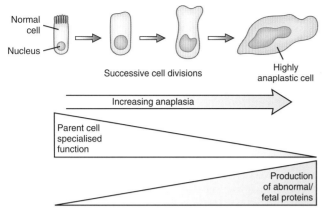

Fig. 3.10 Anaplasia. Increasing degrees of anaplasia causes loss of normal specialised cell function and acquisition of abnormal functions including the production of abnormal proteins.

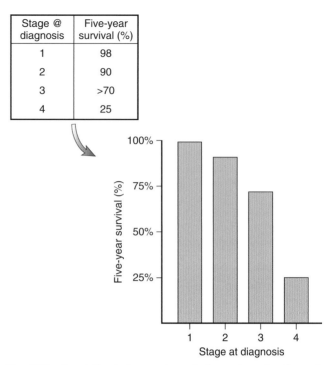

Fig. 3.11 Correlation between stage at diagnosis and outcome in breast cancer. (Data from https://www.cancerresearchuk.org/about-cancer/breast-cancer/survival.)

growths in the vertebrae. If the metastatic cells are not completely de-differentiated and still display some characteristics of breast cells, it informs the medical team of the location of the primary tumour. This in turn determines appropriate treatment. In the most malignant tumours, the cells may be so de-specialised that it is not possible to identify the tissue in which the cancer originated.

De-differentiation also goes hand in hand with drug resistance; tumours showing most de-differentiation are the least likely to respond to drug treatment, and the most likely to exhibit multidrug resistance.

Genetic instability

In healthy cells, preservation and accurate replication of the cell's DNA are essential. Mutations in DNA are either repaired or, if not reparable, the cell is destroyed. Neoplastic cells, however, achieve a semi-independent state of existence in which their accumulated mutations confer additional properties (explained previously), which tend to give them survival advantages over normal cells. As the cancer cell population expands, subpopulations of cells with slightly different genetic makeup appear, and if a new mutation is advantageous (e.g., the production of a new enzyme to break down epithelial basement membranes and allow local invasion, or the disappearance of adhesion molecules on the membrane that normally anchor the cell in place), then that subpopulation prospers and expands within the tumour. The growing tumour therefore undergoes a process of selective evolution, in which successive generations of tumour cells steadily lose normal features and behaviours, and progress in malignancy. Neoplastic cells from an early tumour can therefore be quite different from the same tumour at an advanced stage. The same phenomenon is seen in drug resistance in cancer treatment; using a cytotoxic drug to treat a cancer may kill a significant proportion of the tumour cells, but the cells that remain are those whose genetic variation has made them resistant; these multiply, producing a tumour resistant to that drug (Fig. 3.12).

DIFFERENCES BETWEEN MALIGNANT AND BENIGN NEOPLASMS

Malignant and benign neoplasms can be assessed and compared using a number of key behaviours and features (Fig. 3.13).

It is important to realise that there is significant overlap between normal tissues, benign neoplasms, and malignant neoplasms in this respect, with the exception of metastasis, which is almost exclusively associated with malignancy.

Growth rates

Neoplastic cells tend to divide faster than normal cells, and malignant cells tend to divide faster than benign ones, but this is a big generalisation. The slowest growing malignancies grow more slowly than the fastest growing benign tumours, and some normal tissues (e.g., normal gastrointestinal epithelial cells) grow faster than many benign and the slowest growing malignant tumours.

Local invasiveness

Malignant cells produce enzymes that allow them to break down and actively invade surrounding tissues, including crossing boundaries such as organ capsules and the walls of lymphatic and blood vessels. Cancers are therefore accompanied by varying amounts of local tissue destruction and progressive infiltration. This makes malignant tumours very difficult to remove surgically in their entirety. In addition, benign tumours tend to form well-contained masses with clear boundaries between them and adjacent structures, and they do not infiltrate local tissues.

Presence of a capsule

As the benign tumour grows, it compresses adjacent tissues, which stimulates fibrosis, and so a firm, thickened capsule forms around the expanding mass. The neoplastic cells within do not cross this capsule, which forms a distinctive outer boundary of the tumour and facilitates surgical removal. Malignant tumours do not form this capsule: their

Treatment with drug A
Treatment with drug B
Susceptible to drug A
Susceptible to drug B
Only tumour cells resistant to drugs A and B survive
Expanding tumour now resistant to drugs A and B

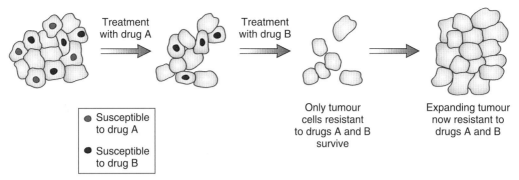

Fig. 3.12 Development of drug-resistant tumours.

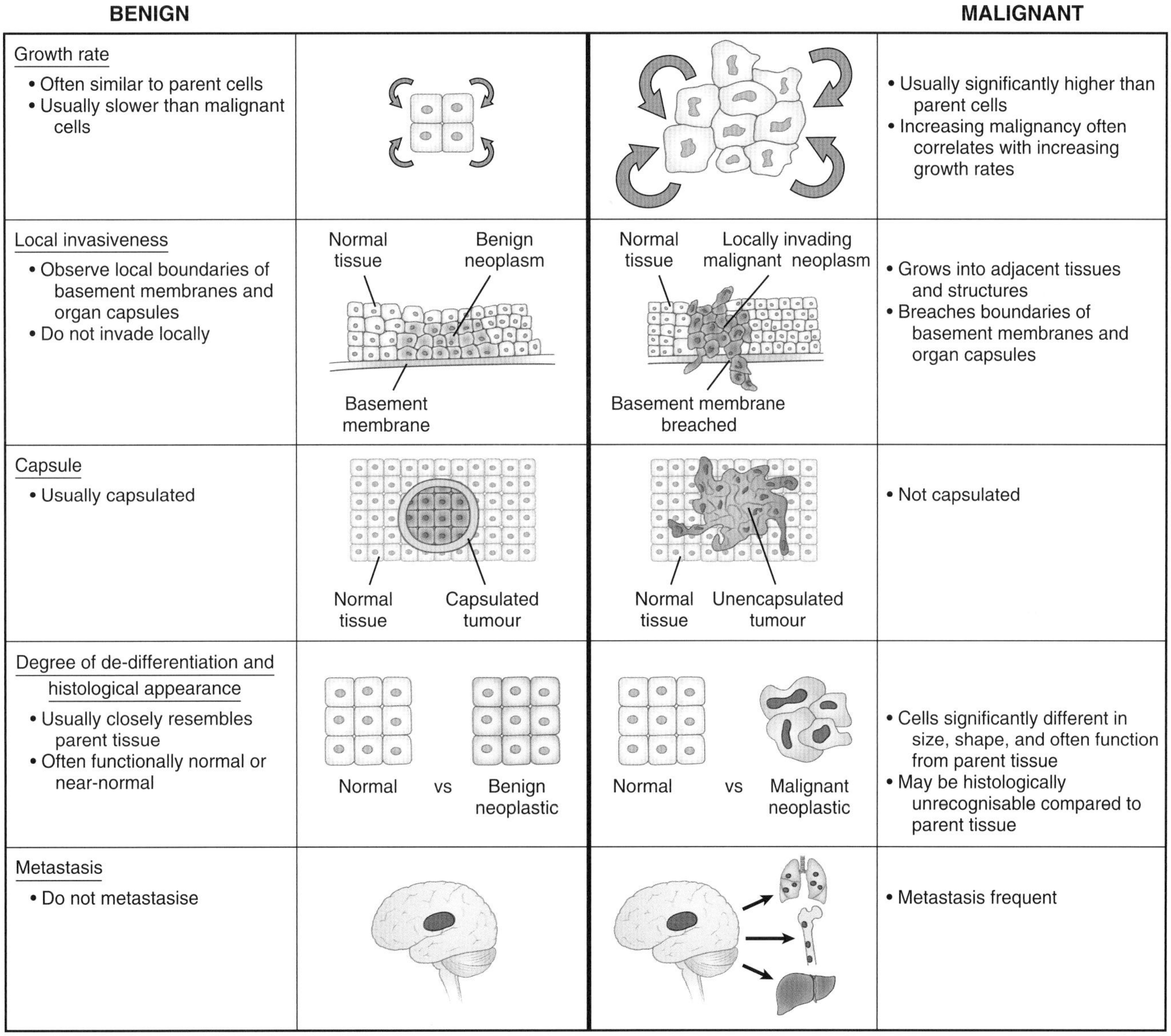

BENIGN
MALIGNANT
Growth rate
• Often similar to parent cells
• Usually slower than malignant cells
• Usually significantly higher than parent cells
• Increasing malignancy often correlates with increasing growth rates
Local invasiveness
• Observe local boundaries of basement membranes and organ capsules
• Do not invade locally
Normal tissue
Benign neoplasm
Basement membrane
Normal tissue
Locally invading malignant neoplasm
Basement membrane breached
• Grows into adjacent tissues and structures
• Breaches boundaries of basement membranes and organ capsules
Capsule
• Usually capsulated
Normal tissue
Capsulated tumour
Normal tissue
Unencapsulated tumour
• Not capsulated
Degree of de-differentiation and histological appearance
• Usually closely resembles parent tissue
• Often functionally normal or near-normal
Normal vs Benign neoplastic
Normal vs Malignant neoplastic
• Cells significantly different in size, shape, and often function from parent tissue
• May be histologically unrecognisable compared to parent tissue
Metastasis
• Do not metastasise
• Metastasis frequent

Fig. 3.13 Distinguishing features of benign and malignant neoplastic cells.

destructive growth habits mean they simply spread into and through neighbouring structures.

Degree of de-differentiation (anaplasia)

Benign neoplasms are characterised by high numbers of cells very similar to the parent cell. In fact, sometimes the cells are indistinguishable histologically from normal, and they usually function normally as well; benign tumours of endocrine glands, such as the thyroid gland, generally respond appropriately to normal signals and produce thyroxine at normal rates. As discussed previously, malignant cells, on the other hand, display a very wide range of de-differentiation.

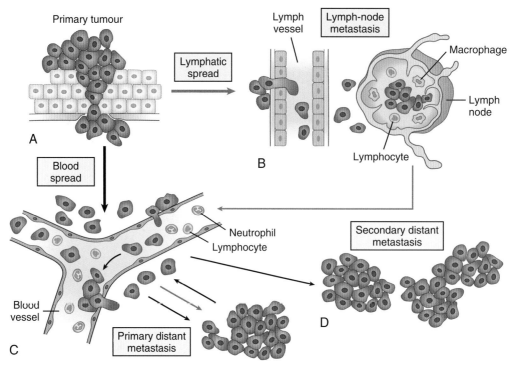

Fig. 3.14 Metastasis.

Histological appearance

Malignant cells are often clearly abnormal when examined under the microscope. They are often large and very variable in size and shape (pleomorphism). Nuclei are usually bigger than normal and may be highly irregular in shape, with very visible nucleoli. The nucleolus is responsible for producing ribosomes, which manufacture proteins for the cell, and integrates important mechanisms that control normal cell growth patterns. Abnormal nucleoli are hallmarks of cancer and may be potential targets for new cancer therapies. The chromosomes are often clumped and more visible than normal. Other cell organelles are also often deformed or absent. Benign neoplastic cells, on the other hand, are usually very similar to their parent tissue.

Metastasis

Malignant tumours are almost universally capable of producing cells that detach from their primary site and travel to a separate site, where they establish a secondary growth. The process of metastasis is described below. Benign tumours do not metastasise.

METASTATIC SPREAD

In metastasis, tumour cells, either singly or in clumps, detach from the parent tumour and travel to a separate, sometimes very distant site, where they establish themselves as a secondary (metastatic) growth. This key behaviour distinguishes a malignant from a benign tumour. Metastatic spread is characteristic of malignancy: nearly one third of solid tumours have metastasised at diagnosis. Because metastatic cancer is usually incurable, this marks an important clinical distinction. It has been estimated that metastatic disease is responsible for 90% of cancer deaths; and despite massive advances in our understanding and treatment of cancer, this statistic has improved very little in the past 50 years.

The stages of metastasis

Metastasis (Fig. 3.14) is a complex multistage process and only a small proportion of malignant cells in a primary tumour are capable of successfully navigating the journey and colonising a distant site. This might seem counter-intuitive because metastasis is such a common event in cancer, implying that it is straightforward and goes hand in hand with malignancy. In fact, many tumours can grow for months or years, producing billions of malignant cells, before some of the cells acquire this potential.

The first step in metastasis is the loosening of cell attachments at the primary site, allowing tumour cells to invade locally. Cancer cells lose the normal cell-surface adhesion molecules such as cadherins responsible for maintaining tissue architecture, and, as described previously, they lose the property of contact inhibition and grow uncontrollably over and through adjacent tissue. They produce proteolytic (protein-digesting) enzymes that dissolve the extracellular matrix supporting local tissues and cut passageways through it. Because they are motile, cancer cells travel through these passageways towards local lymphatic and blood vessels (Fig. 3.14A). Their proteolytic enzymes break down lymphatic and vascular walls, and the cancer cells escape into the lymph (Fig. 3.14B) or the bloodstream (Fig. 3.14C).

Because both blood and lymph are packed with defensive cells, they are unfriendly environments for travelling cancer cells. The vast majority do not survive: more than 99.9% are destroyed by blood and lymph-borne lymphocytes, phagocytic white blood cells like neutrophils and other immune mechanisms. Those that do survive, however, survive because they are best equipped to avoid these dangers: cancer cells are genetically unstable, and cells within a primary tumour are not all genetically identical; some of their genetic alterations will provide the cell with survival advantages, such as the ability to evade immune and defence cells.

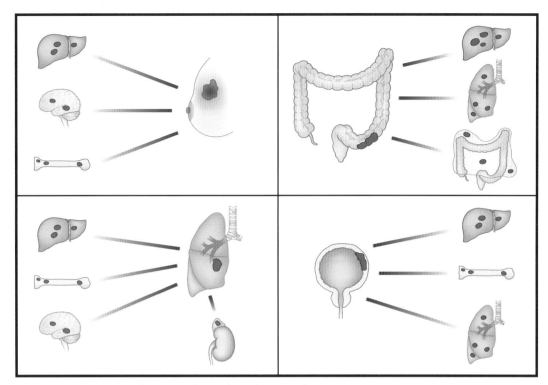

Fig. 3.15   Metastatic preferences of some common cancers.

To produce secondary growths, tumour cells must express adhesion molecules on their plasma membrane that allow them to attach to the endothelium of blood vessels at a new location; otherwise, they would remain circulating in the bloodstream indefinitely. Having anchored at their new site, they break down the blood vessel wall, invade their new tissue, and establish new growth (Fig. 3.14D). To do this, the new tumour must possess the same malignant characteristics as the parent tumour and be able to stimulate angiogenesis and avoid host defences.

Seed and soil: organ-specific metastasis

In 1889, the English surgeon Stephen Paget compared metastasis patterns in breast cancer, uterine cancer, and malignant melanoma. He noted that they were different, contradicting the prevailing view at the time that tumour cells lodged and grew in the first set of capillaries they arrived at after leaving their primary. Breast cancer metastasises preferentially to bone, liver, and ovary, but rarely to the spleen; this cannot be explained by the anatomical pattern of circulation or by the relative blood flow to each organ. Melanoma, on the other hand, metastasises preferentially to the liver, lungs, brain, and some bones. He proposed a 'seed and soil' hypothesis, suggesting that it was not enough just to sow the seed (i.e., the cancer cells) into the circulation; the soil (i.e., the site of secondary growth) had to suit the individual type of cancer; otherwise, distribution of metastases for any cancer would simply directly reflect the route that cell took when travelling from its origin. The 'seed and soil' hypothesis is now widely accepted, recognising that cancer cells show clear preference in their interaction with and metastatic invasion of particular organs (Fig. 3.15). The current view, however, is that anatomical factors also contribute to metastatic patterns (e.g., the liver is a common site for

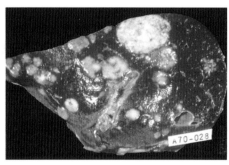

Fig. 3.16   Liver metastases. Multiple pale metastatic tumours are visible. (From Kumar V, Abbas AK, Aster JC, et al. (2010) *Robbins and Cotran pathologic basis of disease*, 8th ed. Philadelphia: Saunders.)

metastasis from gastrointestinal cancers). This is because all cells shedding into the bloodstream from a gastrointestinal tumour travel directly to the liver in the hepatic portal vein, maximising the exposure of the liver to travelling gastrointestinal cancer cells and increasing the likelihood that some will lodge and grow there (Fig. 3.16).

The routes of metastasis

The three main routes taken by tumour cells travelling to distant sites (dissemination) are via the lymphatic network, the bloodstream, or seeding from one area in a body cavity onto another surface in that cavity.

Lymphatic spread

This is generally the first route taken by a metastasising tumour. Lymphatic vessels are thin walled and easily penetrated by cells from invasive tumours growing nearby. From here, dissemination follows through the lymphatic network, passing through the lymph nodes en route. The first lymph node encountered by tumour cells travelling from the primary is called the *sentinel node*. It is important for the sentinel node to be identified and biopsied in assessing any possible spread of a cancer. If the sentinel node is clear of tumour cells, there is a good chance that the disease has not spread this far, considered a positive prognostic factor. However, the lymph nodes are packed with defensive lymphocytes and macrophages (Fig. 3.14), which may delay the further spread of the cancer, and so even if tumour cells are found in local lymph nodes, it does not necessarily mean the cancer has spread to distant sites.

Blood (haematogenous) spread

Blood vessels are thicker walled than lymphatic vessels and are harder to penetrate. Veins have thinner walls than arteries and so are more commonly invaded. Once in the venous system, cancer cells are carried in the blood back to the right side of the heart, through the lungs, and back to the left side of the heart, from where they can be distributed to any body tissue. However, as discussed earlier, metastasis does not occur randomly; individual cancers are generally associated with characteristic patterns of secondary tumours (Fig. 3.15).

Cavity seeding

A cancerous growth expanding within an organ will eventually break through its surface layers and can release tumour fragments into the relevant body cavity. These fragments can attach to and grow on the membranes lining the cavity and penetrate into the organs below. This is called *seeding*. It is commonly seen in the peritoneal cavity, where the peritoneum is a frequent site for secondary growths from ovarian and gastrointestinal tumours (Fig. 3.17).

Identification of tumours most likely to metastasise and/or recur

Currently, the best hope of cure lies in early detection, while the cancer is still confined to its primary location. Identifying tumours at high risk of recurrence—both at the primary site and as new secondary growths—is very important when making treatment decisions. Cancers predicted to have a high metastatic potential require more aggressive treatment, including more extensive surgery, than those assessed as being less likely to recur with secondary tumours. However, unless these patients can be accurately identified, some will be missed and not receive the best treatments

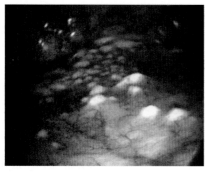

Fig. 3.17 Peritoneal metastases from pancreatic cancer. (From Parks RW, Paterson-Brown S, Garden OJ, et al. (2023) *Hepatobiliary and pancreatic surgery*, 7th ed, Fig. 3.4. Edinburgh: Elsevier Ltd.)

available, whereas others may be inappropriately included in a high-risk category and receive unnecessarily aggressive treatment, increasing treatment-associated risks. The use of clinical staging (p. 81) and tumour size can predict the malignancy of a tumour, and biomarkers such as prostate-specific antigen (PSA) in prostate cancer and HER2 expression in breast cancer are also in routine use.

In 1988, a gene was isolated from experimentally induced rat and mouse tumours that suppressed the ability of a tumour cell to metastasise. Multiple metastatic suppressor genes have now been identified, which prevent the cancer cells from spreading by inhibiting one or more of the steps involved in metastasis. In most primary tumour cells over the lifetime of the primary, these genes effectively block their ability to spread, although they do not slow the growth of the primary tumour. However, as malignant cells are by definition genetically unstable, in some primary cells these metastasis suppressor genes eventually become damaged, permitting the cells to complete the steps required to spread elsewhere in the body. Identifying tumours containing cells whose metastasis suppressor genes have been deactivated promises earlier identification of patients at increased risk of early spread and disease recurrence and may also yield new treatments.

CARCINOGENESIS: THE DEVELOPMENT OF CANCER

Although the term *cancer* is habitually used in the singular, cancer is actually a collection of hundreds of diseases affecting different tissues and organs and is caused by a wide range of genetic mutations, with different prognoses, signs and symptoms, and requiring different treatments. All forms of the disease, however, have one thing in common: they originated as a single mutation in a gene in a single body cell, which is passed to the daughter cells when that cell divides.

THE GENETICS OF CANCER

Each nucleated body cell contains about 20,000 genes (although this figure is still under dispute) packaged into chromosomes and found mainly in the cell nucleus (some genetic material is also located in mitochondria). Each gene codes for a protein, and although every nucleated body cell has a complete set of genes, body tissues only express (i.e., activate) those genes that are required for their specialised function. For example, beta cells in the pancreas express the gene for insulin production, but muscle cells do not.

Hundreds of genes have been identified as candidates in the generation of cancer, and most types of cancer are associated with mutations in a wide range of genes (Fig. 3.18). Although the term *breast cancer* is conventionally used in the singular, it is a group of diseases caused not by a single genetic mutation, but by a wide range of mutations that vary from patient to patient. Cancer-associated genes normally regulate cell growth and division, so when they mutate, some element in the control of cell proliferation is impaired. Some of these mutations are stable and inherited, and they can be passed from generation to generation. Between 5%

and 10% of cancers arise in this way. A wide range of environmental factors also trigger mutations and are associated with cancer, and these are considered later. Other mutations occur spontaneously: a case of random bad luck.

TUMOUR SUPPRESSOR AND TUMOUR PROMOTER GENES

Two important groups of genes commonly mutated in cancers are the growth promoter genes, sometimes called **proto-oncogenes**, and the **tumour suppressor genes**, which restrain cell proliferation. In healthy cells, both groups of genes interact to drive cell division when required, and to stop cell division when it is not. Damage to a gene of either type can initiate uncontrolled proliferation of the cell and is the first step in cancer.

Tumour suppressor genes

In healthy tissues, tumour suppressor genes act as gatekeepers of the cell cycle, switching off cell division by blocking progression of cells from G_1 (see Fig. 3.4). When one or more of these key genes is damaged, genetically abnormal cells can be allowed to replicate. A single mutation in a single tumour suppressor gene can be enough to allow a cell to escape normal controls and begin multiplying independently. Mutations in tumour suppressor genes are almost universal in cancer.

The *p53* tumour suppressor gene
The *p53* tumour suppressor gene, found on chromosome 17 (Fig. 3.18), is a hugely important brake on cell division and is faulty in most malignancies. When a normal cell is stressed (e.g., in hypoxia), if DNA is damaged, or the cell reaches the end of its replicative lifespan, the *p53* gene is activated and produces a protein called TP53. In turn, TP53 protein, sometimes called the *guardian of the genome* because of its central role in preventing old or damaged cells from dividing, activates other genes that trigger senescence, apoptosis, cell cycle arrest at the G_1/S restriction point, and DNA repair. It follows that if p53 is mutated, normal suppression of cell division is lost, and abnormal cells are permitted to proceed through the cell cycle.

Inheriting one functioning copy of a *p53* gene from one parent and a faulty copy from the other greatly increases an individual's risk of developing a range of cancers in early adulthood, including breast, bone, and muscle cancers. However, familial inheritance is much less common than non-inherited (spontaneous) mutations. The widespread occurrence of *p53* mutations in nearly all tumour types has stimulated interest in developing cancer treatments that target mutant *p53* activity: this is a very active and highly promising avenue of research.

The *RB* tumour suppressor gene
The *RB* tumour suppressor gene, the first tumour suppressor gene to be discovered, is located on chromosome 13 (Fig. 3.18). The protein product of the *RB* gene is called pRB, sometimes called the cell's *master governor*. It is a key regulator of the cell cycle and prevents cells from proceeding through the G_1/S restriction point by interfering with cyclin activity. Children inheriting a mutation in this gene

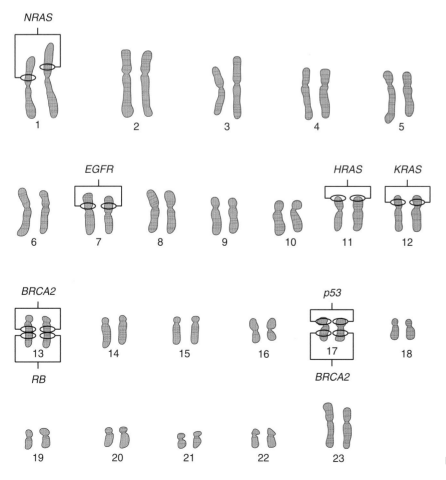

Fig. 3.18 Some key genes involved in cancer.

are at increased risk of developing hereditary retinoblastoma, a malignant tumour of the retina (see p. 48). Although inheritance of a faulty *RB* gene increases the individual's risk, provided the second copy of the gene on the matching chromosome is healthy, cancer does not develop. However, if the paired gene acquires a spontaneous mutation during the multiple cell divisions made during growth and development of the eye, cancer follows. Defects in the *RB* gene can be inherited, as in the example of hereditary retinoblastoma, but more frequently can occur spontaneously in an individual's lifetime. Like p53, *RB* mutations are associated with multiple cancers, including lung, bladder, bone, malignant melanoma, and some leukaemias.

Tumour promoter genes

Just as a healthy cell needs mechanisms to interrupt or switch off cell proliferation, it also requires mechanisms to trigger cell division when required. Genes that produce proteins involved in cell growth signalling are called *proto-oncogenes* and are normally very tightly controlled. When a proto-oncogene mutates, it can become an **oncogene**, functioning independently of normal controls and with the potential to trigger uncontrolled proliferation. The products of oncogenes can stimulate cell growth in several ways, including by activating the cell cycle, by acting as growth factors or growth factor receptors, or by blocking normal cell death processes. Whatever their mechanism, the emergence of oncogenes in a cell's DNA leads to cell proliferation and cell autonomy. As with tumour suppressor genes, mutations in tumour promoter genes are very common in cancer.

The *RAS* oncogene

In 1982, RAS protein, the product of the *RAS* oncogene, was the first oncoprotein identified in human cancer. There are three *RAS* oncogenes—*NRAS*, *KRAS*, and *HRAS*—each producing a related RAS protein. Normal RAS protein is a small peptide that, when activated, pushes a cell through the G_0/S restriction point of the cell cycle into mitosis and cell division. In healthy cells, this stimulates division for normal tissue growth and repair, and RAS protein is deactivated when no longer needed. Mutated RAS, however, remains active, and so the cell is continuously receiving progrowth signals.

RAS oncogenes are involved in most types of cancer but are more important in some than in others. For example,

mutated RAS protein is found in 90% of pancreatic adenocarcinomas but only 30% of lung adenocarcinomas. Because it is such an important procarcinogenic factor, a great deal of research money and time have been spent on the hunt for a drug that would inactivate one or all three RAS oncoproteins. RAS has been referred to as an 'undruggable' protein because of the difficulties scientists have encountered in trying to find, or design, a drug that specifically targets it; new RAS initiatives in the United States are finding some success and igniting optimism that this area will yield a new class of anti-cancer drugs highly effective against RAS-positive cancers. Because this includes some cancers with the poorest survival rates, developments in this area would be highly significant.

The *EGFR* oncogene

Normal cells require the action of one or more of a wide range of growth factors to stimulate normal cell division. In addition to the growth factors themselves, the cells must also produce cell surface receptors for the growth factors to bind and respond to them. In some cancers, the genes that produce either the growth factor or its receptor mutate and become deregulated, and the cell produces much more of either or both growth factor and/or its receptor, meaning it is exposed to an enhanced progrowth signal.

The *EGFR* gene, located on chromosome 7 (Fig. 3.18), produces receptors for epidermal growth factor (EGF), an important stimulant of cell division in normal epithelial tissues. When mutated, the *EGFR* oncogene increases the production of growth factor receptors, increasing the ability of the cell to respond to EGF signals, and stimulating cell division. The EGFR oncogene is involved in a wide range of cancers, including breast, lung, melanoma, and oesophagus. The discovery of the importance of EGF in breast cancer has stimulated the development of specific anti-growth factor receptor drugs, which block binding of EGF to its receptor and significantly improves life expectancies in the cancers involved. For example, one of the growth factor receptors involved, called the *HER2 receptor*, is overproduced in about 20% of breast cancers. These cancers, called *HER2-positive*, respond strongly to EGF, which promotes their growth and division. The drug **trastuzumab** (Herceptin) was designed as an antibody that specifically targets HER2 receptors, blocking EGF binding and depriving the tumour of this potent growth-promoting signal (Fig. 3.19). Trastuzumab

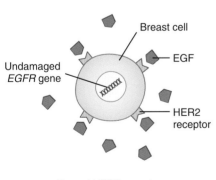

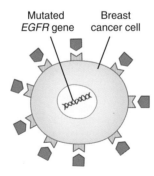

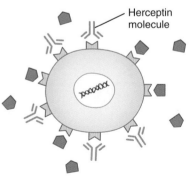

A   Normal HER2 receptor numbers. Cell growth and division control normal

B   HER2 receptors over expressed due to mutated *EGFR* gene. Cell exposed to excessive growth stimulation

C   Herceptin blocks HER2 receptors, reducing the EGF growth stimulus

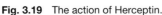

Fig. 3.19   The action of Herceptin.

is now routinely used in women with HER2-positive cancers, and a 2014 meta-analysis of over 4000 women with breast cancer showed trastuzumab to increase 10-year disease-free survival from 62.2% to 73.7%.

THE PROCESS OF CARCINOGENESIS: INITIATION AND PROMOTION

As mentioned previously, some mutations are inherited and some develop spontaneously as a random and unlucky event. However, many mutations develop after exposure of the cell to one or more events known to cause mutation.

The first event that sets the cell on the road to cancer is called the **initiating mutation**. This is permanent and so is usually inherited by all the cells in the tumour that subsequently grows from that single damaged cell, but the initiating mutation is generally not enough to cause a cell to turn cancerous. The second event in carcinogenesis is **promotion**, which does not in itself cause tumours. Instead, promoters increase the rate of cell division, which in turn increases the number of cells carrying the initiating mutation. Because many mutations occur during cell division, this also increases the likelihood that the dividing cells will accumulate additional mutations, called *promoter* or *driver mutations*, each of which increases the risk that the cell line will become frankly malignant. This process of accumulating mutations is believed to take a very long time, probably years, during which the transforming cell manages to escape patrolling immune cells and avoids triggering its own apoptotic genes. To illustrate the concept of initiation and promotion, consider the fact that radiotherapy or cytotoxic drug treatment for cancer exposes all body cells, healthy cells, and tumour cells to significant doses of toxic agents that will hopefully kill the tumour cells and contribute to curing the cancer, but which also damages the DNA in many healthy cells. This is equivalent to an initiating mutation in the healthy cells, which, after a period of possibly many years acquiring additional driver mutations, may then become malignant themselves. Hence, anti-cancer treatment for one form of malignancy increases the risk of unrelated cancers, often of the blood, at some point later in life. Fig. 3.20 shows the relationship between initiation, promotion, and tumour development.

Initiators

Initiators damage cellular DNA. A wide range of environmental and manmade chemicals has been implicated in tumour initiation. Some initiators (e.g., polycyclic hydrocarbons) have both initiation and promoter activity and are sometimes called *complete carcinogens*.

Promoters

Promoters facilitate tumour development by increasing the rate of cell division in a tissue. Factors that stimulate proliferation including hormones (e.g., oestrogen in female reproductive tissues) and a chronic inflammatory condition can act as promoters. Radiation and some viral infections are also important promoters.

Radiation

Sunlight contains three types of ultraviolet radiation—UVA, UVB, and UVC—of which UVB is implicated in a range of

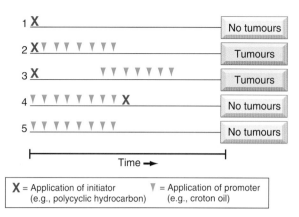

Fig. 3.20 Initiation, promotion, and tumour development. Exposure to initiator alone (1) does not increases tumour risk. Exposure to initiator followed by immediate (2) or delayed (3) promoters increase tumour risk. Exposure to promoter alone (4) or promoter followed by initiator (5) does not increase risk. (Modified from Kumar V, Abbas A, Aster J (2017) *Robbins & Cotran pathologic basis of disease: general pathology, vol 1: First Bangladesh edition*, Fig. 7.43. New Delhi: Elsevier India.)

skin cancers. UVB damages the DNA in skin cells, increasing the rate of cell division as the skin repairs itself. Ionising radiation from X-rays, radiotherapy, or exposure to radioactive chemicals all damage DNA and act as promoters in a cell that has already suffered an initiation mutation.

Infection

Several viruses are directly associated with cancer. Viruses replicate by inserting viral DNA into the DNA of a host cell. The host cell then begins to produce viral proteins, which may disturb the growth control processes of the host cell and increase the likelihood of neoplastic change. Human papilloma virus (HPV) exists in over 70 forms; some HPV forms cause benign warts but some, including HPV16 and HPV18, are sexually transmitted and cause cancers of the cervix, anogenital region, and head and neck (see Ch. 14).

Other significant viruses that cause cancer include the Epstein-Barr virus (EBV), which infects B cells and is associated with lymphoma, including Burkitt's lymphoma and Hodgkin lymphoma. The viruses that cause hepatitis B and C are together thought to account for up to 85% of hepatocellular carcinomas worldwide; the inflammation they cause in the liver of infected people is thought to be the promoting factor in the development of malignancy.

The only bacterium so far associated with cancer is *Helicobacter pylori*, a common stomach resident in gastric ulcer disease. *H. pylori* causes chronic inflammation, increasing the turnover of gastric epithelium and therefore increasing the likelihood of mutation and malignancy. Table 3.2 lists some important initiators and promoters in carcinogenesis.

RISK FACTORS FOR CANCER

The lifetime risk of developing cancer, in both sexes, is one in three. Factors that increase the risk of cancer (Fig. 3.21) are listed below:

Table 3.2   Important initiators and promoters in carcinogenesis

Initiators (i.e., inflict the initial genetic mutation)	Promoters (i.e., stimulate cell division of an initiated cell)
Alkylating agents, including anti-cancer drugs such as the nitrosureas and cyclophosphamide	UVB radiation in sunlight
Some metals e.g., chromium, nickel, cadmium	*Helicobacter pylori*
Some dyes, fungicides, and insecticides	Some viruses
Polycyclic hydrocarbons from, for example, burning fossil fuels, and produced in meats and fish after some cooking and preservation methods	Polycyclic hydrocarbons
Benzopyrene in e.g., soot and cigarette smoke	Hormones e.g., oestrogens
Nitrosamines in e.g., cosmetics, rubber, tobacco, fertilisers and used as food preservatives in pickling and curing foods	Chronic inflammation
Polychlorinated biphenyls: although their manufacture is now banned, they were widely used till the 1970s as refrigerants, lubricants, and insulators, and because they are so stable are still present in the environment.	Ionising radiation from, for example, X-rays, radiotherapy, or exposure to radioactive agents

Age

The incidence of most cancers rises with age, increasing most rapidly in middle age and often declining after the age of 70. Although age is sometimes considered a non-modifiable risk factor, age-related factors such as managing chronic conditions and maintaining a healthy lifestyle reduce risk, even in the high-risk, middle-aged group.

Lifestyle choices

Smoking causes about 90% of lung cancers and contributes to cancers of the upper respiratory tract and oesophagus. High alcohol intake causes cancers of the upper gastrointestinal tract and of the liver. High-fat diets, highly processed diets, pickled or high-preservative foods, and diets with low levels of fresh fruit and vegetables increase the risk of colorectal cancers.

Obesity

Obesity increases the risk of cancer. It has been estimated that 20% of deaths in American women and 14% of deaths in American men are directly caused by obesity. There seems to be several reasons why obesity increases cancer risk. Levels of insulin and its related cytokine insulin growth factor-1 (IGF-1), which increase cell division, are higher in obese people. Oestrogen is produced by adipose tissue and increases the risk of breast and endometrial cancers. Additionally, obesity is associated with a low-grade systemic inflammatory state, which, as mentioned earlier, is procarcinogenic.

Exposure to environmental carcinogens

The list of natural and man-made carcinogens is long (Table 3.2). This can translate into occupation-related risks

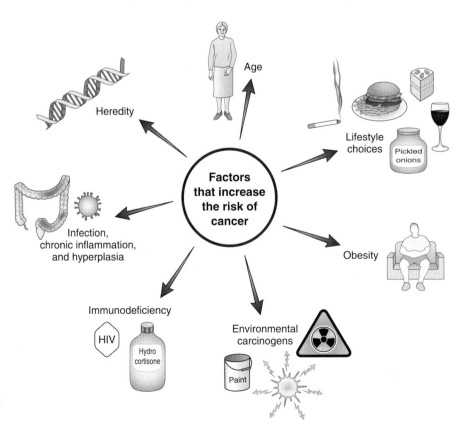

Fig. 3.21   Factors that increase the risk of cancer

(e.g., bladder cancer in hairdressers, who are chronically exposed to hair dyes) or increased rates of leukaemia in workers in the nuclear industry. Painters, agricultural workers, workers in chemical manufacturing, and miners may also experience higher risks associated with their lifetime exposure to carcinogens.

Immunodeficiency

Individuals with an incompetent immune system lose the protective function performed by immunosurveillant T cells (p. 90), which constantly patrol the body, hunting and destroying mutated or damaged cells that may become malignant. Compared with those with healthy immune function, cancer risk is increased in chronically immunosuppressed individuals. For example, in HIV infection, the risk of anal cancer is increased 19-fold, and the risk of the relatively rare Kaposi sarcoma is increased by a factor of 500. Long-term corticosteroid treatment is also immunosuppressant.

Infection, inflammation, and hyperplasia

As mentioned previously, certain viruses are strongly associated with particular cancers because of their ability to interfere with the structure of DNA. Chronic inflammation e.g., chronic bronchitis secondary to cigarette smoking or gastritis associated with *H. pylori* infection increases the risk of lung and stomach cancers, respectively. A high lifetime exposure to oestrogen is a risk factor for endometrial cancer because it stimulates the endometrium and causes thickening and proliferation.

Heredity

This is a complex issue because so many genes are usually involved in any one individual cancer. Most cancers arise sporadically; that is, they result from mutations acquired during an individual's lifetime. A small proportion of cancers are attributable to a faulty, heritable gene transmitted from one generation to the next. Such inherited genes increase the likelihood of cancer within families, but even inheriting a faulty gene does not guarantee that cancer will develop. For example, inheriting the faulty *BRCA1* or *BRCA2* tumour suppressor gene greatly increases the risk of developing breast or ovarian cancer but does not guarantee it. For an affected individual, how that risk plays out will depend also on the interaction between environmental and lifestyle factors. Likewise, the lack of a family history does not mean that there is no inherited component to an individual's cancer; cancer-free close relatives may still have a cancer-related gene that has not produced the disease because of the influence of other factors.

ASSESSMENT AND TREATMENT OF CANCER

Because cancer represents a spectrum of diseases and can arise in almost any organ, the tools used to assess its progress, malignancy, and extent are tailored to the type of cancer involved. Likewise, the signs and symptoms vary from cancer to cancer. Treatment options and prognoses vary widely, from rapid decline and death in highly malignant disease to complete cure. Increasingly, as our knowledge of the molecular biology of cancer improves, the development of tailored treatments is extending life and improving cure rates. The stage in their disease at which people seek medical help is usually crucial to their longer-term prospects.

THE TUMOUR BURDEN AND EFFECTS ON THE BODY

In the early stages of the cancer, which can last for years, the relative size of a tumour to overall body mass is very small and usually causes no or few signs and symptoms. Early indications of disease can seem vague or insignificant and may well be ignored. Because this is the phase of the disease when diagnosis is most likely to result in a complete cure, screening programmes in higher-risk groups for common cancers have been established in most developed countries, and developing countries are beginning to invest in them. Screening increases the chances of detecting a cancer when it is still too small to be symptomatic. For example, colorectal cancer can cause bleeding into the intestinal tract too insignificant to be visible in the stool but shows up in sensitive faecal tests for haemoglobin.

Initial signs and symptoms generally reflect the local effects of the tumour. In more advanced stages, systemic effects are seen. Common signs and symptoms include the following:

Anorexia and weight loss

The growing tumour has an elevated metabolic rate and higher-than-average energy requirements, which may contribute to the unintentional weight loss frequently seen even prior to diagnosis. In addition, appetite changes and nausea are common, and so nutritional factors can play a part. Muscle breakdown is usually a significant feature in cancer-related weight loss, even if the quantity and quality of the diet is good. The chronic inflammatory state induced by cancer favours breakdown of body tissues, partly by releasing multiple cytokines including tumour necrosis factor alpha (TNFα) and interleukin-1 (IL-1). TNFα suppresses the appetite control centre in the hypothalamus of the brain and stimulates breakdown of fat and protein stores. IL-1 also suppresses appetite by increasing serotonin levels in the hypothalamus; serotonin induces a feeling of satiety and reduces food intake. Other reasons for reduced appetite in cancer include low mood and depression, altered taste sensitivity, and reduced physical activity. Once treatment with radiation and/or chemotherapy begins, appetite is likely to be even further suppressed by their associated side effects.

Bleeding

Growing tumours erode local blood vessels. Initially, blood loss may be unnoticed, although the patient might develop anaemia. Bleeding into the airways, the digestive tract, the bladder, or the reproductive tract can all be signs of cancer of these organs. It is worth noting that benign neoplasms can also cause significant bleeding.

Pain

Pain may be a late sign in cancer because many body tissues lack pain receptors. Neoplasm-induced pain may be caused by the growing tumour compressing or invading nerves, or by stretching sensitive organ capsules or linings. Inflammation or infection of affected tissues also causes pain. Tumour growth in confined spaces (e.g., bony tissue) is very painful.

Compression and obstruction

Growing tumours can grow into, compress, and obstruct local passageways and vessels. Compression of the spinal cord causes back pain and sensory and motor changes, depending on the cord level involved. Blockage of a respiratory passageway can cause lung collapse and reduced gas exchange and predisposes to infection in the airways beyond the obstruction. Compression of major arteries or veins reduces blood flow through the tissues. If the gastrointestinal tract is affected, this leads to nutritional compromise.

Immunosuppression

Extensive evidence shows that malignant cells suppress host immunity as part of their self-protection activity. Tumours produce a range of factors, including tumour growth factor beta (TGFβ) and interleukin-10 (IL-10), which inhibit a range of normal immune cell defences, including the ability of T cells (p. 91) to trigger apoptosis in the cancer cells. Additionally, cancer cells can trigger cell death mechanisms in T cells, leading to a reduction in lymphocyte numbers. Cancer therefore increases the risk of infection and developing other cancers and can reactivate latent infections such as herpes. Also, cancer treatments are often profoundly immunosuppressive, increasing the risks even further.

Paraneoplastic syndromes

Paraneoplastic syndromes are collections of signs and symptoms associated with cancer, but not because of the local effects of tumour growth. Cancer cells release a range of chemicals that, circulating in the bloodstream, can have profound effects on body function. For instance, a tumour may begin secreting hormones not secreted by the parent tissue. Some sarcomas (for instance, in the lung or liver) secrete insulin and may cause hypoglycaemia. Some liver or brain tumours secrete erythropoietin, leading to polycythaemia. Some tumours release inflammatory mediators such as bradykinin or serotonin, triggering inflammatory symptoms like flushing or bronchoconstriction.

Cachexia

Cachexia is a malnutrition syndrome characteristic of advanced cancer. It is associated with significant weight loss, anorexia, muscle wasting, and serious metabolic disturbances. As with many paraneoplastic syndromes, cachexia is caused by the release of cytokines and other mediators into the bloodstream by the tumour itself.

ASSESSMENT OF CANCER

Initial assessment of the signs and symptoms of a cancer is followed up with more sophisticated evaluation of the tumour's location, size, genetic makeup, and biochemical activity.

Tumour markers

The use of immunoassays to detect tumour-derived factors circulating in the bloodstream is increasingly important in diagnosis and is a reliable way of assessing response to treatment.

Some important tumour markers include **prostate-specific antigen** (PSA), released by 95% of prostate tumours; **calcitonin**, released by thyroid carcinomas; and **cancer antigen 125** (CA125), released by 75% of ovarian epithelial cancers. However, tumour markers are sometimes released by normal tissues, which can confuse the picture—the presence of a marker does not guarantee the presence of cancer. In addition, the absence of a marker does not guarantee that no cancer is present. Measurement of markers is therefore always used in conjunction with other diagnostic tools.

Imaging

Standard X-rays can visualise tumours and tumour tissue, but more sophisticated approaches are usually much more informative and give details of the extent, structure, size, and metabolic activity of the tumour. Computed tomography (CT) scanners use multiple X-ray images taken from different angles to construct a three-dimensional image of internal organs. Radiosensitive dyes can also be injected or given orally to visualise specific areas. Magnetic resonance imaging (MRI) scans use a strong magnetic field to generate very high-quality, detailed three-dimensional images and are very good at visualising soft tissues (Fig. 3.22). Positron emission tomography (PET) uses radiolabelled substances that are taken up and concentrated within the organ being studied. For instance, radiolabelled glucose (a tracer called fluorodeoxyglucose, or FDG) is used to assess the metabolic activity of a tissue of interest, demonstrating hotspots in metabolically active areas, including tumours and their metastases. Combination of PET and CT imaging techniques (PET-CT) is particularly useful, giving information about tumour structure and its biochemical activity.

Histological examination

Examination of stained thin slices of tissue (or blood or marrow smears for haematogenous cancers) under the light

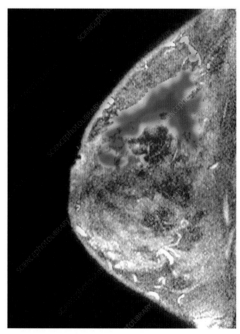

Fig. 3.22   MRI scan showing infiltrating breast cancer. (From Science Source/Science Photo Library.)

microscope is a long-standing tool in cancer assessment. Determining whether a neoplasm is benign or malignant is of critical importance. The histologist looks for evidence of de-differentiation, abnormalities in cell shape, size, and chromosomal content, and any indication of invasive behaviour. When assessing how abnormal the sample is, the histologist will assign a numerical value to it, higher values indicating increasing degrees of abnormality. This is tumour grading (see below).

In addition to basic histological staining, specialised immunological techniques can demonstrate specific chromosomal abnormalities characteristic of particular cancers. Identification of tumour-specific antigens on the cell surface can help identify the tissue of origin when assessing a secondary growth whose primary is not known. Identifying tumour markers is increasingly important in deciding which cytotoxic drugs are likely to be effective. For example, if a breast cancer tests positive for the HER2 receptor, then it will respond to the drug trastuzumab (Herceptin), an antibody that targets this receptor (Fig. 3.19).

Staging and grading

Tumour staging assesses the degree of advancement of a cancer. One of the commonest staging tools is the TNM (**T**umour; i.e., the primary, **N**odal involvement and **M**etastases evident) system. Each category can be subdivided, to indicate in significant detail how advanced the tumour is. Table 3.3 summarises the TNM system as applied to breast cancer. Note that this is a concise summary and, in clinical practice, many more subdivisions within the system are used.

Tumour grading is a histological assessment of the tumour's degree of de-differentiation. On microscopic examination, the cancer is assigned a number, usually between 1 and 4. Individual cancers may have grading schemes tailored specifically to their characteristics and may have more than 4 grades, but the higher the grade assigned, the more abnormal the cells are and usually the higher the growth rate. Some schemes use a combination of staging and grading in tumour assessment. Applying such protocols as part of the clinical evaluation informs treatment decisions and the overall management plan.

Gene profiling

Cancer represents a wide spectrum of diseases in which a combination of damaged genes, from a range of hundreds or possibly thousands of candidates, releases a cell from normal growth constraints. The biology of individual cancers is therefore varied, and two tumours with apparently similar clinical profiles might actually have significant genetic and molecular differences, meaning that, although one tumour might respond well to one drug, the other might be resistant. Identifying these differences holds the key to the development of individualised treatment, increasing the chances of success and reducing patient exposure to damaging therapies that might work poorly or not at all. On the basis of genetic profiling, patients can be allocated to clinical trials that are most likely to benefit them, and patients at the highest risk of relapse can be identified and managed appropriately. The 'one size fits all' approach to cancer management is on its way out.

MAJOR TREATMENT APPROACHES

Surgery

Surgery may aim to completely remove a tumour. This is often easier with benign tumours, which are likely to be capsulated, but most solid malignancies are curable if surgically completely removed at an early enough stage in their development. Malignant tumours may, however, have infiltrated local tissues and have irregular and poorly defined margins, and it is more difficult to ensure that all cancer cells at the site have been removed. Even careful histological examination of the excised tissues to check that an adequate safety margin of normal tissue has been removed along with the tumour does not guarantee that the tumour has not left tendrils of malignant cells behind. Sometimes palliative surgery is performed with no expectation of cure. This may be because the primary tumour is extensive or metastasis has already occurred, but debulking it will ease certain symptoms, or increase the effectiveness of later chemotherapy or radiotherapy.

Cytotoxic therapy

The use of cytotoxic drugs to treat cancer was developed in the 1940s after the recognition that nitrogen mustard gas

---

Table 3.3   Subdivisions of the TNM staging system of tumour assessment in breast cancer

T0: no evidence of tumour	N0: there is no evidence of local nodal involvement	M0: there is no evidence of distant spread
T1: the tumour is less than 2 cm across	N1–N3 and their subdivisions reflect increasing degree of lymph node involvement and identify the specific nodes involved and the number of cancer cells found in each node	cMo(1+): although there is no sign of metastatic growths on scans, X-rays, or on physical examination, cancer cells have been found in distant lymph nodes or in the blood or bone marrow
T2: the tumour is over 2 cm but less than 5–cm across		M1: metastases seen
T3: the tumour is over 5 cm across		
T4: the tumour has invaded locally, including the chest wall and/or the skin, and may have caused significant breast inflammation		

used in chemical warfare in World War 2 caused serious bone marrow suppression in soldiers who had been exposed. Nitrogen mustard suppresses cell division by alkylating cellular DNA, preventing DNA replication. In general, anti-cancer drugs block cell division or trigger cell death and affect both healthy cells and tumour cells, although tumour cells are generally more susceptible because their growth rates are usually higher than normal. As such, side effects are common, especially in fast-growing tissues such as bone marrow, epithelial linings including that of the gastrointestinal tract, and hair follicles.

Radiotherapy
Radiation damages DNA and is itself a risk factor for cancer. Because cancer cells tend to have higher growth rates than normal cells, radiation-induced DNA damage affects them disproportionately and arrests or slows tumour growth.

Immunotherapy
Immunosuppression is common in cancer and is caused by systemic release of tumour-derived immunosuppressant factors. Immunostimulants like interferons and interleukins can activate anti-tumour mechanisms, although such treatments have not been universally effective. Probably the most successful development in this area is **rituximab**, an antibody to a B-cell surface protein called *CD20*. When rituximab binds to CD20 on malignant B cells, it triggers a number of cell-signalling changes in the B cell, leading to growth arrest and increased rates of cell death. Rituximab is therefore used in a range of B-cell malignancies, including non-Hodgkin lymphoma.

Hormone therapy
In 70% to 80% of breast cancers, oestrogen is a powerful growth stimulant important in the pathology of the cancer. Testing breast cancer cells for the presence of oestrogen receptors (i.e., identifying them as ER-positive or ER-negative) is now routine in breast cancer assessment. For ER-positive tumours, an oestrogen receptor antagonist such as **tamoxifen** is an effective treatment, delaying disease progression and prolonging life. Other hormone-dependent cancers include some prostate cancers that grow in the presence of testosterone, and some uterine and ovarian cancers need oestrogen and/or progesterone. Anti-hormone therapies are standard treatments in such cancers.

THE MAJOR CANCERS

LUNG CANCER

Lung cancer is the commonest cancer globally in men and the third commonest in women. Typically, patients present at a fairly advanced stage, and so the prognosis is often poor. Only about 10% of patients are still alive 5 years post-diagnosis, although, as more is learned about the genetic and molecular subtypes of lung cancer, improved survival rates are emerging in some groups.

Risk factors for lung cancer
The main risk factor for lung cancer is tobacco smoking. Tobacco smoke contains at least 60 known carcinogens, both initiators and promoters, plus hundreds more noxious substances that inflame and irritate the airways, interfere with gas exchange in the alveoli, and paralyse the mucociliary escalator. About 90% of lung cancers occur in smokers or ex-smokers. The pathological consequences of tobacco use are not limited to lung cancer, but as with all tobacco-induced effects, the greater the tobacco use, the higher the risk of lung cancer. This is usually quantified in terms of pack-years. A pack year is calculated by multiplying the average number of packs smoked per day by the number of years the individual has been smoking. One pack year is therefore equivalent to smoking one pack a day for a year, or half a pack a day for 2 years, and so on. There is a direct relationship between pack-years and lung cancer incidence. Unsurprisingly, in countries where smoking rates are falling, the incidence of lung cancer is also falling.

Although exposure to tobacco smoke greatly increases the risk of lung cancer, an individual's genetic makeup affects predisposition as well. Some smokers produce metabolising enzymes that increase the risk of activating carcinogens in cigarette smoke, and so their risk of lung cancer is further increased. Exposure to inhaled carcinogens such as asbestos and air pollution are additional risk factors. The rates of lung cancer are slightly higher in city dwellers than in rural residents. Some substances known to increase risk are associated with the workplace (e.g., diesel fumes in mechanics and silica dust in workers in the glass industry).

TYPES OF LUNG CANCER
Lung cancers are classified into several groups. Identification of the type of cancer and molecular profiling of the tumour is essential for best treatment. Metastatic deposits most often occur in bone, brain, adrenal gland, skin, and liver. The lung itself is a common site for secondary growths in cancers originating in other organs. The main types of primary lung cancer are described below.

Small cell lung cancer
Small cell lung cancer accounts for 10% to 15% of lung cancers. It is the most aggressive, tends to metastasise early, is strongly related to cigarette smoking, and carries the poorest prognosis. The cell of origin is a specialised neuroendocrine cell found in the bronchial epithelium lining the airways. Because of their endocrine origin, small cell lung cancers frequently secrete hormones, commonly ACTH and ADH. Nearly all patients have genetic mutations in the *p53* and *RB* tumour suppressor genes.

Squamous cell carcinoma
Like small cell lung cancer, this type of lung cancer is also strongly associated with cigarette smoking and accounts for about 20% of all lung malignancies. It usually develops in the large airways, close to the hilum of the lung. There are multiple genetic abnormalities in the cancer cells, including *p53* and *RB* gene mutations, with a consequent loss of their tumour suppressor activity. Tumour promoter genes are also amplified, including the gene *FGRF1*, which produces a receptor on the cell membrane for fibroblast growth factor and allows cells to respond to this growth signal. Squamous cell carcinomas originate in the bronchial epithelium as a patch of dysplastic cells that transforms into a localised carcinoma in situ. As the tumour grows, it invades and destroys

normal lung tissue, fills and obstructs airways, and may grow through the outer surface of the lung and the pleura and into the thoracic cavity itself.

Adenocarcinomas

About 38% of lung cancers arise from the bronchial epithelium and show glandular features. The commonest genetic mutations here relate to the amplification of growth promoting factors, including the *EGFR* gene. One factor important in normal lung development, thyroid transcription factor-1 (TTF-1), is produced in most types of lung cancer but most strongly in adenocarcinomas. Expression of TTF-1 is associated with well-differentiated tumours with a good prognosis, and multiple studies suggest that examining tumours for this growth factor would contribute usefully to decision making in treatment.

MANIFESTATIONS OF LUNG CANCER

Lung tumours are often asymptomatic for a considerable period of time, and by the time they start producing symptoms that send the patient to a doctor, metastatic growth is usually present, and the outlook is dismal. The overall 5-year survival is in the region of 15%. Dry cough is usually the presenting symptom, and because most patients are either smokers or ex-smokers, many already have a regular cough and ignore it, even if it has changed. There may be haemoptysis (blood in the sputum), particularly common in central tumours; breathlessness; weight loss; and finger clubbing. Tumours growing into an airway can block it, preventing air from flowing in or out of the airways beyond the obstruction. Over time, the trapped air beyond the blockage is absorbed into the bloodstream, and the alveoli collapse (atelectasis). Even a partial blockage can be problematic because it causes breathlessness and wheeze and traps secretions, increasing the risk of infection. There can be pain if there is nerve compression (e.g., of the intercostal nerves running along the inferior and lateral surface of the ribs). If growing at the tip of the lung, a tumour can compress or destroy spinal nerves C8 and T1, which supply the shoulder, arm, and nerves of the sympathetic chain running in the region of the root of the neck, which supply the face. Symptoms relating to impaired or lost function in these nerves include pain, drooping of the eyelid on the affected side, and muscle wasting in the affected arm. Pleural involvement also causes pain because the pleura are rich in pain nerve endings. Once the tumour breaches the lung surface and invades the mediastinum, compression and/or destruction of other structures can lead to major problems: oesophageal involvement restricts swallowing, and compression of the superior vena cava restricts blood return to the heart and increases venous pressure. Lung cancers, especially small cell lung cancers, secrete a wide range of hormones, including ACTH, ADH, insulin, parathormone, calcitonin, and gonadotrophins. The side effects from these can be severe, adding to the burden of the disease and increasing the complexity of disease management. There may also be symptoms associated with metastatic disease. Fig. 3.23 shows the main signs and symptoms of lung cancer.

MANAGEMENT AND PROGNOSIS

Because this cancer is usually not diagnosed until metastasis has occurred, treatment options may be limited. Surgery

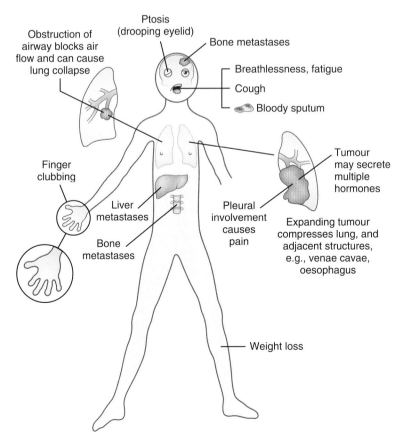

Fig. 3.23 The main signs and symptoms of lung cancer.

offers the best hope for a cure but depends on complete removal of the tumour and affected lymph nodes. Radiotherapy may be more helpful than chemotherapy in prolonging life and palliating symptoms, but it depends on the type of tumour involved. Chemotherapy needs to be carefully chosen to match the tumour profile; for example, some adenocarcinomas, usually in non-smokers or those with a low pack-year history and in those of Asian extraction, express high levels of epidermal growth factor receptor (EGFR) and respond well to the EGRF antibody **afatinib**, which blocks the receptor and prevents EGF from exerting its growth stimulant effect.

BREAST CANCER

This is the commonest female cancer globally and the second commonest cancer overall. A diverse range of genetic mutations is associated with breast cancer, meaning that there is also a wide range of carcinogenic pathways and significant variation between individual tumours. Identifying the molecular profile of an individual's cancer is therefore very important in deciding appropriate treatment, and the development of more aggressive, drug-resistant tumour cell subclones after a course of treatment is a major clinical problem.

Risk factors for breast cancer

Increasing age is the main risk factor for breast cancer. UK statistics show that about 25% of new cases occur in people over 75 years old. Increased lifetime exposure to reproductive hormones, including oestrogen, prolactin, and progesterone, increases risk. These hormones stimulate breast development, increase cell proliferation, and regulate apoptosis. They control the reproductive cycle, including the monthly changes in breast size associated with the menstrual cycle. In addition, breast tissue experiences intense hormone-stimulated periods of growth, including at puberty, during pregnancy, and in breastfeeding. Factors that increase exposure to these hormones include the use of the combined oral contraceptive, post-menopausal hormone replacement therapy, an early menarche and a late menopause, and having naturally high hormone levels. Obesity and overweight are thought to account for 8% of breast cancer cases in the UK, probably because adipose tissue in post-menopausal women produces oestrogen. Risk increases with alcohol consumption, low physical activity, and tobacco smoking, which are all associated with high plasma sex steroid levels.

Multiple pregnancies at a young age and breastfeeding have a protective effect. Lactation suppresses the reproductive cycle and keeps the levels of circulating oestrogen and progesterone low. Interestingly, full-term pregnancies after the age of 35 increase risk, probably because they increase the length of time over which the breast tissue remains functionally active and responsive to oestrogen.

There are also genetic factors involved, although this is complex. Having a first-degree relative (mother, sister) with the disease increases risk, especially if the relative is young. Most cases of breast cancer occur in women with no family history.

BRCA1 and BRCA2 genes

These two genes are located on chromosomes 17 and 13, respectively (see Fig. 3.18). When they are working correctly,

they produce proteins that suppress tumour growth by repairing damaged DNA. Multiple mutations in both the *BRCA1* and *BRCA2* gene have been identified, but they all lead to loss of this important anti-tumour mechanism. The mutant forms are permanent and therefore are passed from parent to child, greatly increasing the likelihood of early development of cancer. Note that mutated *BRCA1* and *BRCA2* genes are involved in other cancers, including prostate and pancreatic malignancy, and that they are not the only gene family involved in heritable breast cancer.

TYPES OF BREAST CANCER

The normal breast is composed of glandular lobules that produce milk, which open into a system of ducts carrying it to the skin surface at the nipple. These structures are supported by a stroma made of fibrous connective tissue and fat. Nearly all (95%) breast cancers develop in the glandular tissue of the lobules and are therefore adenocarcinomas. The commonest site is in the upper outer quadrant.

Ductal carcinoma in situ (DCIS)

One of the identified values of breast screening by mammography is the increased identification rate of breast cancer at an early stage. Screening identifies even small aggregations of malignant cells, visible on the mammogram usually because they have become calcified, and well before they are large enough to be palpable or symptomatic. DCIS is localised and has not yet breached its local basement membrane. Complete cure is possible with surgical removal and adjuvant radiotherapy, and only a very small percentage (1%–3%) of women with a diagnosis of DCIS die of invasive breast cancer. However, fewer than 30% of cases are diagnosed at this stage; most tumours have broken through the basement membrane and invaded adjacent tissues when they are found.

Classification of invasive breast cancers

Most (>95%) are adenocarcinomas, arising from glandular stem cells in the milk duct/lobule system. Breast cancers present as a very wide range of histologically, clinically, and genetically different forms. Identifying the molecular markers on the cancer cell membranes and the growth signals to which the cancer cells respond are key in deciding treatments. The most useful subdivisions relate to expression of oestrogen and EGF (HER2) receptors on the cancer cell surface.

ER-positive, HER2-negative. Tumours expressing cell surface oestrogen receptors (ER-positive) but not HER2 receptors (HER2-negative) constitute 50% to 65% of all invasive breast cancers. There are two main subgroups—low proliferation and high proliferation—and differentiating between them is important because the prognosis is better in the slow growing subgroup. These tumours tend to occur in older women and in men, often respond well to hormone therapy with anti-oestrogenic drugs, and are often associated with good survival times.

HER2-positive. Tumours that express HER2 receptors (about 20% of all invasive breast cancers) are usually found in premenopausal women. They tend to be fast growing and metastasise early. However, the antibody trastuzumab (Herceptin), which targets the HER2 receptor and blocks EGF from binding to the cancer cell (see Fig. 3.19) and stimulating its growth, has enormously improved the prognosis and life expectancy for women with this type of cancer.

ER-negative, HER2-negative. Tumours that express neither oestrogen nor HER2 receptors are usually associated with younger and non-white women and are strongly associated with *BRCA1* mutations. These cancers are also sometimes referred to as the triple-negative group because they are usually negative for progesterone receptors as well. They often metastasise early, and survival times in metastatic disease are the poorest of all types of metastatic breast cancer. However, subgroups of this type can respond completely to treatment, highlighting the relevance of molecular subtyping when making therapeutic decisions.

MANIFESTATIONS OF BREAST CANCER

Unless identified early by screening, the initial sign is usually a painless lump within the breast. There may be dimpling of the skin ('orange peel'; Fig. 3.24) or the nipple above the tumour as the growing tumour distorts the tissue, and the axillary lymph nodes may be palpable if they have become involved. Sometimes the area is inflamed, painful, and swollen, and there may be discharge from the nipple or local ulceration.

MANAGEMENT AND PROGNOSIS

Patients with breast cancer will almost always be offered surgery, which may be limited to lumpectomy or extend to complete mastectomy and axillary lymph node clearance. Radiotherapy is usually offered as well to reduce the incidence of recurrence at the site. Drug treatment is determined by molecular profiling; for example, tumours that express oestrogen receptors (ER-positive) will likely respond to anti-oestrogenic agent such as tamoxifen.

Good prognostic factors include small tumour size, no local lymphatic involvement, and ER-positive status. Breast cancer treatment represents a medical success story, with survival rates improving steadily year on year. UK statistics show that in 1970, only 40% of women diagnosed with breast cancer would still be alive 10 years later. In 2011, nearly 80% survived 10 years or more, despite a steady rise in incidence, reflecting massive improvements in early diagnosis and treatment.

COLORECTAL CANCER

Colorectal cancer is the third commonest cancer worldwide. Globally, the incidence is variable, and there is significant correlation with diet. Developed countries, whose populations typically consume high quantities of processed and high-fat foods, have the highest incidence. Developing countries, whose indigenous people eat more traditional diets, usually based on plants and fish, have much lower incidence (although survival rates are usually poorer). The genetic mutations associated with these cancers are diverse and include deactivation of tumour suppressor genes and abnormalities in genes producing DNA repair enzymes. Most sporadic cases (i.e., with no clear hereditable links) occur in the distal colon and rectum. Metastasis most often occurs to the liver, lung, and peritoneum.

Risk factors for colorectal cancer

Increasing age increases the risk of developing colorectal cancer. Other non-modifiable risk factors include

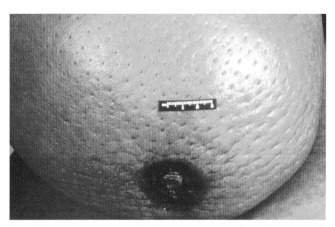

Fig. 3.24 Peau d'orange skin in breast cancer. (From Gunderson L and Tepper J (2007) *Clinical radiation oncology*, 2nd ed, Fig. 61.3. Philadelphia: Churchill Livingstone.)

inflammatory bowel disease and a personal or family history of colorectal cancer or colorectal polyps. About 20% of cases are associated with inherited syndromes such as familial adenomatous polyposis (FAP). However, colorectal cancer is strongly associated with unhealthy lifestyle choices including obesity/overweight, low levels of physical activity, smoking, high alcohol intake, and a diet high in fat, red meat, and processed foods and low in fruit and vegetables. Incidence would be reduced by over 50% if individuals made healthier choices.

The relationship between diet and colon cancer is indisputable, but the reason high-fat diets increase tumour risk remains unclear. It is probably multifactorial. Colonic epithelial stem cells, both in experimental animal studies and grown in cell culture, show increased proliferation, activity, and tumour development when exposed to high levels of fatty acids, probably by deactivating a tumour suppressor gene called *APC*. A 2018 cohort study which followed over 120,000 individuals for 26 years found a clear correlation between consumption of foods associated with the triggering of inflammatory changes in the colon and the incidence of cancer. Such pro-inflammatory foods include highly processed foods and foods high in fats and sugar. The relevance of a pro-inflammatory environment and its pro-cancer effect was discussed previously and is probably important in the pathogenesis of colorectal cancer. It is worth noting here the relationship between inflammatory bowel disease and increased risk of bowel cancer, further supporting the link between inflammation and the triggering of malignant change. A link has also been suggested between diet and altered intestinal flora, and that high saturated fat, high sugar, and highly processed foods alter the normal bacterial population of the intestine to one that is less protective and that may increase cancer risk. In addition, cooking, preserving, and processing foodstuffs such as red meat and fish produce known carcinogens. On the other hand, high-fibre foods decrease colon transit time, reducing exposure of the epithelium to potential carcinogens. Also, fruit and vegetables contain protective anti-carcinogens.

Type 2 diabetes is another predisposing factor. Evidence suggests that high blood sugar, the use of insulin in diabetes management, and the inflammatory environment associated with disturbed metabolism may all predispose to colorectal cancer. Hyperglycaemia increases cell proliferation and reduces apoptosis, both of which contribute to neoplastic growth. In addition, insulin is mitogenic; it is essential in human embryonic development and has growth factor functions in normal tissues and stimulating the growth of some cancer cells.

Cyclo-oxygenase (COX-2) inhibitors like aspirin, which reduce tissue levels of pro-inflammatory prostaglandins, can be protective. COX-2, the enzyme that produces prostaglandins from arachidonic acid, is produced in significantly increased amounts in adenomas and adenocarcinomas compared with normal colon tissues. It increases angiogenesis, reduces apoptosis, and promotes cell proliferation, all of which supports a growing tumour. Large-scale epidemiological studies confirm the protective effect: use of non-steroidal anti-inflammatory drugs (NSAIDs; aspirin is the main one studied) consistently reduces risk by between 30% and 50%. The relationship between COX inhibition and tumour inhibition is not confined to colorectal cancer; many cancers, including breast and prostate, produce abnormally high levels of COX-2. If regular low-dose NSAID treatment proves to be effective in cancer prevention, it could be an immensely useful strategy, especially in high-risk groups.

TYPES OF COLORECTAL CANCER

The commonest gastrointestinal malignancy is adenocarcinoma of the large intestine, originating from glandular tissue stem cells in the intestinal mucosa and appearing anywhere along the length of the colon. Most adenocarcinomas develop from colonic adenomas, benign neoplasms of glandular epithelium that sometimes become malignant. These adenomas may attach to the colon wall with a stalk; these growths are called polyps (Fig. 3.25). Others lie flat against the colon wall and do not protrude into the lumen. Polyps are common, especially in people over 60 years old, and although most (80%–90%) remain benign, many health systems recommend regular screening and removal of polyps in people over 50 years old.

MANIFESTATIONS OF COLORECTAL CANCER

The growth of these tumours is often insidious, with diffuse and non-specific symptoms initially, including bloating, abdominal discomfort, and changes in bowel habits that may be ignored for an extended period before the individual seeks help. If the tumour is in the descending colon/rectal area, there may be rectal bleeding. There may be iron deficiency anaemia caused by a combination of blood loss and reduced iron absorption. The expanding mass may block the colon; obstruction is commoner with tumours affecting the descending colon than the ascending colon.

MANAGEMENT AND PROGNOSIS

The main factors at diagnosis determining survival are the tumour thickness and whether there is local lymph node involvement. The greater the degree of invasion of the gut wall, the poorer the prognosis; additionally, lymphatic involvement is a poor sign. Only 10% of patients present with a localised tumour confined to the epithelium and submucosa; these patients have a 5-year survival rate of over 90%. In contrast, patients who present with established metastasis (e.g., of the liver) have only a 5% chance of being alive 5 years later. Surgery is usually the keystone of treatment and

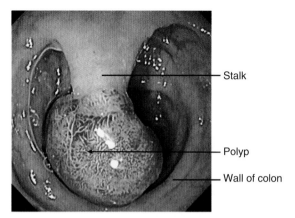

Fig. 3.25 Large colonic polyp. (From Feather A, Randall D, and Waterhouse M (2017) *Kumar and Clark's clinical medicine*, 9th ed, Fig. 13.52. Edinburgh: Elsevier Ltd.)

is curative if the tumour is excised completely before metastasis. Radiotherapy and chemotherapy are used to manage lymphatic spread (up to 40% of patients have lymphatic involvement at diagnosis) or to debulk a tumour before surgery. Even if incurable, palliative surgery may be appropriate to clear an obstruction or relieve pain.

BIBLIOGRAPHY AND REFERENCES

Allemani, C., Matsuda, T., Di Carlo, V., et al. (2018). Global surveillance of trends in cancer survival 2004–14 (CONCORD-3): Analysis of individual records for 37,513,025 patients diagnosed with one of 18 cancers from 322 population-based registries in 71 countries. *Lancet, 391,* 1023–1075.

Aoyagi, T., Terracina, T., Raza, K,P., et al. (2010). Cancer cachexia, mechanism and treatment. *World Journal of Gastrointestinal Oncology* 7 (4), 17–29.

Arnold, M., Sierra, M. S., Laversanne, M., et al. (2017). Global patterns and trends in colorectal cancer incidence and mortality. *Gut, 66,* 683–691.

Beyaz, S., Mana, M. D., Roper, J., et al. (2016). High-fat diet enhances stemness and tumorigenicity of intestinal progenitors. *Nature, 531,* 53–58.

Bussard, K. M., Mutkus, L., Stumpf, K., et al. (2016). Tumor-associated stromal cells as key contributors to the tumor environment. *Breast Cancer Research, 18*(84). https://www.ncbi.nlm.nih.gov/pmc/articles/PMC4982339/.

Campisi, J. (2013). Aging, cellular senescence, and cancer. *Annual Review of Physiology, 75,* 685–705.

DePalma, M., Biziato, D., & Petrova, T. V. (2017). Microenvironmental regulation of tumour angiogenesis. *Nature Reviews Cancer, 17,* 457–474.

Jafri, M. A., Ansari, S. A., Alqahtani, M. H., et al. (2016). Roles of telomeres and telomerase in cancer, and advances in telomerase-targeted therapies. *Genome Medicine, 8,* 69. https://genomemedicine.biomedcentral.com/articles/10.1186/s13073-016-0324-x.

Joerger, A. C., & Fersht, A. R. (2016). The p53 pathway: Origins, inactivation in cancer, and emerging therapeutic approaches. *Annual Review of Biochemistry, 85,* 375–404.

Langley, R. R., & Fidler, I. J. (2011). The seed and soil hypothesis revisited: The role of tumor-stroma interactions in metastasis to different organs. *International Journal of Cancer, 128*(11), 2527–2535.

Lee, W.-C., Kopetz, S., Wistuba, I. I., et al. (2017). Metastasis of cancer: When and how? *Annals of Oncology, 28*(9), 2045–2055.

Mikula-Pietrasik, J., Uruski, P., Tykarsk, A., et al. (2018). The peritoneal 'soil' for a cancerous 'seed': A comprehensive review of the pathogenesis of intraperitoneal cancer metastases. *Cellular and Molecular Life Sciences, 75,* 509–529.

Perez, E. A., Romond, E. H., & Suman, V. J. (2014). Trastuzumab plus adjuvant chemotherapy for human epidermal growth factor receptor 2-positive breast cancer: Planned joint analysis of overall survival from NSABP B-31 and NCCTG N9831. *Journal of Clinical Oncology, 32*(33), 3744–3753.

Ribatti, D. (2017). A revisited concept: Contact inhibition of growth: From cell biology to malignancy. *Experimental Cell Research, 359,* 17–19.

Rigden, H. M., Alias, A., Havelock, T., et al. (2016). Squamous metaplasia is increased in the bronchial epithelium of smokers with chronic obstructive pulmonary disease. *PLoS One, 11*(5). https://journals.plos.org/plosone/article?id=10.1371/journal.pone.0156009.

Rivlin, N., Koifman, G., & Rotter, V. (2015). p53 orchestrates between normal differentiation and cancer. *Seminars in Cancer Biology, 32,* 10–17.

Seager, R. J., Hajal, C., Spill, F., et al. (2017). Dynamic interplay between tumour, stroma and immune system can drive or prevent tumour progression. *Convergent Science Physical Oncology, 3*(3).

Unwith, S., Zhao, H., Hennah, L., et al. (2015). The potential role of HIF on tumour progression and dissemination. *International Journal of Cancer, 136,* 2491–2503.

Vinay, D. S., Ryan, E. P., Pawalec, G., et al. (2015). Immune evasion in cancer: Mechanistic basis and therapeutic strategies. *Seminars in Cancer Biology, 35,* S185–S198.

Zhang, Y., & Lozano, G. (2017). p53: Multiple facets of a Rubik's cube. *Annual Review Cancer Biology, 1,* 185–201.

Useful Websites

American Cancer Society: https://www.cancer.org

Cancer Research UK: https://www.cancerresearchuk.org

Global Cancer Observatory: An interactive web-based platform with international cancer statistics: https://gco.iarc.fr

International Agency for Research on Cancer (IARC): The specialised cancer agency of the World Health Organisation: https://www.iarc.fr

4 Disorders of Immunity

CHAPTER OUTLINE

INTRODUCTION
Innate immunity
Acquired immunity
IMMUNODEFICIENCY
   Primary immunodeficiency
   Secondary immunodeficiency
Complement deficiencies
   Hereditary angioneurotic oedema (HAE)
   Secondary complement deficiencies
Phagocyte deficiencies
   Chronic granulomatous disease (CGD)
   Secondary phagocyte deficiencies
T- and B-lymphocyte deficiencies
   Severe combined immunodeficiency (SCID)
   DiGeorge syndrome
   Antibody deficiencies
   Secondary lymphocyte-related deficiencies
HYPERSENSITIVITY
The four types of hypersensitivity

Type I hypersensitivity
Type II hypersensitivity
Type III hypersensitivity
Type IV hypersensitivity
Allergy
   Anaphylaxis
   Food allergy
   Allergic rhinitis
   Atopic dermatitis
   Penicillin allergy
   Contact dermatitis
Autoimmunity
   Systemic sclerosis (scleroderma)
   Systemic lupus erythematosus (SLE)
   Sjögren disease
   Sarcoidosis
Tissue rejection
   Blood transfusion reactions
   Organ/graft rejection

INTRODUCTION

The body's defence systems provide protection from infection by pathogenic organisms, dispose of mutated and abnormal body cells, and promote the processes of healing and repair. Many body defences—including the skin, the mucociliary escalator in the respiratory tract, the mononuclear phagocyte system, and the secretion of antimicrobial body fluids—protect against a wide range of potential threats. Collectively, these mechanisms are sometimes referred to as **innate** or **non-specific** immunity. In addition to these general mechanisms, the body possesses a collection of defensive structures and cells that mount focussed, targeted responses to specific threats, such as a particular bacterial infection, and attempt to destroy the threat that activated them. These mechanisms are sometimes referred to as **acquired** immunity. Innate and acquired immunity work together to safeguard the body. Innate immunity can be thought of as the body's first line of defence and is usually adequate for protection against the range of physical and infective insults met daily. For example, most minor injuries heal without the development of infection because non-specific phagocytic cells at the injury site destroy any invading organisms and promote wound repair,

and minor contamination of food and drink does not lead to food poisoning because gastric acid kills microbes and destroys toxins. However, if infection is significant, cells of the innate defence system activate acquired immunity, in which lymphocytes and antibodies are directed specifically against the invading organism, mounting a powerful, targeted response. Defective or failed function of any components of the innate or acquired defence mechanisms can increase the risk of infection and/or cancer, and impaired or abnormal healing.

INNATE IMMUNITY

Innate immunity includes physical barriers between the body's internal environment and the external environment: intact skin and mucous membranes are excellent defences, and most pathogenic organisms cannot penetrate them. Body fluids contain antiseptic and antibacterial substances: for example, tears contain **lysozyme**, a bacteriocidal enzyme that destroys bacterial cell walls, and **sebum**, secreted by glands in the skin, is rich in lipids that waterproof the skin and also has antimicrobial properties. Gastric fluids, vaginal secretions, and urine are all acidic, discouraging bacterial growth.

Cells of the mononuclear phagocyte system include non-specific phagocytes, which consume and digest foreign cells like bacteria but are also important in healing and repair by clearing away dead and dying cellular debris from areas of injury. The inflammatory response (p. 11) is a key part of innate defence.

Complement

Complement is a collection of over 30 plasma proteins produced by the liver. It is essential for a normal inflammatory response and also for stimulating increased antibody levels to combat infection (complement is so called because it complements antibody function). Its significance is clearly seen in individuals with inherited deficiencies of one or more complement proteins, who may develop repeated, frequently severe, bacterial infections early in life.

Complement proteins are named using C and a number (e.g., C1, C2). Some complement proteins are enzymes, which circulate in plasma and in body fluids in inactive forms and are activated mainly by contact with pathogens and immune complexes. Activated complement proteins are indicated with the addition of 'a' to their name (e.g., C3a is the active form of C3). Activation of complement enzymes in turn activates large quantities of other complement proteins. In this way, even a small initial stimulus triggers an escalating, significant inflammatory response. Other complement proteins act as regulators, controlling the activation pathways.

The complement pathways

The key event in complement function is the activation of a protein called *C3*. Three different pathways lead to C3 activation: the **classical pathway**, the **lectin pathway**, and the **alternative pathway**, and although all produce the active form of C3, each is initiated by different triggers (Fig. 4.1). From an evolutionary point of view, the most recent is the classical pathway, which is activated by antibody attachment to the antigen. Antibody production is a relatively recent development in human evolution. More ancient are the lectin and alternative pathways, which do not require the presence of antibody; they are directly activated by the presence of pathogens in the body.

Irrespective of the activating pathway, C3 is converted to C3a and C3b, which in turn accelerate the production of other complement components. Ultimately, complement activation leads to three main functional consequences:

- Assembly of five complement proteins into the **membrane attack complex** (MAC), which inserts itself into bacterial cell walls, forming a pore and causing lysis and cell death
- Production of active inflammatory proteins that attract white blood cells and promote the inflammatory response
- Production of active complement proteins that attach themselves directly to the surfaces of pathogens, marking them clearly for destruction by the body's circulating phagocytes. This process is called **opsonisation** and makes it much easier for phagocytes to detect and destroy pathogens.

Control of complement activation. The complement system is carefully controlled, not only to prevent excessive activation and consequent damage to host cells, but also to maintain adequate reserves of inactive complement components in body fluids so that, in the event of infection, there are enough complement proteins present to mount an effective response. The complement system is continuously active at a very low level, providing constant surveillance of body fluids, and essential inhibitors normally keep it in check. One important regulator is C1 inhibitor (C1INH), which blocks conversion of C1 to C4, a key step in classical and lectin pathways (Fig. 4.2). Additionally, there are multiple inhibitors involved in regulating the different steps in the complement pathways.

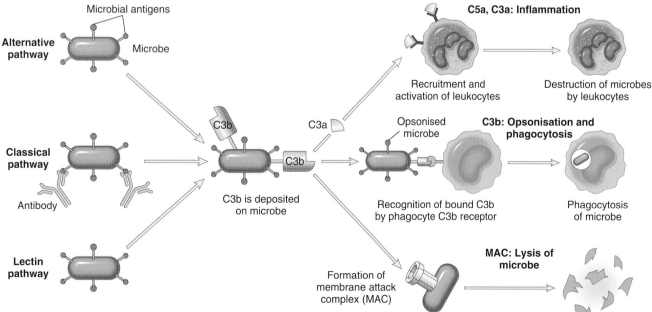

EFFECTOR FUNCTIONS

C5a, C3a: Inflammation

Recruitment and activation of leukocytes

Destruction of microbes by leukocytes

C3b: Opsonisation and phagocytosis

Opsonised microbe

Recognition of bound C3b by phagocyte C3b receptor

Phagocytosis of microbe

MAC: Lysis of microbe

Formation of membrane attack complex (MAC)

Alternative pathway

Microbial antigens

Microbe

Classical pathway

Antibody

Lectin pathway

C3b

C3b

C3a

C3b is deposited on microbe

Fig. 4.1 The complement system. (Modified from Kumar K, Abbas A, Aster JC, et al. (2021) *Robbins essential pathology*, Fig. 4.4. Philadelphia: Elsevier Inc.)

Natural killer (NK) cells

NK cells are lymphocytes and constitute about 10% of the total lymphocyte count. Unlike the remaining 90%, the T- and B-cell populations described below, these cells are not programmed to target a single antigen. Instead, they patrol the body tissues, looking for abnormal cells. They have a key role in detecting mutated cells that may be precursors to malignancy and destroying them before cancerous growth can be established. This is called *immunological surveillance*.

Phagocytes

This collection of defence cells, including neutrophils and macrophages, is important in protection against invading bacteria and other pathogens. **Phagocytosis** (Fig. 4.3) is the process of engulfing and destroying foreign cells and materials and is an integral part of host defence and post-injury clearing of damaged tissue as part of wound healing. It is the most important mechanism for clearing bacteria from body fluids. The phagocyte engulfs the target and internalises it within a vesicle called a phagosome. Lysosomes containing digestive enzymes and toxic chemicals fuse with the phagosome, the target is digested, and the waste is excreted through the cell membrane.

Neutrophils

Neutrophils are small, motile, granular leukocytes and are normally the most abundant type of white blood cell in the body, usually accounting for between 40% and 70% of the total white cell count. They are aggressive scavengers and roam body tissues looking for antigenic particles or cells to engulf and destroy.

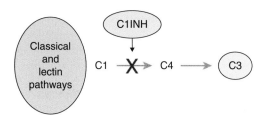

Fig. 4.2　Role of C1INH in inhibiting complement activation.

Their lifespan is short: average survival in the bloodstream is only about 7 hours, which reduces to minutes once actively engaged in phagocytosis because their destructive lysosomal contents, once released, destroy them and their target cells.

Neutrophils and the oxidative burst. The internal environment within the neutrophil is highly toxic: to rapidly destroy their targets, their granules are equipped with an array of digestive enzymes, and with antimicrobial proteins and biochemical pathways to generate very short-lived but highly toxic reactive oxygen species (ROS) via processes collectively termed the **oxidative burst** (sometimes referred to as the respiratory burst). ROS—which include the highly reactive superoxide radical (O_2^-), hydrogen peroxide, and hypochlorous acid (HOCl)—are rapidly lethal to microbial cells because they are so reactive that they damage key enzymes and disrupt essential microbial metabolism. The production of ROS is of major importance to the killing action not only of neutrophils but also of macrophages and other phagocytes.

Macrophages, antigen presentation, and acquired immunity

Macrophages are larger than neutrophils and are distributed widely throughout body tissues. They are part of the mononuclear phagocyte system and are derived from monocytes, large white blood cells found circulating in the bloodstream. Fixed populations of macrophages are strategically located around the body at sites potentially vulnerable to microbial entry, for example the respiratory tract (dust cells), the gastrointestinal tract and in the skin (Langerhans cells).

Macrophages and other phagocytes ingest foreign materials indiscriminately: they are not selective about their targets, and they consume anything they recognise as being foreign. After ingesting a target (e.g., a bacterial cell), the phagocyte digests it, releasing bacterial proteins, which are transported to the phagocyte's plasma membrane and displayed on its surface. When the bacterial load in the body is high, and a high proportion of the body's macrophages is displaying bacterial proteins, this is detected by the body's population of T-lymphocytes, key cells in acquired immunity. T-lymphocytes (usually referred to as *T cells*) respond to this signal, triggering an immune response specific to the foreign proteins detected

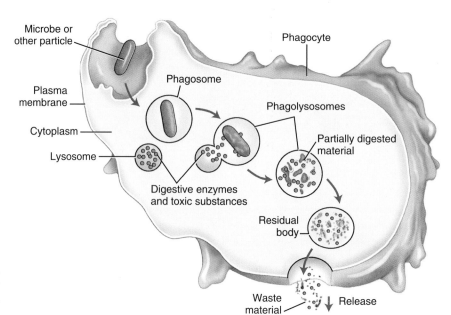

Fig. 4.3　Phagocytosis. (Modified from Van-Meter K and Hubert RJ (2016) *Microbiology for the healthcare professional*, 2nd ed, Fig. 13.18. St Louis: Elsevier.)

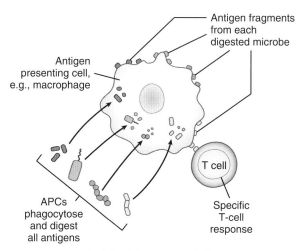

Fig. 4.4   Antigen presentation.

(and hence specific to the invading bacteria) on macrophage surfaces. This key link between innate defences and acquired immunity is called **antigen presentation**. Phagocytes that fulfil this role are called **antigen presenting cells** (APCs) and are essential for activating T cells and antibody production, essential elements of acquired immunity. In Fig. 4.4, an APC has phagocytosed a number of microbes and is presenting antigen from all of them, but the T cell shown is specific to the light blue-coloured microbe, can detect only those antigen fragments, and will ignore the others.

ACQUIRED IMMUNITY

Lymphocytes are produced from lymphoblast precursor cells in the bone marrow during fetal development, where individual cells are equipped with antigen-specific receptors on their plasma membranes so that each individual lymphocyte can recognise and respond to only one antigen. In acquired immunity, exposure to a specific antigen triggers a defensive response driven by T and B cells.

Acquired immunity is associated with immunological memory. This gives the individual a huge survival advantage. The first time an individual comes into contact with a specific antigen, the immune response, including antibody (immunoglobulin, Ig) production, is slow and delayed. Assuming that the individual survives this initial infection, their response to subsequent exposures to the same antigen is much faster and much more powerful than the first time. We would say that the individual is now immune to that infection. Immunity depends on the production of memory cells (described below), formed as a result of the initial infection, which act as a rapid response force whenever the individual comes into contact with the same infection again.

HLA (MHC) proteins

It is critically important that defensive cells differentiate between self-cells and proteins and foreign cells and proteins. Their array of defence mechanisms, which includes phagocytosis (described previously) and the release of a range of highly toxic chemicals, also damages and kills body cells. It is essential that this collateral damage is as limited as possible and that the immune system is not activated inappropriately. For this purpose, all nucleated body cells produce and display 'self' markers on their cell membranes, which act as

'identity cards' and indicate to immune cells that the cell belongs to the body. These markers are proteins, coded for by a collection of genes on chromosome 6. The genes are collectively called the HLA (human leukocyte antigen) complex, or sometimes referred to as MHC (major histocompatibility complex) genes. HLA proteins provide what is called **immunological self-tolerance**, ensuring that body cells are protected from immunological aggression.

HLA proteins are unique to the individual, except for identical siblings, whose HLA proteins are identical because their genetic makeup is identical. This means that, in health, an individual's immune system can accurately differentiate between self and non-self. The system is remarkably efficient but does sometimes malfunction. Mutations in HLA genes are almost always found in autoimmune disorders, in which the immune system mistakes body components as foreign and attacks them.

T cells and immunity

After release from the bone marrow, immature T cells migrate to the thymus gland, which lies behind the sternum and in front of the heart. Within the specialised tissues of the thymus, the T cells are exposed to a range of normal body proteins, including HLA proteins. T cells that cannot identify HLA proteins, and therefore cannot tell the difference between cells of the body and foreign cells, are killed. In this way, the thymus eliminates T cells that would attack body cells. T cells that successfully demonstrate self-tolerance are allowed to develop and differentiate, and when fully mature, they leave the thymus and enter the circulation. These cells patrol body tissues searching for the antigen that matches the antigen-specific receptor they carry on their surface. They cannot respond directly to free antigen, for example, to bacteria in the bloodstream or viral proteins in tissue fluid. Instead, the T-cell response is activated by APCs such as macrophages, which have digested microbial proteins and present these fragments on their cell surface as described previously (Fig. 4.4). When a T cell finds an APC displaying its target antigen on its plasma membrane, it is stimulated to divide, producing a huge population of identical T cells in a very short time (clonal expansion), all bearing the same antigen-specific receptor and all dedicated to clearing that antigen from the body. This is called *clonal expansion.*

T cell subtypes

When stimulated by antigen, the proliferating population of T cells generates four key subtypes. All possess the same cell surface receptor for the original antigen, so all are dedicated to destruction of that antigen, but each subtype has specialised functions to perform. Fig. 4.5 summarises the process of T cell activation.

Helper T cells (Th cells). Helper T cells (Th cells) are also called CD4 cells because they express a protein called CD4, which is important in identifying cell surface HLA (self) proteins and is therefore important in protecting body cells from the immune response. Th cells are key co-ordinating cells in the immune response. They release multiple cytokines, including interleukins and interferons, which promote the activity of other immune cells, including Tc cells (see below) and macrophages. Th cells also activate the B-cell response and trigger antibody production (see below).

Cytotoxic T (Tc) cells. Cytotoxic T (Tc) cells are also called CD8 cells because of their cell surface protein CD8. Like CD4, CD8 proteins identify the MHC (self) proteins that the T cell

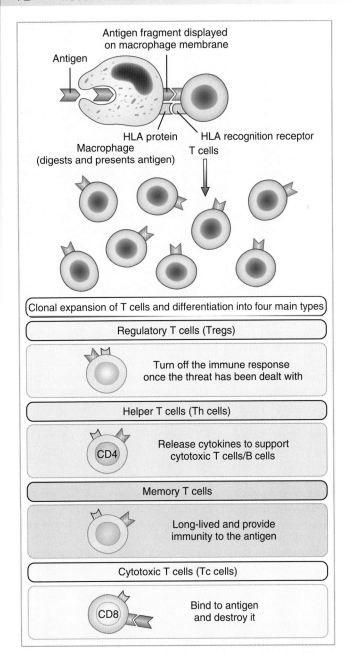

Fig. 4.5 T-cell activation and clonal expansion. (Modified from Waugh A and Grant A (2018) *Ross & Wilson anatomy and physiology in health and illness*, 13th ed, Fig. 15.3. Oxford: Elsevier Ltd.)

checks and so are important in protecting body cells from the immune response. Tc cells are direct killing cells. They are equipped with an array of intracellular toxins and enzymes that, when released in the close vicinity of a target cell, destroy it. Tc cells kill abnormal or stressed body cells, destroy bacteria and initiate apoptosis, programmed cell suicide (p. 65).

Regulatory T cells (Tregs). Regulatory T cells (Tregs) suppress the immune response and are instrumental in preventing autoimmune disease and in protecting the fetus during pregnancy. Because the fetus is genetically different to the mother, the mother is actively immunosuppressed while pregnant to prevent her from mounting an immune response against her baby. Tregs switch the immune response off once an infection has been resolved.

Memory T cells. Memory T cells cells are formed after the first exposure to a particular antigen. Initial exposure to a par-

ticular infection in a non-immune person makes the individual ill. However, after a healthy immune response and resolution of the infection, the individual is left with a population of memory cells, which respond quickly and powerfully in the event of later exposures to the same infection. This is the basis of immunity.

B cells and immunity

B-cell activation follows the T cell response because Th cells are required to initiate it. B cells are found mainly in lymphoid tissue, such as lymph nodes, and like T cells are programmed to respond to only one antigen. Although they detect free antigen in body fluids, this is not enough to activate them. Activation depends on interaction with Th cells. Once activated by this T-B-cell co-operation, B cells proliferate, producing a huge population of B cells, which differentiate into plasma cells. Plasma cells live for only about 24 hours, but each plasma cell produces thousands of antibody molecules per second. This antibody, directed against the same antigen that triggered the initial immune response, leads to antigen destruction in five main ways (Fig. 4.6):

- Activation of complement
- Stimulation of the inflammatory response
- Opsonisation of the antigen, making it easier for phagocytes to detect and destroy it. The structure formed when antibody binds to its antigen is called an *immune complex*. Circulating immune complexes are very good at activating complement and other inflammatory mechanisms, but if they are not cleared effectively from the circulation, they can deposit in blood vessel walls, triggering inflammation and tissue damage.
- Clumping antigens together, which increases their visibility to phagocytes and increases phagocytosis of antigen
- Binding to, and neutralising, bacterial toxins

After resolution of the infection, B cell (and plasma cell production) stops, but, as with the T cell response, a population of memory B cells remains in the body as rapid responders ready to deal with any future reinfection.

Antibody subtypes

There are five types of antibodies, all with a fundamental Y-shaped molecular structure (Fig. 4.7). Each antibody molecule is made up of four chains, two heavy and two light chains, held together with disulphide bonds. The tips of the arms of the Y are called *variable segments* because these are the parts of the molecule responsible for binding antigen. They are therefore different depending on the antigen against which they are directed. The structure and function of the five types of antibody are summarised in Table 4.1.

IMMUNODEFICIENCY

In immunodeficiency, one or more functional aspects of the innate or acquired immune response is inadequate or absent.

PRIMARY IMMUNODEFICIENCY

Congenital (inherited) immunodeficiencies are called *primary immunodeficiencies*. Advances in genetic technology have identified over 130 primary immunodeficiency disorders, which are usually inherited as recessive traits. The affected gene may

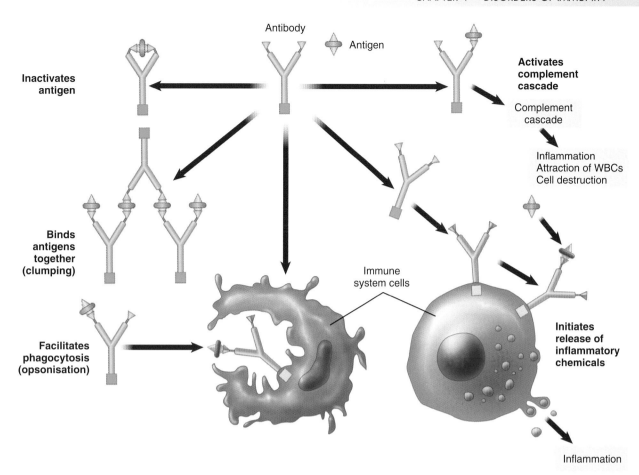

Fig. 4.6 **Antibody action in immunity** (Modified from Patton K and Thibodeau G (2019) *Structure & function of the body*, 16th ed, Fig. 14.7. St. Louis: Elsevier Inc.)

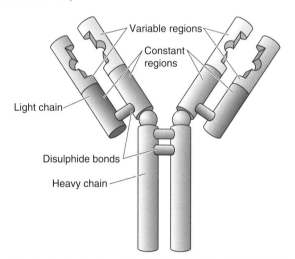

Fig. 4.7 **Antibody structure.** (Modified from Gartner L (2017) *Textbook of histology*, 4th ed, Fig. 12.2. St. Louis: Elsevier Inc.)

be either X-linked or autosomal. The clinical presentations of primary immunodeficiencies are variable, but most cause at least a moderate increase in susceptibility to infection.

SECONDARY IMMUNODEFICIENCY

In secondary immunodeficiency, the immune system is compromised by an infection, toxic agent, or disease. For example, HIV infection progressively destroys Th cell populations, with progressive loss of immune function and increasing susceptibility to infection and malignant disease. Cancer is immunosuppressive, as are some drugs (e.g., corticosteroids and cytotoxic drugs). Malnutrition also depresses immunity. Secondary immunodeficiency is much more common than primary immunodeficiency.

COMPLEMENT DEFICIENCIES

Although primary complement deficiencies are rare (estimated at about 3 in 10,000 of the general population), genetic abnormalities involving all the complement proteins and many of their regulators have been identified. There are significant racial differences; reduced C2 levels is the commonest complement deficiency in people of Caucasian origin, and in Japanese people, more than 1 in 500 have C9 deficiency. Complement deficiency is associated with repeated bacterial infection and with some autoimmune disorders, including systemic lupus erythematosus.

HEREDITARY ANGIONEUROTIC OEDEMA (HAE)

This is the commonest primary complement deficiency and is inherited as an autosomal dominant trait, meaning that a child of an affected parent has a 50% chance of inheriting the disease. The faulty gene is located on the long arm of chromosome 11. Global prevalence varies but has been estimated between 1 in 10,000 and 1 in 150,000.

Table 4.1   The function of the five classes of immunoglobulin

Antibody type	Location	Function
IgM	Body tissues/fluids	Produced early in the immune response; less effective than IgG but very good at activating complement and neutralising toxins
IgG	Body tissues/fluids	Characteristic of mature, well-developed immune responses; the predominant and most effective type of antibody; effective against most types of antigen
IgD	Expressed on B cells	B cells use IgD to detect the presence of their antigen in body fluids
IgE	Coats mast cells	Involved in the release of histamine and allergic responses
IgA	Coats epithelial surfaces	Protects membranes and surfaces, e.g., in the skin, the respiratory tract and the gastrointestinal tract

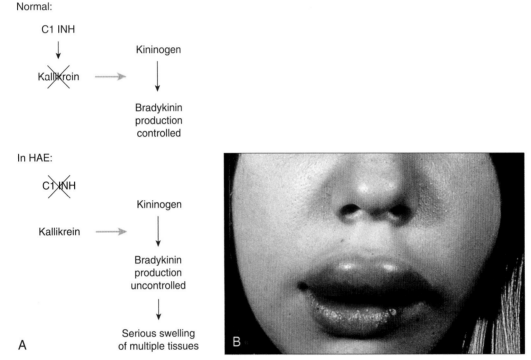

Fig. 4.8   Hereditary angioneurotic oedema. (A) C1INH deficiency leads to continuous production of bradykinin. (B) Facial swelling in HAE. (From Male D, Brostoff J, Roth D, et al. (2013) *Immunology*, 8th ed, Fig. 16.14. Oxford: Elsevier Ltd.)

Pathophysiology

In HAE, C1 inhibitor (C1INH) is deficient. C1INH regulates the lectin and classical pathways of complement activation, but it also blocks production of the inflammatory mediator bradykinin from its precursor kininogen by inhibiting the enzyme kallikrein (Fig. 4.8A). When C1INH activity is reduced, bradykinin production is uncontrolled and greatly increases vascular permeability, leading to repeated bouts of severe swelling (**angioedema**) in different parts of the body, including the skin, gastrointestinal tract, hands, feet, face, and trunk (Fig. 4.8B). Frequency of attacks varies from person to person. In mild or well-controlled disease, attacks can be more than a decade apart, whereas in more severe or poorly controlled cases, attacks can occur every few days.

Signs and symptoms

Diagnosis can be delayed because the condition is rare, although symptoms usually begin in childhood. The course of the disease is usually characterised by recurrent attacks of variable severity, often interspersed with long symptom-free periods. In some women, trigger factors include oestrogen exposure, pregnancy, and hormone replacement therapy, and the use of oestrogen-containing contraceptives can worsen the disease. This is because through an indirect pathway, oestrogen increases bradykinin production. Other trigger factors that may precipitate attacks include cold, emotional stress, and infection. Abdominal pain and other gastrointestinal symptoms such as vomiting and diarrhoea are common and caused by oedema of the gastrointestinal wall. Upper respiratory tract swelling can cause life-threatening respiratory obstruction.

Management and prognosis

Because the swelling of HAE is caused specifically by overproduction of bradykinin, standard anti-inflammatory treatments like antihistamines and anti-inflammatory glucocorticoids are ineffective. Treatments include the bradykinin receptor antagonist icatibant. The disorder cannot be cured.

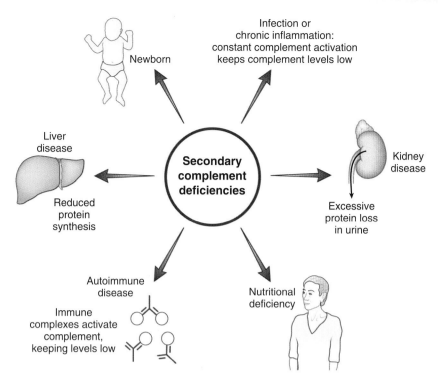

Fig. 4.9 Some causes of secondary complement deficiency.

SECONDARY COMPLEMENT DEFICIENCIES

There is a wide range of causes, some associated with acute conditions such as infection, and others with chronic conditions or autoimmune disease. Transient complement deficiency is normal in newborn babies, but normally corrects itself as the child grows. Any disorder that impairs protein synthesis, including liver disorders or malnutrition, can reduce the level of circulating complement and reduce complement effectiveness. Also, in nephrotic syndrome, excessive protein loss in the urine depletes complement. Conditions characterised by chronic inflammation and constant complement activation keep complement levels low, reducing the body's ability to mount an effective complement response. In autoimmune conditions associated with production of autoantibodies, there may be high circulating levels of immune complexes, which are important activators of complement. An example of such a condition is systemic lupus erythematosus, in which antibodies are produced against constituents of the cell nucleus, including DNA and nuclear proteins. When these antibodies bind to their target, the immune complexes they form circulate in the bloodstream, activating complement, keeping levels too low to meet other challenges. Levels of complement are often useful indicators of the status of this disease because they are reduced when it is more active (Fig. 4.9).

PHAGOCYTE DEFICIENCIES

Failure or deficiency of the body's phagocyte population leads to repeated, severe bacterial infections because of the key role these defence cells play in the destruction of invading organisms. Most phagocyte deficiencies are secondary to other causes, and primary deficiency is rare. For example, primary autoimmune neutropenia, in which antibodies are made to neutrophil proteins and which affects boys and girls equally, occurs in fewer than 1/100,000 live births.

A rare group of inherited disorders, called *leukocyte adhesion deficiency* (LAD), impairs the ability of circulating leukocytes to adhere to vascular endothelium and therefore prevents them from leaving the bloodstream and entering damaged or inflamed tissues. LAD is usually diagnosed early because of recurrent, severe infection. Without leukocyte recruitment into infected tissue, pus cannot be formed, and the inflammatory response is hampered, allowing infection to progress and significantly impairing healing.

Myeloperoxidase (MPO), an enzyme found in neutrophils and monocytes (the precursors of macrophages), is essential for phagocyte production of toxic reactive oxygen species, including hypochlorite (the active ingredient in household bleach!). MPO deficiency is a relatively common finding, in 1 in 4000 individuals. Although it can sometimes increase the risk of infection (e.g., in diabetes) in otherwise healthy people, it usually does not cause problems, presumably because production of other degradative substances in the phagocytes can compensate.

Note that, although individuals with severe phagocytic deficiencies may be severely immunocompromised, many also have reasonably effective acquired immune function, produce effective levels of antibody and cope adequately with exposure to many infections.

CHRONIC GRANULOMATOUS DISEASE (CGD)

This rare (1 in 250,000 live births) disorder was first described in 1954. There are five different genetic mutations associated with CGD, four associated with autosomal inheritance (affecting girls and boys equally), but the most common form is X-linked, therefore affecting mainly males. The underlying fault is with phagocyte levels of key lysosomal toxins, which are deficient, meaning that phagocyte killing is much less effective than normal. The disorder is generally diagnosed in early childhood, with repeated deep-seated infections, including respiratory infections, organ abscesses, osteomyelitis, and non-specific bowel inflammation. The commonest pathogen is *Staphylococcus aureus*, but many other organisms can be involved, notably the fungus *Aspergillus*. Lack of phagocytic activity allows a characteristic range of atypical organisms to establish infections, which can help enormously in the rapid diagnosis of CGD.

Extensive formation of granulomatous tissue is a feature of the disorder. Granulomas (Fig. 1.15) are formed when an agent or process that is difficult to eradicate or resolve causes chronic inflammation in tissues, and the body's response is to try and seal off the area in a walled-up granuloma. Granulomas contain macrophages and T cells and can cause significant damage to adjacent normal tissue. In CGD, expanding granulomas commonly block passageways, often in the gastrointestinal (GI) tract, but also in other body systems such as the ureters and the urethra.

Management and prognosis

Aggressive antimicrobial therapy is used, both prophylactically and in treatment of ongoing infection, to reduce the incidence and severity of bacterial and fungal infections. Life expectancy varies depending on the severity of the disorder but has risen dramatically since the disorder was initially identified, when sufferers usually died in childhood, because treatment has improved greatly. However, repeated infections shorten life and often reduce quality of life, especially with the rise in antimicrobial resistance. Bone marrow transplant can be curative because it replaces the genetically abnormal phagocyte stem cells with healthy stem cells, leading to production of healthy phagocytes.

SECONDARY PHAGOCYTE DEFICIENCIES

There are many causes of secondary neutropenia (low circulating neutrophil levels). Bone marrow failure, leukaemia, certain viral infections (e.g., cytomegalovirus and human immunodeficiency virus), chemotherapy or radiation therapy for cancer, nutritional deficiency (e.g., vitamin B_{12} or folate deficiency), and chemical toxins (e.g., benzene) can all reduce or suppress neutrophil production.

T- AND B-LYMPHOCYTE DEFICIENCIES

T- and B-cell deficiencies impair the body's ability to mount targeted responses to specific pathogens. T-cells are particularly important in protecting against abnormal cells and extracellular pathogens and are essential in activating the antibody response to infection by B cells, so failure of any aspect of normal T cell function leads to combined immunodeficiency (i.e., T- and B-cell deficiency). B cells produce antibodies, so B-cell deficiency compromises this essential arm of the immune response.

SEVERE COMBINED IMMUNODEFICIENCY (SCID)

This group of disorders, caused by a range of genetic defects, is characterised by failure of one or more critical aspects of T cell development, function, or survival. Irrespective of the specific biochemical abnormality, all lead to significant immunocompromise. SCID is rare, affecting 1 to 2 births per 100,000, but it is life-threatening and life-limiting because it causes repeated, persistent, and serious infections, often opportunistic in nature. B-cell production is often normal, but its function is not because without interaction with T cells it cannot produce antibodies. T cells also contribute to the function of NK cells (p. 90), so there may also be a higher-than-normal risk of malignancy.

Some cases of SCID are inherited, whereas others arise from spontaneous mutations, with no previous family history. The commonest form of SCID, accounting for up to 60% of cases, is called *X-SCID*. It is X-linked and is therefore only seen in boys. In X-SCID, T cells lack a key growth factor receptor on their plasma membranes and so cannot respond to normal growth and maturation signals. T cell numbers are very low as a result, although B-cell numbers are unaffected.

The second commonest form of SCID is caused by the deficiency of an enzyme called *adenosine deaminase* (ADA), which plays a part in biochemical pathways essential for DNA breakdown. Without ADA, a toxic metabolite of DNA accumulates within lymphocytes, leading to cell death. In this form of SCID, T-cell, B-cell, and NK cell numbers are all very low. This form is not X-linked and so affects both boys and girls equally.

Management and prognosis

The clinical presentation can vary depending on the underlying genetic abnormality, but diagnosis is usually made early in life because affected children suffer from recurrent, often fungal, infections, and fail to thrive. Death at a young age is inevitable without treatment. Treatment depends on the form of SCID present, but bone marrow transplant is the mainstay. Gene therapy is also under development, where the patient's own lymphocytic stem cells are removed, a healthy gene is inserted, and cells are then transfused back into the patient.

DIGEORGE SYNDROME

In DiGeorge syndrome, the third and fourth pharyngeal pouches fail to develop normally during early embryonic life, and because the thymus gland develops as part of this process, children with DiGeorge syndrome have varying degrees of thymic underdevelopment. Because the thymus gland is the site of the final stages of T-cell maturation, affected individuals have reduced T-cell numbers. In 1% to 2% of cases, the thymus gland is completely absent, and the child has no T cells at all (complete DiGeorge), a life-threatening condition causing a form of SCID. However, the degree of thymic underdevelopment varies considerably between individuals, and the affected child may have little or no immunocompromise. In addition to thymic hypoplasia, there are characteristic facial features: low-set ears, an underdeveloped chin, and wide-set eyes because of the abnormal embryological development (Fig. 4.10). Because the parathyroid glands and parts of the heart and great vessels also develop from the affected embryonic tissues, there may be cardiac abnormalities and problems with regulation of blood calcium levels. The incidence of psychiatric, behavioural, and communication problems is higher than average. Most cases are thought to arise from a spontaneous deletion of a portion of chromosome 22 and are therefore

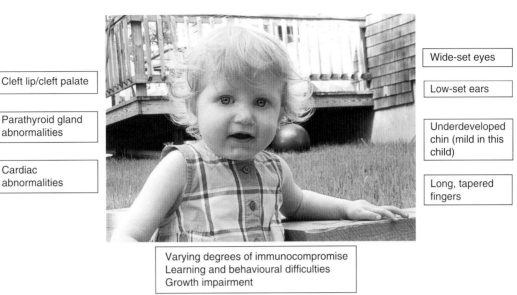

Cleft lip/cleft palate

Parathyroid gland abnormalities

Cardiac abnormalities

Wide-set eyes

Low-set ears

Underdeveloped chin (mild in this child)

Long, tapered fingers

Varying degrees of immunocompromise
Learning and behavioural difficulties
Growth impairment

Fig. 4.10 Features of DiGeorge syndrome. (Modified from Kaban L and Troulis M (2004) *Pediatric oral and maxillofacial surgery*, Fig. 2.5. St. Louis: Elsevier Inc.)

not inherited; the condition is also called chromosome 22q11.2 deletion syndrome. The condition affects around 1 in 6000 live births.

Management and prognosis

There is no cure, but individual issues can be managed, such as correction of hypoparathyroidism with hormone replacement, surgical correction of cardiac defects, and prevention/treatment of infection. The condition is frequently life-limiting because of immunocompromise and the associated congenital heart defects.

ANTIBODY DEFICIENCIES

Antibody deficiency disorders are commoner than T cell deficiencies (about 70% of primary immunodeficiencies are in this category). They may be caused by faulty B-cell development or function, but because B-cell activation depends on the preceding T cell response, T cell disorders can also depress or abolish antibody production. For example, in HIV infection, although the virus invades and destroys the Th cell population, the antibody response is progressively eliminated as well.

The clinical presentation of individuals with antibody deficiency is very variable. Although the conditions usually present with recurrent infections, often of the respiratory system, some people with severe antibody deficiency do not experience an increased incidence of infection and the reason for this is not clear.

Selective IgA deficiency

This is the commonest primary antibody deficiency, with a prevalence of 1 in 500 in people of European descent, although it is much less common in Asian and African peoples. In this disorder, levels of circulating IgA are reduced or almost absent, although many people with very low levels remain asymptomatic. In symptomatic people, common features are frequent infections and increased incidence of autoimmunity and/or allergy. It can present at any age, and only 20% have a family history; in other patients, the disease

might have been acquired as the result of an earlier viral infection. The cause is unknown.

Common variable immunodeficiency

This common disorder (estimated 1/25,000 of the population) is usually not diagnosed until young adulthood, and males are more frequently affected than females. It is a group of disorders associated with deficiency in more than one antibody class, and a deficient antibody response to vaccination. B-cell numbers are often normal, but their genetic abnormality prevents normal differentiation into plasma cells, and so antibody production is also impaired. It is a complex disorder associated with multiple gene defects, giving a wide spectrum of clinical presentations. These range from mild deficiency in B-cell function and minimal hypogammaglobulinaemia to a complete lack of memory B cells. Presenting symptoms include recurrent eye, sinus, and respiratory tract infections, and bronchiectasis is a frequent development. Granuloma formation (p. 16) is common in people of African American descent, but in individuals of European descent occurs in less than a fifth of patients. These granulomas, usually found in the lungs, lymph nodes, liver, and skin, may resolve spontaneously. There is also an increased risk of cancers, particularly of the GI tract and lymphoid tissue. Paradoxically, given that antibody levels are low or absent in these patients, autoimmune disease is often present.

Management and prognosis

Infections must be aggressively treated. The mainstay of treatment is lifelong administration of IgG.

X-linked agammaglobulinaemia

This disorder, also called *Bruton's agammaglobulinaemia*, was named in 1952, but the gene that causes it, which codes for an enzyme called tyrosine kinase, was not discovered until 1993. The gene is found on the X-chromosome, and the tyrosine kinase it produces is essential for B-cell maturation. It is rare, affecting about 1 in 200,000 live male births. When

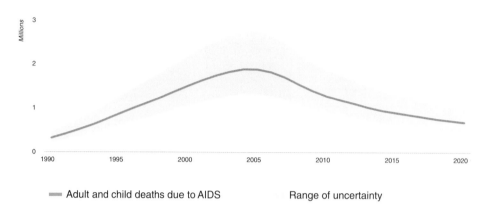

Adult and child deaths due to AIDS   1990–2020

Fig. 4.11   Trends in HIV-related deaths. (From UNAIDS epidemiological estimates, 2022: https://aidsinfo.unaids.org/.)

the gene is faulty, B-cell development is blocked and therefore antibody production is impaired. Mature B-cell numbers are low, and there is panhypogammaglobulinaemia (deficiency in all classes of antibody). Children usually present after about 6 months of age with recurrent infections because by then the baby's circulating levels of IgG obtained from his mother have fallen to ineffective levels.

Management and prognosis

Infections must be aggressively treated and protecting the lungs from the consequences of frequent infection is a clinical priority. The mainstay of treatment is lifelong administration of IgG.

SECONDARY LYMPHOCYTE-RELATED DEFICIENCIES

Secondary lymphocyte deficiencies are commoner than primary diseases. Bone marrow failure or disease, or removal of lymphoid tissue, including the spleen, reduces lymphocyte numbers because these tissues are essential for lymphocyte production, maturation, and residence. Important causes of bone marrow failure include cytotoxic drugs used to treat cancer and systemic steroid treatment. Bone marrow/lymphoid tissue malignancy, such as Hodgkin disease, impairs their production of lymphocytes. Infection (e.g., HIV), which targets Th cells, also reduces lymphocyte populations. Secondary causes of antibody deficiency include excessive loss of antibody in urine in kidney disease (e.g., in nephrotic syndrome) or via the GI tract in disorders where chronic diarrhoea is a feature.

Worldwide, the commonest cause of reduced immunity is poor nutrition.

Co-existing infection and malnutrition is a particularly potent immunosuppressant combination.

Human immunodeficiency virus (HIV) infection

Although the number of new cases of HIV infection is falling worldwide, and although death rates have fallen dramatically since 2000 (Fig. 4.11), it remains the second commonest global cause of secondary immunodeficiency. Globally, at the end of 2020, 37.7 million people were living with HIV. HIV is a retrovirus (p. 21) that originated in primates in Africa. It was transmitted to humans probably over 100 years ago, likely initially to hunters. HIV transmission is via sexual contact, exposure to contaminated blood, other body fluids

or blood products, or vertically from mother to baby. Although high-risk groups include those participating in anal sex and intravenous drug users, most new cases are infected through heterosexual sex.

Pathophysiology

HIV infects immune cells carrying the CD4 protein (see Fig. 4.5), including Th cells and macrophages. Because Th cells are central both to the T cell immune response and also to activating the B-cell response and antibody production, untreated HIV infection progressively disables both arms of the immune system. Over time, as immunosuppression becomes increasingly profound, opportunistic infections and characteristic malignancies develop. The progression of untreated HIV infection is shown in Fig. 4.12.

Signs and symptoms

Initial infection causes a viral-like illness that normally resolves within 2 weeks. Commonly, this involves fever, myalgia, malaise, headache, and arthralgia. At this point, the diagnosis can be missed, but symptoms suggestive of a primary HIV infection include a transient fall in circulating CD4 lymphocyte numbers, a maculopapular rash (p. 376), and the presence of mucosal ulcers. The diagnosis is confirmed if anti-HIV antibodies are detected in the blood, indicating exposure to HIV. An extended asymptomatic period follows resolution of the initial illness, during which the virus insidiously infects and destroys the body's population of CD4 cells. This stage of clinical latency can last for years, but eventually, with increasing viral load and critically low levels of functional immunity, the person begins to suffer from repeated, often severe infections. This final stage of illness is referred to as AIDS (acquired immunodeficiency syndrome) and is associated with weight loss, fever, a very low CD4 cell count (below 200 cells/mm^3), and/or the appearance of one or more AIDS-defining conditions.

HIV affects all body organs and tissues, so the range of infections and associated pathological changes is wide and very variable between patients. Because of the patient's profoundly immunosuppressed state, organisms that are normally non-pathogenic can establish themselves and cause opportunistic infection. Viral and fungal infections are frequent.

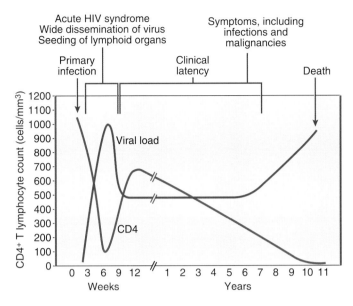

Fig. 4.12 Disease progression in untreated HIV infection. (Modified from Walker BR, Colledge NR, Ralston SH, et al. (2014) *Davidson's principles and practice of medicine*, 22nd ed, p. 394, Fig. 14.3. Churchill Livingstone Elsevier.)

Respiratory infections are common, including tuberculosis, the commonest cause of death worldwide in people who are HIV positive. Skin and mucous membranes are frequently involved, with a range of infective, ulcerative, and malignant conditions. Nervous system manifestations include central nervous system (CNS) infections and peripheral neuropathy, which arises because HIV damages nerve axons. Cardiomyopathy, arthritis, renal failure, and suppressed blood cell production are all seen.

One significant effect of HIV-associated immunosuppression is the development of HIV-related malignancies. The progressive loss of lymphocytes, including NK and Th cells, causes failure of immunological surveillance, and mutated, potentially precancerous, body cells are not killed. A characteristic of HIV infection (and an example of an AIDS-defining condition) is Kaposi's sarcoma, an otherwise rare cancer of skin and mucous membranes caused by a herpes virus. HIV-mediated immunosuppression leads to a failure to combat the virus, which establishes itself in epithelial progenitor cells and initiates the mutation that leads to the cancer. The patient develops tumours of the skin, genitals, hands, feet, and the linings of the gastrointestinal tract and lungs. The incidence of Kaposi sarcoma is 3600 times more frequent in HIV infection compared with the general population. Other HIV-associated cancers include non-Hodgkin lymphoma and cervical cancer. Cervical cancer is usually associated with human papilloma virus infection, and as with the Kaposi herpesvirus, the immunosuppression associated with HIV allows the virus to proliferate.

Management and prognosis
In 2020, AIDS-related deaths worldwide had fallen to 680,000 from the peak of 1.9 million deaths in 2004 because of the combined effects of improved treatment, wider access to treatment, and effective health education campaigns, reducing the spread of infection. When the global threat of the AIDS epidemic was recognised in the 1980s, life expectancy was only about 12 years post-infection. Provided effective antiretroviral treatment (ART) is begun early, life expectancy in HIV infection is now considered to be near normal. Current ART is very effective in suppressing viral activity. It can reduce viral load to near undetectable levels and eliminate the risk that a person who is HIV positive will transmit the infection to an uninfected sexual partner.

The onset of HIV-related complications is earlier in those with lower CD4 cell counts, in increased viral load, and in older age. Antiretroviral drugs are used in combination to reduce the development of drug resistance in the HIV virus. Current practice is to commence treatment at diagnosis, using three antiretroviral agents.

HYPERSENSITIVITY

Hypersensitivity is an inappropriate or excessive immune response, either to an infecting organism or to a harmless antigen. The main manifestations of hypersensitivity are **allergy** and **autoimmunity**. Hypersensitivity reactions also account for tissue transplant rejection and blood transfusion reactions.

THE FOUR TYPES OF HYPERSENSITIVITY

The two main weapons in the immune armoury are cytotoxic T cells and the production of antibodies, and hypersensitivity reactions involve one or both. In 1963, Gell and Coombs categorised the four types of hypersensitivity, summarised in Table 4.2 and shown in Fig. 4.13. Some hypersensitivity disorders may involve pathological processes that fall into more than one of Gell and Coombs' sections.

TYPE I HYPERSENSITIVITY

This is sometimes called *immediate hypersensitivity* because symptoms occur within minutes of exposure to the antigen. An antigen that causes allergy is called an **allergen**. Allergic responses are usually associated with type I hypersensitivity. In type I hypersensitivity, initial exposure to an allergen, which is usually in itself harmless, triggers production of IgE antibodies to that allergen. These antibodies have very high affinity for mast cells and attach themselves to mast cells membranes, displaying their allergen-binding sites and awaiting re-exposure to the allergen. When the allergen enters the tissues

Table 4.2   The Gell and Coombs classification of hypersensitivity

	Type I immediate hypersensitivity	Type II antibody-mediated hypersensitivity	Type III immune complex-mediated hypersensitivity	Type IV delayed hypersensitivity (cell-mediated)
Onset	Minutes	Minutes-hours	12–36 h	2–4 days
Immune agent	IgE	IgG	IgG	T cells
Example	Allergic rhinitis	Some drug allergies, e.g., penicillin	Serum sickness	Contact dermatitis
	Some food allergies	Blood transfusion reactions	Systemic lupus erythematosus	Rheumatoid arthritis
	Asthma	Autoimmune haemolytic anaemia	Post-streptococcal glomerulonephritis	Type 1 diabetes mellitus
	Anaphylaxis			Multiple sclerosis
				Graft rejection

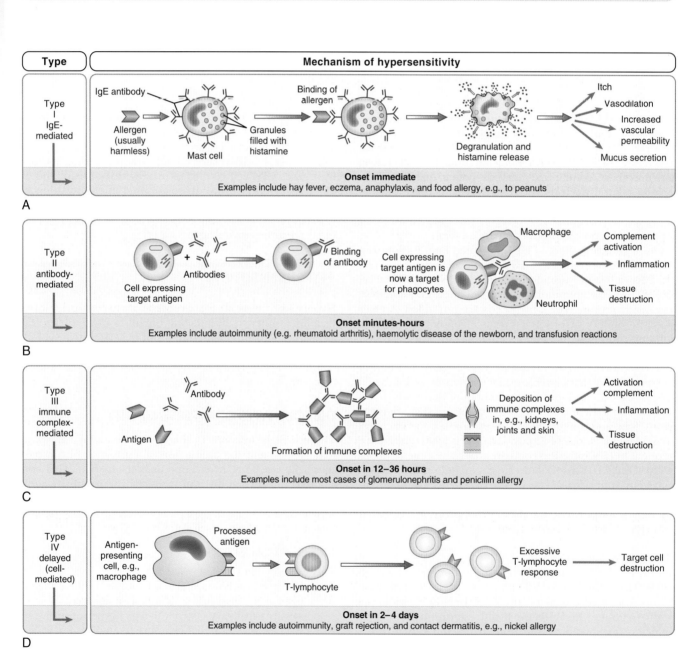

Fig. 4.13   The four mechanisms of hypersensitivity. (A) The mechanism of IgE-mediated hypersensitivity. (B) The mechanism of type II-mediated hypersensitivity. (C) The mechanism of type III-mediated hypersensitivity. (D) The mechanism of type IV-mediated hypersensitivity. (Modified from Waugh A and Grant A (2018). *Ross & Wilson anatomy and physiology in health and illness*, 13th ed, Fig 15.9. Oxford: Elsevier Ltd.)

again, it binds to the IgE on the mast cells, which respond immediately by degranulating and releasing huge amounts of histamine into body tissues (Fig. 4.13A). Histamine, an important inflammatory mediator, causes local inflammation with increased vascular permeability, vasodilation, mucus secretion, oedema, smooth muscle spasm, and itch. Mast cells are located throughout body tissues, but tissues exposed to the external environment, particularly the skin and the respiratory and gastrointestinal tracts, have dense mast cell populations and allergic reactions often involve cutaneous, respiratory, and gastrointestinal symptoms. Reactions can be localised (e.g., an insect bite or sting) or systemic if histamine levels rise in the bloodstream, affecting cardiovascular and respiratory function, and leading to the development of anaphylactic shock (see Anaphylaxis below).

TYPE II HYPERSENSITIVITY

Type II hypersensitivity is also called *antibody-type hypersensitivity* because the body produces IgG or IgM antibodies against a target molecule, often on one of the body's own cells, but sometimes to an antigenic protein on a foreign cell or in body tissues (Fig. 4.13B). By attaching to the cell-surface antigens, the antibody makes the cell a target for phagocytes, activates complement, and triggers a local inflammatory response. This form of hypersensitivity develops within minutes to hours of allergen exposure. Transfusion reactions to incompatible erythrocytes are an example of a type II hypersensitivity response. Some drug allergies (e.g., penicillin) also fall into this category.

TYPE III HYPERSENSITIVITY

This is also called *immune complex mediated hypersensitivity* and, like type II, it involves the action of IgG and IgM antibodies against a target molecule. The antibodies bind to the target, forming an immune complex. If the target molecule is fixed in the tissues, immune complexes build up at the site, activating complement and triggering inflammation and tissue destruction in the targeted tissues. If the target is travelling in the bloodstream, for example, a drug molecule, the immune complexes develop in the bloodstream and are carried in the circulation to other tissues, where they are deposited and trigger an inflammatory response there (Fig. 4.13C). Type III hypersensitivity reactions usually take about 12 hours to develop after antigen exposure. The glomerular capillaries of the kidney are common sites for immune complex deposition because the blood pressure here is four times higher than in other capillary beds, and so renal involvement is common in type III hypersensitivity conditions. Immune complexes can, however, deposit in blood vessels anywhere in the body, and cause an immune-mediated vasculitis, seen for example in systemic lupus erythematosus, systemic scleroderma or after type III drug reactions.

TYPE IV HYPERSENSITIVITY

This is also called *cell-mediated hypersensitivity* because it is characterised by the production of T cells directed against the antigen (Fig. 4.13D). It is also sometimes called *delayed-type hypersensitivity* because it is the slowest of the four types and can take days to develop because that is the time needed to activate the T cell population. Substances like nickel, household chemicals such as laundry products, dyes, some drugs, and plant substances are known sensitisers in type IV

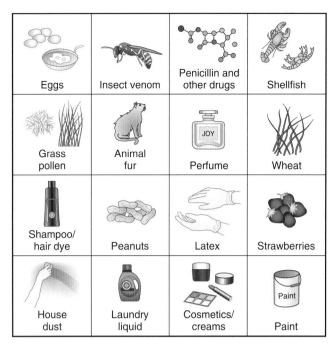

Fig. 4.14 Some common allergens.

hypersensitivity. Type IV reactions are part of the body's response to hard-to-clear infections, and many chronic inflammatory and infective disorders involve T-cell activation; they include tuberculosis and Crohn disease.

ALLERGY

Allergy is common, affecting up to 20% of the general population. Most allergy is caused by type I hypersensitivity (i.e., is IgE-mediated), but some allergies (e.g., nickel allergy, a form of contact dermatitis; see below) are type IV and are associated with T cell activation. Some other hypersensitivity reactions commonly referred to as 'allergy' (e.g., penicillin allergy; see below) can also involve type II, III, or IV responses.

Type I hypersensitivity is associated with higher-than-average levels of IgE and/or increased sensitivity to IgE. Such individuals are said to be atopic. Atopy has a strong genetic component (allergies 'run in families'). The child of two parents with allergy has a 75% chance of themselves being atopic.

Most allergens are proteins, and a wide range are associated with allergic disease: pollen, animal fur and dander (skin flakes), fungal spores, some food proteins, atmospheric pollutants, and some drugs, such as aspirin and penicillin (Fig. 4.14). Allergic disorders include asthma, food allergy and hay fever (seasonal rhinitis). Management of allergy centres on allergen avoidance and the use of antihistamines. Desensitisation therapy can be very successful, and adrenaline is used in anaphylactic emergencies (see below).

ANAPHYLAXIS

Anaphylaxis (Fig. 4.15) is severe type I hypersensitivity, usually after injection, inhalation, or ingestion of the allergen. There is respiratory compromise because histamine release causes swelling and narrowing of the respiratory passageways and swelling of the epiglottis. In addition, histamine

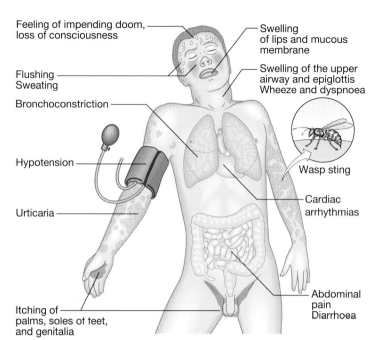

Fig. 4.15 Signs and symptoms of anaphylaxis. (Modified from Ralston S, Penman I, Strachan M, et al. (2018) *Davidson's principles and practice of medicine*, 23rd ed, Fig. 4.9. Edinburgh: Elsevier Ltd.)

contracts the smooth muscle in airway walls, causing severe bronchoconstriction. Circulating histamine causes systemic vasodilation and increased vascular permeability, so blood pressure falls rapidly as the vascular space expands and fluid leaves the bloodstream and enters the tissues. In severe cases, this cardiorespiratory compromise leads to the development of anaphylactic shock, which may be fatal if not treated. Histamine also causes a widespread itchy rash (urticaria). Treatment with adrenaline supports heart function, causes vasoconstriction, and dilates the airways.

FOOD ALLERGY

A relatively small number of food proteins, including peanuts, soy, shellfish, milk, and egg, are associated with food allergy. Peanut exposure is a particular problem because peanuts and peanut proteins are widely used in food production, and accidental exposure is common. Worldwide, food allergy is becoming more common, and current estimates suggest the incidence of food allergy is up to 10%, with the highest prevalence occurring in younger children. Risk factors include male sex and a family history of allergy.

It is not known why the incidence of food allergies, especially in children, is rising. Although the predisposition to allergy has a strong hereditable component, the rapid increase in recent decades suggests some lifestyle or environmental influence. The route by which young children are initially exposed to food antigens may be important. The immune system is programmed to tolerate antigens introduced into the gastrointestinal tract (e.g., eaten or drunk) and early oral exposure to peanut protein protects against peanut allergy. On the other hand, allergens introduced through the skin induce an immune response. Exposure to food allergens, including peanut and wheat proteins, in skin creams and in household dust increases the risk of allergy and may be a factor in the rise in peanut allergy. Other lifestyle factors affect the incidence of allergy: growing up in a family with several siblings and in the presence of pets reduces risk, and there is evidence that children who eat a

nutritionally diverse diet and who possess a diverse range of intestinal bacteria are protected against the development of food allergy.

Symptoms of food allergy include diarrhoea, intestinal cramping, nausea, and vomiting. Tingling, itching, and swelling of the lips, mouth, and throat result from the direct contact of the allergen with these tissues. If the allergen is absorbed into the bloodstream, it can cause systemic effects including skin rashes. Most seriously, anaphylaxis (Fig. 4.16) can be life threatening.

ALLERGIC RHINITIS

Depending on the allergen involved, allergic rhinitis can be either seasonal (hay fever) or perennial, which occurs all year round. Hay fever, caused by airborne grass pollen, is worse in spring and summer when the pollen count is high. Pollen is deposited on the membranes of the eye and the upper respiratory tract and triggers histamine release. Symptoms include nasal congestion and increased nasal secretions, sneezing, loss of the sense of smell, sinusitis, and itchy, runny eyes. Allergy to other airborne substances, such as animal dander, house mite faecal pellets, house dust, and fungal spores, causes similar symptoms, but all year round.

ATOPIC DERMATITIS

This is also called *atopic eczema* and is mediated by a type I hypersensitivity reaction. It may be caused by direct contact with the allergen e.g., the itchy rash from nettle stings or consumption of e.g., a food allergen.

PENICILLIN ALLERGY

The penicillin family of antibiotics is widely used, and penicillin allergy is fairly common. The allergenic portion of the molecule is the **beta lactam ring**, which also happens to be the part of the molecule essential for its antibacterial action, so all penicillins (and the related group of antibacterials, the cephalosporins) possess it. Penicillin allergy can be a type I, II, III, or IV hypersensitivity

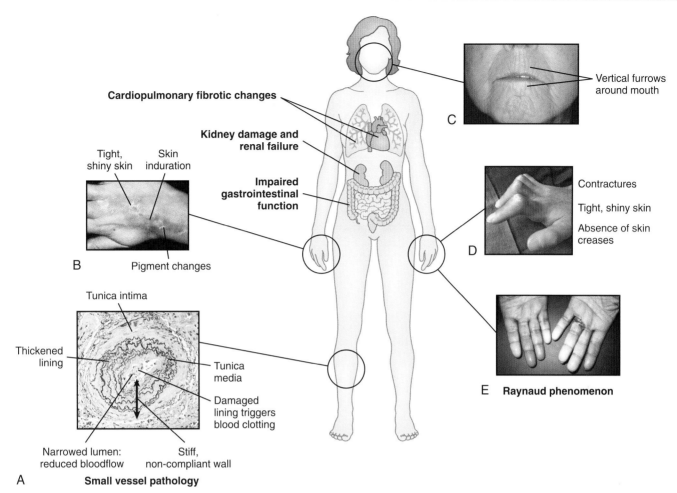

Fig. 4.16 Signs and symptoms in systemic sclerosis. (A) Blood vessel changes. (B) Skin changes. (C) Vertical furrows around the mouth. (D) Contractures. (E) Raynaud phenomenon. (Modified from (A) Silman A, Smolen J, Weinblatt M, et al. (2019) *Rheumatology*, 7th ed, Fig. 151.6. Philadelphia: Elsevier Ltd; (B) James WD, Elston D, Treat JR, et al. (2020) *Andrews' diseases of the skin*, 13th ed, Fig. e8.26. Oxford: Elsevier Inc; (C) Goldman L and Ausiello D (2004) *Cecil textbook of medicine*, 22nd ed. Philadelphia: Saunders; (D) Melone CP and Dayan E (2018) Articular surgery of the ischemic hand in systemic scleroderma: a vascular basis for arthrodesis and arthroplasty, 43(6): 574.e1–574.e9; (E) Firestein G, Budd R, Gabriel SE, et al. (2021) *Firestein & Kelley's textbook of rheumatology*, 11th ed, Fig. 89.2. San Francisco: Elsevier Inc.)

reaction. Type I hypersensitivity, caused by IgE-mediated release of histamine from mast cells, is characterised by the immediate, severe, and life-threatening anaphylactic reactions to penicillin. It is, however, relatively rare, occurring in less than 0.05% of the population. Although up to 10% of patients report penicillin allergy, the great majority of these hypersensitivity reactions are not type I, but types II, III, or IV, where the body produces IgG or IgM antibodies or targeted T cells to the beta lactam ring in the penicillin molecule. Antibody binding to the penicillin molecule triggers an inflammatory reaction, including activation of complement and phagocytic cells. Common manifestations of non-type I hypersensitivity reactions to penicillin include skin reactions, haemolytic anaemia, and kidney damage. Generally, however, these responses are not life threatening.

CONTACT DERMATITIS

Contact with any one of a whole group of otherwise harmless environmental substances can trigger a type IV (delayed hypersensitivity) reaction, causing contact dermatitis. Included in this collection are nickel (a constituent in cheap jewellery), ingredients in cosmetics, latex rubber, and plants such as poison ivy. Symptoms include the development of a red, raised, itchy rash at the contact site.

AUTOIMMUNITY

Autoimmune disorders are a group of diseases in which the immune system loses self-tolerance and produces T cells and/or antibodies to proteins and other cellular components of the body's own tissues. Mutations in HLA genes (p. 91) are almost always found in autoimmunity. It is normal to produce a certain level of autoantibodies, but in healthy people, they are found in very small quantities. Autoantibody levels increase naturally with age and are usually higher in women than men. Autoimmune disorders are usually chronic and affect a wide spectrum of body tissues and organs. Some autoimmune disorders are considered below, and others are described in chapters, but with key elements of their immunology presented in Table 4.3. Autoimmune disorders are generally commoner in females than males.

Table 4.3 Some common autoimmune disorders

	Hypersensitivity type	Key immunological effector	Effect
Diabetes mellitus (p. 257)	IV	Autoreactive T cells against the insulin-producing beta cells of the pancreas	Progressive destruction of pancreatic beta cells, eliminating the production of insulin
Myasthenia gravis (p. 328)	II	Autoantibodies target the acetylcholine (ACh) receptor at the neuromuscular junction	Progressive destruction of ACh receptors on skeletal muscle leaves it unable to respond to nerve stimulation, with weakness and paralysis afterward
Rheumatoid arthritis (p. 338)	IV	Autoreactive T cells against the synovial membrane lining synovial joints	Progressive destruction of the synovial membrane, with progressive destruction of associated bone and other joint tissues
Graves disease (p. 265)	II	Autoantibodies to the TSH receptor on the thyroid gland	The autoantibodies simulate the action of TSH, stimulating the thyroid gland to produce thyroxine, leading to hyperthyroidism
Coeliac disease (p. 298)	IV	Autoreactive T cells produced to the protein gluten, found in wheat, rye and barley	Inflammation and destruction of intestinal epithelium
Multiple sclerosis (p. 212)	IV	Autoantibodies to myelin	Patchy destruction and inflammation of the myelin sheath and associated nerves
Immune-mediated glomerulonephritis (p. 306)	III	Autoantibodies react with circulating antigens, forming immune complexes that deposit in the glomeruli	Circulating immune complexes, irrespective of the antigen involved, tend to deposit in glomerular capillary walls because of the relatively high pressure here. This triggers inflammation in the glomeruli and progressive destruction of glomerular tissues

SYSTEMIC SCLEROSIS (SCLERODERMA)

As the name suggests, this type III autoimmune disorder affects organs and tissues throughout the body. The skin is usually affected, giving the disorder the name *scleroderma*, but the term *systemic sclerosis* is preferred because a wide range of systems may be involved. It is rare, affecting 2 to 3 people per 10,000 of the population, and is much more common in females than males. People of African origin have increased susceptibility and tend to develop more serious disease. The peak incidence occurs between 50 and 60 years of age.

Pathophysiology

Both autoreactive T cells and autoantibodies have been found, although the antigen stimulating their production is not known. However, this autoimmune mechanism triggers inflammation and fibrosis in connective tissue throughout the body. Blood vessels are usually affected early in the disease, with arterioles and small arteries preferentially attacked, and they become leaky and fibrosed, and are eventually destroyed (Fig. 4.16A). The damaged endothelium of affected vessels behaves abnormally and becomes pro-thrombotic instead of anti-thrombotic. Eventually, the vessels become so damaged that blood flow is badly compromised, and tissue ischaemia and necrosis follow. Progressive, widespread inflammation leads to deposition of collagen and other fibrotic materials throughout body tissues,

frequently involving the gastrointestinal tract, heart, lungs, and kidneys.

Signs and symptoms

The presentation can be very variable (Fig. 4.16), depending on the organs involved, but skin involvement is very common, including increased or decreased pigmentation, thickening and loss of elasticity, atrophy, induration (thickening), and ulceration (Fig. 4.16B). Vertical furrows round the mouth (Fig. 4.16C) and contractures (Fig. 4.16D) may be seen. Raynaud phenomenon is common (Fig. 4.16E). Inflammation, fibrosis, and atrophy in the gastrointestinal tract lead to loss of peristalsis, with gastric reflux, constipation, and malabsorption caused by loss of villi. More than half of patients have respiratory complications, and the lungs become fibrotic and lose compliance. The work of breathing therefore increases, and the person becomes dyspnoeic. Stiffening of the lung tissue, and its blood vessels, obstructs lung blood flow and pulmonary hypertension is frequent. Over 60% of patients have renal involvement, which progressively reduces renal function and leads to serious hypertension.

Management and prognosis

There is no cure, and treatment is aimed at alleviating symptoms and reducing complications; for instance, hypertension caused by damaged kidneys should be aggressively managed. Immunosuppressants like methotrexate and, more recently, cytokine inhibitors can be useful. Although survival rates have improved, severe forms of the disease can be life-limiting, and death usually occurs from pulmonary fibrosis, pulmonary hypertension, or renal failure.

SYSTEMIC LUPUS ERYTHEMATOSUS (SLE)

This type III hypersensitivity disorder is found in all races, but there is a clear geographical and racial distribution. It is commoner in African American women (406 per 100,000) than Caucasian American women (164 per 100,000). In European countries, African and Asian women are more susceptible than whites. Of all cases, 90% are in women, and the disease usually manifests itself before the age of 40. It often follows a relapsing/remitting course and is very variable in severity between patients; some people have very mild disease, whereas at the other end of the spectrum, SLE can be life threatening.

Pathophysiology

In SLE, autoantibodies are produced against components of the cell nucleus, including DNA itself and the histones associated with it. Normally, immune cells do not come into contact with intracellular components because, protected within cells, these components are not present in body fluids or at cell surfaces. Immune cells therefore do not recognise intracellular proteins and other materials as 'self' and treat them as foreign if exposed to them. How immune cells are exposed to these intracellular materials is not fully understood, but it is believed that individuals with SLE have ineffective clearance of the cellular products of apoptosis. Apoptosis (p. 65)—programmed cell death—releases intracellular substances from within the dying cell as the cell disintegrates, but normal phagocytic mechanisms clear these materials rapidly, before immune cells have the chance to detect and respond to them. Scavenging macrophages in people with SLE are less effective, giving immune cells the opportunity to detect and react to intracellular antigens exposed on apoptotic cell fragments.

The antibodies produced form immune complexes with their target antigens. These immune complexes can be deposited almost anywhere in the body, activating complement and triggering inflammation and destruction of affected tissues. This explains why SLE affects such a wide range of organs and can present with a wide range of signs and symptoms.

Signs and symptoms

Commonly affected tissues include the skin (85% of patients), joints (90% of patients, usually the hands and wrists), and the nervous system (60%). Typical of SLE is a butterfly-shaped rash (called a *malar rash*) across the bridge of the nose and spread across the cheeks. There may be photosensitivity, a discoid rash (coin-shaped lesions), mucus membrane ulceration, and alopecia. Deposition of immune complexes in the renal glomerular capillaries causes renal failure, fluid retention, and hypertension. Immune complex deposition in the brain leads to seizures, headache, meningitis, and serious psychiatric illness, including psychosis. Inflammation of peripheral nerves can cause sensory or motor loss. Inflammatory changes in the lungs, blood vessels, heart, and gastrointestinal system cause a wide range

of signs and symptoms because function is progressively impaired (Fig. 4.17).

Management and prognosis

There is no cure for SLE, but improved care and management of the disease means that most people (80%–90%) have a normal life expectancy. Treatment focuses on anti-inflammatory therapy and newer drugs specifically targeting cytokines and B cells, suppressing antibody production.

SJÖGREN DISEASE

The aetiology of this multisystem inflammatory condition is not known, but there is evidence of altered immune function, and it frequently occurs with other autoimmune diseases, in which case it is referred to *Sjögren syndrome*. It was first described in 1933 by Dr. Henrik Sjögren and affects all known racial groups. It is relatively common, affecting up to 4% of the population, and there is a 9:1 female:male ratio. It is usually diagnosed in middle age.

Pathophysiology

What causes the chronic inflammation of this disorder is not known, but it has a known autoimmune component, and sufferers produce a wide range of autoantibodies. The trigger for the development of autoimmunity has not been identified, but one suggestion is viral infection, which leads to host cell death and damage. This in turn generates antigens that activate immune responses and sets a chronic inflammatory process in train that potentially affects all body organs. Frequently involved, however, are the salivary glands and the lacrimal glands of the eye, which become infiltrated with inflammatory cells and progressively lose their secretory function. Antibodies to acetylcholine receptors destroy the receptors and render the gland unable to respond to parasympathetic nerve stimulation (secretion of saliva is a parasympathetic function).

Extraglandular symptoms may relate to specific autoantibodies; for example, many patients have circulating rheumatoid factor (RF; p. 338), which is associated with joint disease. Formation of circulating immune complexes once the autoantibody has bound to its antigen is followed by deposition in widespread body tissues with associated inflammation.

Signs and symptoms

Very common symptoms are dry eye and dry mouth, with eye and mouth infections and dental caries frequent. However, the clinical picture is quite varied because the disorder can affect such a wide range of organs. Fatigue is a common presenting symptom, and Raynaud phenomenon and other vascular symptoms, osteoarthritis, and glomerulonephritis may occur.

Management and prognosis

There is no cure, so management is directed at providing symptomatic relief in the form of eye lubricants, adequate oral hygiene, and prompt treatment of infections.

SARCOIDOSIS

The aetiology of this multisystem inflammatory disorder is not understood. The disease is characterised by an excessive immune response to an unknown antigen. There is a

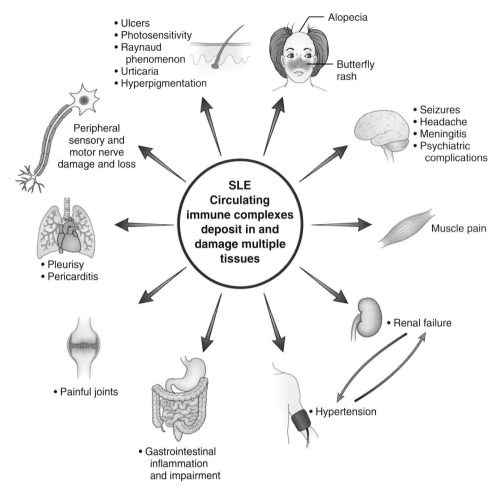

Fig. 4.17 Signs and symptoms in systemic lupus erythematosus.

seasonal variation, with more cases presenting in the spring and summer, which has led to speculation about a possible infective cause triggering the abnormal immune response. Although the condition occurs worldwide, there are significant population differences in prevalence. In Sweden, the incidence is 20 per 100 000 people, but only 1.3 per 100,000 in Japan. The incidence in black African Americans is three times higher than white Americans. Twice as many women as men are affected, and the disease tends to run a more severe course in females. There are two incidence peaks, one at 25 to 35 and another at 45 to 65 years.

Pathophysiology

Overactive T cells and activated macrophages are fundamental to the pathophysiology of this disorder. These immune cells collect in large numbers in affected tissues, and levels of cytokines associated with these cells, such as TNF and IL-2, are higher than normal. B-cell activation also occurs, and there may be increased levels of antibody. This excessive immune response triggers inflammatory changes in multiple body tissues. The lungs are involved in 90% of cases, but other tissues affected include the skin, eye, and joints. Within the lung, granulomas form, with cavitation and fibrosis.

Signs and symptoms

Pulmonary involvement gives signs and symptoms of interstitial lung disease (p. 189). There is often fatigue, fever,

and anorexia. Other symptoms depend on the tissue affected by the ongoing inflammatory response. One common feature is erythema nodosum, a form of panniculitis, which is inflammation of subcutaneous fat. It arises as red, painful, swollen nodules under the skin, usually on the shins, is associated with some autoimmune conditions, and can be caused by infections and neoplastic disease. Other systemic features include splenomegaly, arthropathies, granuloma formation in the liver, uveitis (inflammation of the uvea of the eye), and peripheral neuropathy.

Management and prognosis

Sarcoidosis is a disease of relapses and remissions, and patients may go into remission spontaneously. If inflammatory changes are troublesome, non-steroidal anti-inflammatory drugs and/or the anti-inflammatory and immunosuppressant glucocorticoids can be used.

TISSUE REJECTION

Transplanted tissues and organs, unless from a genetically identical sibling, carry cell-surface HLA antigens foreign to the recipient. This activates the immune response in the same way that entry of any foreign substance into the body does. A **graft** is defined as healthy tissue or organ transferred from one part of the body to another to replace a diseased or damaged tissue or organ, but it is also used to refer to a

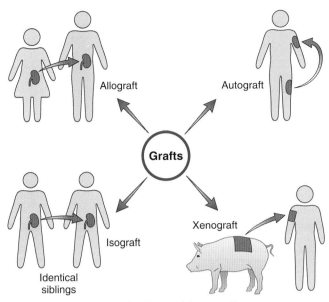

Fig. 4.18 Types of tissue graft.

healthy tissue or organ transplanted from one individual to another (Fig. 4.18). An autograft is the grafting of one part of the body to another part of the same body; a skin graft taken from the patient's thigh to cover a burn site elsewhere is an example. An allograft is a tissue or organ transplanted between two members of the same species (e.g., human to human), and the specific term *isograft* refers to transferring a tissue or organ between two genetically identical individuals. A xenograft is a tissue or organ transplanted from one species to another. The history of medicine describes multiple attempts, dating from the 18th century, to transplant skin, corneas, blood, and blood vessels, among others, from pigs, chimpanzees, and baboons, again among others, into humans. The recipients rarely survived more than a few hours. Research interest is ongoing, however, because, if the rejection problem can be overcome, xenograft technology could provide at least a partial solution towards meeting the current huge demand for transplanted tissues and organs in the treatment of, for example, liver, kidney, and heart failure.

BLOOD TRANSFUSION REACTIONS

These are type II hypersensitivity reactions. The recipient of an incompatible transfusion reaction makes IgG and IgM antibodies to non-self proteins on the surface of transfused red blood cells. Erythrocytes do not possess HLA antigens on their surface, but they do display a wide range of other surface proteins, which trigger immunological rejection in an incompatible transfusion. There are at least 30 different groups of proteins on erythrocyte membranes, but those most commonly involved in transfusion reactions are the ABO system and the Rhesus antigen.

The ABO system

This was first described by the Viennese doctor, Karl Landsteiner, who received the 1930 Nobel Prize in Physiology or Medicine for the discovery of blood groups and identifying and categorising blood into A, B, AB, or O. This is based on the distribution of two proteins, A and B, on red blood cell membranes. These proteins are referred to as *antigens* because they cause immunological rejection in incompatible transfusions. Individuals with the A antigen are blood group A, individuals with the B antigen are blood group B, individuals with A and B are blood group AB, and individuals with neither are blood group O. The presence of A and B antigens is genetically determined (i.e., they are inherited from the parents) and can be used in paternity disputes to disprove parentage. The key to understanding any blood transfusion reaction is understanding that individuals produce antibodies to foreign blood antigens but are tolerant of their own and therefore do not produce antibodies to self-antigens. Therefore, individuals with blood group A do not produce anti-A antibodies because the A antigen is a self-protein, but as antigen B is a foreign antigen, they produce antibodies to any blood cells carrying B antigens; this includes both blood groups B and AB. This is summarised in Fig. 4.19. Anti-A and anti-B antibodies, like A and B antigens, are genetically determined and naturally produced in the body and do not require T cell involvement. This explains why transfusion reactions occur so quickly.

The commonest ABO group worldwide is O⁺ (the + refers to the Rhesus antigen; see below), but as blood types are genetically inherited, there are significant population differences. So, for example, O⁺ is the commonest in the UK and in the United States, but in Denmark the commonest is A⁺ and in India it is B⁺.

Haemolytic transfusion reactions. Introducing incompatible blood into a recipient triggers rapid production of IgM antibodies to the foreign antigens on the red cell surface. The antibodies attach to erythrocyte membranes and clump the red cells together, which activates complement and destroys the clumped cells in the circulation. This leads to anaemia, and in severe cases can cause shock. In addition, clumps of partially haemolysed erythrocytes block blood flow through capillary beds, including the glomeruli in the kidney.

The rhesus antigen

Although the Rhesus antigen is conventionally named in the singular, it is actually a complex group of many proteins, of which the most important is the D protein. Individuals with the Rhesus antigen on their red cells are described as Rhesus positive, indicated by a superscript [+] over their ABO indicator. An individual with A, B, and Rhesus antigens on their red cells is therefore described as AB⁺. The absence of the Rhesus antigen is designated with a [−] superscript. Hence, an individual with A and B antigens but no Rhesus antigen is described as AB⁻. Rh⁺ status is much more common than Rh⁻.

Rhesus incompatibility. This may be the consequence of a poorly matched blood transfusion, when an Rh⁻ individual is transfused with Rh⁺ blood and produces anti-Rhesus antibodies to destroy the foreign cells. As medical systems the world over now routinely match blood transfusions, this is relatively uncommon. Much more frequently, a potential problem arises in pregnancy, when an Rh⁻ mother is carrying an Rh⁺ fetus. There is very high risk that some of the baby's blood cells may cross the placenta and enter the mother's circulation, stimulating the production of maternal anti-Rh IgG antibodies. The mother is now said to be sensitised, and these antibodies persist for life.

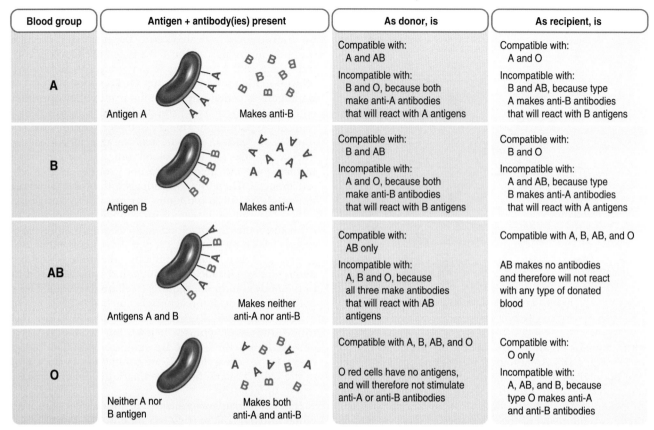

Blood group	Antigen + antibody(ies) present	As donor, is	As recipient, is
A	Antigen A / Makes anti-B	Compatible with: A and AB Incompatible with: B and O, because both make anti-A antibodies that will react with A antigens	Compatible with: A and O Incompatible with: B and AB, because type A makes anti-B antibodies that will react with B antigens
B	Antigen B / Makes anti-A	Compatible with: B and AB Incompatible with: A and O, because both make anti-B antibodies that will react with B antigens	Compatible with: B and O Incompatible with: A and AB, because type B makes anti-A antibodies that will react with A antigens
AB	Antigens A and B / Makes neither anti-A nor anti-B	Compatible with: AB only Incompatible with: A, B and O, because all three make antibodies that will react with AB antigens	Compatible with A, B, AB, and O AB makes no antibodies and therefore will not react with any type of donated blood
O	Neither A nor B antigen / Makes both anti-A and anti-B	Compatible with A, B, AB, and O O red cells have no antigens, and will therefore not stimulate anti-A or anti-B antibodies	Compatible with: O only Incompatible with: A, AB, and B, because type O makes anti-A and anti-B antibodies

Fig. 4.19   Antigens and antibodies in ABO blood grouping. (Modified from Waugh A and Grant A (2018) *Ross & Wilson anatomy and physiology in health and illness*, 13th ed, Fig. 4.8. Oxford: Elsevier Ltd.)

Nearly always, the mixing of fetal and maternal blood occurs at delivery when the trauma of the placenta detaching from the uterine wall tears the placental membranes that separate the maternal and fetal circulations. With a first pregnancy, the baby is safely delivered by the time anti-Rh antibodies rise in the mother's circulation, and the baby is unharmed. However, subsequent pregnancies with an Rh⁺ fetus are affected. Anti-Rh antibodies cross the placenta from the mother's bloodstream and attach to the fetal erythrocytes, triggering haemolysis. The baby therefore becomes anaemic and may die in the womb or suffer from varying degrees of anaemia at birth. The condition is called *haemolytic disease of the newborn* (Fig. 4.20). It may be mild, but in severe cases the strain on the baby's heart associated with the anaemia may cause cardiovascular failure and shock. Haemolysis releases large amounts of haemoglobin, which is converted to bilirubin in the liver, causing jaundice in the baby. Deposition of bilirubin in the central nervous system damages the brain and may cause permanent developmental impairment or death of the child.

The severity of Rh incompatibility varies. Many Rh⁻ individuals fail to produce anti-Rh antibodies, even after challenge. However, anti-Rh antibodies rise with each subsequent Rh⁺ pregnancy, and a Rhesus incompatibility is more likely to be serious if the mother and fetus also have different ABO blood groups.

ORGAN/GRAFT REJECTION

The kidney was the first organ to be transplanted into a human recipient. In 1954, after decades of failed attempts, a kidney transplant was performed in Boston, Massachusetts, USA, between two identical twins, and the recipient twin survived for 8 years, eventually dying of a cardiac event. In all transplant attempts before this, the grafted kidneys had always rapidly failed, even if they had functioned normally immediately post-operatively. The immunology behind organ rejection was not understood, although the 1954 medical team had reasoned that, whatever the biological barriers to transplant were, they were likely to be much lower in identical twins. The use of immunosuppressants to delay or prevent the onset of rejection only began in the 1960s and was a major step in improving survival after transplantation. Our understanding of transplant biology is largely based on the body of work done in kidney transplant research because the kidney is the most frequently transplanted organ.

Pathophysiology

T cells are central to graft rejection, which is classified as a type IV hypersensitivity reaction. Graft rejection is a much more powerful reaction than the immune response to pathogenic organisms because there are large numbers of allograft-recognising T cells. When cells carrying foreign HLA antigens are transferred to another person, T cells are activated, followed by B-cell activation and antibody production, all against the non-self HLA proteins.

T cells and rejection. Both Tc and Th cells are involved in T cell-mediated graft rejection. Tc cells directly attack and kill the graft cells. Th cells produce a range of cytokines and

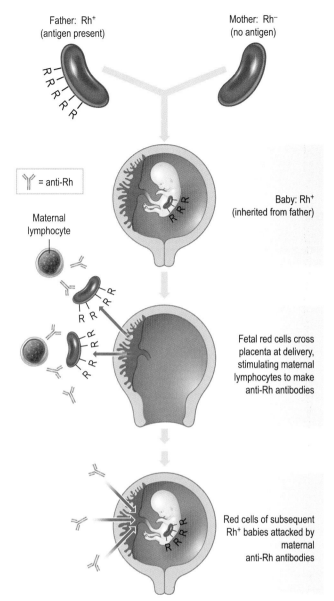

Fig. 4.20 Haemolytic disease of the newborn. (Waugh A, and Grant A, 2018, *Ross & Wilson anatomy and physiology in health and illness*, 13th ed, Oxford, Elsevier Ltd, Fig. 4.18.)

Father: Rh⁺
(antigen present)

Mother: Rh⁻
(no antigen)

= anti-Rh

Maternal
lymphocyte

Baby: Rh⁺
(inherited from father)

Fetal red cells cross
placenta at delivery,
stimulating maternal
lymphocytes to make
anti-Rh antibodies

Red cells of subsequent
Rh⁺ babies attacked by
maternal
anti-Rh antibodies

immune stimulants, which recruit and activate defence cells and inflammation at the transplant site.

Antibody-mediated rejection. Antibodies are also important in rejecting a foreign graft. Whereas the T cell response usually takes 2 or 3 days to manifest itself, if the graft recipient already has circulating antibodies to the transplanted tissue, rejection begins at once. Blood transfusion reactions are an example because antibodies to foreign red blood cell antigens are genetically determined and do not depend on pre-sensitisation. Therefore, for example, an individual with type A blood naturally produces anti-B antibodies

(see above), which attack any foreign erythrocytes displaying the B antigen as soon as transfusion begins. If a mother is exposed to fetal antigens during pregnancy or during birth, she will make antibodies to those antigens. If later in life she receives a graft from that child, her pre-formed antibodies lead to rapid graft destruction. This rapid rejection is rare nowadays because of careful cross-matching before transplantation; potential antibody-mediated rejection is picked up in advance, and the graft identified as incompatible.

Signs and symptoms

Acute rejection occurs days or weeks after transplant. T cells directed against the graft attack it and its associated blood vessels, causing ischaemia and necrosis. Activation of complement and macrophages cause swelling, infiltration of the graft with inflammatory cells, and progressive cell death. Chronic rejection can occur over a period of months to years. An important feature of this is progressive destruction of the graft's blood supply, with inflammation and thickening of blood vessel walls, and eventual obstruction of blood flow. The graft therefore becomes ischaemic and necrotic. Unlike acute rejection, which can often be significantly delayed with modern immunosuppressant treatment, chronic rejection is difficult to manage and there is little that currently can be done to prevent it.

Management and prognosis

Careful pre-transplant screening to ensure as close a match as possible between the host and donor HLA proteins improves the survival prospects of grafts. Immunosuppressant treatment is always required (except in isografts, where the HLA proteins are identical in both donor and recipients). In time, however, the graft almost always fails as chronic rejection processes destroy it. Graft and patient survival times have been steadily increasing over the past 60 years and vary according to the health of the patient at time of transplant and the closeness of the graft match. Sometimes graft failure occurs because the disease that caused the original organ to fail affects the transplanted organ.

BIBLIOGRAPHY AND REFERENCES

Arnold, D. E., & Heilmall, J. R. (2017). A review of chronic granulomatous disease. *Advances in Therapy, 34,* 2543–2557.

Helbert, M. (2017). *Immunology for medical students* (3rd ed.). Elsevier.

Legendre, D. P., Muzny, C. A., Marshall, G. D., et al. (2014). Antibiotic hypersensitivity reactions and approaches to desensitization. *Clinical Infectious Diseases, 58*(8), 1140–1148.

Loh, W., & Tang, M. L. K. (2018). The epidemiology of food allergy in the global context. *International Journal of Environmental Research and Public Health, 15*(9), 204–20.

Male, D., Peebles, S., & Male, V. (Eds.). (2020). *Immunology* (9th ed.) Elsevier.

McCusker, C., & Warrington, R. (2011). Primary immunodeficiency. *Allergy, Asthma and Clinical Immunology, 7*(Suppl. 1), S11–S20.

Rich, R. R., Fleisher, T. A., Shearer, W. T., et al. (Eds.). (2019). *Clinical immunology principles and practice* (5th ed.) Elsevier.

Sicherer, S. H., & Sampson, H. A. (2018). Food allergy: A review and update on epidemiology, pathogenesis, diagnosis, prevention and management. *The Journal of Allergy and Clinical Immunology, 141*(1), 41–59.

Disorders of Blood

CHAPTER OUTLINE

INTRODUCTION
  Plasma
The developmental tree of blood cells
  Erythrocytes
  Platelets
  Leukocytes
MALIGNANCIES OF WHITE BLOOD CELLS
The leukaemias
  Acute myeloid leukaemia (AML)
  Chronic myeloid (myelogenous) leukaemia (CML)
  Acute lymphoblastic leukaemia (ALL)
  Chronic lymphocytic leukaemia (CLL)
The lymphomas
  Hodgkin lymphoma (HL)
  Non-Hodgkin lymphoma (NHL)
Myeloma (multiple myeloma)
RED BLOOD CELL DISORDERS

Proliferative erythrocyte disorders
  Polycythaemia vera
The anaemias
  Haemolytic anaemias
  Anaemias secondary to reduced erythrocyte production
CLOTTING DISORDERS
Thrombotic disorders
  Arterial thrombosis
  Venous thrombosis
  Disseminated intravascular coagulation (DIC)
Inherited coagulation deficiencies
  von Willebrand disease (vWD)
Acquired coagulation deficiencies
  Coagulopathy of acute trauma
  Vitamin K deficiency
  Acquired platelet deficiencies

INTRODUCTION

Blood cell formation (**haemopoiesis**) begins in the first few weeks of embryonic development with the production of haematopoietic stem cells located initially in the liver and shifting to the bone marrow in the fourth month of pregnancy. In children, red bone marrow rich in haematopoietic stem cells is located throughout the skeleton, but by adulthood its distribution is restricted to the ends of long bones and within flat and irregular bones. Total blood in the average adult is in the order of about one eighth of body weight, so larger people usually have a larger blood volume than smaller people. On average, total blood volume in a healthy adult is around 5 L.

Blood is an essential transport medium, carrying oxygen and nutrients to body cells and removing wastes. It transports hormones, drugs, antibodies, and white blood cells for protection and immunity. Blood regulates the water concentration of extracellular and intracellular fluids because water in the blood exchanges freely across capillary and cell membranes. Blood samples can be separated by gravity or by centrifugal force in a laboratory into two discrete phases: a fluid phase, called **plasma**, which is mainly water with dissolved and suspended substances; and the **cellular** phase, containing erythrocytes, leukocytes, and platelets.

PLASMA

Plasma is 90% water. It is clear and pale yellow. Plasma proteins, mainly produced in the liver, account for 7% of plasma volume. **Albumins** are the most abundant plasma proteins (60%) and are the main contributors to the maintenance of plasma colloid osmotic pressure. They also act as transport proteins, binding and transporting drugs, bilirubin, hormones, and fatty acids. **Globulins**, accounting for about 35% of the total, are mainly immunoglobulins (antibodies, p. 92), produced by B cells. Other important plasma proteins are the clotting proteins, of which **fibrinogen** is the most abundant, and some specialised transport proteins, including **transferrin**, which carries iron and hormone specific transport proteins (e.g., **thyroid-binding protein**, which carries thyroxine).

THE DEVELOPMENTAL TREE OF BLOOD CELLS

At birth, red bone marrow contains a large population of pluripotent stem cells: non-specialised cells that continually divide, constantly replenishing themselves. Some of these stem cells differentiate into myeloid stem cells, which in turn commit to one of several developmental pathways to become erythrocytes, megakaryocytes (which produce platelets), granulocytes, or monocytes. Other stem cells differentiate into lymphoid progenitor cells, which divide and produce cells committed to becoming B cells, T cells, or natural killer (NK) cells (Fig. 5.1).

ERYTHROCYTES

Erythrocytes (red blood cells) are small (7 μm diameter), flattened discs with no nuclei but which are packed with haemoglobin, the blood's oxygen transport protein. The normal erythrocyte count in whole blood is 4.5 to 6.5 million/mm³ in adult males and 3.8 to 5.8 million/mm³ in females. Having no nucleus, they cannot divide, so red cell numbers are kept within the normal range by balancing production (about 2 million new red cells are produced every second) with destruction. Old and worn-out red cells are trapped in specialised tissues in the spleen and liver, removed from the circulation and broken down.

The life cycle of red blood cells is shown in Fig. 5.2. The process of erythrocyte production from a stem cell takes about 7 days. When released into the bloodstream, the erythrocyte is still not fully mature and is called a **reticulocyte**, which completes its maturation during its first week or so in the bloodstream.

Haemoglobin production

Each erythrocyte contains approximately 280 million molecules of **haemoglobin** (Hb, Fig. 5.3A). The haemoglobin molecule is made of four protein chains (two α and two β chains) wrapped in a specific three-dimensional structure. Each protein chain incorporates an iron atom, which binds an oxygen molecule; therefore each haemoglobin molecule can bind up to four molecules of oxygen. Iron in haemoglobin is in the ferrous state (Fe^{2+}) state, which is essential to its capacity to bind oxygen. The ferrous ions are prevented from oxidising to the physiologically inactive ferric (Fe^{3+}) form by the enzyme glucose-6-phosphate dehydrogenase in red blood cells (Fig. 5.3B).

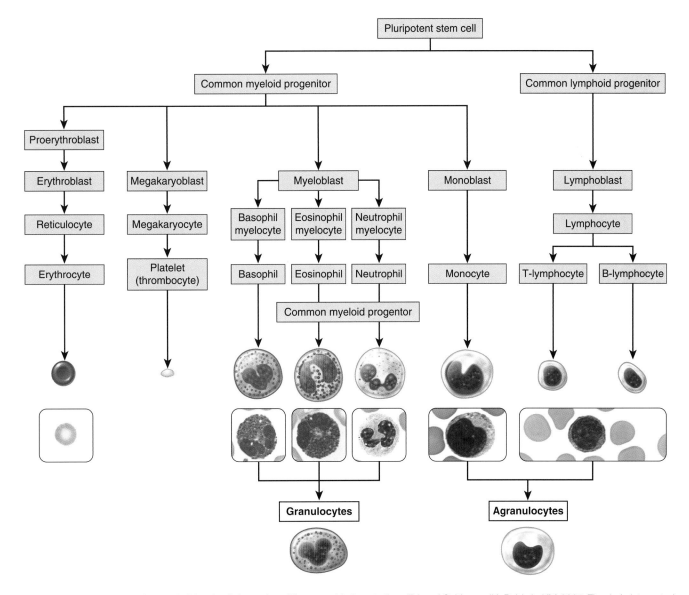

Fig. 5.1 Development pathways in blood cell formation. (Photographic inserts from Telser AG, Young JK, Baldwin KM 2007 *Elsevier's integrated histology*. Mosby: Edinburgh; and Young B, Lowe JS, Stevens A et al. 2006 *Wheater's functional histology: a text and colour atlas*. Edinburgh: Churchill Livingstone. Reproduced with permission.)

Iron absorption and metabolism

The haemoglobin in circulating erythrocytes contains 70% of the body's iron; 5% is found in **myoglobin**, the oxygen-binding protein found in muscle, and the remaining 25% in storage sites, mainly liver and bone marrow. Iron is absorbed by specific carrier mechanisms in the small intestine and is transported to the liver and bone marrow bound to **transferrin**. The body has no specific mechanisms for excreting iron, so iron levels are regulated by controlling absorption, which in turn is regulated according to the body's needs. In iron deficiency, iron absorption increases, and when iron levels are adequate, iron absorption is reduced.

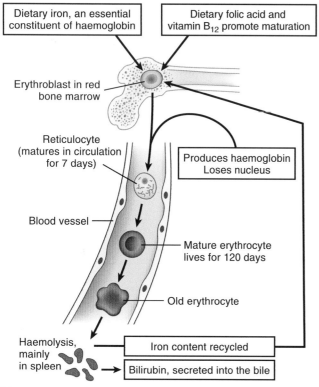

Fig. 5.2 The life cycle of the erythrocyte. (Modified from Waugh A and Grant A (2018) *Ross & Wilson anatomy and physiology in health and illness*, 13th ed, Fig. 4.5. Oxford: Elsevier Ltd.)

Control of erythrocyte production

As mature erythrocytes have no nucleus, they cannot divide, so erythrocyte numbers in the blood are regulated by controlling the rate at which they are produced in the bone marrow. Key to this mechanism is the kidney, which contains specialised oxygen-sensitive cells that detect hypoxia. When oxygen levels in the renal blood flow fall, the kidney responds by producing the hormone **erythropoietin** and releasing it into the bloodstream. In the bone marrow, erythropoietin increases the rate at which reticulocytes are released into the bloodstream.

PLATELETS

These small, irregularly shaped cell fragments are released from megakaryocytes in the red bone marrow. They have no nucleus but are packed with dense granules containing clotting factors: adenosine diphosphate and serotonin. The platelet also contains actin and myosin filaments, which actively contract after clot formation to expel fluid and promote sealing of the wound. After tissue injury, platelets are activated and accumulate at areas of blood vessel damage, where their function is to form a clot and control bleeding. Activation of clotting factors, including fibrinogen, contributes to the clotting cascade and clot formation. Serotonin is a vasoconstrictor, reducing blood vessel diameter and blood flow through injured tissues, and ADP triggers platelet activation, promoting the positive feedback loop in the clotting cascade. The normal platelet count in healthy adults is 200,000 to 350,000/mm^3. At the end of their lifespan (8–9 days), old and worn-out platelets are removed from the circulation by the spleen.

Blood clotting

The clotting cascade is driven by positive feedback, so once it has been initiated, it is self-perpetuating. Table 5.1 lists the clotting factors involved, and their main roles in clotting. Many of these clotting factors are proenzymes, meaning that they are enzymes circulating in their inactive form. When clotting is activated, these proenzymes activate each other in a controlled and predictable sequence. Clotting can be described in three stages: the vascular stage, the platelet stage, and the coagulation stage.

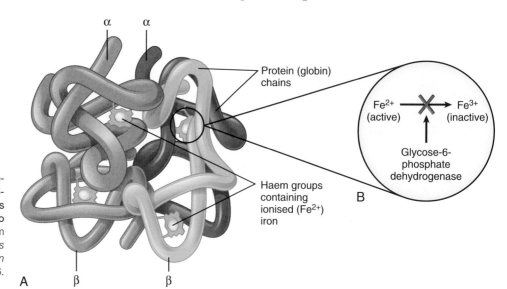

Fig. 5.3 Haemoglobin. (A) The haemoglobin molecule. (B) Glucose-6-phospate dehydrogenase prevents the conversion of ferrous ions to inactive ferric ions. (Modified from Waugh A and Grant A (2018) *Ross & Wilson anatomy and physiology in health and illness*, 13th ed, Fig. 4.6. Oxford: Elsevier Ltd.)

Table 5.1 Clotting factors

Factor	Remarks
I/Ia	*Fibrinogen/fibrin*
II/IIa	*Prothrombin/thrombin (proenzyme/enzyme).* Prothrombin, the inactive form of the enzyme, is made in the liver and its synthesis requires vitamin K. Thrombin converts fibrinogen to fibrin.
III	*Tissue factor (TF).* This is a glycoprotein in cell membranes of tissue cells and is required to activate FVII in the extrinsic pathway.
IV	Ca^{2+} *ions.* These are required as cofactors in converting some of the clotting proenzymes to enzymes.
V	*Labile factor.* This is made in the liver and is one of the clotting factors released by platelets when they are activated.
VII/VIIa	*Stable factor.* FVII is made in the liver and its synthesis requires vitamin K. FVIIa is an enzyme of the extrinsic pathway that activates FX.
VIII/VIIIa	*Anti-haemophilic factor.* FVIIIa is an enzyme that works with FIXa in the intrinsic pathway to activate FX.
IX/IXa	*Christmas factor.* FIX is made in the liver and its synthesis requires vitamin K. FIXa is an enzyme that works with FVIIIa in the intrinsic pathway to activate FX.
X/Xa	*Stuart factor.* FX is made in the liver and its synthesis requires vitamin K. FXa is an enzyme that converts prothrombin to thrombin, the first step in the final common pathway.
XI/XIa	FXI is released by platelets in the clotting cascade. FXIa activates FIX in the intrinsic pathway.
XII/XIIa	*Hageman factor.* FXIIa activates FXI in the intrinsic pathway.
Von Willebrand factor	Found in platelets and released when the platelet is activated. Stabilises FVIIIa in the intrinsic pathway.

Those clotting factors present in both inactive and active forms are indicated. The suffix 'a' indicates the active form.

The vascular stage. When tissue injury damages blood vessels, the smooth muscle in the tunica media constricts in response to substances released by the damaged tissues. This reduces blood flow and is an immediate mechanism by which blood loss is minimised. The endothelial cells lining the vessel release pro-coagulation substances, including von Willebrand factor, which together attract and activate platelets.

The platelet stage. Platelets do not stick to normal healthy endothelium. However, blood vessel injury damages the endothelium and exposes platelets to the deeper tissues of the blood vessel wall, including collagen. Platelets adhere to collagen, are activated, and release their pro-clotting contents, including serotonin, von Willebrand factor, and ADP. They also release growth factors, including platelet-derived growth factor, which support healing and repair. Activated platelets stick to each other, so a fast-growing platelet mass accumulates at the site of injury. This platelet plug is soft and easily disrupted, but it provides a short-term seal and is the foundation for the sturdier clot that begins to form within minutes of injury.

The coagulation stage. Activated platelets bind fibrinogen, which is the precursor of fibrin that forms the framework of the final clot. Conversion of fibrinogen to fibrin is the final event in the clotting cascade and happens in the coagulation stage as clotting factors activate each other in a pre-set sequence. Fibrinogen is converted to fibrin via one of two pathways: the **intrinsic** and the **extrinsic** (Fig. 5.4). The intrinsic pathway, which is slower but more effective than the extrinsic, is triggered within the bloodstream (hence 'intrinsic') when Factor XII is activated by contact with platelet membranes. Activated Factor XII is an enzyme, which actives the proenzyme Factor XI, which in turn activates Factor IX, which, along with activated Factor VIII, activates Factor X. The extrinsic pathway is activated when Factor III (tissue factor) activates Factor VII, which in turn activates Factor X. Calcium is an essential cofactor in both pathways.

The result of activation of either clotting pathway is activation of Factor X. It is the first event in the **final common pathway**, which culminates in the conversion of fibrinogen to fibrin. Factor X activates a proenzyme called *prothrombin* and converts it to the active enzyme thrombin, which converts fibrinogen to fibrin. Fibrin threads are insoluble and sticky; they adhere to one another, the blood vessel wall, and to blood cells, glueing the components of the platelet plug together and producing the much stronger clot, a dense network packed with trapped platelets and red blood cells that seals the injured blood vessel wall. The actin and myosin in the platelets then contract, squeezing excess fluid from the clot and helping to pull the wound edges closer together, promoting healing.

Clotting is, therefore, a complex affair. The major advantage to cascade systems like this is the progressive amplification of the response at each stage of the cascade. Small quantities of active Factor XII, for example, rapidly generate large quantities of active Factor XI, which in turn rapidly generates even larger quantities of Factor IX, and so on.

Clotting control and fibrinolysis

The smooth, low-friction endothelial lining of blood vessels is important in preventing inappropriate clotting. Blood flow over healthy endothelium is smooth and non-turbulent. Endothelial damage, for example in trauma or atherosclerosis, may trigger clotting at the site. The clotting cascade is self-perpetuating to ensure as rapid a halt to bleeding as possible, but it still needs to be controlled so that it is terminated when appropriate. Endothelial cells at the site of injury release anticoagulants such as **antithrombin** that act as brakes on the clotting cascade. Activation of other key inhibitors of clotting, such as protein C and protein S, also dampen down clotting activity. The finished clot needs to be stable enough to provide a strong seal in the blood vessel wall, but as healing begins within a few hours of injury, there must also be mechanisms to break it down and remove it as tissues regenerate and repair. The main enzyme responsible for controlled dissolution of the clot is **plasmin**. Plasmin is released from its inactive precursor, plasminogen, by plasminogen activators such as tissue plasminogen activator.

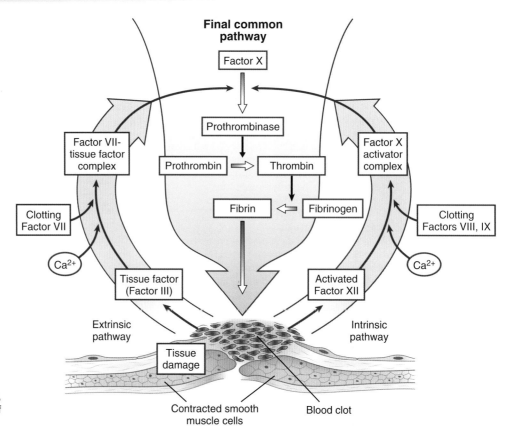

Fig. 5.4 The intrinsic, extrinsic, and final common pathways of clotting.

LEUKOCYTES

Leukocytes (leuko = white, cyte = cell), or white blood cells, are essential components of the body's defence and immunity systems (see also Chapter 4). They are broadly classified into the granulocytes (these cells contain granules in their cytoplasm: neutrophils, eosinophils, and basophils) and agranulocytes (with no granules: monocytes and lymphocytes).

MALIGNANCIES OF WHITE BLOOD CELLS

As with other cancers, white blood cell cancers are a result of malignant transformation of a single white blood cell precursor or, sometimes, of a mature cell. This cell then proliferates, producing an expanding population of cancer cells. The cell of origin may be in the bone marrow, where most white cells are produced, or in lymphoid tissue, where some white cells are produced and where many are resident. Often, but not always, the cancerous cells show up in the bloodstream.

The classification system for malignant diseases of white blood cells is complex and based on the cell of origin, its stage of development at the point of malignant transformation, and the timescale involved in disease development (acute or chronic). **Lymphoid malignancies** arise from precursor cells in T-cell, B-cell, or NK cell development; and **myeloid malignancies** arise from precursors of granular white blood cells, platelets, or erythrocytes. Additionally, descriptive terminology identifies whether the neoplastic cells are found mainly in the blood (**leukaemias**) or form solid tumours in lymphatic tissues, including lymph nodes (**lymphomas**). The boundaries between the classifications can be fluid, and disease that is initially chronic and slow

developing may transform into a rapidly progressive acute form. Presentations can be very variable; for example, some lymphomas, presenting as solid tumours in lymphoid tissue, have significant leukaemic features (i.e., with many abnormal cells in the peripheral blood), whereas in other lymphomas, the peripheral blood picture may be close to normal.

Multiple genetic abnormalities are associated with blood malignancies, mainly translocation abnormalities of chromosomes (p. 54) containing key genes regulating blood cell differentiation, growth or survival. Some disorders associated with genetic instability (e.g., Down syndrome and Fanconi anaemia) increase the risk of developing acute leukaemia. Key genetic markers may be so characteristic of a particular leukaemia or lymphoma that they give the diagnosis. They are also useful in monitoring the response to therapy: checking for the presence of residual cancer cells bearing the genetic abnormality is done with cytogenetic analysis and determines the efficacy of treatment and identifies periods of remission. Some viral infections (e.g., HIV and Epstein-Barr virus) increase the risk of certain lymphomas. Viruses replicate by inserting their DNA into the genome of the infected cell, leading to mutation and genetic instability, and increasing the risk of malignant transformation. Other factors, such as chronic inflammation and exposure to carcinogenic stimuli (smoking, radiation, carcinogenic chemicals, chemotherapeutic agents), increase the general risk of cancer, including blood malignancies.

THE LEUKAEMIAS

The leukaemias are not common forms of cancer, accounting for less than 3% of all new cases globally, and their

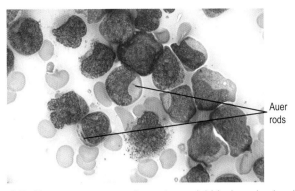

Auer rods

Fig. 5.5 Bone marrow smear in acute myeloid leukaemia showing large abnormal blast cells, some with Auer rods. (Modified from Rozenberg G (2011) *Microscopic haematology*, 3rd ed, Fig. B6-18. Sydney: Elsevier Australia.)

incidence is low in most populations. Distinguishing between acute and chronic leukaemias, and the cell of origin (myeloid or lymphoid) is the basis of the traditional classification system. Acute leukaemias are generally associated with a white cell population in the blood or bone marrow containing over 20% immature blast cells, and although they tend to arise rapidly and follow an aggressive course, they often respond better to treatment than chronic leukaemias. Chronic leukaemias develop slowly and may cause only minor signs and symptoms over extended periods of time (years). Acute myeloid leukaemia is much commoner than acute lymphoblastic leukaemia in adults, but it is the other way round in children, in whom acute lymphoblastic leukaemia is much more common. Common to both acute and chronic forms is bone marrow failure and white cell infiltration of many body organs, including the liver, brain, and testes.

ACUTE MYELOID LEUKAEMIA (AML)

AML is not a single disease, because of the complexity of the differentiation pathways of myeloid cells, and is divided into a number of subtypes according to genetic changes and histological features present. It is more common in men than women, the risk increases with age, and it is more common in white than non-white people. The peak age for presentation is 80 years. Most patients present with no known risk factors, so the underlying cause in these people is not identified. Known risk factors include pre-existing bone marrow disease, pre-existing genetic disorder (e.g., Down syndrome), and exposure to known carcinogens (e.g., smoking, benzene, chemotherapeutic drugs, and radiation). This latter includes therapeutic radiation, so people treated with radiotherapy for other malignancies have an increased risk of AML in later life. AML is a rare disease, with prevalence across all ages, genders, and ethnicities estimated as between 0.2 to 13 per 100,000 of the population.

Pathophysiology

The affected cells—myeloid progenitors—are arrested in their development early in the developmental pathway. Recall that myeloid precursors give rise to granulocytes, erythrocytes, and megakaryocytes (see Fig. 5.1) so that the production of these cells stops, leading to anaemia, neutropenia, and thrombocytopenia. In addition, the abnormal myeloblasts proliferate even though their progress down their developmental pathways is blocked, so that they accumulate in the bone marrow and cause bone marrow failure. They spill into the blood and collect in and damage the liver and spleen. They do not undergo normal apoptosis (p. 65), contributing to the great expansion in their numbers.

Several genetic abnormalities have been associated with AML. The commonest involve chromosomes 8 and 16 and cause the loss of a key protein essential for normal myeloid development. Knowledge of the genetic abnormality present is essential when making treatment decisions because different subtypes respond differently to different treatment regimens. It also informs prognosis: some of the most significant genetic abnormalities—such as deletions of entire chromosomes—are associated with very poor outcomes.

Diagnosis depends on the presence of at least 20% blast cells in the bone marrow. Blast cells are large, immature, and clearly abnormal when viewed under the microscope. AML blast cells are characterised by Auer rods, distinctive dark-staining linear structures in the cytoplasm (Fig. 5.5).

Signs and symptoms

The bone marrow fails as the malignant myeloblasts proliferate and fill the bone spaces, replacing all normal haematopoietic tissue. This leads to anaemia, neutropenia, and thrombocytopenia. Anaemia causes fatigue, breathlessness, and dyspnoea as body tissues become hypoxic. Neutropenia leads to increased risk of infections (Fig. 5.6). Thrombocytopenia causes inappropriate bleeding and an inability to clot after blood vessel injury. Tissues become infiltrated with the proliferating myeloblasts, causing pain, swelling, and damage in the affected organ; for example, the liver can enlarge and become tender, and accumulation of myeloblasts in the central nervous system can compress nerves—impairing their function—or cause headache. Expansion of bone marrow can cause bone pain.

Management and prognosis

If not treated, AML is always rapidly fatal. The prognosis with treatment varies considerably, depending on the patient's age and state of health, their white cell count at presentation, and the subtype of AML present. Relapse is common. Children have a better outlook than adults; two thirds of patients under 20 survive for at least 5 years. Five-year survival in the 20- to 64-year-old age group is less than 40% and falls to 5% in those over 65. Decisions are made at diagnosis regarding the likely success of treatment. Curative treatment (including chemotherapy and stem cell transplant) is offered if cure is considered possible, but it is aggressive, extended and itself carries a significant risk of death. If cure is not deemed likely, palliative treatment to manage symptoms is the alternative course.

CHRONIC MYELOID (MYELOGENOUS) LEUKAEMIA (CML)

This form accounts for up to 20% of all cases of leukaemia. It is twice as common in males than females, and the peak age for presentation is 55 years. As with AML, the affected cell is a myeloid precursor, so production of erythrocytes, granulocytes, and platelets is affected, although granulocyte production is most significantly reduced.

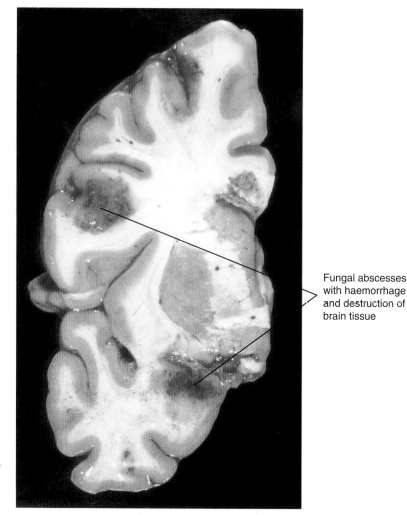

Fungal abscesses with haemorrhage and destruction of brain tissue

Fig. 5.6 Multiple fungal brain abscesses in acute myeloid leukaemia. (Modified from Cross S (2013) *Underwood's pathology: a clinical approach*, 6th ed, Fig. 23.31C. Oxford: Elsevier Ltd.)

Pathophysiology

CML is an acquired disorder associated with exchange of material (translocation, p. 54) between chromosomes 9 and 22. The terminal sections of the long arms of these two chromosomes swap over. These sections are not of equal length. The section of chromosome 22 that becomes attached to chromosome 9 is longer than the section of chromosome 22 that attaches to chromosome 22 so that chromosome 9 becomes longer than it should be and chromosome 22 becomes shorter. The abnormal, shortened chromosome 22 is called the **Philadelphia chromosome**, after the city where it was first described (Fig. 5.7). The result of this exchange creates a new fusion gene called the bcr-abl gene on chromosome 22, which codes for a new fusion protein that causes the development of CML, although the mechanism is not understood. The presence of the Philadelphia chromosome is diagnostic for CML. The initiating factors creating the abnormal Philadelphia chromosome are not known, although radiation is likely to be one because the incidence of CML increased in survivors of the Nagasaki and Hiroshima atomic bombs.

Signs and symptoms

There are three stages in CML progression. In the first, the chronic stage, there may be no symptoms, although anaemia may cause fatigue, weight loss, and reduced exercise tolerance. Neutropenia may cause fevers and infections. Platelet deficiency is fairly uncommon in these early stages, and therefore bleeding times are usually normal. There may be abdominal discomfort if the liver or spleen is infiltrated with myeloblasts. The chronic stage can last several years. However, if it is not recognised and treated, or if treatment is ineffective, it always progresses, sometimes through an accelerated phase, with evidence of more malignant change, to the third stage of blast crisis. Blast crisis is the transformation into acute leukaemia; most (70%) are AML and the remaining 30% acute lymphoblastic leukaemia. At this point, prognosis becomes significantly poorer.

Management and prognosis

Although the early stage of CML is often characterised by the non-specific signs and symptoms described previously, or may indeed be asymptomatic, it requires treatment to prevent development into blast crisis. The most significant treatment advance in recent years is the development of several biological drugs, including **imatinib**, that specifically target the fusion protein produced by the abnormal fusion gene on chromosome 22. Blocking the effect of this protein produces complete remission in over 95% of patients. Once blast crisis has occurred, stem cell transplant is the only useful option. Blast crisis is usually fatal.

NORMAL   **AFTER TRANSLOCATION**

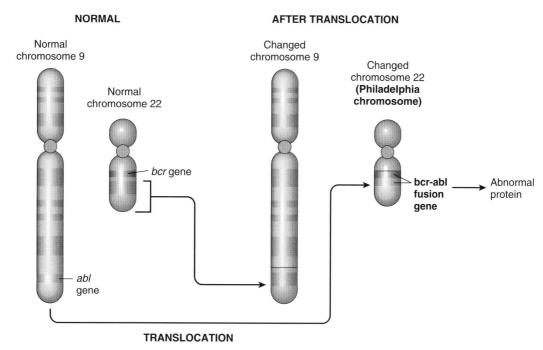

Fig. 5.7   Formation of the Philadelphia chromosome. (Modified from Chabner DE (2021) *The language of medicine*, 12th ed, Fig. 19.5. St Louis: Saunders.)

ACUTE LYMPHOBLASTIC LEUKAEMIA (ALL)

ALL is the commonest cancer in children (75% of cases occur under the age of 6 years) and is characterised by the production of large number of immature B or T cells, whose development has been arrested at the lymphoblast stage. B-cell leukaemias account for 85% of all ALLs and generally appear in childhood; both sexes are equally affected. T-cell ALLs are commonest in adolescent males. The presentation can be variable; sometimes the abnormal cells are present primarily in the bone marrow and in the blood (leukaemic presentation), but there may also be solid tumours, commonly a mediastinal mass caused by the involvement of the thymus gland in T-cell ALL (lymphoma presentation).

Pathophysiology

The malignant lymphoblasts proliferate in the bone marrow, eliminating normal haematopoietic tissue; therefore, as with other forms of leukaemia, there is anaemia, neutropenia, and thrombocytopenia. A range of genetic abnormalities has been found in the malignant cells, usually involving genes that direct the differentiation pathways of T and B cells.

Signs and symptoms

The clinical picture can be very similar to AML because the disease involves bone marrow failure, and there is anaemia, thrombocytopenia, and neutropenia. The lymphoblasts can accumulate in other body organs, such as the liver and the central nervous system.

Management and prognosis

As with other cancers, identifying the underlying mutation where possible is important because it may be relevant in choosing treatments and may inform on prognosis. The outlook in younger patients is significantly better than in older people. As

few as 20% of adults with ALL are cured, whereas paediatric ALL is almost always curable, with up to 85% cure rate. However, ALL is the commonest cause of cancer deaths in children.

CHRONIC LYMPHOCYTIC LEUKAEMIA (CLL)

This is the commonest leukaemia, and the commonest leukaemia in adults. It most commonly presents in people in their 60s and is commoner in males than females.

Pathophysiology

The cell of origin, a B cell, is further along the differentiation pathway than the affected cells in AML, ALL or CML, and under the microscope these cells are very similar to fully mature B cells. A range of genetic abnormalities have been associated with CLL, the commonest being deletion of the short arm of chromosome 13. As with other leukaemias, identifying the specific genetic abnormality is important because it informs treatment decisions and can relate directly to prognosis. B cells in CLL produce less antibody than normal, leading to hypogammaglobulinaemia and reduced protection against infection.

Signs and symptoms

The onset of disease is usually slow and insidious, and about a quarter of cases are discovered only through tests being done for other reasons. Enlarged lymph nodes are common, caused by B cells proliferating within them. There may be hepatomegaly and splenomegaly, and non-specific symptoms such as fatigue. About 10% of patients develop an autoimmune haemolytic anaemia.

Management and prognosis

Prognosis is variable and may relate directly to the genetic abnormality present: for example, aberrations in chromosome 13 carry a good prognosis, whereas mutations in chromosomes 11 or 17 are associated with rapid progression and a poorer outlook. In general, CLL is not curable. In patients with milder forms of the disease, especially in older people, no treatment may be indicated, and life expectancy may be normal. Occasionally, the disease may transform into a progressive, more aggressive phase called Richter's transformation, which is hard to treat and is significantly life shortening.

THE LYMPHOMAS

As explained previously, the boundary between leukaemia and lymphoma is blurred, with some white cell malignancies possessing features of both. The cell of origin in most lymphomas is the B cell.

HODGKIN LYMPHOMA (HL)

The incidence of HL is about 3 per 100,000 population, but its occurrence varies from country to country. In the United States, incidence is falling, whereas in the UK it is rising. Globally, it is commoner in males than females, and there are two peaks across the age range, one in young adults (15–34 years old) and another in older adults (over 55 years).

Pathophysiology

The origin of HL is in a single lymph node or group of nodes, and initially it spreads predictably from an affected node to adjacent nodes through lymphatic channels connecting the nodes. The World Health Organisation describes five types of HL (Box 5.1). The first four are considered the 'classic' HL and share key characteristics, whereas the fifth, nodular

---

BOX 5.1 WHO subtypes of Hodgkin lymphoma

Classic HL:

- Nodular sclerosis classic HL
- Lymphocyte-rich classic HL
- Mixed cellularity classic HL
- Lymphocyte-depleted classic HL

Nodular lymphocyte-predominant HL

---

lymphocyte-predominant HL is pathologically distinct and managed differently.

The cell of origin in HL is almost always an early form of B cell, which transforms into a giant neoplastic cell called a *Reed-Sternberg cell*, first described in 1898. Reed-Sternberg cells typically comprise less than 2% of the tumour mass, but they release a range of chemicals, including growth factors and interleukins, responsible for driving tumour development. The chemical factors attract macrophages and a range of other inflammatory cells including lymphocytes, which make up the bulk of the tumour (Fig. 5.8) Once recruited into the growing mass, and under the direction of the Reed-Sternberg cells, these inflammatory cells, called *reactive cells*, maintain an environment that supports cell division and survival of the neoplastic Reed-Sternberg cells and the expansion of the tumour. The neoplastic cells protect themselves against attack by T cells by releasing immunosuppressant factors, further promoting their own survival.

Signs and symptoms

The patient usually seeks medical help because of swollen lymph nodes (lymphadenopathy), usually in the neck (Fig. 5.9), but sometimes in the armpit or groin. In the initial stages of the disease, the affected nodes are localised because the cancer spreads from affected nodes to neighbouring nodes through linking lymph channels. Splenomegaly and hepatomegaly occur because of white cell infiltration. Generalised itch (pruritis) occurs in up to a quarter of patients, although the reason why is not known. Non-specific symptoms include weight loss, fatigue, loss of appetite and anorexia, night sweats, and fever.

Management and prognosis

The prognosis, in general, is often excellent, and 85% of patients are cured using a combination of radiotherapy and cytotoxic drugs. Long-term complications from the treatment are, however, significant and include sterility and increased risk of secondary cancers, for example, lung and breast cancer and acute leukaemia. Prognosis depends on age (older people tend to have a poorer outlook) and the stage of disease at diagnosis. Clinically, Hodgkin lymphoma is assigned

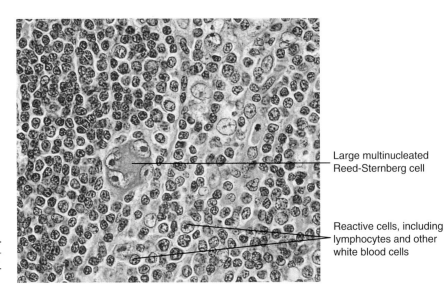

Large multinucleated Reed-Sternberg cell

Reactive cells, including lymphocytes and other white blood cells

Fig. 5.8 The histology of Hodgkin lymphoma. (Modified from Cross S (2013) *Underwood's pathology: a clinical approach*, 6th ed, Fig. 22.7. Oxford: Elsevier Ltd.)

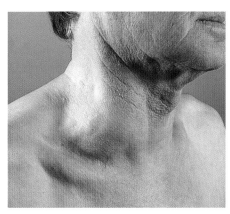

Fig. 5.9 Cervical lymph node swelling in Hodgkin lymphoma. (From Howard MR and Hamilton PJ (2013) *Haematology: an illustrated colour atlas*, 4th ed. London: Churchill Livingstone.)

BOX 5.2 Staging of Hodgkin lymphoma

Stage	Key features
I	Disease confined to a single lymph node or site
II	Disease involves two or more lymph nodes on one side of the diaphragm or lymph nodes plus one other site on one side of the diaphragm
III	Disease involves two or more lymph nodes or sites on both sides of the diaphragm
IV	Disseminated disease

---

to stage I, II, III, or IV at diagnosis, depending on the extent of organ involvement (Box 5.2).

NON-HODGKIN LYMPHOMA (NHL)

NHL is an umbrella term encompassing many lymphoid tumours, including diffuse large B-cell lymphoma (the commonest form worldwide), Burkitt's lymphoma, hairy cell leukaemia, and mantle cell lymphoma, although the list is long. No definite cause has been described, but some subtypes are associated with viral infection e.g., Epstein-Barr virus (Burkitt lymphoma), hepatitis C (several NHL subtypes), and HIV (Burkitt lymphoma). *Helicobacter pylori* infection (p. 288) is associated with primary gastrointestinal lymphomas. Other risk factors include chronic inflammatory states; for example, thyroid lymphomas are strongly associated with Hashimoto thyroiditis. Some chemicals, maternal smoking, increasing age, and immunodeficiency are also linked to certain forms of NHL.

The incidence of NHL is generally increasing worldwide, although there are population differences. It is commoner in economically developed countries than in developing countries. Other risk factors include male sex and increasing age.

Pathophysiology
Ninety percent of NHL cases involve cells from the B-cell lineage, and 10% are derived from T cells. Unlike HL, NHL usually presents with a range of lymph nodes affected. Because NHL is a group of diseases, there is a range of genetic abnormalities associated with different subtypes. For example,

Burkitt's lymphoma is strongly associated with a translocation abnormality (p. 54) of chromosome 8 that increases the activity of a growth-promoting gene called *MYC*. As a result of this, the growth rate of Burkitt lymphoma is the fastest of all human cancers. Fortunately, Burkitt lymphoma is rare. The specific genetic abnormality in mantle cell lymphoma upregulates cyclin D1, which drives the cell cycle from G1 to S (p. 63) and promotes cell division and proliferation. High-grade, aggressive tumours are associated with proliferation of actively dividing early T- or B-cell precursors, but low-grade, indolent tumours are associated with mature T or B cells, which have reached the end of their differentiation journey, are fully specialised, and have stopped dividing.

Signs and symptoms
The presentation is variable. Aggressive tumours, such as diffuse large B-cell lymphoma, Burkitt lymphoma, and mantle cell lymphoma, are usually well advanced at diagnosis, with widespread lymph node involvement and often marrow involvement as well. Expanding tumours can compress blood vessels and body organs, and the malignant cells can invade other tissues, including bone marrow, skin, the gastrointestinal tract, brain, and testis. Whether high grade or low grade, non-specific symptoms include fever, weight loss, fatigue, and night sweats.

Management and prognosis
Both vary enormously, depending on the type of lymphoma involved. The staging system used is the same as for HL (Box 5.2), but patients are often not diagnosed until stage III or IV. Some NHL subtypes are relatively benign and respond well to chemotherapy; an example is hairy cell leukaemia, which generally takes a protracted course, and treatment-induced remissions are generally long lasting. Although survival rates in many forms of NHL have improved substantially in recent decades, some remain currently incurable, for example, mantle cell lymphoma, or are rapidly fatal unless treated, for example, diffuse large B-cell lymphoma. Generally, prognosis is poorer in older patients and in those who present with more advanced disease.

MYELOMA (MULTIPLE MYELOMA)

This is a malignant proliferation of plasma cells, the terminally differentiated form of B cells produced in the innate immune response and responsible for antibody production (p. 92). It is mainly found in older people, generally over the age of 60, with males having a higher risk than females (a 3:2 ratio) and black people at higher risk and lower average age of onset than whites.

Pathophysiology
The malignant plasma cells proliferate and fill the bone marrow, replacing normal haematopoietic tissue, leading to anaemia, infections, and sometimes bleeding problems. As their population expands, the bone tissue itself is progressively destroyed, leading to pain, fractures, vertebral collapse, and hypercalcaemia because calcium released when bone is lysed accumulates in the blood. The hypercalcaemia contributes to the kidney injury seen in multiple myeloma, and measures must be taken to rapidly reduce blood calcium levels. The neoplastic plasma cells produce large

quantities of immunoglobulin (antibody) protein, usually light chain protein (p. 93), called **paraprotein**. Because all the malignant plasma cells are descendants of one single mutated plasma cell, the immunoglobulin released is all of one type only (referred to as monoclonal) and is usually of IgG type. High immunoglobulin levels may increase the viscosity of the blood and is frequently associated with kidney injury because it deposits in the renal glomeruli. Fig. 5.10 summarises the pathophysiology of multiple myeloma.

Signs and symptoms
Infections and anaemia are seen because of bone marrow failure. Backache is a frequent presenting symptom because of vertebral damage as bone damage progresses, but bone pain may be experienced elsewhere. The bone lesions are clearly visible on X-ray. Kidney function may deteriorate, for the reasons given previously. Paraprotein can spill into the urine and is detected as Bence-Jones protein.

Management and prognosis
Prognosis is better in younger patients and when diagnosis is made at an early stage of the disease. Survival times are increasing, and some patients now survive 10 years or more. Radiotherapy and chemotherapy are used to destroy the neoplastic cells, and additional symptomatic management is used as required, for example, pain control, prevention and treatment of bone fractures, and correction of anaemia and electrolyte imbalances.

RED BLOOD CELL DISORDERS

Erythrocytes transport oxygen and carbon dioxide in the blood, so disorders associated with their deficiency or reduced function may lead to hypoxia, which, if chronic, can place undue strain on the heart and cause heart failure. An increased erythrocyte count increases blood viscosity, likewise increasing the workload of the heart.

PROLIFERATIVE ERYTHROCYTE DISORDERS

Erythrocytes develop from myeloid precursors in the red bone marrow (see Fig. 5.1). Polycythaemia (high red cell count) itself is not necessarily an abnormal finding: it is a normal physiological response to hypoxia (e.g., at altitude) or may be a temporary state associated with loss of fluid from the bloodstream in dehydration. However, erythrocyte numbers are pathologically elevated in some myeloproliferative disorders. The commonest such disorder is polycythaemia vera.

POLYCYTHAEMIA VERA

This is a relatively rare condition, with prevalence estimated worldwide at 0.6 to 1.6 cases per 1,000,000 people. It occurs worldwide in all population groups, and there is no sex preference. It generally presents in people between 50 and 70 years.

Pathophysiology
This condition is actually a panmyelotic disease; that is, there is increased stem cell activity in the bone marrow, and all three blood cell types are increased: erythrocytes, leukocytes, and platelets. However, the most significant aspect of the disorder is the increase in erythrocyte numbers, which greatly increases blood viscosity, haemoglobin content, and total blood volume. The abnormal stem cells in the bone marrow do not respond appropriately to growth signals, and the myeloid progenitors that produce erythrocytes continue to divide even in the absence of erythropoietin, their normal growth signal. The underlying genetic mutation is in a gene called *JAK2*. Normal *JAK2* codes for a protein called JAK2, which stimulates blood cell production. When it mutates, it produces abnormal and overactive JAK2 protein, promoting haemopoiesis (Fig. 5.11).

Signs and symptoms
The risk of clotting is increased because of the increased viscosity and sluggish flow of the thickened blood. Increased blood volume causes splenomegaly, hepatomegaly, and hypertension. The increased blood volume and slow blood flow cause venous congestion. The person is cyanotic because, despite the high levels of haemoglobin in the blood, blood is not circulating adequately through the lungs and is stagnating in the tissues. There is frequently pruritis and gastric ulceration, possibly because histamine levels are high as a result of release from the increased number of basophils in the blood.

Perhaps counterintuitively, given that platelet numbers are high and the increased blood viscosity increases the risk of intravascular clotting, bleeding is a feature of this disorder. This is because the platelets are dysfunctional and their von Willebrand factor function is reduced.

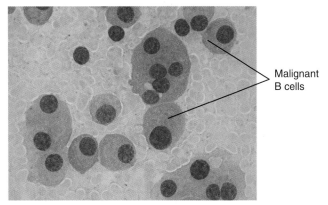

Fig. 5.10 The pathophysiology of multiple myeloma. (Modified from Hudnall SD (2023) Hematology: a pathophysiologic approach. St. Louis: Elsevier.)

Malignant B cells

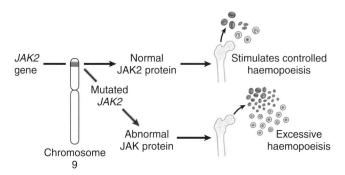

Fig. 5.11 *JAK2* and polycythaemia vera.

BOX 5.3 Some key terms relating to erythrocyte structure

Normochromic	Normal colour
Normocytic	Normal size
Hypochromic	Paler than normal
Microcytic	Smaller than normal
Macrocytic	Larger than normal
Poikilocytic	Abnormal shape
Megaloblastic	Large and immature

BOX 5.4 Erythrocytes: normal values

Measure	Normal values
Erythrocyte count—number of erythrocytes per litre, or cubic millilitre (mm^3), of blood	Male: 4.5×10^{12}/L to 6.5×10^{12}/L (4.5–6.5 million/mm^3)
Packed cell volume (PCV, haematocrit)—the volume of red cells in 1 L or mm^3 of blood	0.40–0.55 L/L
Mean cell volume (MCV)—the volume of an average cell, measured in femtolitres (1 fL = 10–15 L)	80–96 fL
Haemoglobin (Hb)—the weight of haemoglobin in whole blood, measured in grams/100 mL of blood	Male: 13–18 g/100 mL Female: 11.5–16.5 g/100 mL
Mean cell haemoglobin (MCH)—the average amount of haemoglobin per cell, measured in picograms (1 pg = 10–12 g)	27–32 pg/cell
Mean cell haemoglobin concentration (MCHC)—the weight of haemoglobin in 100 mL of red cells	30–35 g/100 mL of red cells

Source: From Waugh A and Grant A (2018) *Ross & Wilson anatomy and physiology in health and illness*, 13th ed, Table 4.1. Oxford: Elsevier Ltd.

Management and prognosis

Repeated venesection is used to reduce blood volume. Cytotoxic drugs reduce activity of the proliferating stem cells in the bone marrow. Newly developed *JAK2* inhibitors block the activity of the faulty gene. Polycythaemia vera can transform into a more aggressive myeloproliferative disorder such as acute leukaemia. The incidence of thrombotic events is high, with up to 60% of patients experiencing stroke or coronary artery thrombosis. The prognosis is poor (up to 3 years) without treatment, but depending on age and general health, survival times now may be up to 20 years.

THE ANAEMIAS

The term *anaemia* is defined as the inability of the blood to carry enough oxygen to meet the body's needs. This may be a consequence of increased erythrocyte destruction (haemolytic anaemias), bone marrow failure, inadequate or abnormal haemoglobin synthesis, or premature release from the bone marrow before erythrocytes are appropriately mature. Anaemia may also result from blood loss. Chronic kidney disease can cause anaemia because erythropoietin, the hormone that stimulates erythrocyte synthesis, is produced in the kidney.

Box 5.3 lists some key terms used to describe the structure of erythrocytes, and Box 5.4 gives some key normal values relating to erythrocytes.

Physiological adaptations to chronic anaemia

Whatever the reason underlying the anaemia, tissue hypoxia follows, and key physiological compensatory mechanisms are activated (Fig. 5.12). The kidney increases erythropoietin release, and over a period of weeks and months, the erythrocyte count rises to restore total blood oxygen levels towards normal; however, this increases blood viscosity, which increases the pumping effort required by the heart, makes blood flow more sluggish, and predisposes to clots. In response to hypoxia, the heart rate rises, also increasing cardiac workload. The respiratory rate rises, and there may be fatigue and reduced exercise tolerance. The skin, conjunctiva, and nailbeds may become pale.

HAEMOLYTIC ANAEMIAS

Haemolytic anaemias are associated with increased rates of erythrocyte breakdown, meaning that red cells have a reduced lifespan and are removed from the bloodstream and destroyed prematurely. The number of mature erythrocytes in the circulation therefore falls. Some of these disorders are acquired and others are inherited.

Pathophysiology

Erythropoietin levels rise to restore the red cell count to normal, and red cell production by the bone marrow may increase as much as eightfold. There is hypoxia and fatigue. As a result of excessive haemoglobin breakdown, bilirubin levels rise in the blood, causing jaundice. Haemoglobin levels in the urine rise, and the excess iron released from haemoglobin breakdown can deposit in and damage renal tubules. In most haemolytic anaemias, haemolysis occurs in the spleen, liver, and bone marrow; but in others, erythrocytes are haemolysed while still in the circulation. If the spleen is involved in the removal and destruction of erythrocytes, it enlarges because it becomes congested with the phagocytes that perform this function.

Acquired haemolytic anaemias

Some infections, including malaria (described below), lead to erythrocyte haemolysis. Other infections that cause haemolytic anaemia include some *Clostridium* species, the intracellular parasite *Babesia*, and the bacterium *Bartonella*.

Malaria

Malaria is responsible for between 1 and 3 million deaths annually. The condition is common in rural subtropical regions of the world, but it is not restricted to these areas (Fig. 5.13). The risk of death from malaria is increased in the very young, in pregnancy (especially the first pregnancy), with co-existing infection (e.g., HIV), and in non-immune travellers. Malaria is caused by species of the intracellular parasite *Plasmodium*, which spend part of their lifecycle in the Anopheles mosquito, and the other part in the human red blood cell (Fig. 5.14). Initial infection follows a mosquito bite (1), when the mosquito injects contaminated saliva into the bloodstream. The form of parasite transmitted at

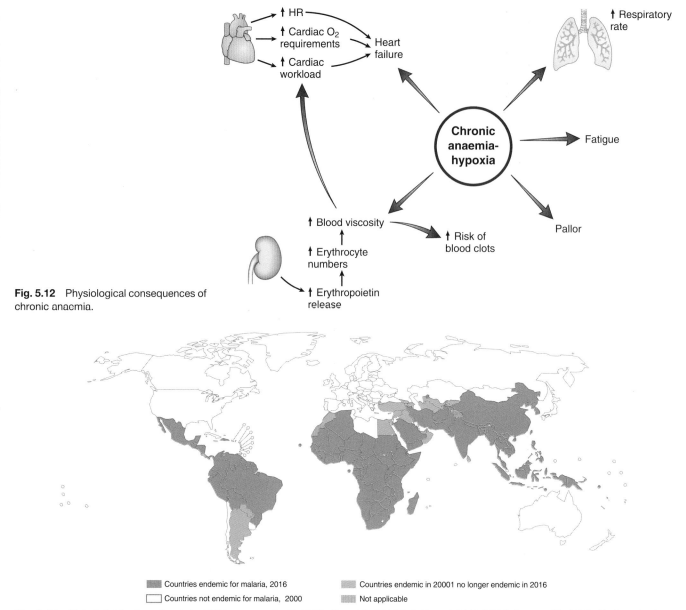

Fig. 5.12 Physiological consequences of chronic anaemia.

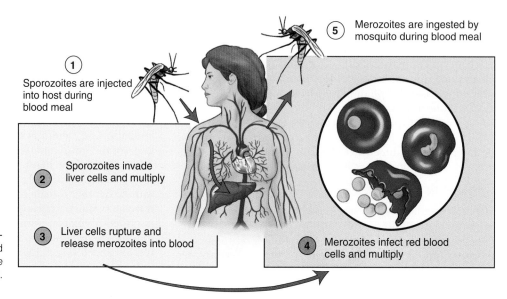

Fig. 5.13 Global distribution of malaria, 2016 compared with 2000. (From *World Malaria Report 2016* (2016) Geneva: World Health Organization. License: CC BY-NC-SA 3.0 IGO.)

Countries endemic for malaria, 2016

Countries not endemic for malaria, 2000

Countries endemic in 20001 no longer endemic in 2016

Not applicable

① Sporozoites are injected into host during blood meal

② Sporozoites invade liver cells and multiply

③ Liver cells rupture and release merozoites into blood

④ Merozoites infect red blood cells and multiply

⑤ Merozoites are ingested by mosquito during blood meal

Fig. 5.14 The life cycle of *Plasmodium.* (Modified from VanMeter K and Hubert R (2022) *Microbiology for the healthcare professional*, 3rd ed, Fig. 18.9. St Louis: Elsevier Inc.)

infection are called sporozoites, and they travel to the liver (2), where they establish themselves and begin to divide, releasing individual parasites (merozoites) into the bloodstream (3). The merozoites enter red blood cells and start dividing (4). Eventually, the red blood cell bursts, releasing large numbers of merozoites, which in turn infect other red blood cells. When another mosquito bites and takes a blood meal from the infected person, they ingest the merozoites (5), which migrate to the mosquito's salivary gland and are transmitted to the next bite victim, propagating the cycle of infection. *P. falciparum* and *P. vivax* are the commonest *Plasmodium* species infecting humans, but others include *P. ovale*, *P. malariae*, and *P. malariae*.

Malaria causes haemolytic anaemia, partly because of the parasite-mediated red cell destruction, but also because uninfected erythrocytes pick up parasitical proteins shed by *Plasmodium* and become a target for the body's immune defences. Other symptoms include fever and chills. Infected erythrocytes adhere to the capillary endothelium in capillary networks supplying body organs, including the brain, liver, lung, heart, and skin, triggering an inflammatory and immune response that damages the blood vessels and impairs blood flow through the organ. In severe malaria, there is splenomegaly and hepatomegaly, shock from the severe anaemia, and central nervous system involvement including headache, convulsions, and coma. Even with treatment, 10% to 20% of infected people die. Treatment is with quinine and quinine related drugs. In 2021, the first approved malaria vaccine was released, the product of three decades of collaboration between the Bill and Melinda Gates Foundation and GlaxoSmithKline. Compared with other vaccines, its efficacy is modest, preventing about 30% of severe disease after four doses in children under five. However, because of the high prevalence of the disease—malaria killed 411,000 people in 2018—this could still save tens of thousands of lives a year if made available in the worst affected areas.

Immunologically mediated haemolysis

Red blood cells carry large populations of proteins on the outer surface of their membranes. These proteins are referred to as antigens. If these proteins are not carefully cross-matched before transfusion into a recipient, the recipient's immune system recognises them as foreign and mounts an immune response against them (a transfusion reaction), resulting in haemolysis of the donated cells. The process of identifying the proteins on the blood cells of a prospective donor is called blood typing. There are at least 30 different families of proteins on the surface of erythrocytes, any of which can in theory provoke a transfusion reaction if given to a recipient whose own erythrocytes do not possess those proteins, and whose immune system would therefore attack and destroy them, causing a haemolytic anaemia. The two protein groups most likely to cause problems are the ABO group and the Rhesus protein (p. 107).

In addition, some haemolytic anaemias are caused by the production of autoantibodies against red blood cells. About half of these cases have no identified cause and are referred to as primary autoimmune haemolytic anaemias. They are commoner in women than men, and the incidence increases with age. In the remaining 50%, haemolysis is associated with pre-existing autoimmune disease, such as systemic lupus erythematosus.

Sometimes the immune response is caused by the binding of certain drugs to red blood cells, which then triggers an immune reaction in which the drug/erythrocyte combination is targeted and destroyed. Drugs associated with drug-induced haemolytic anaemia include penicillin.

Miscellaneous causes of acquired haemolytic anaemia

Drugs and poisons can cause haemolysis; for example, sulphonamide antibiotics, arsenic, copper, chlorates, and nitrobenzenes are all recognised causes. Prosthetic heart valves, especially of synthetic materials, produce significant shear stresses for erythrocytes passing through and are associated with reduced red cell survival times and haemolysis. Disorders of the microvasculature (e.g., in hypertension, also subject erythrocytes to increased physical stress) damage them and shorten their lifespan.

Hereditary haemolytic anaemias

There is a wide range of hereditary haemolytic anaemias.

Hereditary spherocytosis

This is usually inherited as an autosomal dominant condition and is found worldwide. It affects approximately 1 in 3000 people of Northern European ancestry but is much less common in other population groups; for example, prevalence in China is between 1 and 1.5 people per 100,000 people. A range of genetic abnormalities can cause this disorder, but whatever the underlying fault, it produces defective erythrocyte membranes, and the red cells are smaller than usual and rounded rather than biconcave. They are also less flexible than normal and so are rapidly removed from the circulation and destroyed, leading to anaemia. Severely affected people may need transfusions to restore red cell counts, and because the spleen is an important site of red cell breakdown, splenectomy usually significantly improves erythrocyte survival. Mild cases may need no day-to-day treatment.

Glucose-6-phosphate dehydrogenase deficiency

This is the commonest enzyme deficiency in humans and affects 400 million people worldwide. Glucose-6-phospate dehydrogenase (G6PD) has multiple functions in cellular biochemistry, preventing oxidation of a range of key ions and molecules, and deactivating toxic oxygen products released in certain circumstances including infection. Neutrophils, for example, release oxygen free radicals to destroy bacteria in infection, but the free radicals also damage body cells by oxidising and denaturing cellular chemicals. This includes ferrous (Fe^{2+}) iron found in haemoglobin. Ferrous ion binds oxygen, but its oxidised ferric form (Fe^{3+}) is unstable and degrades (see Fig. 5.3B). In G6PD deficiency, key red blood cell molecules including the ferrous form of iron in haemoglobin and some membrane proteins are oxidised and denatured. Denatured haemoglobin collects in aggregated clumps called Heinz bodies within erythrocytes (Fig. 5.15).

G6PD deficiency is a sex-linked recessive trait, so the disorder is expressed mainly in males. Most people are asymptomatic most of the time, but at times of oxidative stress, such as infection and the use of oxidant drugs (e.g., antimalarial drugs and some antibiotics), G6PD levels are inadequate to reduce and detoxify the toxic oxygen free radicals produced by body cells. G6PD deficiency in red blood

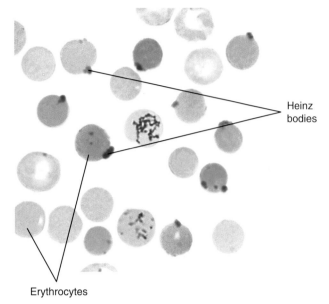

Fig. 5.15   Heinz bodies in erythrocytes in glucose-6-phosphate dehydrogenase deficiency. (Modified from Keohane E, Otto C and Walenga J (2020) *Rodak's hematology*, 6th ed, Fig. 11.12. St Louis: Elsevier Inc.)

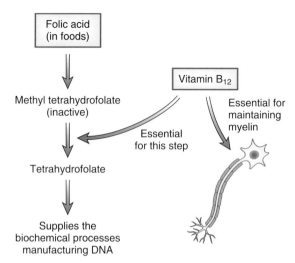

Fig. 5.16   The role of vitamin B_{12} and folate in DNA synthesis.

cells damages the membrane and denatures haemoglobin. These cells are rapidly removed from the circulation and destroyed, giving rise to the episodes of haemolytic anaemia characteristic of the disease.

Thalassaemia

The thalassaemias are a group of inherited disorders associated with impaired synthesis of the α or β chains of the haemoglobin molecule. They are discussed in more detail on p. 51.

Sickle cell disease

Sickle cell disease, an inherited disorder, is associated with the production of abnormal haemoglobin, deforming erythrocytes, and increasing their fragility. It is discussed in more detail on p. 48.

ANAEMIAS SECONDARY TO REDUCED ERYTHROCYTE PRODUCTION

Anaemia is very common in chronic disease, such as cancer, chronic infections, and chronic inflammatory diseases (e.g., rheumatoid arthritis). It is thought that one effect of systemic inflammation is to prevent the liver from exporting its stored iron to the bone marrow for erythrocyte synthesis. This anaemia may be worsened by chronic bleeding, cachexia, poor-quality diet, or other factors associated with chronic disease.

Vitamin B_{12} and folic acid deficiency anaemia

Human cells acquire folic acid (vitamin B_9) and vitamin B_{12} from the diet. Folic acid is found in green leafy vegetables, pulses, red meat, some fruits, and fortified foods. Vitamin B_{12} is found mainly in eggs, meat, and dairy products, so deficiency is particularly likely in strict vegans. Other people at higher risk are pregnant women, those with excessive alcohol intake, and individuals with impaired gastrointestinal absorption.

Pathophysiology

Both these micronutrients are required for adequate erythropoiesis. Vitamin B_{12} (cytocobalamin) is essential for converting the inactive form of folic acid, 5-methyl tetrahydrofolate, to the biologically active tetrahydrofolate, which in turn is an essential catalyst for DNA synthesis (Fig. 5.16). The bone marrow is highly sensitive to agents that interfere with DNA synthesis because the rate of stem cell division and blood cell production is extremely high. Deficiency of either of these essential micronutrients causes megaloblastic anaemia, with large numbers of large, immature erythrocytes in the circulation. However, other aspects of the clinical picture differ depending on which micronutrient is deficient, so it is very important to identify which one is involved.

Vitamin B_{12} deficiency. As described previously, this produces megaloblastic anaemia. However, this vitamin is also essential for the maintenance of myelin in the nervous system, and deficiency leads to irreversible neurological damage, causing numbness and tingling of the fingers and toes, balance and walking problems, personality changes, and even psychotic illness. It is therefore essential to identify and treat any B_{12} deficiency.

Pernicious anaemia. This is caused by a lack of intrinsic factor (IF), which is produced by parietal cells in the stomach. IF binds to vitamin B_{12} in the duodenum, forming a B_{12}-IF complex, the form in which the vitamin is absorbed in the ileum (Fig. 5.17A). In pernicious anaemia, autoantibodies destroy the parietal cells and reduce IF secretion. There are also autoantibodies to IF itself, reducing IF levels even further (Fig. 5.17B). Because parietal cells also secrete gastric acid, the disorder also increases gastric pH, which has other consequences, including an increased risk of gastric cancer.

Folic acid deficiency. As described previously, this produces megaloblastic anaemia. Treatment with folic acid supplements cures the anaemia, even in the presence of ongoing vitamin B_{12} deficiency, as the role of vitamin B_{12} here is to activate folic acid (Fig. 5.16). Vitamin B_{12} deficiency may therefore be masked until the neurological symptoms appear, which are irreversible. Care must be taken when examining the aetiology of a megaloblastic anaemia so that a vitamin B_{12} deficiency diagnosis is not missed.

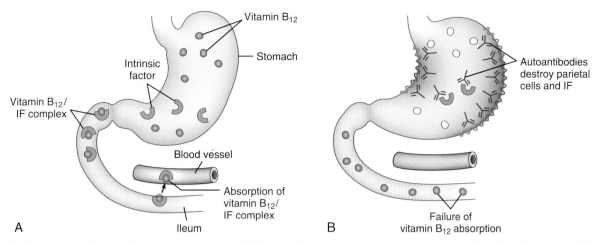

Fig. 5.17 The pathophysiology of pernicious anaemia. (A) Normal. (B) Antibody destruction of parietal cells and intrinsic factor (IF) prevent absorption of vitamin B$_{12}$.

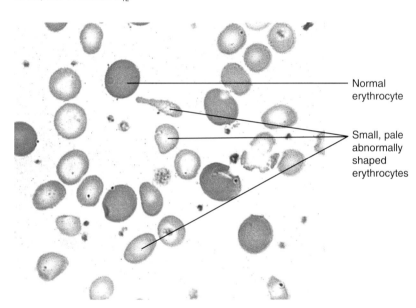

Fig. 5.18 Red blood cells in iron-deficiency anaemia undergoing treatment with iron supplements. Both normal and abnormal erythrocytes are seen. (Modified from Cross S (2019) *Underwood's pathology: a clinical approach*, 7th ed, Fig. 23.13. Oxford: Elsevier Ltd.)

Iron deficiency anaemia

Globally, this very common disorder can be caused by a wide range of factors, which may be secondary to insufficient dietary iron intake, reduced iron absorption from the small intestine, or chronic blood loss.

Insufficient intake. In 2019, the World Health Organisation estimated that about half of the global burden of anaemia is caused by iron deficiency anaemia. The average daily iron intake in the Western world is 10 to 20 mg, from meat products, vegetables, supplemented cereals, and other foodstuffs, but in low- and middle-income countries intake can be significantly lower. Worldwide, 97% of deaths from iron deficiency anaemia occur in developing countries. Iron requirements are higher in children, especially very young children, pregnant women, and menstruating women, and these groups are very prone to iron deficiency. Individuals with normal requirements but poor diets (the elderly, teenagers, alcohol-dependent people, those on calorie restricted weight loss diets) are also at increased risk.

Impaired absorption. Individuals with reduced intestinal absorption (e.g., from chronic diarrhoea or gastrointestinal infection) have increased risk. Gastrectomy reduces iron absorption because the acid pH of the stomach contents increases absorption in the duodenum.

Chronic blood loss. In the Western world, this is the commonest cause of iron deficiency anaemia. Even small amounts of blood lost regularly can cause deficiency in the medium to long term. Heavy menstrual periods, or chronic bleeding from gastrointestinal ulcers or tumours of the urinary or gastrointestinal tracts, may result in iron deficiency.

Pathophysiology

Iron deficiency anaemia develops slowly because in the initial stages, erythropoiesis can usually proceed normally because there are iron stores in the liver and bone marrow. Once iron reserves are used up, iron from circulating transferrin in the blood is extracted, which supports normal red cell production for another period of time. Once both these reservoirs are exhausted, haemoglobin synthesis is reduced, and the signs and symptoms of anaemia start to appear. Erythrocytes are microcytic and of varying sizes, and hypochromic because they contain less haemoglobin than normal. Fig. 5.18 shows a blood smear in iron deficiency anaemia being treated with iron, showing mainly small, pale erythrocytes but several normal erythrocytes for comparison. Signs and symptoms are as described previously for anaemia. In addition to its role in haemoglobin, iron is required for enzyme function in other body tissues, and additional symptoms include hair loss, a sore, swollen and red tongue (glossitis), and degeneration of the gastric mucosa.

Management and prognosis

Iron supplements are the standard treatment to replace iron stores, but it is essential to identify and treat the underlying cause of the anaemia.

Aplastic anaemia

This is a general term referring to a collection of conditions associated with complete failure of the bone marrow. It therefore causes not just anaemia, but also leukopenia and thrombocytopenia. The bone marrow loses marrow tissue (i.e., becomes hypocellular). Aplastic anaemia usually follows some insult (i.e., is acquired), accounting for 80% of cases. There is a range of causes, summarised in Box 5.5. The remaining 20% are classified as primary aplastic anaemia because there is no identified cause. It is a rare condition: the incidence in European populations is 2 per 1,000,000 people; it is higher in Asian populations, between 4 and 6 per million people. No significant difference between the sexes has been shown.

Pathophysiology

Aplastic anaemia is not associated with neoplastic change. The haematopoietic bone marrow tissue is reduced to less than 25% and is replaced with adipose tissue. The

haematopoietic tissue that remains does not respond normally to growth factors. Acquired aplastic anaemia is generally considered to be an autoimmune disorder, mediated by cytotoxic T cells that progressively destroy the bone marrow. The autoantigen that they are attacking has not yet been identified.

Fanconi anaemia. This inherited disease of the bone marrow was first described in 1927. Of all patients, 75% have additional birth defects, including short stature, skeletal abnormalities, and developmental delay, although most affected people are of normal intelligence. There is a wide range of presentations because at least 15 different genes may be involved. Inheritance is autosomal recessive in 99% of cases, with the remaining 1% being sex-linked. The disorder is linked to chromosomal instability, and affected people have a significantly increased risk of cancer. The aplastic anaemia usually appears in childhood, with easy bruising (low platelet count), anaemia (low erythrocyte count), and repeated infections (low leukocyte count). The disease is life-limiting, with a median survival of around 30 years.

CLOTTING DISORDERS

Blood clotting is a complex process, requiring effective platelet function and adequate levels of clotting factors. Within the blood, a delicate balance needs to be struck between maintaining fluidity of the blood, while ensuring that any injury triggers almost instant clotting. Disturbing this equilibrium in either direction (i.e., either increasing clotting times or triggering inappropriate clotting) causes problems.

Measurement of clotting parameters

Assessment of the clotting ability of the blood is made using standard screening tests (Table 5.2).

THROMBOTIC DISORDERS

In health, microthrombi are continually being formed in the bloodstream and are continually being dissolved. Inappropriate or excessive clot formation in the bloodstream follows when normal physiological control mechanisms governing clotting are disturbed in some way. A thrombus is a semisolid mass of clotted blood in the bloodstream. If it is dislodged, either in its entirety or as fragments, the travelling masses are referred to as emboli (singular, embolism). A predisposition to clotting is called *thrombophilia*.

BOX 5.5 Causes of acquired aplastic anaemia

Infection (e.g., Epstein-Barr virus, HIV, tuberculosis)	Pregnancy
Ionising radiation, including therapeutic radiation	Severe folic acid or vitamin B_{12} deficiency
Toxic chemicals (e.g., benzene, toluene)	Some drugs (e.g., chloramphenicol, gold, phenylbutazone, chemotherapeutic agents)
Acute lymphoblastic leukaemia	Insecticides and pesticides

Table 5.2 Standard tests of blood clotting

Test	Basis of the test	Normal values
Thrombin time (TT)	Thrombin is added to a plasma sample. If there is inadequate fibrinogen, the TT will be prolonged.	Plasma should clot within 14–16 s.
Prothrombin time (PTT)	Tissue factor is added to a plasma sample. If any of the enzymes involved in the extrinsic pathway (FVII, FX, FV, prothrombin and fibrinogen) are deficient, the PTT will be prolonged.	Plasma should clot within 10–14 s.
Platelet count	Low platelet counts are associated with aplastic anaemia, bone marrow failure caused by haematological malignancies, pregnancy.	200,000–350,000/mm³
Activated partial thromboplastin time (APTT)	If any of the factors involved in the intrinsic pathway (FXII, FXI, FIX, FX, FVIII, prothrombin, fibrinogen) are deficient, the APTT will be prolonged.	Plasma should clot within 30–40 s.

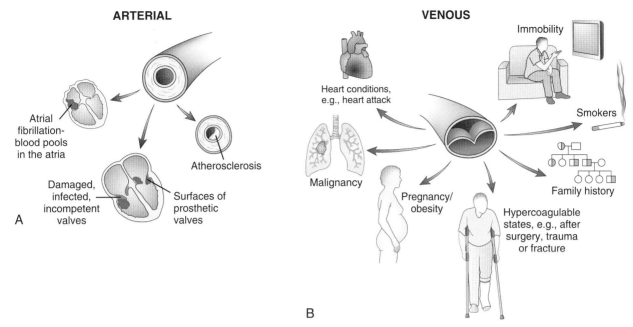

Fig. 5.19 Some predisposing factors in thrombosis. (A) Arterial thrombosis. (B) Venous thrombosis.

ARTERIAL THROMBOSIS

Blood flow in arteries is rapid and under high pressure. Arterial walls are therefore predisposed to the development of atherosclerotic changes (p. 158), especially at points where arteries divide, where flow is likely to be turbulent and initiate endothelial damage. Arterial clots can also form in the heart, if blood flow is slowed there, for example, in atrial fibrillation (p. 146), in which the fibrillating atria are not effective pumps and stasis of the blood can occur. Other cardiac factors include infections or damage of the heart valves, which can initiate clot formation, and the surfaces of prosthetic valves (Fig. 5.19A).

VENOUS THROMBOSIS

Blood flow in veins is slower and under less pressure than in the arterial system. Blood returning to the heart from the legs is flowing under such low pressure that these veins need valves to ensure one-way flow, and compression of the veins by adjacent skeletal muscles is an important contributor to maintaining flow back to the heart.

Risk factors for thrombosis

A wide range of factors increases the risk of clotting (Fig. 5.19B). There is a racial component: Hispanic and Asian populations have a lower incidence than white and black people.

Deficiencies of clotting inhibitors. Inherited low levels of antithrombin lead to prolonged clotting because levels of active thrombin remain high for longer than appropriate. There is, additionally, a range of disorders associated with deficiency of specific clotting factor inhibitors. For example, protein C inhibits clotting factors V and VIII, so deficiency of protein C, or any one of a number of other clotting factor inhibitors, removes these essential brakes on the clotting cascade.

Venous stasis and immobility. As mentioned previously, the physical compression of leg veins by nearby skeletal muscles helps 'pump' the blood back to the heart against gravity, and exercise increases heart rate and maintains rapid blood circulation. Reduced activity or frank immobility therefore slows blood flow, leading to pooling of blood in the large veins, and increasing the risk of clotting. Varicose veins (p. 160) are associated with stretched and baggy veins, sluggish blood flow, and thrombosis. Post-operative patients are at high risk because of post-operative immobility and because anaesthetic agents cause vasodilation, reducing pressure and flow in blood vessels. Any condition that impairs effective cardiac pumping reduces the force behind the blood flowing into the circulation and increases the risk of clotting. Such conditions include myocardial infarction and congestive heart failure.

Pregnancy. In pregnancy, circulating progesterone causes vasodilation, which makes blood flow more sluggish. In addition, the expanding uterus can compress the veins returning blood from the legs and abdomen, increasing venous pressures, and causing stasis.

Malignant disease. The increased incidence of thromboembolism in a wide range of cancers is well documented. Many tumours release clotting factors.

Blood disorders. Conditions of the blood that increase viscosity make flow more sluggish and clotting more likely. Polycythaemia and thrombocythaemia of any cause predispose to clotting.

Surgery and trauma. This may follow surgical procedures or physical trauma such as broken bones or crushing injuries, which activate the clotting system as part of the systemic inflammatory response to injury. Endothelial damage caused by insertion of venous catheters also increases risk, particularly peripherally, where blood flow is slower than in central veins.

Age. Predisposition rises with age, but older people with no other risk factors (e.g., non-smokers with no family history) have lower risk than younger people with known risk factors.

Smoking. Smoking increases blood coagulability. Heavy smokers are at higher risk than lighter smokers.

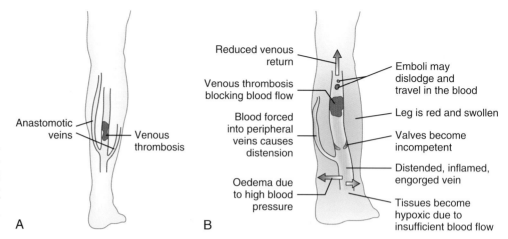

Fig. 5.20 Deep venous thrombosis (DVT) of the calf. (A) With anastomotic vessels, blood returning from the lower leg and foot can bypass the obstruction and the DVT may be asymptomatic. (B) Symptomatic DVT.

Family and personal history. People who have experienced one venous thrombosis are at increased risk of developing more. In addition, if close family members have experienced the condition, the individual's risk is elevated.

Obesity. This is of increasing importance because of the worldwide obesity epidemic. The pathology of obesity and thrombotic predisposition is complex, but obesity is associated with chronic, low-grade systemic inflammation, which activates blood vessel endothelium and increases the activity of pro-clotting mechanisms. In addition, fibrinolytic processes are inhibited.

Pathophysiology

The German physician Rudolf Virchow, who performed a great deal of important early work in the area of thrombosis, proposed in 1856 that three main co-existing factors indicate increased risk of venous thrombosis: slow blood flow, hypercoagulability of the blood, and blood vessel endothelial damage. Now referred to as **Virchow's triad**, its concepts remain a cornerstone in assessing risk of thrombotic events. Thrombus formation usually begins behind valve cusps, or at a branching point in the veins, where flow is slower or more turbulent than usual. Clots forming in the veins may cause local occlusion and block blood flow, causing blood to back up in the veins beyond the obstruction, with associated venous congestion. At the site of the blockage, the venous walls become inflamed. Fragments of the clot can break off from the parent clot and travel to distant sites, most significantly the lungs, and block blood flow elsewhere (pulmonary embolism, p. 191). Most pulmonary embolisms arise from thrombosis in the deep veins of the pelvis or thigh.

Deep venous thrombosis (DVT). Most DVT resolves spontaneously because of the fibrinolytic processes constantly operating in the bloodstream, which dissolve the clot and recanalise the blocked blood vessel. In addition, if there is a collateral circulation, these vessels can expand and help drain the blood from the affected limb, bypassing the obstructed vein and ensuring adequate venous return. In some patients, therefore, a DVT may be asymptomatic (Fig. 5.20A). In other cases, with no collateral veins to take up the slack, the DVT prevents flow through the affected vein, causing congestion and back pressure in the veins feeding it. This causes swelling, pain, redness, and sometimes discolouration in the distal tissues (Fig. 5.21). The valves of the deep veins, subjected to the pressure and inflammation of

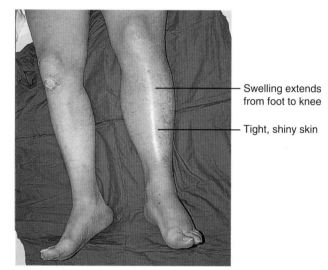

Fig. 5.21 Deep venous thrombosis of the left leg. (Modified from Forbes CD and Jackson WF (2003) *Colour atlas and text of clinical medicine*, 3rd ed. London: Mosby.)

constant engorgement, are damaged and become incompetent. Blood is forced backwards in the venous system and eventually finds its way into the superficial veins, which also become engorged and swollen. Their valves can no longer close properly, further contributing to the venous stasis. The peripheral veins become inflamed, establishing a vicious circle of thrombosis, obstruction, and lower limb congestion (Fig. 5.20B). The venous walls and the valves undergo remodelling, with permanent structural changes, and end up stiffened, permanently dilated, and damaged.

Superficial thrombophlebitis. This is thrombosis in a superficial vein, usually in the leg but occasionally elsewhere, particularly at sites of intravenous catheter insertion. The most commonly involved leg vein is the saphenous vein, the longest vein in the body, which runs a superficial course from the foot up the medial aspect of the leg before emptying into the femoral vein. Thrombosis here is associated with varicose veins (Fig. 6.37). Because the vein and its major branches lie just below the skin, there is no support from the skeletal muscles of the leg, and blood flow is prone to slowing down, pooling, and triggering clot formation. There is significant inflammation of the vein, which becomes raised, red, swollen, and tender and is clearly visible as a ropelike structure below the skin.

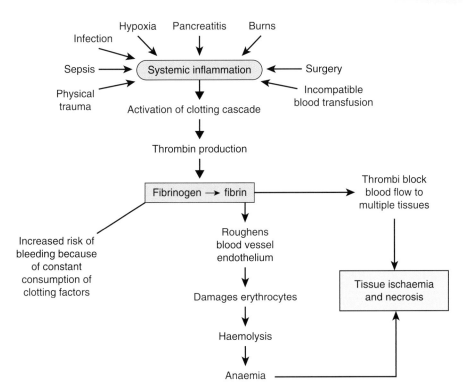

Fig. 5.22 The pathogenesis of disseminated intravascular coagulation.

Treatment and prognosis

The mainstay of treatment is anticoagulant and fibrinolytic drug therapy, along with avoidance or reduction of known risk factors. Depending on the underlying cause, many thrombi can be successfully dissolved and the formation of new clots prevented. However, DVT is a common cause of death in hospitalised patients. The most dangerous complication of progressing DVT is pulmonary embolism.

DISSEMINATED INTRAVASCULAR COAGULATION (DIC)

DIC is inappropriate and widespread activation of the clotting cascade within blood vessels, producing multiple microthrombi throughout the vascular system and obstructing blood flow to body organs and tissues throughout the body.

Pathophysiology

Any factors that trigger a systemic inflammatory response may cause DIC because circulating inflammatory mediators damage vascular endothelium and release multiple chemicals that activate clotting. This further promotes inflammation, so mutual interaction of the two systems enhance each other's activity. A wide range of significant insults (Fig. 5.22) may trigger DIC. Activated thrombin produces large quantities of fibrin and also increases adhesion of white blood cells to blood vessel walls, which further enhances the ongoing inflammatory response. Insoluble fibrin, the end product of the clotting cascade, is deposited throughout body tissues, blocking blood vessels and causing ischaemia and necrosis of the organs they supply. Fibrin deposition in the walls of small blood vessels increases the shear stress on erythrocyte membranes as they squeeze past, damaging them and increasing the rate of their removal in the spleen and liver. There may therefore also be anaemia.

Perhaps counterintuitively, DIC is characterised by bleeding. This is because the clotting factors in the blood are used up by the constant state of coagulation, and the condition is therefore characterised by thrombocytopenia and deficient levels of fibrinogen and other clotting factors. This means the clotting response to any injury is slow and inadequate, and even minor trauma, such as venepuncture, can lead to prolonged bleeding.

Signs and symptoms

Bleeding is a common presenting feature. There may be evidence of impaired organ function, commonly the kidneys, because of blockage of the microvasculature supplying the tissues. The standard measures of clotting times, TT, PTT, and APTT (see Table 5.2) are all prolonged.

Management and prognosis

DIC is an important contributor to mortality rates in patients who are already very ill with another condition, and development of DIC in these patients is a poor prognostic indicator. However, if the underlying condition can be successfully treated, the DIC resolves, the microthrombi are reabsorbed, and there may be complete recovery. There may be some permanent damage in some organs associated with fibrin deposition, and there may be some residual organ dysfunction after ischaemia and/or necrosis sustained during the period of ongoing coagulation.

INHERITED COAGULATION DEFICIENCIES

Any of the individual clotting factors may be deficient if there is a mutation in the gene that codes for their production. Haemophilia A (Factor VIII deficiency) and haemophilia B (Factor IX, Christmas factor deficiency) are described on p. 42.

vON WILLEBRAND DISEASE (vWD)

This is the commonest inherited bleeding disorder. The clotting factor von Willebrand factor (vWF) is found in endothelial cells and in platelets, and it promotes platelet adhesion and activation at sites of vascular damage. It is also a key substance in the extrinsic coagulation pathway (see Fig. 5.4). It was first described in 1924 by a Finnish doctor, from his work caring for a family with a serious bleeding disorder, but vWF itself was not identified until thirty years later. Some degree of deficiency is probably present in about 1% of the population, but the prevalence of symptomatic disease is much lower, at about 1.25 per 10,000 people. It affects males and females equally.

Pathophysiology

Most vWD is inherited as a dominant autosomal disorder. The *vWF* gene, found on the short arm of chromosome 12, codes for the production of vWF. Mutations of this gene may reduce the amount of functional vWF produced or, in the worst mutations, mean that no vWF is produced at all. Depending on how much vWF is present, if any, and the severity of the disease, vWD is categorised into three groups: types I, II, and III. Most (80%) of the cases are type I, with usually mild disease, because there is generally at least some functional vWF. Type II is intermediate, and type III is the most severe because the gene is so badly mutated that no vWF is produced at all. This form is very rare. People with blood group O often have more serious disease. Very occasionally, vWD may be acquired, not inherited. This is usually autoimmune and caused by the production of autoantibodies to vWF.

The disease manifests with periods of prolonged bleeding, easy bruising, and excessive bleeding after even minor injury or dental procedures. Menstruating women may experience heavy, prolonged periods. The spectrum of severity ranges from clinically invisible except in severe trauma to episodes of life-threatening spontaneous bleeding.

Management and prognosis

Generally, the condition is mild and can usually be well managed. Accurate profiling is important to inform best treatment. Clotting times are extended, and measurement of vWF and FVIII show the degree of deficiency. Plasma levels of vWF can increase temporarily in response to physiological stresses including pregnancy, infection, exercise patterns, and sympathetic activity and can reach normal levels, which can confuse diagnosis and management. Repeated testing is therefore important. Treatment options include recombinant vWF administration. Sometimes, anti-fibrinolytic drugs are used to prolong the life of clots and staunch bleeding in mild cases.

ACQUIRED COAGULATION DEFICIENCIES

Acquired coagulation deficiency disorders are more common than inherited ones and usually involve lack of more than one of the clotting factors.

COAGULOPATHY OF ACUTE TRAUMA

Trauma, associated with violence, self-inflicted injury, or accidents, is a major cause of morbidity and mortality worldwide, especially in those under 45 years and particularly in males. Haemorrhage caused by a dysfunctional clotting response is a major contributor to death in these situations.

Pathophysiology

Acute injury activates the clotting cascade to minimise blood loss. However, victims of acute trauma may bleed uncontrollably. The underlying pathology is very complex but seems to be caused by three main factors.

Reduced levels of clotting factors. Physical trauma to blood vessels and tissues activates the intrinsic and extrinsic pathways of clotting as described previously, leading to rapid consumption of clotting factors, including fibrinogen. This reduces the coagulability of the blood. In addition, standard treatments in trauma, including volume replacement with intravenous fluids dilute these levels even further.

Platelet dysfunction. The massive initial hyperactivation of platelets seems to desensitise them so that they become less responsive to clotting signals and fail to clot normally. The hypothermia often associated with trauma also inhibits platelet function. Platelet function is further impaired by the acidosis associated with trauma. Acidosis is secondary to CO_2 accumulation and the production of acidic wastes from tissue injury.

Activation of anticoagulant mechanisms. Proteins C and S are essential components in curbing an ongoing coagulation cascade. In acute trauma, protein C is activated, contributing to the reduced capacity of the blood to clot.

Management and prognosis

Platelet and/or plasma transfusions replace the missing coagulation components, but the outlook for the individual depends on the degree of trauma, any underlying medical conditions, and the speed of treatment.

VITAMIN K DEFICIENCY

This group of fat-soluble vitamins is found in green leafy vegetables, meat, and dairy products, and is also synthesised by colonic bacteria. It is needed for the synthesis of several clotting factors so that deficiency manifests as haemorrhagic disorders. Deficiency in adults is rare because the daily requirements are low—90 mcg in women and 120 mcg in men—but it does occur in people with a poor diet (e.g., alcohol-dependent people), in conditions that reduce absorption (e.g., coeliac disease), in pregnancy, or when taking drugs that inhibit vitamin K absorption (e.g. some antibiotics, cholestyramine, warfarin, aspirin, and some anticonvulsants). Conditions where bile production or bile delivery into the small intestine is reduced may also cause deficiency because bile is needed for the absorption of fats and fat-soluble vitamins. Deficiency is commonest in newborn babies, whose gastrointestinal tracts are sterile with no microbial production of the vitamin; in addition, little is absorbed across the placenta or from breast milk. This is called *haemorrhagic disease of the newborn* but is relatively rare in most healthcare systems because vitamin K is routinely given to neonates at birth.

Pathophysiology

Vitamin K acts as a cofactor in the production of clotting factors VII, IX, X, and prothrombin in the liver, so deficiency interferes with the intrinsic, extrinsic, and final common pathway of clotting (Fig. 5.23). It is also needed for the production of proteins C and S, anticoagulant proteins important in the regulation of the clotting cascade. PTT and APTT (see Table 5.2) are both prolonged.

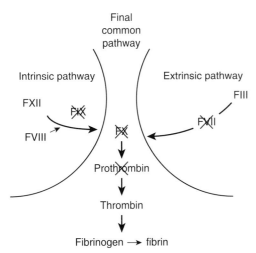

Final
common
pathway

Intrinsic pathway   Extrinsic pathway

FXII   FIII

FXX

FVIII   FXII

FX

Prothrombin

Thrombin

Fibrinogen → fibrin

Fig. 5.23 Clotting factors affected in vitamin K deficiency.

Signs and symptoms
Bleeding is the predominant feature: from the gums, into the skin or body cavities, or into the gastrointestinal or genitourinary tracts.

Management and prognosis
Prevention is the ideal and is accomplished by identifying people at risk and providing vitamin K supplementation. Once vitamin K levels are restored, there are usually no long-term consequences, unless there have been significant bleeding events such as massive intracranial haemorrhage.

ACQUIRED PLATELET DEFICIENCIES

Thrombocytopenia may be a result of reduced platelet production, as in bone marrow failure (aplastic anaemia, and the leukaemias, p. 114), or increased platelet destruction, which can happen in splenomegaly. Autoantibodies produced to platelets can cause autoimmune thrombocytopenia. Platelet deficiency can occur even when total platelet numbers are normal because of haemodilution for any reason; for example, there is a relative thrombocytopenia in pregnancy because blood volume increases and dilutes the platelets. A wide range of drugs cause thrombocytopenia, including quinine, gold, and carbamazepine. In these cases, the drugs are thought to attach to the platelets and trigger antibody formation, which is followed by destruction of the drug-platelet-antibody complex by macrophages. The condition resolves when the drug is withdrawn.

Autoimmune thrombocytopenic purpura
This may be primary, with no identified cause, or follow a recognised initiating event, such as infection. Whether primary or secondary, autoantibodies to platelets attach themselves to the platelet membrane, activating phagocytosis and destruction by macrophages. It may be acute or chronic. Acute disease usually affects children, frequently follows an infection, and generally resolves spontaneously within 6 months. Chronic disease usually affects women under 40 years and may be part of an ongoing autoimmune syndrome such as systemic lupus erythematosus.

There is a low platelet count and increased tendency to bleed. The PT and PTT times are normal because levels of clotting factors in the plasma are normal. Steroid therapy suppresses the immune system and reduces the production of autoantibodies, but with significant side effects such as increased risk of infections, hypertension, and bone fracture among others.

BIBLIOGRAPHY AND REFERENCES

Blokhin, I. O., & Lentz, S. R. (2013). Mechanisms of thrombosis in obesity. *Current Opinion in Hematology, 20*(5), 437–444.

Brodsky, R.A., & Jones, R.J.. (2020). Acquired aplastic anaemia. In N. R. Rose, & I. R. Mackay (Eds.), *The autoimmune diseases* (6th ed., pp. 923–934). Elsevier.

George, J. N., & Aster, R. H. (2009). Drug-induced thrombocytopenia: Pathogenesis, evaluation and management. *Hematology: The American Society of Hematology Education Program*, 153–158. https://www.ncbi.nlm.nih.gov/pubmed/20008194.

Malard, F., & Mohty, M. (2020). Acute lymphoblastic leukaemia. *The Lancet, 395*(10230), 1146–1162.

Filho, A., Pineros, M., Ferlay, J., et al. (2018). Epidemiological patterns of leukaemia in 184 countries: A population-based study. *The Lancet Haematology, 5*(1), PE14–PE24.

Piris, M. A., Medeiros, L. J., & Chang, K.-C. (2020). Hodgkin lymphoma: A review of pathological features and recent advances in pathogenesis. *Pathology, 52*(1), 154–165.

Rokak, B. F., Fritsma, G. A., & Keohane, E. M. (2019). *Hematology clinical principles and applications* (6th ed.). Elsevier.

Simmons, J. W., & Powell, M. F. (2016). Acute traumatic coagulopathy: Pathophysiology and resuscitation. *British Journal of Anaesthesia, 117*(S3) iii31–iii43.

Swerdlow, S. H., Campo, E., Pileri, S. A., et al. (2016). The 2016 revision of the World Health Organisation classification of lymphoid neoplasms. *Blood, 127*(20), 2375–2390.

6 Disorders of Cardiovascular Function

CHAPTER OUTLINE

INTRODUCTION
THE HEART
   The coronary circulation
   The myocardium and its conducting system
   The cardiac cycle
   Cardiac output and stroke volume
   Control of cardiovascular function
Ischaemic heart disease (IHD)
   Pathophysiology
   Risk factors
   Angina
   Acute coronary syndrome
   Management and prognosis
Heart failure
   Pathophysiology
   Causes of heart failure
   Management and prognosis
Conduction abnormalities
   Atrial arrhythmias
   Ventricular arrhythmias
   Heart block
   Wolff-Parkinson-White syndrome
Valve disorders
   Mitral valve disease
   Aortic valve disease
Congenital heart disease

   The fetal circulation
   Ventricular septal defect
   Patent foramen ovale (atrial septal defect)
   Patent ductus arteriosus
   Transposition of the great arteries
   Coarctation of the aorta
Infective and inflammatory conditions of
   the heart
   Infective endocarditis
   Rheumatic heart disease
   Pericarditis
BLOOD VESSELS
   Arteriosclerosis and atherosclerosis
   Peripheral vascular disease (PVD)
   Peripheral venous disease
   Thromboembolism
SHOCK
   Compensatory mechanisms in shock
   The pathophysiology of shock
   Signs and symptoms
   Management and prognosis
DISORDERS OF BLOOD PRESSURE
Regulation of blood pressure
Hypertension
   Classification of hypertension
Pulmonary hypertension

INTRODUCTION

The role of the cardiovascular system, which is composed of the heart and the extensive system of vessels that spreads throughout almost every tissue of the body, is to supply body cells with blood and remove wastes. Specific functions of the blood are discussed in Chapter 5, but in general terms, blood flow supplies tissues with nutrients, oxygen, antibodies, defence cells, clotting substances, hormones, drugs, and other key substances, and carries away wastes. Water and electrolyte balance in the tissues also depend on blood flow, and blood distributes heat from heat-generating tissue like muscle and liver to less metabolically active areas, maintaining core body temperature.

The muscular heart generates the power to propel blood through blood vessels, which in turn regulate blood flow, blood pressure and exchange of substances depending on the structure of the vessel wall.

World Health Organisation data show that, globally, cardiovascular disease (CVD) is the leading cause of death. In 2019, 17.9 million people died from CVD worldwide, representing 32% of global deaths. Most were in developed countries and showed a roughly 53:47 male:female ratio. Many of these deaths are considered preventable because many risk factors in CVD are modifiable, including smoking, high alcohol intake, diets rich in high sugar and fatty foods but low in fresh fruit and vegetables, physical inactivity, obesity, diabetes, and hypercholesterolaemia.

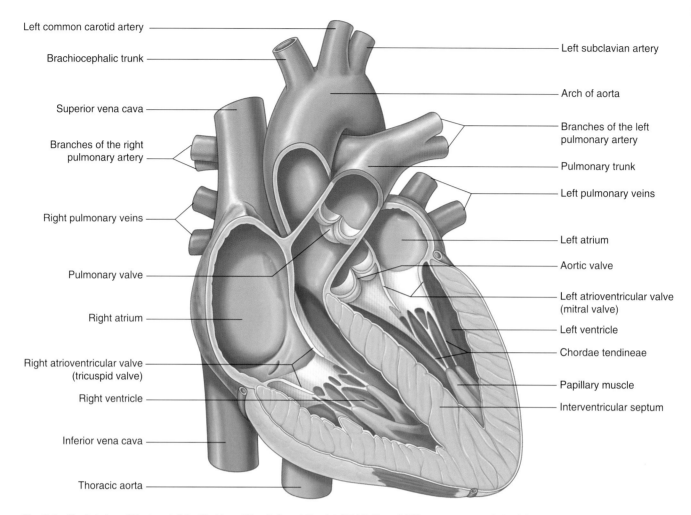

Left common carotid artery

Brachiocephalic trunk

Superior vena cava

Branches of the right pulmonary artery

Right pulmonary veins

Pulmonary valve

Right atrium

Right atrioventricular valve (tricuspid valve)

Right ventricle

Inferior vena cava

Thoracic aorta

Left subclavian artery

Arch of aorta

Branches of the left pulmonary artery

Pulmonary trunk

Left pulmonary veins

Left atrium

Aortic valve

Left atrioventricular valve (mitral valve)

Left ventricle

Chordae tendineae

Papillary muscle

Interventricular septum

Fig. 6.1 The interior of the heart. (Modified from Waugh A and Grant A (2018) *Ross & Wilson anatomy and physiology in health and illness*, 13th ed, Fig. 5.11. Oxford: Elsevier Ltd.)

Over an average lifespan, the workload of the heart is immense. A person who dies at age 70 has enjoyed in the region of 2 billion heartbeats. There is significant cardiac reserve, so disease may be well advanced before symptoms start to appear. However, once heart function is so poor that it affects its ability to supply body tissues, there are consequences for all body systems.

THE HEART

The heart contains four chambers: two smaller atria above and two larger ventricles below. The heart is divided into left and right by a wall of muscle and fibrous tissue, called the **septum**, and is therefore essentially two pumps. The right side of the heart supplies deoxygenated blood to the pulmonary circulation for oxygenation, and the left side of the heart pumps blood to the systemic circulation. Fig. 6.1 shows the internal structure of the heart, including the valves that ensure one-way flow. The muscle of the heart, the **myocardium**, is specialised for its key functions, and the cells are connected with gap junctions (p.10) to ensure that when the cardiac pacemaker fires, they contract in a synchronised and co-ordinated manner to generate the

pumping action required. Myocardium is the thickest of the three layers of the heart wall and is built around an internal framework of fibrous tissue called the *fibrous skeleton*, which supports it. The left ventricle has the most muscular wall of all four chambers because it needs to generate enough force to push the blood to distant tissues. The heart chambers and their valves are lined with a very smooth, single-cell thick layer of **endocardium**, continuous with the endothelium of the arteries and veins that enter and leave the heart, allowing blood to flow through the heart with as little friction and turbulence as possible. The outermost layer of the heart wall, the **pericardium**, encloses a potential space (the pericardial space), which contains a few millilitres of pericardial fluid to lubricate the pumping action of the heart. The fibrous pericardium, the outermost layer, is tough and inelastic for protection, and anchors the heart to adjacent structures in the mediastinum.

The valves ensure one-way flow of blood. They are formed from two or three cup-shaped folds of fibrous tissue covered in endothelium. The atrioventricular valves are anchored to the inside of the ventricles with string-like tendons called the **chordae tendineae**. The valves open and close in response to pressure differences on their upper and lower surfaces. When the atria contract, the pressure on the atrioventricular valves increases from above, and the valve flaps are pushed downwards into the ventricles, the valve opens and blood flows through. When the ventricles contract, the pressure rises below the valves, and the flaps are pushed upwards, fitting together and sealing the channel between the atria and the ventricles. They cannot prolapse into the atria because the chordae tendineae secure them, like guy ropes on a tent. Likewise, the aortic valve and pulmonary valve open and close according to intracardiac pressures. When the ventricles contract, pressure behind the valves increases and opens them, allowing blood to flow from the heart into the vessels. However, when the ventricles relax and the pressure within them starts to fall again, the pressure in the aorta and pulmonary artery is now higher than in the ventricles, and push the valves shut, preventing blood from re-entering the heart.

THE CORONARY CIRCULATION

The coronary arteries supplying the myocardium with blood arise directly from the arch of the aorta, very close to the aortic valve, where the aorta emerges from the left ventricle (Fig. 6.2). The left coronary artery splits into the left anterior descending (LAD) artery and the left circumflex artery (CX). The LAD supplies most of the left ventricle and the interventricular septum, and the CX supplies posterior and inferior regions of the left ventricle. The right coronary artery (RCA) supplies the right atrium and the right ventricle and a small part of the left ventricle. The posterior descending artery supplies the posterior and inferior interventricular septum.

THE MYOCARDIUM AND ITS CONDUCTING SYSTEM

The heart possesses **autorhythmicity**; that is, provided that it is supplied with adequate oxygen and glucose and its wastes are removed, it contracts independently of nerve or hormonal stimulation. Within the upper outer wall of the right atrium lies a small area of electrically unstable tissue called the **sino-atrial (SA) node**. Because it is unstable, it depolarises spontaneously at a rate somewhere between 60 and 100 times a minute, setting the basic heart rate. Under the influence of the autonomic nervous system and circulating

hormones and other chemicals, this intrinsic rate is adjusted upwards or downwards, depending on the body's needs. The action potentials fired by the SA node spread throughout the heart via a network of specialised conducting fibres (Fig. 6.3A).

The fibrous skeleton of the heart does not conduct electricity, and because the upper and lower chambers are separated by a ring of fibrous tissue, the electrical activity of the atria cannot spread to the ventricles except at one point, the atrioventricular (AV) node. Here, the fibrous skeleton is

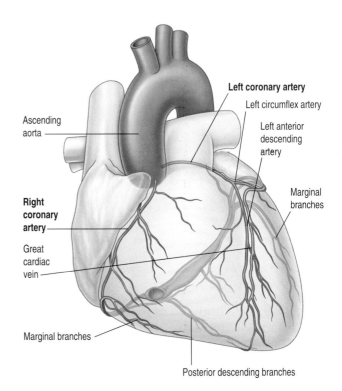

Fig. 6.2 The coronary circulation. (Modified from Waugh A and Grant A (2018) *Ross & Wilson anatomy and physiology in health and illness*, 13th ed, Fig. 5.15. Oxford: Elsevier Ltd.)

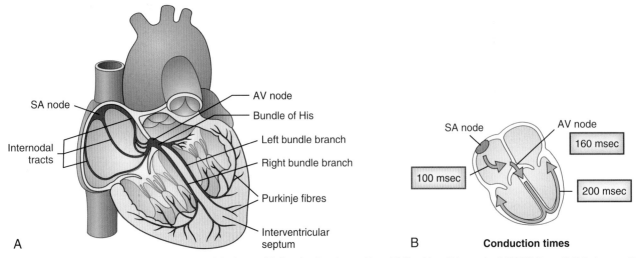

Fig. 6.3 (A) The electrical conducting system of the heart. (B) Conduction times. (From Phillips N and Hornacky A (2022) *Berry & Kohn's operating room technique*, 14th ed, Fig. 43.5. St Louis: Elsevier Inc.)

penetrated by a ribbon of conducting tissue, which carries the atrial impulse through to the interventricular septum and into the interventricular bundle (of His). The impulse, which spreads through the atria via a number of internodal tracts in the space of about 100 ms, is slowed by about 160 ms as it passes through the AV node (Fig. 6.3B). This allows the atria to finish contracting and ejecting their blood into the ventricles below.

Once the impulse arrives at the bundle of His, conduction rate increases again and it passes through the right and left bundle branches and into the Purkinje fibres, the tiny fibres in direct contact with individual myocytes, and triggers ventricular contraction. The ventricular phase of electrical activation takes place in less than 200 ms. Because electrical impulses spread through healthy conduction pathways following exactly the same route with each heartbeat, the myocytes act as a co-operative unit, and their co-ordinated contraction produces the effective pumping action of the heart chambers. Disease of, or damage to, any part of the conduction pathways interrupt the conduction pathway and can lead to abnormal spread of electrical activity, irregular and unco-ordinated contraction of the myocytes, and impaired or absent pumping action of the heart.

THE CARDIAC CYCLE

The average resting heart rate (HR) in a healthy young adult is usually between 60 and 80 beats per minute (bpm). The activity of each part of the heart during each heartbeat is summarised in the cardiac cycle (Fig. 6.4) In a cardiac cycle of 0.8 seconds, the heart spends about 0.4 seconds completely resting (complete cardiac diastole; see Fig. 6.4A). During diastole, although the myocardium is resting, the heart chambers are continuously, passively filling: circulation of the blood is continuous. The atria are filling because pressure within them is lower than the venous pressure of blood flowing back to the heart in the veins. The ventricles are also filling because, as blood flows into the atria above, it pushes the atrioventricular valves open and blood flows from atria to ventricles. About 70% to 80% of the blood in the ventricle when it begins to contract has flowed passively into the chamber; atrial contraction only tops it up.

Cardiac contraction (systole) begins with the atria (Fig. 6.4B). In response to an impulse from the SA node, the atria contract (almost) simultaneously. This period of atrial systole lasts about 0.1 seconds. While the atria are contracting and atrial pressure is high, the atrioventricular valves are pushed open to allow blood to flow into the ventricles, but the aortic and pulmonary valves, which control inflow to the atria, are pushed shut to prevent backflow. After atrial systole, the atria relax (atrial diastole), and the ventricles begin to contract. As the pressure inside the ventricles rises, the atrioventricular valves are pushed shut to prevent backflow into the atria, but the aortic and pulmonary valves are pushed open to permit blood flow into the systemic and pulmonary circulations. This period of ventricular systole lasts about 0.3 seconds (Fig. 6.4C) and is followed by ventricular diastole. As the atria are also relaxed at this point, this takes the cycle back into complete cardiac diastole.

Tachycardia and bradycardia

Tachycardia means a heart rate of over 100 bpm and may represent the normal response of a healthy heart to stress (e.g., exercise) but is also a feature of a range of systemic and cardiac conditions. Bradycardia, a heart rate less than 60 bpm, is also not necessarily a pathological finding; for example, trained athletes have lower heart rates than the less physically fit because their cardiorespiratory systems and oxygen use are more efficient.

The electrocardiogram (ECG)

The ECG records the spread of electrical activity through the heart with each cardiac cycle. It gives information on the origin of the impulse that initiated the heartbeat, the size of the heart chambers, and the path taken by the impulse as it passes through the myocardium. It is very useful in identifying sites of ischaemia and infarction, the relative size of the heart chambers, and the pathological basis of arrhythmias. The term **sinus rhythm** refers to normal heart rhythm originating from the SA node. Sinus tachycardia and sinus bradycardia indicate a fast and slow heart rate, respectively, but are associated with normal ECG complexes. Fig. 6.5 shows a normal ECG and relates it to the electrical events taking place in the different parts of the heart during one cardiac cycle. The initial wave—the small P wave—is generated by electrical excitation (**depolarisation**) of the atria. It is followed by a larger wave complex called the QRS complex, representing depolarisation of the ventricles. The third and final wave is called the T wave; this is ventricular **repolarisation**, electrical recovery of the ventricular muscle in preparation for the next cardiac cycle. Atrial repolarisation occurs during ventricular depolarisation but is not seen because it is hidden by the electrical signal from the much larger muscle mass of the ventricles.

CARDIAC OUTPUT AND STROKE VOLUME

Each time the ventricle contracts, it ejects a volume of blood called the **stroke volume** (SV) into its receiving artery: the left ventricle pumps blood into the aorta, and the right ventricle pumps blood into the pulmonary artery. The **cardiac output** (CO) is the total volume of blood ejected by one ventricle in 1 minute, so to calculate this volume, the stroke volume is multiplied by the heart rate:

$$\text{cardiac output} = \text{stroke volume} \times \text{heart rate}$$

The SV from both the right and left ventricles is roughly equal and is about 70 mL at rest. Therefore an individual with an SV of 70 mL and an HR of 70 bpm has a CO of 4900 mL or 4.9 L. SV can double in strenuous exercise, and CO can increase more than fivefold.

Preload

The degree of stretch in the walls of a heart chamber just before contraction is called **preload**. Preload is directly related to the volume of blood in the heart chambers at the end of diastole (end-diastolic volume (EDV)). The more blood in the chamber, the more stretched the walls of the heart chambers are, and the higher the preload.

There is a direct relationship between the preload and the volume of blood ejected by the ventricle at systole. The more stretched the myocardium (i.e., the greater the volume of blood at the end of diastole), the more powerfully it contracts, and the greater the stroke volume. This

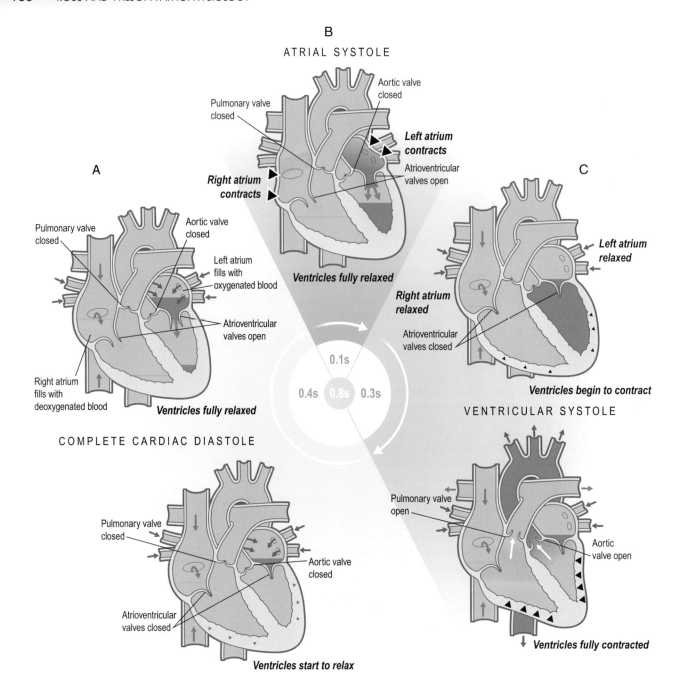

Fig. 6.4   The cardiac cycle. (From Waugh A and Grant A (2018) *Ross & Wilson anatomy and physiology in health and illness*, 13th ed, Fig. 5.19. Oxford: Elsevier Ltd.)

relationship ensures that the ventricles eject the blood that is returned to them, even when that volume increases, and is called **Starling's law** (Fig. 6.6). It is a key element in increasing CO in the healthy heart (e.g., during exercise) when increased heart rate and increased venous return significantly increase the volume of blood collecting in the ventricles during cardiac diastole. Preload also increases during sympathetic stimulation in bradycardia (because the heart has longer to fill between beats), in increased central venous pressure (which increases the filling pressure of the atria), or in obstructed outflow from the heart, such as in aortic

stenosis (because less blood is ejected and pressure in the chambers starts to rise).

Afterload

Afterload represents how hard the heart has to work to eject blood from the ventricle and is controlled mainly by blood vessel diameter. The resistance offered to ejected blood by the blood vessels is called **peripheral resistance**. If there is generalised constriction in the arterial tree or an obstruction, or if the normally elastic aorta is stiff and does not expand to accept ejected blood, then the pressure resisting the

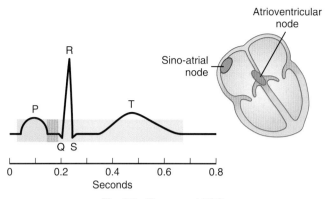

Fig. 6.5   The normal ECG.

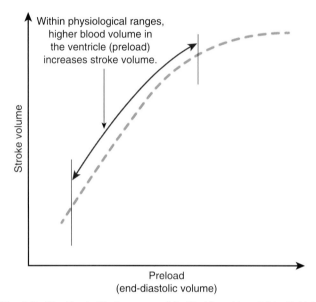

Fig. 6.6   The Frank-Starling curve. (Modified from Ungerleider R, Nelson K, Cooper D, et al. (2019) *Critical heart disease in infants and children*, 3rd ed, Fig. 13.11. Philadelphia: Elsevier Inc.)

ejected blood is high: this is high afterload. In this circumstance, the heart has to work harder to push blood into the arterial tree and the stroke volume is likely to be reduced. If, however, the aorta is healthy, stretchy, and compliant, and if the arterial system is adequately dilated, then resistance to ventricular contraction is low: this is low afterload. This reduces the ventricular workload and tends to increase stroke volume.

CONTROL OF CARDIOVASCULAR FUNCTION

The cardiovascular centre (CVC) is a collection of specialised nerves located in the medulla oblongata of the brainstem. It receives constant information from multiple inputs regarding the body's cardiovascular status and controls the activity of the heart and the diameter of the blood vessels to maintain blood pressure and tissue perfusion in response to changing situations.

The CVC receives input directly from baroreceptors in the carotid and aortic bodies, relating to the pressure in these arteries, via the glossopharyngeal nerve and the vagus nerve, respectively. The baroreceptors are simple stretch receptors embedded in the artery walls. When flow (and therefore blood pressure) is high, the arterial walls are

stretched and the rate of baroreceptor firing goes up. When flow and pressure are lower, the rate of firing decreases. In this way, the CVC is kept constantly informed regarding systemic blood pressure and maintains moment-to-moment control. This important regulatory mechanism is called the **baroreceptor reflex**.

The CVC also receives direct input from peripheral chemoreceptors in the carotid arteries, aorta, and central chemoreceptors in the brain. These chemoreceptors continuously monitor blood pH, blood CO_2, and blood O_2. Additionally, it receives input from the hypothalamus, which allows it to respond to acute emotional or psychological states and changes in body temperature, such as the increased body temperature of exercise.

The CVC responds to these multiple inputs by making appropriate adjustments, via its sympathetic and parasympathetic output, to the activity of the heart and blood vessel diameter. It also directly supplies the adrenal medulla and so controls adrenaline output from this gland (Fig. 6.7).

ISCHAEMIC HEART DISEASE (IHD)

In 2019, 9.1 million people worldwide died from IHD, one of the leading life-shortening illnesses in both men and women. Although its incidence is falling in many developed countries, it is increasing in parts of the developing world, where traditional diets and lifestyles are changing in response to Western influences. In IHD, oxygen supply to the myocardium is reduced, usually because of narrowing or obstruction of the coronary arteries, which in turn is usually caused by atheroma and is sometimes referred to as coronary artery disease (CAD). The most frequently affected artery is the left anterior descending, and so most infarctions occur in the anterior wall of the left ventricle.

PATHOPHYSIOLOGY

Coronary artery blood flow may be obstructed when blood vessels are narrowed by atheroma or by a blood clot formed as a result of the atheromatous changes in the blood vessel wall. This is by far the commonest cause of IHD. Other causes include blockage by travelling embolism, such as a blood clot that may have formed in one of the leg veins. Occasionally, the coronary arteries may be diseased by non-atheromatous changes, such as arteritis associated with autoantibodies in systemic lupus erythematosus. Even if the coronary arteries are healthy, the myocardium may become ischaemic if its oxygen supply is reduced, as in anaemia or in hypotension.

Coronary artery atherosclerosis

The term *atheroma* refers to pathological changes in the blood vessel wall, involving inflammatory changes and the formation of a lipid-rich plaque covered with a rough, fibrous cap. Atherosclerosis is the condition produced by atheroma formation in the blood vessel wall, and is characterised by thickening and stiffening, along with narrowing of the vessel lumen. The characteristic changes of atheroma formation are shown in Fig. 6.34 and are described in more detail on p.158. Although this section considers atheroma formation specifically in the coronary arteries, the same process occurs elsewhere, for example, in the renal and cerebral arteries, with potentially disastrous consequences for

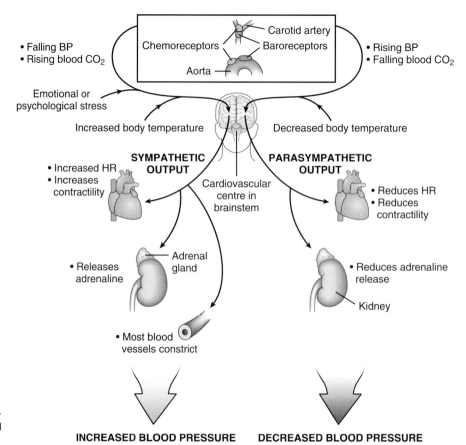

Fig. 6.7 Summary of input into the cardio-vascular control centre and control of blood pressure.

the organs supplied. Individuals with coronary artery disease are at increased risk of stroke and peripheral vascular disease because it is likely the disease process is developing at more than one site.

RISK FACTORS

The risk factors for IHD are shown in Box 6.1. Clearly, non-modifiable factors such as family history, sex, and age are fixed, but the long list of modifiable risk factors suggests that much IHD is preventable. This is supported by the evidence that in many developed countries, where public education has reduced smoking and improved diet, the incidence of IHD is falling.

ANGINA

Angina (the term means 'strangling' in Greek) is commonly used to refer to the pain associated with ischaemic myocardium. It is more accurately referred to as angina pectoris (pectoris = chest) and is usually described as crushing, squeezing, or burning. It is caused when myocardium, deprived of oxygen, switches from aerobic to anaerobic metabolism and becomes damaged and inflamed.

The damaged muscle releases algesic (pain-producing) substances like bradykinin, adenosine, and potassium. These chemicals irritate sensory nerve endings in the myocardium, generating signals along sympathetic nerves to the brain. In general, the brain maps sensory information from the viscera (internal organs including the heart) very loosely and interprets its origin very imprecisely. This is because the sensory nerves carrying pain signals to the brain from the heart also carry sensory information from tissues

Box 6.1	Risk factors for IHD
Non-modifiable risk factors	**Modifiable/potentially modifiable risk factors**
Male sex Increasing age Family history	Cigarette smoking, obesity, hyperlipidaemia, diabetes, low physical activity levels, hypertension, high alcohol consumption

elsewhere, which can make it hard for the brain to identify the exact origin of the pain. For example, pain signals from the left ventricle are carried into the brain on nerves entering the spinal cord at levels T1 to T5, which also serve the left arm, shoulder, and neck. The brain is unable to tell that the signals are coming from the heart and interpret the origin of the pain as coming from the distal sites. Anginal pain is therefore characteristically referred to the jaw, the left shoulder, and down the left arm.

Stable and unstable angina

In people with compromised myocardial blood flow, ischaemia and ischaemic pain occur when the oxygen supply to the heart muscle is insufficient to meet its needs. In the early stages, therefore, when compromise is mild, the heart is likely to become ischaemic only during exercise or other periods of extreme stress, when the demands on the heart rise significantly. In more developed IHD or other causes of compromised blood flow, the heart becomes hypoxic at lower levels of stress and so angina develops perhaps with gentle exercise, or during emotional responses, or on exposure to cold, when skin arterioles constrict, increasing afterload. In the most serious cases, when coronary artery obstruction is severe and very little blood gets through, the heart is constantly hypoxic, even at rest. **Stable angina** refers to the situation where pain severity correlates directly with the level of activity and can be predicted according to exercise levels.

Unstable angina, on the other hand, is not predictable, and pain can arise unexpectedly even at rest. The underlying cause of this is rupture of an atheromatous plaque, with local thrombus formation, inflammation and ulceration of the plaque and spasm of the artery wall. Unstable angina is associated with fluctuating symptoms because ongoing thrombosis can cause a sudden, complete blockage and myocardial cell death, or alternatively the developing clot can break up and symptoms improve. However, unstable angina is a dangerous condition, and a frequent precursor to complete blockage and myocardial infarction.

ACUTE CORONARY SYNDROME

Acute coronary syndrome is an umbrella term including unstable angina and myocardial infarction (MI, or heart attack), the death of myocardium because of inadequate oxygen supply. Acute coronary syndromes are associated with cardiac pain, breathlessness, panic and anxiety, massive sympathetic activation (tachycardia, pallor, sweating), hypotension, nausea, and vomiting. An ECG reading usually confirms diagnosis and can be used to track the evolution of the infarction, as hypoxic heart muscle initially becomes ischaemic and finally necrotic. The location of the infarction depends on which coronary artery is affected (Fig. 6.8). Most infarctions occur in the left ventricle.

Pathophysiology of MI

Only 1 or 2 minutes after sudden and complete occlusion of its blood supply, an affected area of heart muscle, deprived of oxygen, switches from aerobic to anaerobic metabolism and becomes unable to generate adenosine triphosphate (ATP). ATP is its key cellular energy source, so there is a rapid decline in contractility of that area. Anaerobic waste products such as lactate accumulate. The Na^+/K^+ pump in the muscle membranes, which needs ATP to function, fails. The muscle cell becomes unable to regulate the movement of ions in and out of the cell, and so the electrochemical gradient (high intracellular potassium and high extracellular sodium) essential for contraction is lost. Within half an hour, the myocytes swell as intracellular sodium rises, accumulate calcium and may lyse. At this stage, the damage is irreversible. The consequence of these events reduces or abolishes contractility of the affected area (Fig. 6.9).

Surrounding this central area of dead muscle is a region of ischaemic tissue, which may be salvaged if the blood supply can be restored quickly enough. Infarction occurs fastest in the part of the affected muscle closest to the ventricular lumen (i.e., lying below the endocardium) because its blood vessels are only fully open during cardiac diastole; in systole, the contracting myocardium compresses them and temporarily completely obstructs blood flow. This leaves the muscle they supply more vulnerable to ischaemia and necrosis when blood supply is compromised in disease.

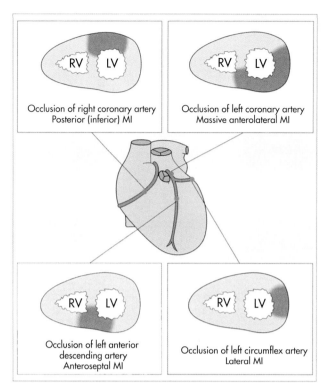

Fig. 6.8 Location of infarctions associated with blockage of the main coronary arteries. (Modified from Stevens A and Lowe J (2009) *Core pathology*, 3rd ed, Fig. 10.39. Edinburgh: Mosby Ltd.)

The area of muscle that has lost its direct blood supply is most badly damaged. This is the zone of infarction itself, and myocytes may die (necrosis). Adjacent muscle is progressively injured as the infarction evolves according to how close it lies to the zone of infarction and the degree of obstruction (Fig. 6.10), and its chances of survival increase the further away it is. If the spreading infarction eventually affects the full thickness of the ventricle wall, it is described as **transmural**.

In the hours and days after the initial insult, the area of infarcted muscle undergoes fairly predictable changes. The first few days are characterised by a particular type of tissue death called **coagulative necrosis**, in which the tissue retains its fundamental structure and stays firm, even though the cells are dead. Coagulative necrosis is almost always caused by ischaemia. As always happens after tissue damage, inflammatory cells including macrophages and neutrophils migrate into the infarction, and after 3 or 4 days phagocytosis of the necrotic myocardium begins. After about 2 weeks, much of the dead muscle has been removed and replaced with a fibrous granulation tissue, and after about 6 weeks, the area is replaced with a dense fibrous scar, which of course is electrically inactive and incapable of conducting electrical impulses or contraction.

Biochemical markers in the blood

Intracellular proteins released by damaged cardiac myocytes spill into the bloodstream, and measurement of their levels can indicate the degree of cardiac damage and give some prognostic information.

- **Creatinine kinase MB** is an enzyme found mainly in heart muscle. After infarction, its levels rise steeply

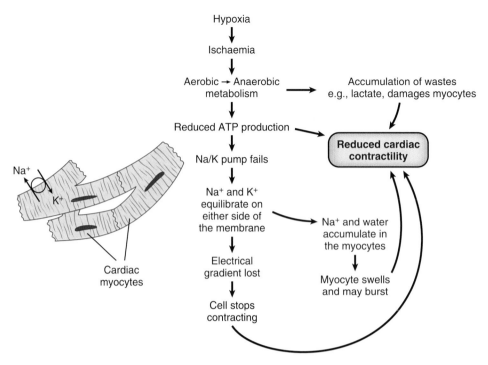

Fig. 6.9 Pathophysiology of myocardial ischaemia.

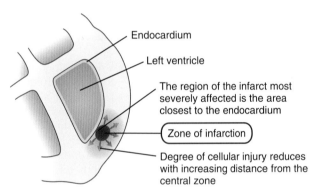

Fig. 6.10 Myocardial ischaemia spreading from zone of infarction.

in the blood, peak at around 24 hours, and then fall to normal. If they rise again after that, it indicates a reinfarction.

- **Cardiac troponins** are part of the actin-myosin complex found in skeletal and cardiac muscle. There are three of these small proteins, troponin C, troponin I, and troponin T, and the cardiac forms of troponin T and troponin I are different enough from the skeletal muscle forms to make them very sensitive indicators of cardiac muscle infarction. Troponin levels peak in the blood about 24 hours post-injury and remain high for 7 to 10 days. Troponin levels have an important prognostic value: the higher they are, the higher the risk of death.

STEMI and non-STEMI

This classification of MI is based on ECG changes of the ST segment. In STEMI (ST-elevation MI), the ST segment is elevated (sometimes called the 'current of injury' because it is thought to represent acute cellular injury and ischaemia) in the early stages after the event (Fig. 6.11). STEMI is usually caused by complete blockage of a major coronary artery and carries a poorer prognosis than non-STEMI. In non-STEMI, the ST segment is not elevated and may be depressed. It is caused by partial occlusion of a coronary artery, and the degree of cardiac ischaemia is less than in STEMI. If caused by an unstable plaque, which may progress and cause full occlusion of the vessel, it may progress to STEMI.

Post-MI complications

The incidence of post-infarct complications is high. About 8% of patients suffering an acute MI die in the 30 days post-event from evolving complications.

Sudden cardiac death

Infarcted muscle can no longer pump. If a large section of the heart muscle loses its blood supply and infarcts, the heart may no longer be able to pump effectively, and death follows swiftly from circulatory collapse. Other causes of death in the immediate post-infarction period include fatal arrhythmias, caused by damage to the heart's conduction system.

Arrhythmias

Arrhythmias are very common post-MI because the fibrous scar tissue left after healing does not conduct electricity, interfering with the heart's conduction pathways. Both ventricular and atrial arrhythmias may occur, including ventricular fibrillation, which is rapidly fatal without intervention.

Ventricular rupture

Infarcted muscle is weak and can tear or rupture completely. The effect on cardiac function depends on the site of the infarction, but always worsens the prognosis, and contributes to mortality in up to 30% of post-MI deaths. If the mitral valve papillary muscle (Fig. 6.1) ruptures, and the mitral

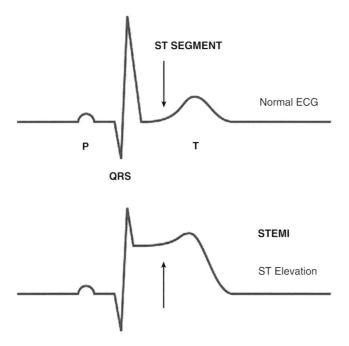

Fig. 6.11 ST-segment elevation in STEMI. (From © 2022, Bayer AG, www.thrombosisadviser.com.)

valve fails, then regurgitation during ventricular contraction quickly leads to pulmonary congestion. Rupture of the ventricular wall can lead to either tamponade (bleeding into the pericardial sac) or the creation of a shunt between the right and left ventricles.

Heart failure

The infarcted muscle is replaced during healing with non-contractile, inelastic fibrous tissue. Small areas of fibrous tissue may not significantly interfere with cardiac contractility, but the more scar tissue is present, the more difficult it is for the myocardium to function effectively as a pump. In addition, the infarcted area is often thinner and weaker than before, which can lead to the development of an aneurysm in the ventricular wall. Over time, the increased workload of the scarred heart can lead to progressive heart failure.

Thromboembolism

Clotting is stimulated when blood comes into contact with roughened infarcted tissue. A thrombus formed in this way usually leaves the heart and heads into the systemic circulation, where it can cause a stroke, a pulmonary embolism, or block peripheral circulation.

MANAGEMENT AND PROGNOSIS

People with risk factors for IHD can be treated prophylactically with lipid-lowering drugs (e.g., statins) and antithrombotic drugs (e.g., aspirin) to reduce their risk of suffering a cardiovascular event like a myocardial infarction. In patients with angina caused by coronary artery disease, vasodilators such as glyceryl trinitrate and calcium channel blockers are also used to reduce peripheral resistance and therefore the heart's workload. Stents are inserted to keep an atherosclerotic artery open, or the diseased artery can be bypassed in a procedure called coronary artery bypass graft (CABG). For this, a section of blood vessel from the patient, usually from the saphenous vein or mammary artery, is stitched in place to directly link the aorta to the damaged coronary artery distal to the blockage (Fig. 6.12). Although this is a high-risk procedure, with a 1.5% average mortality, it is usually highly successful, and nearly 60% of patients remain angina-free 5 years later.

Management of acute MI focuses on pain control, antithrombotic treatment to reduce the risk of stroke, and reperfusing the infarcted tissue. This can be done using clot-dissolving (thrombolytic) drugs like alteplase, to clear an obstructing clot from an affected coronary artery, and/ or percutaneous coronary intervention, a procedure where a fine catheter bearing an inflatable balloon is passed into the affected coronary artery. Once at the site of blockage, the balloon is inflated, disrupting the clot, opening the artery, and restoring blood flow.

HEART FAILURE

The definition of heart failure is the inability of the heart to meet the body's demands for oxygen. In mild heart failure, the heart may cope when the individual is at rest or in gentle exercise but does not cope with more strenuous activity or other stressors requiring increased cardiac output, such as overwhelming emotion or exposure to cold. The incidence of heart failure increases with age.

Heart failure is not a single disease; it is a syndrome that can develop in the later stages of almost any form of heart disease. In that respect, it is essential to identify the underlying cause so that appropriate treatment can be given.

Compensatory mechanisms in increased cardiac workload

When a healthy heart is stressed, for example, in physical exercise, it responds by increasing the rate of contraction (**positive chronotropy**) and the strength of contraction (**positive inotropy**). The CVC detects falling blood pH (because lactate and CO_2 levels rise) and immediately increases sympathetic drive to the heart via sympathetic nerves supplying the myocardium, and triggers adrenaline release from the adrenal medulla. Adrenaline has both a positive

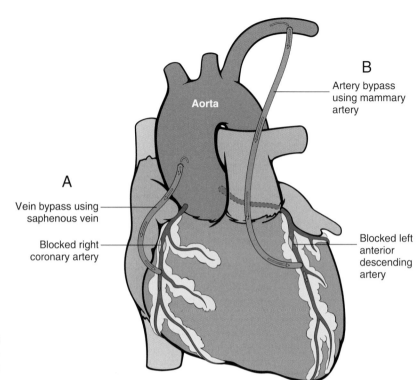

Fig. 6.12 Coronary artery bypass graft. (Modified from Lovaasen K (2016) *ICD-10-CM/PCS coding: theory and practice, 2016 edition*, Fig. 15.22. St Louis: Saunders.)

chronotropic effect and a positive inotropic effect. The heart's workload therefore rises, but in health its additional oxygen needs are met by increased respiratory activity and its nutritional needs are met by sympathetically mediated rising blood glucose levels. In addition, adrenaline causes vasoconstriction in non-essential blood vessel beds (e.g., the gastrointestinal tract) to divert blood to working skeletal muscle. In the short term, then, these compensatory mechanisms form an integral part of the body's response to exercise. In the early stages of heart failure, this increased sympathetic drive maintains cardiac output and tissue perfusion, but in the medium to longer term, the increased stress it places on the heart causes deterioration of heart function.

In addition, increased cardiac workload stimulates the myocytes to enlarge (hypertrophy), a standard response of any muscle to increased workload. The heart chambers enlarge, and the myocardium thickens. This initially supports cardiac function, but eventually the thickening ventricular walls begin to reduce the space within the ventricle itself and interfere with effective contraction.

Clearly, normal compensatory mechanisms come at a price to the failing heart because, although they support cardiovascular function in the short to medium term, they increase the heart's oxygen demands and workload, interfere with normal contractile function, and increase peripheral resistance. Ultimately, they become maladaptive (i.e., they do more harm than good) and accelerate heart failure.

PATHOPHYSIOLOGY

Functionally, the heart possesses significant physiological reserve. This means that, according to Starling's law (Fig. 6.6), it adjusts the force of contraction to match preload, and increasing venous return or blood accumulating in the

ventricles stretches the myocardium and stimulates more powerful ventricular contraction. In heart failure, the compensatory mechanisms outlined previously have become exhausted, and heart function begins to fail. The ventricle can no longer generate enough power to clear the blood being returned to it, and cardiac output starts to fall. Blood begins to accumulate in the ventricle, increasing pressure; this backs up into the atria, and so atrial pressure rises; and then finally, the rising pressure in the heart backs up into the veins bringing blood into the atria: the pulmonary vein supplying the left atrium and the venae cavae supplying the right atrium. From here, as congestion worsens, pressure rises in the pulmonary circulation and in the systemic venous circulation respectively (Fig. 6.13).

Left ventricular failure

The chamber of the heart most likely to fail is the left ventricle. This chamber has the greatest workload because it pumps blood against arterial blood pressures into the systemic arterial network. It is more likely than the right ventricle to be affected by infarction, and the left atrioventricular valve is more likely to be diseased than the right.

Left ventricular failure and the lungs

As the left ventricle fails, congestion develops initially in the left ventricle, then back through the left atrium, through the pulmonary vein and eventually into the pulmonary capillaries (Fig. 6.13). Blood pressure in the lungs is normally low (40/15 mm Hg compared with 120/80 mm Hg in the systemic circulation) to prevent fluid in the pulmonary capillaries from being pushed into the alveoli. When blood (hydrostatic) pressure in the pulmonary capillary, pushing fluid out of the blood and into the alveoli, is greater than colloid osmotic pressure pulling fluid back into the capillary, there is net

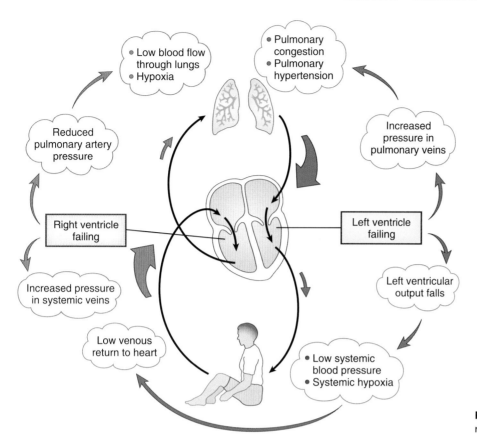

Fig. 6.13 Changing vascular pressures in right- and left-sided heart failure.

movement of fluid out of the bloodstream, which accumulates first in the interstitial spaces of the lung tissue, and then in the alveoli themselves. This is called *pulmonary oedema* and can rapidly reduce gas exchange across alveolar walls, causing severe hypoxia and retention of carbon dioxide (Fig. 6.14).

Left ventricular failure and systemic blood supply

Cardiac output from a failing left ventricle is reduced. Consequently, pressure and perfusion to organs and tissues throughout the body are reduced. The resultant fall in blood pressure is detected by central baroreceptors in the aortic and carotid bodies, which stimulate the cardiovascular centre in the medulla oblongata to increase sympathetic output. Sympathetic nerve stimulation of the heart and increased circulating adrenaline increase heart rate and initially increase the force of contraction and cardiac output even though the ventricle is failing. However, this increases the failing heart's workload and inevitably, eventually, worsens its function, establishing a vicious circle and driving cardiac output progressively down.

The left ventricle hypertrophies as it tries to adapt to its increased workload. Although the walls of the ventricle thicken, the heart can only expand so far because it is contained within its inelastic pericardium, so eventually the thickening walls impinge on the ventricular space, and the volume of the left ventricle begins to fall, further increasing pressure. This also impairs the ability of the myocardium to contract efficiently, reducing cardiac output even further.

Another consequence of poor systemic perfusion is activation of the renin-angiotensin system (see Fig. 6.43). Falling pressure in the renal arteries stimulates renin release,

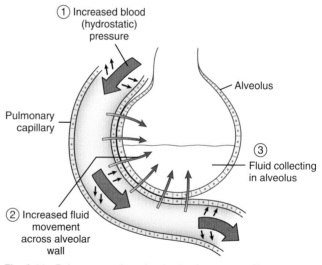

Fig. 6.14 Pulmonary oedema in raised pulmonary capillary pressure.

and the ultimate consequence of that is increased sodium and water retention, increasing blood volume and preload. In addition, angiotensin II is a potent vasoconstrictor, and significantly increases peripheral resistance and therefore afterload. Although this may initially improve perfusion pressures and help restore systemic blood pressure, as with increased sympathetic stimulation of the heart, it places increasing strain on the already failing heart, which deteriorates faster. Fig. 6.15A illustrates the main consequences of left ventricular failure.

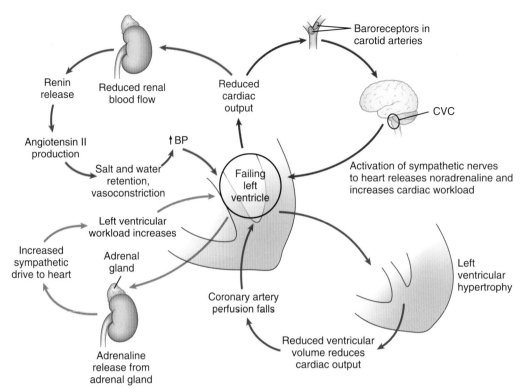

Fig. 6.15   Consequences of left ventricular failure.

Signs and symptoms of left ventricular failure (Fig. 6.16A)

As pulmonary oedema develops, it causes dyspnoea and cough, especially when the individual is lying down, because in this position blood held in the large veins of the legs by gravity is returned to the heart, increasing blood volume and pressure in the pulmonary circulation. Increased pulmonary venous pressure can cause pleural effusion (p. 195). Systemic blood pressure may be low; there is also tachycardia, and there may be pallor, cyanosis, and cool extremities, evidence of a low cardiac output. There may also be peripheral oedema if the renin-angiotensin system has been activated causing fluid retention.

Right ventricular failure

When the right ventricle fails, congestion backs up through the right atrium and into the venae cavae, which return blood from the systemic circulation to the heart.

Signs and symptoms of right ventricular failure (Fig. 6.16B)

As the pressure rises in the systemic veins, jugular venous pressure increases; the jugular veins may be prominent and distended. Backpressure into the systemic venous system causes swelling and oedema, leading to liver distension, ascites, and peripheral oedema.

CAUSES OF HEART FAILURE

Any heart disorder may eventually lead to heart failure, but non-cardiac disorders that place excessive strain on the heart can also be the underlying cause. For example, hyperthyroidism increases cardiac workload because thyroxine stimulates cardiac contraction. If untreated, it causes sustained tachycardia, increased stroke volume, and cardiac

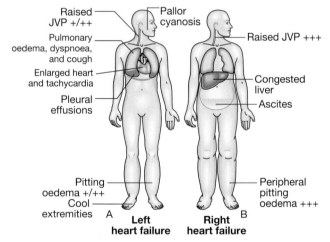

Fig. 6.16   The signs and symptoms of left- and right-sided heart failure. (Modified from Walker B, Colledge NR, Ralston S, et al. (2014) *Davidson's principles and practice of medicine*, 22nd ed, Fig. 18.24. Oxford: Churchill Livingstone.)

output, and causes heart failure because of the constantly high cardiac workload.

Significant causes of heart failure include the following:

- *IHD and MI*. These are the commonest causes of heart failure. Up to 40% of cases are associated with IHD. Cardiac muscle deprived of its oxygen supply loses strength and bulk. After MI, if a significant portion of the heart wall is replaced with non-functional scar tissue, heart function can be significantly impaired and heart failure follows.

- *Systemic hypertension.* This is the second most frequent underlying cause of heart failure. When systemic blood pressure is consistently high, the workload of the left ventricle is greatly increased. Once normal compensatory mechanisms are exhausted, the ventricle begins to fail.
- *Pulmonary hypertension.* When pressure in the pulmonary circulation is high, the afterload of the right ventricle is increased, and it may start to fail. Lung disease, including chronic obstructive pulmonary disease and pulmonary fibrosis, which scar or destroy lung tissue and pulmonary blood vessels, increases the right ventricular afterload.
- *Arrhythmias.* Examples of arrhythmias associated with heart failure include atrial fibrillation (AF), which is associated with prolonged periods of tachycardia and excessive cardiac workload. In complete heart block (p.149), the heart rate falls to match the intrinsic firing rate of the AV node, usually about 40 bpm. This bradycardia allows the heart chambers long filling times and they become overfilled, increasing preload and the work of contraction.
- *Congenital heart defects.* For example, in ventricular septal defect, there is a hole in the interventricular septum (Fig. 6.25). Because the pressure in the left ventricle is higher than in the right, blood is shunted into the right ventricle when pressure rises during ventricular systole. This increases the workload of the right ventricle, which may then start to fail.

MANAGEMENT AND PROGNOSIS

Addressing any identified cause is essential. Lifestyle changes to improve cardiac health are also essential: stopping smoking, maintaining a healthy weight, taking regular exercise, moderating alcohol consumption, and eating a healthy diet are all important. Useful drugs include diuretics to reduce fluid load, vasodilators to reduce afterload and improve coronary artery blood flow and angiotensin converting enzyme (ACE) inhibitors to block activation of the renin-angiotensin system are all standard treatments. The prognosis is often poor, with only 50% of sufferers still alive 5 years post-diagnosis.

CONDUCTION ABNORMALITIES

Arrhythmia is a general term referring to any disorder of normal heart rate or rhythm. Abnormalities of the sinoatrial or atrioventricular nodes, or the specialised conduction pathways of the heart, may cause arrhythmia. Arrhythmias can be discussed according to their origin: atrial arrhythmias originate in the atria, and ventricular arrhythmias originate in the ventricles. Heart block is a general term used for conduction abnormalities originating in the AV node or within the ventricular bundles. Some arrhythmias (e.g., Wolff-Parkinson-White (WPW) syndrome) can involve both chambers.

Re-entry circuits

Many arrhythmias are secondary to what are called *re-entry circuits*. In normal cardiac conduction tissue, activation is followed by an extended refractory period, which means that the myocardium cannot be reactivated until it has recovered from the refractory period. This is essential for normal cardiac function because it prevents electrical impulses from travelling back along pathways they came from (**retrograde conduction**) and prevents the heart from going into sustained and prolonged contraction (tetanus). Tetanus is an essential feature of normal skeletal muscle function but would be disastrous in the heart, disrupting the normal cardiac cycle and halting normal cardiac pumping activity. An extended refractory period also means that adjacent areas of conduction tissue cannot stimulate each other, even if one area is stimulated very slightly ahead of the other. Impulses can therefore only spread through the heart along one-way, pre-determined, consistent pathways, essential for co-ordinated pumping activity (Fig. 6.17).

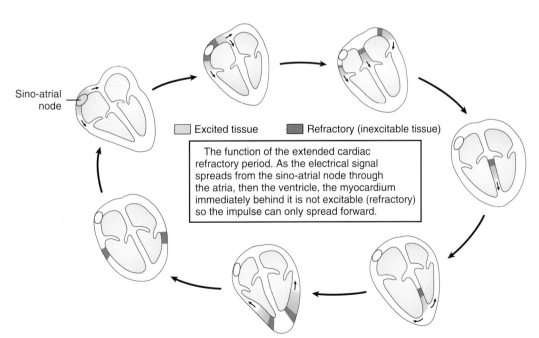

Sino-atrial node

Excited tissue   Refractory (inexcitable tissue)

The function of the extended cardiac refractory period. As the electrical signal spreads from the sino-atrial node through the atria, then the ventricle, the myocardium immediately behind it is not excitable (refractory) so the impulse can only spread forward.

Fig. 6.17 The importance of the extended refractory period in myocardium in preventing backward (retrograde) conduction.

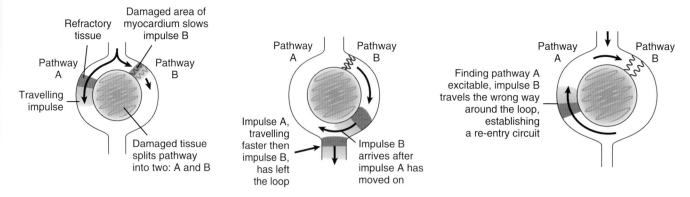

Fig. 6.18   Re-entry circuits.

Problems arise when the speed of impulse conduction or the pathways of conduction are changed because of damage or disease. An impulse travelling along a pathway that splits in two should not be able to spread from one branch of the pathway to the other because the refractory period blocks re-excitation of the myocardium. This holds true if both branches are conducting, and recovering, simultaneously. However, if one branch of the pathway is damaged, for example, with scar tissue from a heart attack, and conducts more slowly than the other, it can reactivate the other branch once the refractory period of the normal branch has passed. This activation spreads back upwards along the normal branch to the junction point between the two branches, establishing an endless circuit of activation: a **re-entry circuit**, and the basis of many arrhythmias (Fig. 6.18).

ATRIAL ARRHYTHMIAS

Disorders of atrial conduction generally have less impact on cardiac function than ventricular arrhythmias because most ventricular filling is done passively and the atrial contribution to ventricular filling can be relatively small.

Atrial fibrillation (AF)

The main risk factor for this common arrhythmia is age; 80% of people with AF are over 65, and it is commoner in men than women. Although it can occur in the absence of identified underlying causes (so-called *lone* or *idiopathic AF*), it is usually associated with other cardiac pathologies (e.g., coronary artery disease, valvular disease, hypertension, sinoatrial node abnormalities, pericardial disease, and cardiomyopathy). Other associated risk factors include chronic obstructive pulmonary disease, hyperthyroidism (thyroid hormones stimulate the heart), and alcohol abuse. AF may be continuous or paroxysmal, in which episodes of fibrillation are interspersed with periods of normal sinus rhythm.

Idiopathic AF can appear before the age of 40. There is a familial association, and mutations in key genes associated with cardiac development have been demonstrated in lone AF with young age onset. Although by definition lone AF is not associated with any identified cardiac abnormality, this evidence points to some genetically determined cardiac mechanism that is still to be identified.

The incidence of AF is rising worldwide because improved management of CVD is increasing survival times. This means that more people are living longer with CVD, a key risk factor for AF.

Pathophysiology

AF is characterised by ectopic impulses originating in atrial tissue, often the junctional area where the pulmonary veins enter the right atrium. These abnormal impulses enter self-propagating re-entry circuits within the atrial myocardium, generating continuous electrical activity that does not trigger normal atrial contraction. On the ECG, the P waves are therefore absent, although the baseline between QRS complexes may be irregular, indicating chaotic fibrillation activity in the atria (Fig. 6.19A). Continuous transmission of atrial signals through the AV node usually cause ventricular tachycardia, but the ventricular rate is irregular because not all impulses get through.

Signs and symptoms

AF may be asymptomatic and only picked up incidentally when investigating something else or on a routine check-up. However, the tachycardia experienced by many patients can lead to enlargement of the atria and ventricular overwork. Not all people have reduced cardiac output, because passive ventricular filling may be adequate to maintain stroke volume despite the lack of effective atrial contribution, but there can be breathlessness, palpitations, and dizziness, particularly on exercise. If the tachycardia is excessive, it can cause myocardial ischaemia and chest pain.

Management and prognosis

The main hazard in AF is increased likelihood of stroke. It has been estimated that one in five strokes in the UK are associated with untreated AF. This is because, with ineffective atrial pumping, blood stagnates within the atria and forms clots. Emboli from these clots cause stroke if they travel to the cerebral circulation and block cerebral arteries. Early intervention is important because it improves prognosis. Re-entrant circuits become more strongly established the longer they are allowed to operate, and the AF becomes progressively more troublesome. Anticoagulants reduce the risk of emboli forming in the blood pooling in the non-pumping atria. Anti-arrhythmic drugs can suppress the re-entry circuits, and catheter ablation is used to target and destroy the areas of heart muscle generating the ectopic beats.

Atrial flutter

Atrial flutter is often associated with atrial fibrillation, and risk factors include increasing age, male gender and pre-existing heart disease. About 30% of people have no

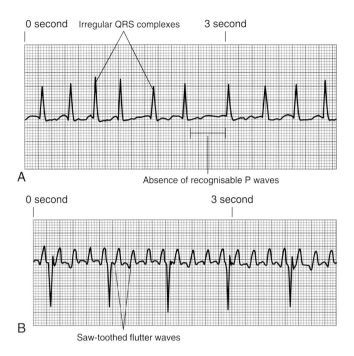

Fig. 6.19 ECG traces in atrial arrhythmias. (A) Atrial fibrillation. (B) Atrial flutter. (Modified from (A) Urden LD, Stacy KM, and Lough ME (2022) *Critical care nursing*, 9th ed, Fig 13.63. Philadelphia: Elsevier Inc; (B) Urden LD, Stacy KM, and Lough ME (2022) *Critical care nursing*, 9th ed, Fig. 13.62B. Philadelphia: Elsevier Inc.)

underlying heart disease, but other conditions associated with atrial flutter include diabetes, chronic obstructive pulmonary disease, alcohol abuse, and hyperthyroidism.

Pathophysiology
In atrial flutter, a large re-entry circuit drives atrial contraction at excessively high speeds of up to 300 bpm. On the ECG, this shows as saw-toothed flutter waves (Fig. 6.19B). Almost always, only a proportion of these atrial beats are conducted through the AV node to the ventricles (this is a form of heart block; p.148), and there is usually a proportionate relationship between the flutter wave speed and ventricular contraction. For example, if the atrial rate is 300 bpm and only every second beat reaches the ventricles, the pulse is 150 bpm. At this speed, ventricular filling is poor and cardiac output is likely to be low.

Signs and symptoms
Palpitations, dizziness, low exercise tolerance, and feeling faint are common because of low cardiac output. There may be chest pain if the heart rate is very fast, and the myocardium becomes ischaemic.

Management and prognosis
Anti-arrhythmic drugs can interrupt the abnormal conduction circuit and control symptoms. Surgical ablation, creating a line of scar tissue that interrupts conduction of impulses around the re-entrant circuit, is usually curative.

VENTRICULAR ARRHYTHMIAS

Ventricular arrhythmias are more troublesome than atrial arrhythmias because the ventricles are the chambers responsible for ejecting blood from the heart and carry a significant risk of sudden death.

Ventricular ectopic beats

Also called *extrasystoles*, or *premature beats*, these occur when one or more ectopic foci in the ventricles fire irregularly and with no connection to the normal sinus rhythm of the heart. They are common, and their incidence increases with age. They may be associated with underlying heart disease, including heart failure, and are common in the post-MI period.

Pathophysiology
The normal QRS duration is short, between 0.08 and 0.1 seconds, because in the normal heartbeat, both ventricles are stimulated simultaneously. In a ventricular ectopic beat, the QRS complex is wider than normal, because the impulse from the ectopic focus spreads in an abnormal pattern through the ventricle of origin and into the other ventricle through a non-standard route. Thus the spread of excitation takes longer, and the ventricles are stimulated sequentially instead of simultaneously. In addition to the prolonged QRS event, the abnormal conduction routes taken by the impulses generated by the ectopic focus produce bizarrely shaped QRS waves (Fig. 6.20A).

Signs and symptoms
People may notice their irregular pulse and missed beats. The extrasystole beat ejects a low stroke volume because it has come before the normal sinus beat and the ventricle has not completely filled. The beat after that may feel stronger than usual because the heart has then had increased filling time.

Management and prognosis
Many people with extrasystoles need no intervention but underlying cardiac disease should be treated.

Ventricular tachycardia and ventricular fibrillation

Ventricular tachycardia (VT) can frequently develop into ventricular fibrillation (VF).

Pathophysiology
VT is usually associated with significant myocardial damage, such as acute myocardial infarction, or chronic

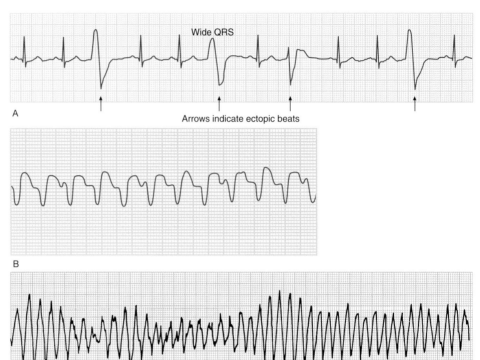

Fig. 6.20 ECG traces in ventricular arrhythmias. (A) Ventricular ectopic beats. (B) Ventricular tachycardia. (C) Torsades de pointes. (Modified from (A) Ralston S, Penman I, Strachan S, et al. (2018) *Davidson's principles and practice of medicine*, 23rd ed, Fig. 16.40. Edinburgh: Elsevier Ltd; (B) Walker B, Colledge NR, Ralston S, et al. (2010) *Davidson's principles and practice of medicine*, 21st ed, Fig. 18.48. Oxford: Churchill Livingstone; (C) Goldberger A, Goldberger Z, and Shvilkin A (2018) *Goldberger's clinical electrocardiography*, 9th ed, Fig. 16.18. Edinburgh: Elsevier Inc.)

myocardial ischaemia associated with coronary artery disease. Normal conduction pathways are damaged and disrupted, and re-entry circuits are established, with continual activation of ventricular muscle. The heart rate is usually somewhere between 120 and 220 bpm. With such a fast heart rate, ventricular filling time is too short, and so stroke volume and cardiac output are low. The QRS complexes are wide and bizarre, for the same reason as given for ventricular ectopic beats (Fig. 6.20B). The risk of deteriorating into ventricular fibrillation, where the chaotic electrical activity no longer stimulates effective ventricular contractions, is high. In VF, the pulse is absent, circulation effectively ceases, there is loss of consciousness, and death is inevitable unless the individual is lucky enough to be close to suitable resuscitation facilities.

VT is sometimes found in individuals with structurally normal hearts, in whom it often causes no problems but can be managed with anti-arrhythmic drugs if necessary.

Torsades de pointes. This form of VT is associated with extended ventricular repolarisation (giving extended QT intervals on the ECG). Torsade means twisting, and in this arrhythmia, there is a gradual change in the size of QRS complexes, giving the impression that the trace is twisting around the baseline. The QT interval, generally between 0.40 and 0.44 seconds, is considered extended if longer than 0.45 seconds in males and 0.47 seconds in females. The lengthened time taken by the ventricles to repolarise allows abnormal depolarising currents to trigger repeated cycles of activation and the tachyarrhythmia to appear (Fig. 6.20C). Generally, episodes of torsades are self-limiting and normal sinus rhythm reasserts itself, but

sometimes they can degenerate into VF. Sometimes the condition is congenital and associated with mutations in genes that code for sodium and potassium ion channels in the heart muscle, which control the ion flows that depolarise and repolarise the myocardium. In other cases, the prolonged QT interval may be caused by certain drugs (e.g., quinidine), some antibiotics (e.g., erythromycin), tricyclic anti-depressants and anti-psychotics, electrolyte imbalances (hypocalcaemia, hypomagnesaemia, or hypokalaemia), or cardiac injury (e.g., post-MI).

Management and prognosis

VT can be managed with anti-arrhythmic drugs, but any underlying cause (e.g., electrolyte abnormalities) needs to be corrected, which may resolve the arrhythmia. VF is a clinical emergency requiring defibrillation and resuscitation.

HEART BLOCK

The term *heart block* refers to a group of disorders in which there is a physical barrier to conduction somewhere in the AV node or the ventricular conducting tissue. Impulse conduction may be slower than normal or blocked altogether. The block may occur as a normal physiological response to rapid atrial contractions, as in AF, where the speed at which the AV node is being stimulated is too high to allow it to transmit all the impulses, and they do not all get through. Other forms of block may be the result of damage to the conducting system, such as non-conducting fibrous tissue replacing healthy heart tissue after MI, inflammatory or infective heart conditions, or electrolyte imbalances that interfere with the ionic gradients required for conduction and contraction.

Atrioventricular (AV) block

AV block, impaired conduction through the AV node, is classified according to the proportion of atrial beats actually getting through to the ventricles (Fig. 6.21).

First-degree AV block

In first-degree block, all atrial impulses reach the ventricles, but only after a delay. The PR interval, normally 0.12 to 0.2 seconds, is extended to over 0.2 seconds, but every P wave is followed by a QRS wave in a 1:1 ratio (Fig. 6.21A). Most first-degree AV block causes no symptoms, but there may be reduced exercise tolerance and fatigue.

Second-degree AV block

In second-degree block, only some atrial beats reach the ventricles. It causes fatigue, low exercise tolerance, breathlessness, light-headedness, and sometimes fainting. There are three main patterns:

- **Mobitz I block.** In this form, the ECG shows increasing PR intervals over several successive beats (indicating the AV conduction is getting slower and slower), until finally a P wave is not conducted at all and there is no QRS seen. The following P wave triggers a QRS as normal, and the pattern repeats.
- **Mobitz II block.** Some P waves do not conduct to the atria, and are therefore not followed by QRS waves, but the PR interval is consistent with every conducted beat.
- **2:1 and 3:1 block.** P waves are conducted in a fixed ratio: so in 2:1 block, every second P wave is conducted and generates a QRS complex (Fig. 6.21B), and in 3:1 block, only one P wave in 3 gets into the ventricles.

Third-degree (complete) heart block

In complete heart block, none of the atrial beats are transmitted to the ventricles. The SA node is firing, triggering atrial contraction and P waves are seen on the ECG, but none are conducted through the AV node. In this case, the AV node assumes the role of cardiac pacemaker, but its intrinsic rate of firing is much lower than the SA node, at only 40 to 60 bpm. On the ECG, therefore, both P and QRS waves are seen, but they bear no relationship to one another because the upper chambers and the lower chambers are now operating independently (Fig. 6.21C). Complete heart block causes bradycardia, breathlessness, light headedness, fainting, poor exercise tolerance, palpitations, and sometimes chest pain.

Management

Inserting a cardiac pacemaker increases heart rate and cardiac output in symptomatic patients for whom heart block is causing troublesome symptoms.

Bundle branch blocks

When conduction in either the left or right bundle branches is impaired, the spread of excitation through the ventricles takes a slow, abnormal route to bypass the non-functional tissue. The QRS complex may therefore be wider than usual and abnormally shaped, but bundle branch blocks often cause no problems for the patient.

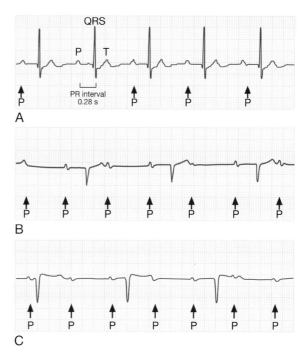

Fig. 6.21 ECG traces in first-, second-, and third-degree heart block. (A) First-degree heart block. Every P wave is followed by a QRS complex, but only after a delay; the PR interval is 0.26 seconds. (B) Second-degree heart block in a fixed 2:1 ratio. (C) Third-degree heart block. There is no relationship between P waves and QRS complexes. (Modified from (A) Ralston S, Penman I, Strachan M, et al. (2018) *Davidson's principles and practice of medicine*, 23rd ed, Fig. 16.44. Edinburgh: Elsevier Ltd; (B) Ralston S, Penman I, Strachan M, et al. (2018) *Davidson's principles and practice of medicine*, 23rd ed, Fig. 16.47. Edinburgh: Elsevier Ltd; (C) Ralston S, Penman I, Strachan M, et al. (2018) *Davidson's principles and practice of medicine*, 23rd ed, Fig. 16.48. Edinburgh: Elsevier Ltd.)

WOLFF-PARKINSON-WHITE SYNDROME

This condition was first identified in 1930 in a group of children with episodes of tachycardia and characteristic ECG changes. It is likely that there is a genetic component, and there is sometimes a clear familial link. There are well-recognised associations with certain myopathies, including inherited familial cardiomyopathy and skeletal muscle myopathy. Incidence is about 1 to 3 people per 1000. It is usually diagnosed in youth and is more common in boys.

Pathophysiology

In this condition, there is an extra conduction pathway (an 'accessory pathway') linking the atria to the ventricles, bypassing the AV node. The accessory pathway may conduct impulses one-way, either from the atria to the ventricles or vice versa, or it may permit two-way conduction. In addition, it usually has a different conduction speed to the AV conduction tissue, meaning that a re-entrant circuit can be set up, causing tachycardia. The manifestations of WPW, and the changes seen on the ECG, therefore depend on the properties of the abnormal accessory pathway, and there is a large degree of variability in signs, symptoms and ECG patterns. If the accessory pathway conducts one way, from the atria to the ventricles (Fig. 6.22A), it pre-excites the ventricles

A   One-way conduction-
     atria → ventricles

B   One-way conduction-
     ventricles → atria

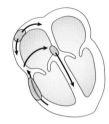

Atrioventricular
node

Sino-atrial
node

Accessory
pathway

• Rapid conduction to ventricles
• Short P-R interval
• QRS may be wider than normal

• Retrograde conduction from
  ventricles to atria
• Atria re-excited
• Sets up re-entrant loop
  and tachycardia

Fig. 6.22 Accessory conducting pathways in Wolff-Parkinson-White syndrome.

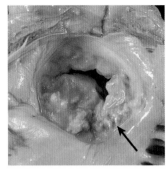

Fig. 6.23 A calcified, narrowed mitral valve. The arrow indicates areas of calcification. (From Kumar V, Singh M, Abbas A, et al. (2022) *Robbins & Cotran pathologic basis of disease*, 10th ed, South Asia Edition, Volume 1, Fig. 12.20. New Delhi: RELX India Pvt. Ltd.)

because it bypasses the AV node, where the signal from the atria is delayed, and broadens the QRS, but the ECG may show almost normal sinus rhythm otherwise. It is also possible to set up a re-entrant circuit where the impulse travels from atria to ventricles down the fast accessory pathway and back up to the atria via the AV pathway. If the accessory pathway only conducts one way, from the ventricles to the atria, then ascending impulses from the ventricles to the atria can lead to atrial tachycardia and atrial fibrillation, which in turn causes tachycardia because the increased activity in the atria transmits signals down the AV node and drives the ventricles at an increased rate (Fig. 6.22B).

Management and prognosis
Catheter ablation of the accessory pathway usually cures the condition. As many patients are asymptomatic with otherwise normal hearts, treatment is not always needed. There is a very small risk of sudden cardiac death as a result of the onset of VF and is usually seen in people with more than one accessory pathway, associated heart disease, or a family history of sudden cardiac death. The condition often improves with age and may even resolve completely. This is thought to be secondary to age-related fibrotic changes in the heart and reduced conductivity of the accessory pathway.

VALVE DISORDERS

The heart valves ensure one-way flow from the atria to the ventricles and from the ventricles into the aorta and pulmonary arteries. If the cusps of a valve are damaged, they may fail to close properly, and allow blood to flow the wrong way (regurgitation). A diseased valve may also be narrowed (stenosed), restricting blood flow through the valve opening. Both situations reduce the efficiency of the heart's pumping action and increase its workload. Heart valve disease is very common, particularly among older people. In the general population, its prevalence is around 2.5%, but this rises to over 10% in the over-75 age group.

MITRAL VALVE DISEASE

The mitral (left atrioventricular) valve has two cusps (bicuspid) and guards the opening between the left atrium

and left ventricle. As pressures in the left side of the heart are higher than the right side of the heart, this valve is under greater mechanical stress than the right atrioventricular valve and is more susceptible to damage. The channel formed when the healthy mitral valve opens is between 4 and 6 cm^2 in area, and symptoms occur when this falls to less than 2 cm^2.

Pathophysiology
The commonest cause of mitral valve disease is post-streptococcal rheumatic heart disease (p.155), which causes calcification, stiffening and fibrosis of both valve cusps (Fig. 6.23). The distorted cusps can no longer close, so they leak and allow regurgitation of blood, and the opening between the atrium and ventricle is narrowed. This restricts blood flow from the left atrium into the left ventricle, so blood accumulates in the atrium, atrial pressure rises, and congestion backs up into the pulmonary circulation, causing pulmonary hypertension and pulmonary oedema. Pulmonary oedema reduces gas exchange, restricting oxygen diffusion into the bloodstream. Because most ventricular filling is done passively, which is seriously reduced when the mitral valve is narrowed, the left ventricle then relies on atrial contraction to fill it up and maintain stroke volume. The left atrium, struggling to pump blood through the narrowed valve, hypertrophies and enlarges.

Signs and symptoms
The first indication that there is a problem is usually reduced exercise tolerance, with increasing breathlessness as cardiac output falls and pulmonary congestion develops. There may be cough with bloody sputum because of the pulmonary oedema. Blood stagnates in the left atrium, increasing the risk of thrombosis and embolism. Sometimes the increased cardiovascular load of pregnancy gives the first indication that there is a problem with the valve. There may be associated arrhythmias, such as atrial fibrillation.

Management and prognosis
Anticoagulants are used to reduce the risk of embolism, and anti-arrhythmic drugs are used to control associated arrhythmias. Statins may slow valvular degeneration. Repair or replacement of the valve can be performed in those at highest risk of embolism or whose cardiac function is particularly poor.

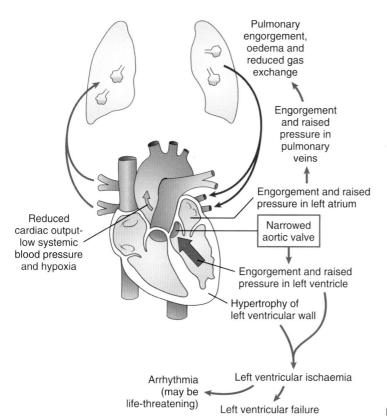

Fig. 6.24 The consequences of aortic valve disease.

AORTIC VALVE DISEASE

The commonest cause of aortic valve disease is age-related progressive stenosis, with calcification, stiffening, and distortion of the valve cusps. It affects up to 40% of the population over 75. The second commonest cause is a congenitally abnormal valve, with only two cusps (bicuspid) instead of the usual three, affecting 1% to 2% of the population. This is the commonest form of congenital heart disease and can be familial. Thirdly, like mitral valve disease, aortic valve damage can be secondary to post-streptococcal rheumatic heart disease.

Pathophysiology
With aortic valve stenosis, the workload of the left ventricle is significantly increased as it struggles to pump blood past the stiffened, unyielding cusps into the aorta. Pressure in the left ventricle therefore rises, and its oxygen requirements increase. The ventricle responds by dilating and with hypertrophy of its muscular walls, but as the aortic valve becomes progressively more obstructed, eventually the enlarged ventricle requires more oxygen than it can receive, and ischaemia develops. The ischaemia can lead to arrhythmias and left ventricular failure, with a falling cardiac output and systemic hypotension. As the stenosis progresses, and the left ventricle becomes more congested, the pressure backs up through the left atrium, the pulmonary veins and into the pulmonary capillaries. Congestion here leads to pulmonary oedema, with compromised gas exchange. Fig. 6.24 shows the consequences of aortic valve disease.

Signs and symptoms
Generally, cardiac output is maintained at normal levels until the aortic valve orifice is less than a third of normal, so up to that point people are generally symptom-free. Typical initial symptoms include angina and reduced exercise tolerance, and exercise-induced fainting (because of low cardiac output and hypotension). Pulmonary congestion, poor gas exchange in the oedematous alveoli, and hypoxia cause dyspnoea.

Management and prognosis
Once symptoms appear, prognosis is poor unless there is surgical repair or replacement of the valve.

CONGENITAL HEART DISEASE

Congenital malformations of the heart may result from faulty embryonic development or from failure of the fetal circulation to adapt to life after birth. They are common, occurring in 1 in 100 live births, and may manifest in childhood or may cause no symptoms until later in life.

THE FETAL CIRCULATION

The fetal circulatory system is significantly different to the circulatory system after birth, mainly because the fetal lungs are non-functional. The unborn child absorbs essential nutrients and oxygen, excretes wastes across the placental membranes, and receives all nutritional support from the mother. The fetal pulmonary circulation is collapsed, and very little cardiac output goes to the fetal lungs.

Blood returning to the fetal heart from the fetal veins is delivered to the right atrium. It is important that this is not then delivered to the non-functional lungs. The pulmonary circulation is largely collapsed, so resistance to blood flow into the pulmonary arteries is very high, and blood can be

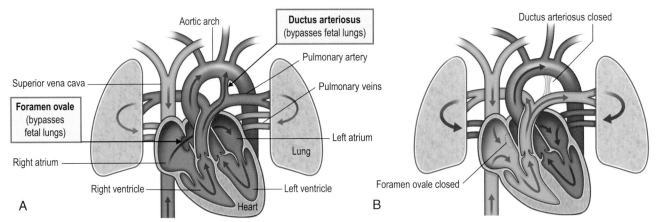

Fig. 6.25 The fetal heart and lungs. (A) Before birth. (B) Changes at birth. (Modified from Waugh A and Grant A (2018) *Ross & Wilson anatomy and physiology in health and illness*, 13th ed, Fig. 5.45. Oxford: Elsevier Ltd.)

readily shunted via alternative routes. The first bypass route is a right-to-left shunt between the atria. When the right atrium contracts, most of the blood within is pushed through a communicating channel into the left atrium, from where it travels into the left ventricle and back into the systemic circulation. This channel is called the **foramen ovale** (Fig. 6.25A). It is covered with a flap which acts as a valve so that blood may travel from right to left but not from left to right. Some blood from the right atrium reaches the right ventricle, and it too must be diverted away from the fetal lungs. Therefore, as the right ventricle contracts and ejects the blood into the pulmonary artery, most of it travels through a small communicating artery called the **ductus arteriosus** (Fig. 6.25A), which links the pulmonary artery directly to the aorta.

After delivery of the baby, pressures within the cardiovascular system change. It is essential that the blood flow through the lungs is established immediately because the baby has lost the placental supply of oxygen. The fetal shunts must be closed down (Fig. 6.25B).

As the baby takes those first breaths, blood oxygen levels surge, which causes vasodilation in the pulmonary circulation. This rapidly reduces resistance in the lungs, so blood begins to flow into the pulmonary blood vessels. Pressure therefore immediately falls in the right side of the heart and becomes lower than pressure in the left side. As pressure in the left atrium exceeds that in the right, the valve between them is pushed shut and the foramen ovale closes. All blood in the right atrium is now pumped into the right ventricle and into the pulmonary artery. The high oxygen levels in the blood constricts the ductus arteriosus, shutting down the shunt between the pulmonary artery and the aorta. With both these bypass mechanisms closed off, the newborn baby's cardiopulmonary circulation is now adapted for extrauterine life.

VENTRICULAR SEPTAL DEFECT

This is the commonest congenital heart defect, occurring in about 1 in 500 live births. The interventricular septum should be fully formed by the end of the first 8 weeks of embryonic life. Incomplete fusion of two key embryonic structures, called the *inferior and superior endocardial cushions*, leaves a communicating channel between the ventricles: the ventricular septal defect. If the defect is very small, it may close naturally within the first few years of life, and even if it persists

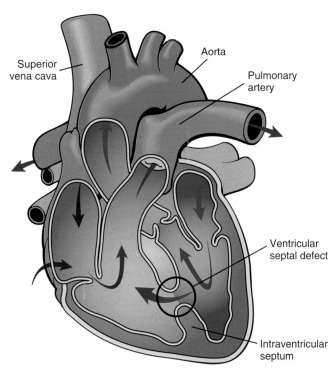

Fig. 6.26 Ventricular septal defect. (Modified from Damjanov I, Perry A, and Perry K (2022) *Pathology for the health professions*, 6th ed, Fig. 7.4. St Louis: Elsevier Inc.)

into adulthood, it may cause no problems. Larger defects are troublesome because they allow blood to flow from the high-pressure left ventricle to the low-pressure right ventricle (Fig. 6.26). This means that the amount of oxygenated blood leaving the left ventricle to supply the systemic circulation is reduced, leading to hypotension and hypoxia. Not only is the systemic circulation undersupplied, but the right ventricle now contains more blood than normal, which is pumped to the lungs, overloading the pulmonary circulation and causing pulmonary hypertension and pulmonary oedema. Surgical repair carries a good prognosis in most cases.

PATENT FORAMEN OVALE (ATRIAL SEPTAL DEFECT)

This is commoner in women than men (about a 2:1 ratio) and represents about 10% of congenital cardiac defects. It

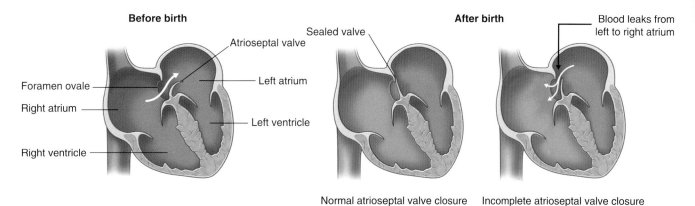

Fig. 6.27 Atrial septal defect. (From Waugh A and Grant A (2018) *Ross & Wilson anatomy and physiology in health and illness*, 13th ed, Fig. 5.59. Oxford: Elsevier Ltd.)

occurs when the flap of tissue covering the foramen ovale between the right and left atria fails to seal properly after birth, leaving a patent channel of communication (Fig. 6.27). Blood shunts from the high pressure left atrium to the lower pressure right atrium, reducing the cardiac output of the left ventricle, reducing systemic blood supply: hypotension and poor organ perfusion. At the same time, the right atrium and the right ventricle are overloaded, so they dilate and hypertrophy. The increased volume of blood entering the pulmonary circulation causes pulmonary hypertension, pulmonary congestion- and pulmonary oedema, which impairs gas exchange. Surgical repair carries a good prognosis.

PATENT DUCTUS ARTERIOSUS

Failure of the ductus arteriosus to close after birth allows oxygenated blood from the high-pressure aorta to shunt into the lower-pressure pulmonary artery, which carries blood under low pressure to the lungs (Fig. 6.28). This decreases delivery of blood to the systemic circulation, causing possible hypotension and poor systemic perfusion, but the main presenting problems usually involve pulmonary congestion and pulmonary hypertension because increased volumes of blood are shunted into the pulmonary artery. The workload of the right side of the heart is increased because of this, so there is right sided dilation and hypertrophy.

The ductus arteriosus normally constricts and closes within 15 hours of birth, and the closure becomes permanent over the first few weeks of life as it becomes fibrotic. As a solitary abnormality, patent ductus arteriosus is often asymptomatic and not diagnosed until adulthood. However, if it causes significant shunting into the lungs, it can cause permanent damage to the lung vasculature and trigger heart failure even in infancy and must be dealt with immediately. Risk factors include low birth weight, prematurity, female sex, and having affected siblings.

TRANSPOSITION OF THE GREAT ARTERIES

In the normal heart, the aorta is connected to the left ventricle and the pulmonary artery to the right ventricle, so blood is circulated alternately between the pulmonary and the systemic circulations. In complete transposition of the great arteries, the aorta is connected to the right ventricle and the pulmonary artery is connected to the left ventricle (Fig. 6.29A). This arrangement completely separates the pulmonary and the systemic circulations (Fig. 6.29B).

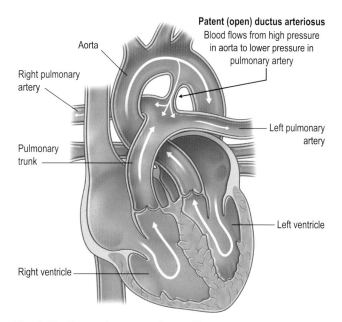

Fig. 6.28 Patent ductus arteriosus. (From Waugh A and Grant A (2018) *Ross & Wilson anatomy and physiology in health and illness*, 13th ed, Fig. 5.58. Oxford: Elsevier Ltd.)

It clearly cannot support life because blood circulating through the lungs has no route for supplying the body's tissues, and blood circulating through the systemic circulation has no route to travel through the lungs for oxygenation. It requires urgent surgical repair early in life. If the condition is picked up by antenatal scans, treatment can be planned and delivered as early as possible, which improves outcomes.

COARCTATION OF THE AORTA

This is a narrowing of the aorta, usually very close to the origin of the left subclavian artery on the aortic arch. This restricts blood flow from the left ventricle into the systemic circulation and increases flow into the arteries supplying the upper body and arms, which arise from the aortic arch proximal to the narrow point (Fig. 6.30) Coarctation of the aorta is commonly associated with other cardiac defects, including a bicuspid aortic valve, patent ductus arteriosus, and mitral valve stenosis. It is twice as common in men as women and is found in 1 in 4000 live births, accounting for 5% to 8% of all congenital heart defects.

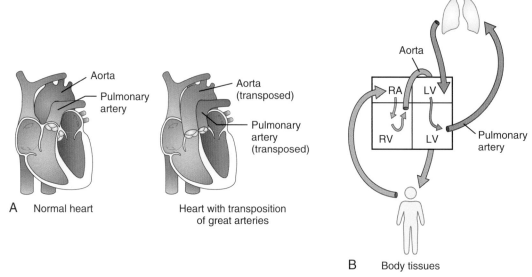

Fig. 6.29 Transposition of the great arteries.

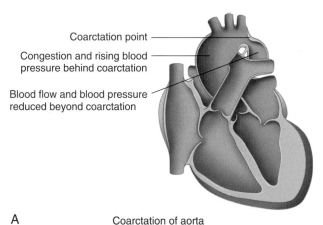

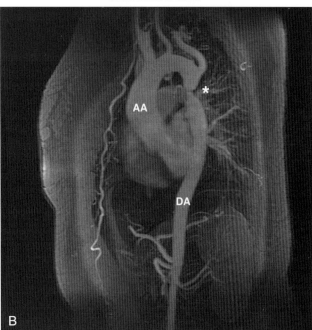

Fig. 6.30 Coarctation of the aorta. (A) Illustration showing the coarctation point. (B) Magnetic resonance image showing coarctation of the aorta (asterisk) in the proximal descending thoracic aorta (DA). AA, Ascending aorta. (Modified from (A) William D. Edwards, MD, Mayo Clinic, Rochester, MN; (B) Lockwood C, Moore T, Copel J et al (2019) *Creasy and Resnik's maternal-fetal medicine: principles and practice*, 8th ed, Fig. 52.11. Philadelphia: Elsevier Inc.)

Mild narrowing may give no symptoms, but with greater degrees of obstruction, the systemic circulation receives less blood, leading to poor perfusion of the legs and feet. With time, collateral vessels develop, which divert some of the aortic blood from the ballooning blocked aorta into other arterial beds and help reduce upper body congestion and improve lower body perfusion. Poor renal blood flow can trigger systemic hypertension (p.165). Hypertension in the upper body and head can cause headaches and aneurysms of the cerebral arteries. The left ventricle has a greatly increased workload as it tries to pump blood through the obstructed aorta. Left ventricular enlargement, hypertrophy, and heart failure all develop quickly in a severely affected child. If the condition is milder and not diagnosed until later in life, the presenting symptom is usually systemic hypertension (because of activation of the renin-angiotensin system; see Fig. 6.43). The condition requires surgical correction.

INFECTIVE AND INFLAMMATORY CONDITIONS OF THE HEART

The heart may be colonised by bacteria circulating in the bloodstream, damaged by circulating inflammatory mediators, or targeted by immunological mechanisms.

INFECTIVE ENDOCARDITIS

This is infection of the endocardium, which lines the heart chambers and covers the valves. It sometimes presents as an acute condition, but if treatment is inadequate, it may become chronic. The infecting organism is introduced by an invasive event such as tooth extraction, intravenous drug use, endoscopy, surgery, or insertion of intravenous lines, and survives and multiplies in the bloodstream. A range of bacteria and other microbes can cause the infection, depending on the nature of the event that introduced the infection in the first place. For example, because the mouth is heavily populated with streptococcal species, they are usually the culprits in infective endocarditis arising from poor oral hygiene or a dental procedure. Staphylococci and enterococci are also frequent causes: *S. aureus* is the commonest causative organism worldwide. The strains associated with

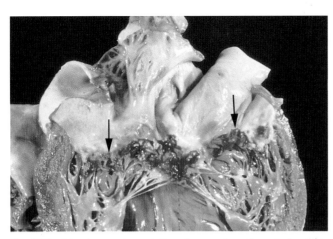

Fig. 6.31 Streptococcal vegetations (arrowed) on the mitral valve in bacterial endocarditis. (From Kumar V, Singh M, Abbas A, et al. (2022) *Robbins & Cotran pathologic basis of disease*, 10th ed, South Asia Edition, Volume 1, Fig. 12.24A. New Delhi: RELX India Pvt. Ltd.)

infective endocarditis are often well equipped to resist body defences and are good at surviving attack by complement and other immune mechanisms. They are therefore more likely to persist, and the infection may become chronic. The incidence of infective endocarditis is higher in older people and three times higher in males than females.

Pathophysiology

Bacteria adhere to the endocardium and establish growth, and it is easier for them to do this if the endocardium is damaged in some way. Within the cardiovascular system, the endocardium is most likely to be damaged at sites of turbulence, such as sites where blood vessels divide, or, within the heart, where blood flows over valves. It is not surprising, then, that infective endocarditis mainly affects the heart valves, especially the mitral and aortic valves, where blood flow and turbulence are highest. Cardiac implants, such as prosthetic valves and pacemakers, can provide a focus for infection.

Bacteria establish colonies on the valve cusps. These colonies trigger platelet activation and fibrin deposition, further roughening the area and making it easier for other bacteria to attach and establish themselves, which in turn attract more platelets and accelerate the formation of a mass of bacteria-rich vegetation at the site (Fig. 6.31). Buried within the vegetation, bacteria are protected from body defences. Vegetation growth triggers local inflammation, which progressively damages the valve and surrounding tissue. The growing vegetation impedes the ability of the valve to open and close normally and causes valvular incompetence. In addition, chunks of the vegetation may break off the main mass and travel as emboli in the bloodstream, blocking distant blood vessels, and possibly establishing sites of infection elsewhere. In chronic infective endocarditis, the immune system produces antibodies to the invading bacteria, generating significant quantities of immune complexes (p. 92) that deposit in tissues throughout the body, leading to systemic effects, such as glomerulonephritis and joint involvement.

Signs and symptoms

These are variable, depend on whether the condition is acute or chronic, and need careful assessment to ensure a diagnosis is not missed. General indicators of infection include fever, sepsis, and the appearance of peripheral abscesses. Blood cultures may grow typical bacteria. Cardiac-related signs and symptoms may develop, including valvular murmurs or indications of heart failure. Small haemorrhagic spots may appear on the palms and the soles of the feet, and on mucous membranes such as the conjunctivae and oral membranes. Renal failure, haematuria and cerebral emboli are also features.

Management and prognosis

Without treatment, mortality is very high. Control/prevention of infection and antibiotic treatment are the cornerstone of management.

RHEUMATIC HEART DISEASE

Rheumatic heart disease follows an episode of rheumatic fever, which in turn is usually secondary to a type A streptococcal throat infection. Rheumatic fever is a multisystem disorder, but the heart is usually the only organ that suffers long-lasting consequences. About 1 in 10 children with rheumatic fever develop cardiac complications. Antibodies are produced to bacterial components as part of the body's response to the infection, but these antibodies cross-react with myocardial proteins and damage the heart. The chronic autoimmune inflammatory process causes scarring and deformity of the affected heart. Acute rheumatic fever usually affects children and is the commonest cause of acquired heart disease in young people. There is a familial component, and a relationship between the development of rheumatic fever and certain types of HLA proteins (p.91) has been demonstrated.

Pathophysiology

Onset of symptoms usually falls 1 to 3 weeks after the sore throat. The anti-streptococcal antibodies bind to cardiac tissues, triggering inflammation and tissue destruction across all three layers of the heart wall (pancarditis), but the endocardium is usually the worst affected. Of the valves, the mitral and aortic valves are much more frequently affected than the pulmonary or tricuspid. The cusps become inflamed, thickened, and distorted, and the valve opening becomes narrowed. Myocardial damage includes scarring and necrosis of the muscle, potentially disrupting parts of the conducting pathway. Pericardial inflammation can lead to pericardial effusions (p.156), which restrict cardiac contractility.

Signs and symptoms

Pancarditis, plus valvular stenosis, can cause heart failure, which in turn causes breathlessness, tachycardia and cardiac enlargement. There may be heart pain. Myocardial damage and scarring can cause arrhythmias.

Management and prognosis

Penicillin is the antibiotic of choice to clear any residual streptococcal infection, and steroids dampen down the inflammatory and autoimmune processes damaging the heart. Heart failure is managed as required, and severe valvular damage might require valve repair or

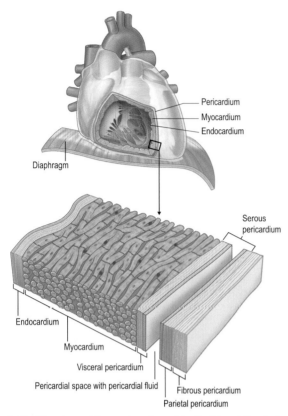

Fig. 6.32 Structure of the pericardium. (Modified from Waugh A and Grant A (2018) *Ross & Wilson anatomy and physiology in health and illness*, 13th ed, Fig. 5.9. Oxford: Elsevier Ltd.)

Table 6.1	The main causes of pericarditis
	Comments
Infective pericarditis	May be a variety of pathogens: bacterial (e.g., *Staphylococcus aureus*), fungal (e.g., *Candida albicans*), viral (e.g., coxsackie virus). Immunocompromised patients may be at higher risk. It may also be caused by tuberculosis.
Malignant pericarditis	Associated with malignant disease, such as breast or lung cancer. Pericarditis in cancer may result from direct infiltration into the pericardium from a local tumour, from the cancer treatment, or from circulating toxins originating from the tumour itself.
Post-myocardial infarction	After a transmural heart attack, pericarditis overlying the area of ischaemia is very common. It usually resolves with healing of the infarction.
Uraemia	Rising blood-borne metabolic toxins in renal failure irritate and inflame the pericardium.
Autoimmune and inflammatory disorders	Pericardial involvement in autoimmune disorders such as systemic lupus erythematosus, rheumatoid arthritis, and scleroderma and rheumatic fever occurs because circulating autoantibodies attack cardiac tissues.
Miscellaneous	Thyroid disease, direct trauma, allergic response to some drugs (e.g., penicillin).

replacement. Once the patient is over the age of 21, further attacks are unlikely.

PERICARDITIS

The pericardium, the outer membranes of the heart, protects the heart and lubricates its contractions within the pericardial sac. The structure of the pericardium is shown in Fig. 6.32. The fibrous pericardium anchors the heart to adjacent structures, and the two layers of the serous pericardium—the visceral and parietal pericardia—enclose the pericardial space, in which 20 to 49 mL of lipid-rich pericardial fluid lubricate the movement of the beating heart. It may be acute or chronic, and can be caused by infection or inflammation, although frequently a cause is not identified (idiopathic pericarditis). Idiopathic pericarditis is likely to be caused by an undiagnosed viral infection, and is seasonal, with spikes in spring and autumn. The main causes of pericarditis are summarised in Table 6.1.

Pathophysiology

Inflamed pericardial membranes become roughened and swollen and secrete non-lubricating inflammatory fluids that may contain pus, blood, or fibrin, depending on the cause of the pericarditis. This is called **pericardial effusion**, and large quantities of inflammatory fluid collecting in the pericardial space can compress the heart and impede its pumping action, a situation called **cardiac tamponade**. Healing can leave the pericardium with significant scar tissue, which can fuse the parietal and serous pericardia together,

eliminating the pericardial space. Scar tissue can also seriously interfere with the pumping action of the heart, leading to constrictive pericarditis.

Signs and symptoms

Fever and chest pain—which may be referred to the neck, back, arm, or shoulder—are common. Under the stethoscope, a characteristic scraping sound (**pericardial rub**) is heard over the inflamed pericardium. If heart function is reduced because of effusion, there may be breathlessness and indications of a falling cardiac output.

Management and prognosis

Most cases of pericarditis follow a self-limiting course and resolve with no long-term complications. Bed rest and anti-inflammatory treatment are usually effective, along with management of any identified factors such as infection. Eighty percent recover completely from a single acute attack, but about 20% progress to relapsing endocarditis with repeated episodes.

BLOOD VESSELS

The vascular system distributes blood to all body tissues. Arteries, which carry blood away from the heart, and veins, which return blood to the heart, possess the same three layers of tissue in their walls (Fig. 6.33). Capillaries, the tiny thin-walled vessels linking the arterial and venous networks, permit exchange of nutrients and wastes between the tissues and the blood. Tiny blood vessels, called the *vasa vasorum*, form a branching network in the walls of thicker blood vessels, to supply their tissues.

Disorders of the vascular network are common. Arteries absorb and transmit the pressure wave generated with each heartbeat. The mechanical and shear stress on their walls, caused by high pressures and rapid blood flow, over time causes a degree of stiffening even in healthy older people. Damage and disease involving blood vessels can have drastic consequences for perfusion and drainage of body tissues. Medium to large veins of the lower limbs are equipped with valves, to promote return of blood to the heart, usually against gravity, and under the low pressures associated with venous blood flow.

ARTERIOSCLEROSIS AND ATHEROSCLEROSIS

Sclerosis derives from the Greek term meaning 'harden'. **Arteriosclerosis** is a general term, meaning hardening of blood vessel walls and usually refers to the age-related thickening and fibrosis seen mainly in muscular arteries of older people, although it can affect all blood vessels. **Atherosclerosis** also causes thickening and stiffening of blood vessel walls but should not be confused with arteriosclerosis because, although both pathological processes often occur together, their aetiologies have important differences.

Arteriosclerosis

With advancing age, blood vessel walls change and deteriorate. This applies particularly to those vessels subjected to high levels of mechanical stress, mainly the arteries. In arteriosclerosis, the wall becomes fibrosed and calcified. The wall is thickened and the lumen is narrowed, so blood flow is reduced. The vessel loses its elasticity, reducing the transmission of the pressure wave towards the distal parts of the body, and increasing the afterload of the heart, which has to work much harder to push blood through the stiffened and narrowed arteries. The related term, **arteriolosclerosis**, refers to sclerotic changes in small arteries (arterioles). Risk factors include increasing age, hypertension, diabetes, and smoking.

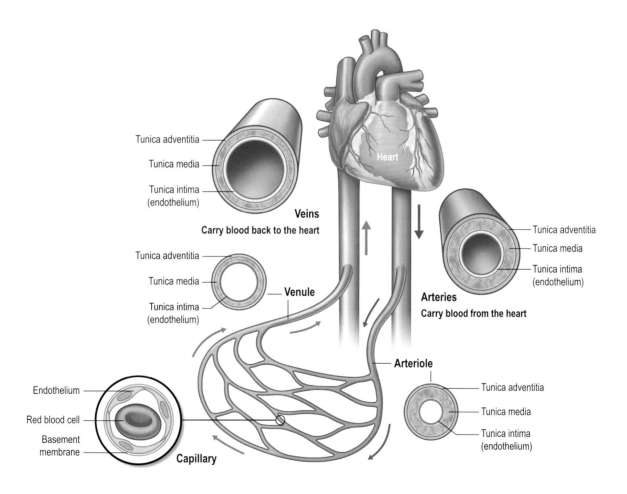

Fig. 6.33 The structure of blood vessel walls. (From Waugh A and Grant A (2018) *Ross & Wilson anatomy and physiology in health and illness*, 13th ed, Fig. 5.2. Oxford: Elsevier Ltd.)

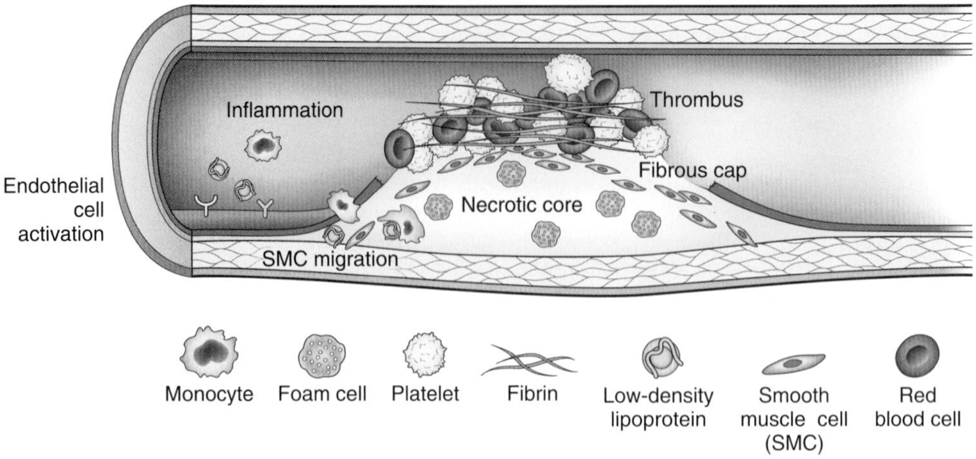

Fig. 6.34 The structure of a mature atherosclerotic plaque. (Modified from Dormont I, Varna M, and Couvreur P (2018) Nanoplumbers: biomaterials to fight cardiovascular diseases, *Materials Today* 21(2): 122–143. https://doi.org/10.1016/j.mattod.2017.07.008.)

Atherosclerosis

The primary event underpinning atherosclerosis is accumulation of low-density lipoprotein within the arterial wall. This activates macrophages and initiates an inflammatory response, forming patches of thickened, remodelled tissue. These patches are called *plaques* and are covered by a rough, fibrous cap that can trigger thrombosis.

Pathophysiology

Fig. 6.34 shows the evolution of an atherosclerotic plaque within the intima. The process is initiated at a site of endothelial damage, often associated with high pressure or turbulent blood flow, for example at arterial branching points. The early stages of atheroma formation are associated with a fatty streak, a yellowish patch on the damaged endothelium, which is the focal area for the development of progressive inflammatory changes within the vessel wall. Damaged endothelium functions very differently to healthy endothelium. Firstly, it becomes increasingly 'sticky' because it produces adhesion molecules, which allow inflammatory cells and other circulating cells (including pathogenic organisms) to adhere to the arterial wall. Secondly, it loses its anti-thrombogenic properties, so that instead of inhibiting clot formation, it now provides a surface that favours it. Thirdly, it becomes increasingly permeable, allowing substances such as plasma proteins and low-density lipoproteins (LDLs) to cross into the subintimal tissues. Here, the accumulating lipoprotein is taken up by macrophages, whose job is to scavenge and destroy unwanted materials. The ongoing influx of LDLs into the arterial wall rapidly bloats the macrophage population with fat, leading to the formation of **foam cells**, macrophages with a cytoplasm packed with bubbles of fat. Foam cells lyse and release their contents into the developing plaque, driving an ongoing inflammatory response and filling the core of the plaque with a yellowish, lipid rich, semiliquid sludge. The tissues of the plaque exist in a complex state of chronic inflammation. Multiple inflammatory cytokines and mediators are involved, including transforming-growth factor beta (TGFβ), promoting an ongoing inflammatory state and the migration of other cell types, including smooth muscle cells and other inflammatory cells, into the area. Over the top of the expanding plaque, fibroblasts lay down a fibrous cap, which supports the plaque and gives it mechanical strength. Its rough surface, however, may activate clotting and trigger thrombus formation. Mature plaques can also show calcification. There is evidence that blood supply to the diseased area via the vasa vasorum is impaired in atherosclerosis, contributing to reduced blood flow and the ongoing inflammatory response.

Plaque formation obstructs the blood vessel lumen, reducing blood flow. As it enlarges, the risk of rupture and thrombosis increases. When the cap ruptures, the blood comes into contact with the lipid-rich material forming the core of the plaque, triggering clotting. The thrombus forming at the site may block blood flow through the affected artery, preventing blood reaching distal tissues. In cerebral arteries, this can cause a stroke, and in coronary arteries this can cause myocardial infarction. If part of the thrombus breaks off and forms a travelling embolus, it will block blood supply to whichever organ bed it eventually lodges in. Risk factors for atherosclerosis are shown in Box 6.2. Atherosclerosis is a systemic condition and can affect blood vessels in any part of the body, although the cerebral and coronary arteries are often affected, causing stroke, angina, and myocardial infarction.

PERIPHERAL VASCULAR DISEASE (PVD)

Damage to arteries compromises blood supply to tissues. Damage to veins compromises blood drainage from tissues.

Peripheral arterial disease

This is usually caused by developing atherosclerotic plaques within the blood vessel wall, progressively obstructing blood flow to the distal tissues, with ischaemia and, if the blood supply is cut off altogether, necrosis. It often affects the lower limbs, the cerebral circulation, the abdominal circulation, and the renal arteries. Peripheral arterial disease is very common in older people, with a prevalence of about 15% in the over-75s. There is a sex imbalance, with males more often affected than women. Other risk factors include smoking, hyperlipidaemia, diabetes, and hypertension, all of which directly damage arterial walls.

Lower limb arterial disease

This is often referred to as *peripheral vascular disease*. Atherosclerotic changes in the large arteries supplying the lower limbs—namely, the aorta, the iliac, and the femoral

Box 6.2 Risk factors for atherosclerosis

Non-modifiable risk factors	Modifiable/potentially modifiable risk factors
Age, male sex, family history	Smoking, diabetes, obesity, high-fat diets low in fruit and vegetables, hypercholesterolaemia, some drugs (e.g., combined contraceptives, high alcohol intake, lack of exercise)

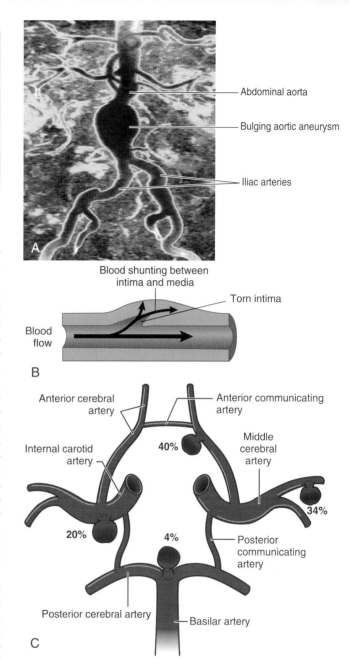

Fig. 6.35 Aneurysms. (A) Aortic aneurysm. (B) Dissecting aortic aneurysm. (C) Berry aneurysms in the circulus arteriosus (circle of Willis). (Modified from (A) Zephyr/Science Photo Library. Reproduced with permission; (B) Aitken L, Marshall A, and Chaboyer W (2016) *ACCCN's critical care nursing*, Fig. 10.16C. Sydney: Elsevier Australia; (C) Banasik J (2022) *Pathophysiology*, 7th ed, Fig. 44.16. St Louis: Saunders.)

arteries—progressively reduce blood supply. Ischaemia, ulceration, and possibly necrosis develop as tissue perfusion worsens.

Signs and symptoms. These depend on how high in the arterial tree the obstruction is, and how complete the blockage. With mild obstruction, the distal tissues may have an adequate oxygen supply at rest and with mild exercise, but symptoms develop during more strenuous exercise as the tissues become ischaemic. Leg pain associated with exercise-induced ischaemia of the muscles is called **intermittent claudication**. It usually occurs in the calf because the artery supplying the calf muscles, the superficial femoral artery, is commonly involved, but if arteries supplying the buttock and thigh are affected, intermittent claudication is felt in those muscles as well. As the atheroma progresses and the obstruction worsens, pain develops with less and less exertion, and eventually occurs constantly, even at complete rest. The limb is cool and may be cyanosed or discoloured, and the skin is dry. Necrosis may appear in the toes, and spread proximally, as the blood supply becomes poorer and poorer. Distal pulses become increasingly hard to find and disappear altogether as the condition progresses.

Management and prognosis. Necrosis of the toes and foot may require surgical removal, but death in these patients is usually related to cardiac or cerebrovascular disease because atheroma is likely to be widespread. Lifestyle adjustments are essential, including smoking cessation and managed exercise programmes. Contributing factors such as diabetes and hypercholesterolaemia must be managed.

Aneurysm

Aneurysm is a permanent ballooning of a blood vessel, causing its diameter to double or more (Fig. 6.35A). It is caused by a weakness in the wall, often associated with hypertension and atherosclerosis, but it may also be secondary to structural abnormality. In Marfan syndrome, for example, an inherited abnormal form of the protein fibrillin produces faulty elastic tissue, weakening the arterial wall. Other rarer causes of aneurysm include bacterial or fungal infections, in which the wall of the artery is damaged when organisms circulating in the bloodstream adhere to the intima and establish growth. This triggers inflammatory and immune responses that cause fibrosis and weakening at the site.

Aortic aneurysm. The aorta is the commonest site of aneurysm because, of all the body's blood vessels, it experiences the highest blood pressures and shear stresses. It is usually associated with atherosclerotic damage and develops most frequently in the abdominal aorta between the origins of the right and left renal arteries. It is common, with a prevalence of 3% of men over 65, particularly those with evidence of atherosclerotic peripheral vascular disease. It usually goes unnoticed until it becomes so large that it begins to cause symptoms, or until it ruptures, which is usually a life-terminating event. As the aneurysm expands, it compresses adjacent structures, which causes pain in the loin, abdomen, or back depending on its location along the aorta. Compression of the vasa vasorum in the aortic wall reduces blood supply, further weakening the vessel wall.

Dissecting aortic aneurysms originate with a tear in the aortic intima, and the high pressure of blood in the aorta haemorrhages blood into this tear, progressively extending it and separating the layers of the aortic wall. This weakens the wall and leads to aneurysm formation (Fig. 6.35B).

Berry aneurysm. These aneurysms arise somewhere along the circulus arteriosus (circle of Willis), the ring-road of blood vessels at the base of the brain from which the brain itself is supplied (Fig. 6.35C). Berry aneurysms arise at points where arteries branch from the circle, which experience high turbulence and mechanical stress. Rupture here causes subarachnoid haemorrhage.

Raynaud phenomenon

Raynaud phenomenon is characterised by intense vasoconstriction, usually of the hands or feet, with perfusion so low that the tissues become strikingly white. It is usually in response to cold and is reversible. The affected areas show a clear line of demarcation and may be painful (Fig. 6.36). Reperfusion causes cyanosis, followed by redness, as rebound hyperaemia brings in extra blood to supply the oxygen-starved tissues. If there is no identified cause or accompanying clinical disease, the condition is called *Raynaud disease* (sometimes also called *primary Raynaud disease*). It affects about 5% of the population and manifests at a young age, and women are more commonly affected than men.

The phenomenon may be part of the clinical picture associated with an identified systemic disease in which case it is referred to as secondary Raynaud disease, or just Raynaud phenomenon. It is important to distinguish between primary Raynaud and secondary Raynaud disease to offer appropriate treatment.

Pathophysiology

It is not certain what the underlying fault is in primary Raynaud disease. Deficiencies in key vasodilator agents, such as nitric oxide and calcitonin gene-related peptide, have been identified. Other studies suggest that vasoconstrictor agents such as endothelin and thromboxane A_2 may be overactive. Some research suggests that central control of blood vessel

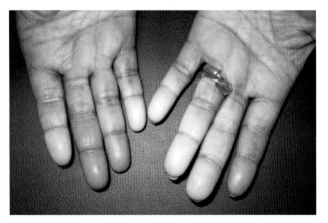

Fig. 6.36 Raynaud phenomenon. (From Firestein G, Budd R, Gabriel SE, et al. (2021) *Firestein & Kelley's textbook of rheumatology*, 11th ed, Fig. 89.2. San Francisco: Elsevier Inc.)

diameter, by the vasomotor centre in the brainstem, may be faulty.

Raynaud phenomenon is seen in various autoimmune connective tissue diseases, including systemic sclerosis (p.104), in which circulating autoantibodies attack blood vessel tissues. It may also develop in some malignancies, in thyroid disease, and after drug treatment with, for example, some cytotoxic agents.

PERIPHERAL VENOUS DISEASE

Veins have thinner, more compliant walls than arteries and venous blood flows at much lower pressures than within the arterial system. Effective venous return from the lower leg relies on the so-called *muscular pump of the calf*, formed from the muscles and connective tissues in which the deep veins are embedded. The deep leg veins are supported by their surrounding tissues and squeezed every time the calf muscles contract. The squeezing action compresses them and pushes the blood towards the heart because the valves are designed to prevent backward flow. Each time the calf veins are compressed, 40% to 60% of the blood they contain is pushed towards the heart. Superficial veins lack this support and rely heavily on effective valve function to keep blood flowing one way.

Blood in the venous system is susceptible to pooling if return of blood to the heart is obstructed in any way, and the veins and their associated valves can become stretched and baggy, with sluggish blood flow and increased risk of thromboembolism, especially in superficial veins.

Varicose veins

Varicose veins are swollen sections of veins, caused by local pooling of blood. Blood pooling can occur because the valves are incompetent, the venous pressure is higher than normal, or the leg muscles are not compressing the veins adequately to help with venous return (or a combination of two or more of these factors). Superficial veins, with less support than deeper veins, are most commonly affected, and their bulging, distended appearance is obvious and often unsightly (Fig. 6.37). They can be painful, itchy, burning, or throbbing. The pooling blood (venous stasis) is at increased risk of clotting, which further obstructs blood flow and can cause stroke, pulmonary embolism, or a myocardial infarction if it dislodges and goes travelling in the bloodstream. As back pressure in the distended veins increases, the pressure on the valves increases and can cause permanent damage. Damaged valves, unable to close properly, permit backflow of blood, worsen venous pooling, and establish a self-perpetuating cycle. Risk factors include female sex, increasing age, increasing weight, spending long periods standing, and pregnancy.

THROMBOEMBOLISM

Blood flow in the venous system is slower than in the arterial system because venous pressure is lower than arterial pressure. Additionally, veins are baggier and hold larger quantities of blood than arteries; about two thirds of the body's total blood volume is normally found in the venous system. This contributes to an increased tendency for blood to pool and for clots to form. Thromboembolism, both arterial and venous, is discussed on p.126.

SHOCK

The term *shock* does not refer to a single disease but to a syndrome and is a possible consequence of a wide range of pathophysiological processes. Irrespective of the cause, shock can be defined as a condition in which the cells and tissues of the body have an inadequate oxygen supply and become hypoxic as a result. Here, shock will be considered in four categories: hypovolaemic shock, cardiogenic shock, distributive shock, and obstructive shock (Fig. 6.38).

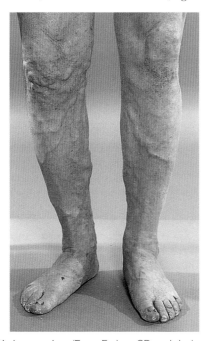

Fig. 6.37 Varicose veins. (From Forbes CD and Jackson WF (2003) *Color atlas and text of clinical medicine*, 3rd ed. London: Mosby.)

Hypovolaemic shock

The underlying haemodynamic problem here is reduced circulating blood volume. This may be caused by haemorrhage or excessive fluid loss associated with gastrointestinal disorders, renal disorders, or burns. Rapid loss of circulating blood volume causes a drastic fall in blood pressure, reduced venous return to the heart, reduced cardiac output, and reduced perfusion and hypoxia in systemic tissues (Fig. 6.38A).

Cardiogenic shock

The underlying haemodynamic problem here is failure of the heart to pump effectively, despite normal blood volume and normal venous return. This might follow a massive myocardial infarction, or in acute heart failure. In cardiac tamponade, blood or serous fluid collecting in the pericardial space compresses the heart and impedes contraction. When the heart cannot beat effectively and clear the blood returning to it from the venae cavae, pressure builds up in the venous system, blood flow through the lungs is reduced, and the output of the left ventricle into the systemic circulation falls, with reduced perfusion and tissue hypoxia. (Fig. 6.38B). The consequences of cardiogenic shock are very similar to those seen in acute heart failure (Fig. 6.13).

Distributive shock

The underlying haemodynamic problem here lies with the inability of the peripheral blood vessels to maintain adequate pressure in the system. An example is **septic shock**, in which an identified or suspected infection triggers an overwhelming and dysregulated response in the host. Another example is **anaphylactic shock**, with widespread and sudden vasodilation. Blood pressure falls rapidly. In anaphylactic shock, the blood vessels also become significantly more permeable, so

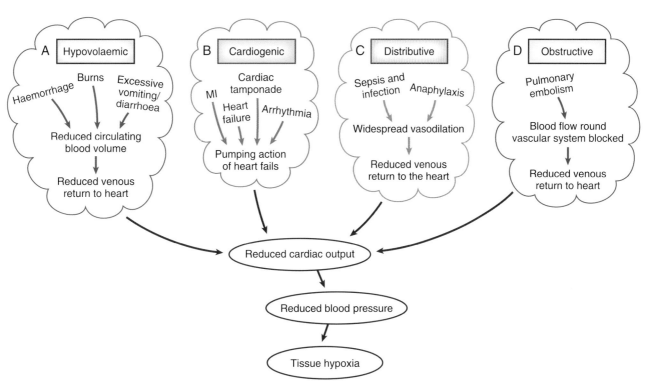

Fig. 6.38 The four types of shock. (A) Hypovolaemic shock. (B) Cardiogenic shock. (C) Distributive shock. (D) Obstructive shock.

not only does the vascular compartment suddenly expand, but the volume within it falls as fluid leaves the bloodstream and enters the tissues. Reduced blood pressure and circulating blood volume rapidly lead to poor tissue perfusion and hypoxia (Fig. 6.38C)

Obstructive shock

The underlying haemodynamic problem here is caused by some mechanical blockage or restriction of blood flow. An example is massive pulmonary embolism, which obstructs blood flow through the lungs, reducing return to the left side of the heart and reducing left ventricular output. This leads to poor tissue perfusion and hypoxia (Fig. 6.38D).

COMPENSATORY MECHANISMS IN SHOCK

With the onset of poor tissue perfusion, hypoxia, and metabolic acidosis from the accumulation of wastes, compensatory mechanisms are rapidly activated. Key mechanisms centre on the sympathetic nervous system, which in turn activates the renin-angiotensin system. The aim of the compensatory mechanisms (Fig. 6.39) is to maintain blood pressure and tissue perfusion, and they give rise to some of the clinical manifestations seen in shock (e.g., tachycardia and fluid retention).

The early stages of all forms of shock reduce blood flow through peripheral tissues. There may or may not be a reduced blood volume, and there may or may not be a metabolic acidosis caused by carbon dioxide retention and lactate production at this stage, depending on how rapidly the shock has developed. Falling blood pressure activates the baroreceptor reflex (p.137), which increases heart rate and contractility and triggers systemic vasoconstriction, both of which increase venous return and cardiac output. This is enhanced by release of adrenaline from the adrenal medulla. Reduced renal perfusion activates the renin-angiotensin system (see Fig. 6.43), which causes widespread vasoconstriction and increases sodium and fluid retention, supporting blood pressure.

Multiple endocrine mechanisms are activated in addition to the renin-angiotensin system. Cortisol is released from the adrenal cortex. This glucocorticoid hormone activates fundamental metabolic mechanisms designed to help the body deal with stress. It increases blood glucose levels and releases free fatty acids from fat stores so that key body tissues have access to sources of energy and increases blood amino acid levels. It stimulates fluid retention by the kidney to maintain blood volume and pressure and suppresses anabolic activity such as bone building so that the availability of raw materials remains high. It also suppresses the inflammatory and immune responses. Other hormones include ADH, which leads to water retention, again with the aim of supporting blood pressure; and endogenous opioids, the body's natural analgesics. If circulating blood volume is low, the spleen contracts to expel its stored blood. The splenic blood reserve is about 350 mL.

THE PATHOPHYSIOLOGY OF SHOCK

The ability of compensatory mechanisms to maintain cardiovascular function is finite. When they are exhausted, or are themselves contributing to the deteriorating situation, shock develops. Multiple mechanisms contribute towards the downward spiralling combination of events in developing shock, with progressive cell injury, hypoxia, ischaemia, and eventual complete circulatory collapse and death.

Increased sympathetic drive

As described previously, activation of the sympathetic nervous system in the early stages of shock from whatever cause supports cardiovascular function by stimulating the heart, increasing fluid retention and blood volume, and causing vasoconstriction to maintain blood pressure. These mechanisms are initially supportive but as shock progresses, they become maladaptive. Increased sympathetic drive to the heart initially increases its performance,

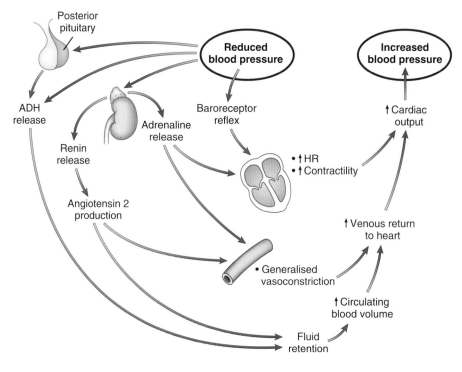

Fig. 6.39 Compensatory mechanisms in shock.

but also its workload and its oxygen demands. Eventually, the heart becomes exhausted and begins to fail. Vasoconstriction initially maintains blood pressure but contributes to the workload of the heart by increasing peripheral resistance and reduces blood flow to the tissues, worsening perfusion and hypoxia.

Release of inflammatory and immune mediators

In septic shock, circulating microbial materials stimulate the inflammatory and immune responses. One important bacterial product—**lipopolysaccharide** (LPS, endotoxin), derived from the cell wall of Gram^{-ve} bacteria—is particularly potent in this respect and stimulates massive release of inflammatory and immune mediators. This worsens cardiovascular insufficiency by causing vasodilation and increased vascular permeability. Activation of phagocytes (e.g., neutrophils) releases their destructive contents, causing tissue damage.

Increased coagulability of the blood

As part of the body's response to stress or injury, the blood becomes hypercoagulable. This reduces the danger of haemorrhage but increases the risk of inappropriate intravascular clotting, which can block blood vessels and contribute to microvascular damage and poor tissue perfusion. In developing shock, whatever its origin, blood flow becomes sluggish: in distributive shock, this is because of vasodilation and a fall in pressure; in cardiogenic shock, because the pressure generated by the heart is reduced; in hypovolaemic shock, because blood volume is falling; and in obstructive shock, because of low blood flow beyond the obstruction. This increases the risk of thrombus formation, which is further increased by the inflammatory response developing as part of the shock pathogenesis.

Shift from aerobic to anaerobic metabolism

All forms of shock are characterised by tissue hypoxia, either because the cells are using more oxygen than normal or because oxygen delivery is reduced. In distributive shock, oxygen delivery is reduced because of massive vasodilation, leading to a fall in blood pressure and poor tissue perfusion. In cardiogenic shock, there is inadequate perfusion because of poor heart function. In hypovolaemic shock, there is inadequate circulating blood to carry enough oxygen to supply the tissues. In obstructive shock, the obstruction to blood flow somewhere in the circulatory system leads to reduced blood supply beyond the obstruction, and tissue hypoxia. With inadequate oxygen, cells shift to anaerobic metabolism, which can only be safely sustained for short periods of time before accumulating waste products begin to affect cellular health. Anaerobic metabolism is a very inefficient way of producing ATP. In the presence of oxygen, 38 ATP molecules can be generated from a single glucose molecule. In anaerobic conditions, that falls to two. Therefore, ATP production in hypoxic cells rapidly falls, and very quickly the cell is unable to make enough ATP to meet its energy needs. When that happens, essential cellular processes begin to fail. Among them is the Na$^+$/K$^+$ pump, responsible for pumping sodium out of the cell and potassium in, keeping sodium levels high outside the cell and low inside, and vice versa for potassium. This ionic gradient is essential for the electrical activity of nerve and muscle, including the heart. Pump failure rapidly depresses the contractility of the heart and worsens its decline. Accumulating lactic acid and other acidic products of anaerobic metabolism reduces cellular pH, deactivating cellular enzyme systems and damaging blood vessel walls. This further increases vascular permeability, reduces blood flow, accelerates tissue damage and hypoxia, and increases blood clotting.

An additional consequence of failure of the Na$^+$/K$^+$ pump is redistribution of body water. When Na$^+$/K$^+$ pump function declines, sodium rapidly accumulates inside cells. This draws water after it, and the proportion of total body water inside cells increases. The interstitial fluids therefore become more concentrated because they have lost water to the intracellular compartment, and to equalise osmolarity, the interstitial fluid draws water out of the bloodstream. Circulating blood volume therefore falls even further, reducing perfusion and increasing the strain on the heart.

Poor perfusion in capillary beds causes microvascular damage. Tiny blood vessels rapidly become blocked by accumulating tissue debris, making perfusion worse. Fig. 6.40 summarises the metabolic impairment that develops in shock.

SIGNS AND SYMPTOMS

Depending on the initiating events, the signs and symptoms of shock can vary (Fig. 6.41). In the early stages, compensatory mechanisms can preserve blood flow, and blood pressure can remain within the normal range until shock is quite well developed.

Hypovolaemic shock

Hypovolaemic shock (Fig. 6.41A) causes tachycardia, pallor, and cool extremities as sympathetic stimulation of the heart and peripheral vasoconstriction attempt to maintain tissue perfusion. Up to 20% of total blood volume can be lost before shock develops. The pulse is thin and thready because blood volume is low. The person is thirsty because activation of the renin-angiotensin system releases aldosterone, which stimulates thirst. Urine production is reduced while the kidneys attempt to conserve water to bolster blood volume. There is confusion, drowsiness, and irritability caused by cerebral hypoxia; and anxiety and sweating caused by sympathetic stimulation. Acidosis caused by carbon dioxide retention and lactate production stimulates respiratory chemoreceptors and increases respiratory rate.

Cardiogenic shock

The signs and symptoms of cardiogenic shock (Fig. 6.41B) are similar to hypovolaemic shock because the amount of blood reaching the tissues is low as a result of low cardiac output. In addition, there may be cardiac pain if there is associated MI, and signs of heart failure, such as pulmonary congestion and raised jugular venous pressure.

Distributive shock

There is widespread vasodilation, so the person is flushed and has warm skin, hands, and feet (Fig. 6.42C). There is tachycardia and increased respiratory rate. In anaphylactic shock, signs and symptoms depend on the nature of the

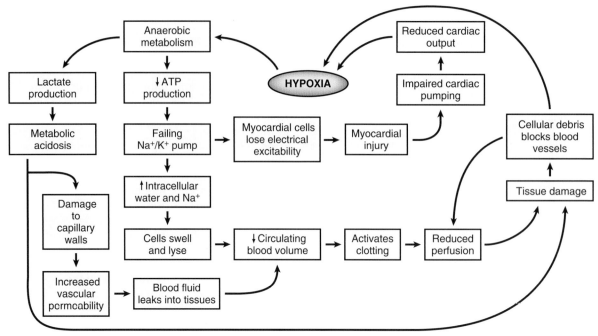

Fig. 6.40   The metabolic changes in shock.

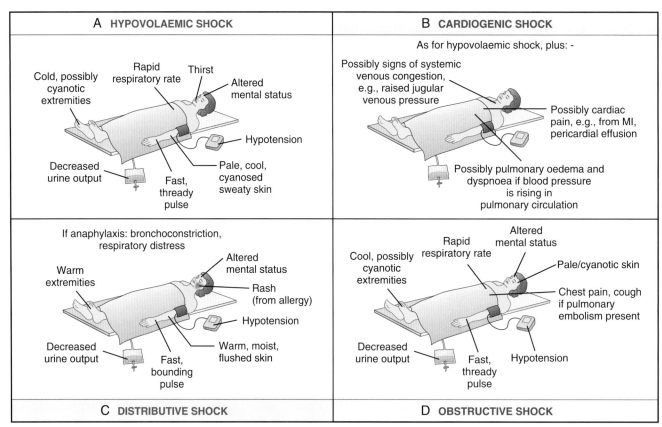

Fig. 6.41   The signs and symptoms of shock.

allergic stimulus: bronchospasm, skin reactions, itch, respiratory distress caused by upper respiratory airway swelling and obstruction, or gastrointestinal symptoms like abdominal pain and diarrhoea. In septic shock, usually secondary to infection, there may be fever, nausea, vomiting, a bounding pulse, rashes, and intravascular coagulation.

Obstructive shock

Signs and symptoms (Fig. 6.42D) are very similar to hypovolaemic shock because the amount of blood reaching the tissues is low because of the obstruction. If the obstruction is caused by a pulmonary embolism (p.191), there may be signs and symptoms associated with that.

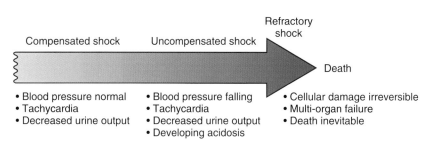

Fig. 6.42   The continuum of shock.

Compensated and uncompensated shock

Shock can be seen as a continuum composed of three stages that merge into one another as it progresses, and it can develop terrifyingly fast. In the early stages of developing shock, compensatory mechanisms as described previously support cardiovascular function and identifying a shocked patient may be difficult. This is called **compensated shock**. Once the capacity of the compensatory mechanisms to maintain tissue perfusion is exhausted, the state of **uncompensated shock** follows, and reflects vicious circles of progressive deterioration in multiple organs. Blood pressure falls, myocardial function is progressively reduced, there is renal failure, pulmonary oedema develops, and central nervous system function depressed. The point at which organ damage is irreversible and death is inevitable marks the beginning of the end stage, refractory shock (Fig. 6.42).

MANAGEMENT AND PROGNOSIS

Identifying and treating the underlying cause is essential; for example, antibiotics in sepsis and fluid replacement in hypovolaemic shock. The earlier the diagnosis is made, the better. Mortality from any type of shock rises substantially the longer the delay in initiating treatment.

DISORDERS OF BLOOD PRESSURE

REGULATION OF BLOOD PRESSURE

With each heartbeat, the heart forces blood into the arterial system, generating a pressure wave that needs to be powerful enough to carry blood to the distal tissues. Blood pressure is the pressure exerted on the walls of blood vessels as the blood surges through them. It does not remain constant throughout the cardiac cycle (Fig. 6.4); it is at its highest at the peak of ventricular contraction and falls to its lowest during cardiac diastole. These two extremes are measured as the **systolic** and **diastolic** pressures, respectively.

Moment-to-moment regulation of blood pressure by the baroreceptor reflex is described earlier in the chapter (Fig. 6.7). Longer-term control is achieved primarily by the renin-angiotensin system (RAS), mediated by the kidney. Renal disorders and disturbances of the RAS are frequently involved in hypertension.

The kidney and blood pressure

Each of the kidney's 1.5 million nephrons possesses a highly specialised structure called the **juxtaglomerular apparatus** (JGA; see Fig. 12.6). The JGA is a bundle of cells lying close to the point where the distal convoluted tubule of the nephron and the afferent arteriole bringing blood into the glomerulus of the nephron lie next to each other. The JGA measures blood pressure in the afferent arteriole. If it detects a fall in blood pressure or a fall in blood sodium levels the kidney responds by releasing the enzyme **renin** into the bloodstream. Renin acts on an inactive precursor—angiotensinogen—in the circulation, and converts it into **angiotensin I**. Angiotensin I is biologically inactive, but as it passes through the pulmonary capillaries, **angiotensin converting enzyme** (ACE) converts it into the highly active **angiotensin II**. This agent increases blood pressure by several mechanisms. Firstly, angiotensin II is a direct vasoconstrictor. Secondly, it triggers aldosterone release from the adrenal cortex. Aldosterone, a mineralocorticoid, increases sodium and water retention in the kidney, increasing the body's water load, blood volume, and blood pressure. ADH levels also rise, stimulating water reabsorption by the kidney, and angiotensin II also stimulates sympathetic nervous system activity with the consequent stimulatory effects on cardiovascular function (Fig. 6.43).

HYPERTENSION

Hypertension, or high blood pressure, is strongly associated with increased risk of cardiovascular, renal, and cerebrovascular disease. It has been described as the leading preventable cause of death worldwide. In 2019 it was estimated that globally, 32% of adults aged between 30 and 79 had hypertension. The burden is not spread evenly; in wealthy countries, hypertension rates are falling, but are rising in economically developing countries. The difference is almost certainly the result of better awareness, detection, and public health management in richer countries. Blood pressure rises naturally with age because of age-related reduction in blood vessel elasticity and compliance. There is no given value that defines hypertension, although 140 mm Hg systolic and/or 90 mm Hg diastolic readings are often used as benchmarks for initiating treatment.

CLASSIFICATION OF HYPERTENSION

Conventionally, hypertension is split into two categories. In **primary (essential) hypertension**, there is no single identifiable cause for the raised blood pressure. In **secondary hypertension**, there is an identifiable condition responsible. Primary hypertension is far more common (90% of cases) than secondary.

Primary hypertension

Although there is no single cause, risk factors for primary hypertension are well recognised: increasing age, male sex, family history, smoking, diabetes, overweight, sedentary

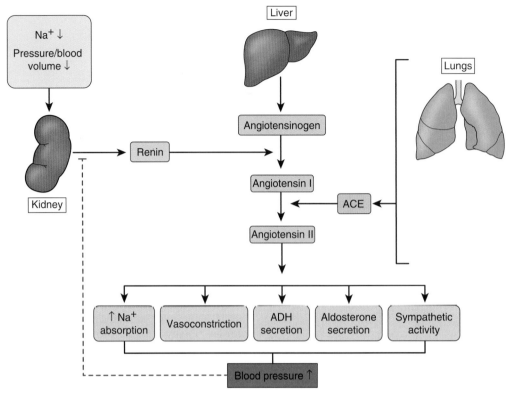

Fig. 6.43 The renin-angiotensin system. (Modified from Sidawy AN and Perler BA (2019) *Rutherford's vascular surgery and endovascular therapy*, 9th ed. Edinburgh: Elsevier Ltd.)

lifestyle, high-salt diets low in fresh foods and high in fats, sugars, processed foods, and alcohol.

Pathophysiology

The aetiology is multifactorial because the regulation of blood pressure in health is complex, depending on a range of hormones and neurological mechanisms.

Sympathetic nervous system overactivity. The sympathetic nervous system is believed to be dysfunctional in many hypertensive patients. Sympathetic overactivity causes increased cardiac output and general vasoconstriction, increasing blood pressure. In response to constantly increased blood pressure, blood vessels become stiff and non-compliant and unable to expand to accommodate ventricular output with each heartbeat. They become damaged, inflamed, and fibrosed, changes that become permanent with time and result in remodelling of the vessel wall. When this happens, many of the treatments used to manage hypertension become ineffective and the condition becomes treatment resistant.

Hypertension and diabetes mellitus. Hypertension is strongly associated with diabetes mellitus (DM): two thirds of DM sufferers are also hypertensive. The connection between these two important chronic disorders is complex and the subject of intense research. Type 2 DM is associated with insulin resistance, a decreased sensitivity of body cells to insulin. Cells that are less sensitive to insulin extract less glucose from body fluids, leading to hyperglycaemia, one of the key clinical problems in DM. Prolonged hyperglycaemia damages blood vessel walls, accelerating atherosclerosis development, leading to abnormal blood vessel function and worsening hypertension.

To restore normal glucose uptake, insulin-resistant people secrete excess insulin (hyperinsulinaemia). Insulin has other functions in the body in addition to increasing cellular uptake of glucose. It stimulates sodium reabsorption in the kidney, which may play a part in diabetes-related hypertension, and it also stimulates the sympathetic nervous system. Insulin is a growth stimulator, and hyperinsulinaemia may contribute to the remodelling and stiffening seen in blood vessels of diabetic hypertensive people. In addition, insulin resistance is associated with impaired vasodilation, which also may help explain the link between the two disorders.

Hypertension and inflammation. The link between a systemic inflammatory state and activation of immune mechanisms and primary hypertension is well established. Low-grade systemic inflammation is characterised by activation of a range of inflammatory cells, which infiltrate and damage the endothelium of blood vessels, including the renal vasculature. They release a range of inflammatory mediators, including interleukins and TNFα. The ongoing inflammatory response causes damage and dysfunction of blood vessels, including fibrosis, stiffening and increased sensitivity to sympathetic nervous system-induced vasoconstriction. Inflammatory changes in renal blood vessels are a major contributor in hypertension because it establishes a vicious circle as deteriorating renal function progressively activates fluid retention and vasoconstriction. Immunologically mediated (T-cell) damage to the kidney has also been implicated in some patients with hypertension.

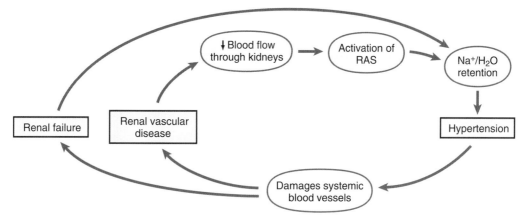

Fig. 6.44 The self-reinforcing relationship between hypertension and renal disease.

Management and prognosis

Lifestyle modification is always important, irrespective of other treatments. Stopping smoking, increasing exercise levels, and eating a healthy diet may be enough in mild cases to bring blood pressure down to acceptable levels. Diuretics to reduce blood volume, vasodilators to reduce peripheral resistance and beta-blockers to slow the heart and reduce cardiac workload are all effective anti-hypertensive agents.

Secondary hypertension

Some common causes of secondary hypertension are described here. Management of the condition is generally directed towards dealing with the underlying condition.

Pregnancy

In pregnancy, water retention and blood volume rise, as does cardiac output. All these factors can increase blood pressure. A reduction in systemic vascular resistance usually causes a slight fall in blood pressure in the first months of pregnancy but raised blood pressure is common in the later stages, especially in older or obese women. It generally resolves when the baby is delivered. Pre-eclampsia, a serious condition that threatens the lives of both baby and mother, is associated with the rapid development of hypertension, proteinuria, and fetal growth retardation.

Renal disease

The kidneys play a central role in the control of blood pressure, through regulation of body fluid load and activation of the renin-angiotensin system. Renal disease is often involved in hypertension, both as a consequence and a cause (Fig. 6.44). In renal artery disease (e.g., caused by atherosclerotic changes) blood flow through the kidney falls. The kidney responds by releasing renin, leading to angiotensin II production and an increase in blood pressure. On the other hand, the kidney is a common casualty in hypertension. High blood pressure damages tiny blood vessels, and the glomerular capillaries in the kidney are frequently targets. Reduced renal blood flow in turn activates the RAS and worsens hypertension.

Hormonal imbalances

Many hormones increase blood pressure, and increased production leads to hypertension. These include thyroxine from the thyroid gland, adrenaline from the adrenal medulla and steroid hormones (cortisol, aldosterone) from the adrenal cortex. Oestrogens are also hypertensive, including those in oral contraceptive preparations. The commonest cause of secondary hypertension is Conn syndrome (primary hyperaldosteronism).

PULMONARY HYPERTENSION

This is high blood pressure in the pulmonary circulation (p. 190). Pulmonary pressure values are significantly lower than systemic pressures. Average mean systemic arterial pressure is about 90 mm Hg. The corresponding pressure in the pulmonary circulation is about 14 mm Hg. This prevents blood fluid from being pushed into the alveoli. Pulmonary blood pressure higher than 25 mm Hg is defined as pulmonary hypertension.

Obstructed blood flow through the lungs increases blood pressure behind the obstruction but left-sided heart disease also causes pulmonary hypertension as blood backs up in the pulmonary veins. Fibrotic lung disorders increase pulmonary blood pressure because lung tissue and the vessels embedded within it become stiff and non-compliant. Disorders that destroy lung tissue also cause pulmonary hypertension because the same volume of blood coming from the right ventricle is forced through fewer vessels. Pulmonary embolism blocks one or both of the pulmonary arteries or their branches and increases pressure in the vessels feeding the blocked vessel.

BIBLIOGRAPHY AND REFERENCES

Berthiaume, J. M., Kirk, J. A., Ranek, M. J., et al. (2016). Pathophysiology of heart failure and an overview of therapies. In L. M. Buja, & J. Butany (Eds.), *Cardiovascular Pathology* (4th ed, pp. 271–339). Elsevier.

Brown, D. L. (2019). Coronary physiology and pathophysiology. In D. L. Brown (Ed.), *Cardiac Intensive Care* (3rd ed, pp. 60–67).

Smith, N., Lopez, R. A., & Silberman, M. (2019). *Distributive shock.* StatPearls. https://www.ncbi.nlm.nih.gov/books/NBK470316/.

Useful websites

Straightforward explanation of the pathophysiology of myocardial infarction: https://www.khanacademy.org/science/health-and-medicine/circulatory-system-diseases/coronary-artery-disease/v/heart-attack-myocardial-infarction-pathophysiology Straightforward explanation of the pathophysiology of myocardial infarction

WHO factsheet on cardiovascular disease: https://www.who.int/health-topics/cardiovascular-diseases/#tab=tab_1

7 Disorders of Respiratory Function

CHAPTER OUTLINE

INTRODUCTION
  Anatomy of the respiratory system
  Gas exchange in the lungs and tissues
  Lung volumes and capacities
  Ventilation-perfusion matching
INFECTIONS OF THE RESPIRATORY TRACT
Viral respiratory tract infections
  Common cold
  Coronavirus infections
  Influenza
Pneumonia
Tuberculosis
MALIGNANCIES OF THE RESPIRATORY TRACT
OBSTRUCTIVE AND RESTRICTIVE LUNG DISEASE
Obstructive airways disease

  Asthma
  Cystic fibrosis
Restrictive lung disease
  Acute respiratory distress syndrome
  Interstitial lung disease
  Non-pulmonary causes of restrictive lung disease
PULMONARY VASCULAR DISEASE
Pulmonary hypertension
  Secondary pulmonary hypertension
Pulmonary embolism
  Pulmonary thromboembolism
PLEURAL DISORDERS
Lung collapse (atelectasis)
  Pneumothorax
  Pleural effusion
Mesothelioma

INTRODUCTION

The primary responsibility of the respiratory system is to provide the body with the means of absorbing atmospheric oxygen into the bloodstream and excreting carbon dioxide. Subsidiary functions include speech and the production of angiotensin II in activation of the renin–angiotensin system Fig 6.43. The upper parts of the respiratory tract are designed for bulk air flow, and they warm and moisten the air as it travels to the deeper structures. In the lower respiratory tract, gas exchange takes place across the fused membranes of the alveoli and the pulmonary capillaries. Bulk flow of air in and out of the respiratory passageways is controlled by co-ordinated contraction of groups of skeletal muscles, mainly the diaphragm and the intercostal muscles, supported by the accessory muscles of respiration such as the scalenes when required.

ANATOMY OF THE RESPIRATORY SYSTEM

Conventionally, the respiratory system is divided into two main parts: **upper** and **lower**, with the upper including respiratory structures in the head and neck, and the lower comprising the thoracic structures. Fig. 7.1 shows the main structures of the respiratory system.

Anatomy of the respiratory passageways

The mouth and nose are the entry and exit points for air travelling in or out of the respiratory system. The oral and nasal cavities open into the **trachea** (the windpipe) via the pharynx, which is shared with the digestive system. The trachea, about 10 to 11 cm in length, is supported by 12 to 20 incomplete rings of cartilage and lined with ciliated pseudostratified epithelium containing goblet cells. Goblet cells produce mucus, which traps inhaled particles, and is then cleared from the respiratory tract by the beating action of the cilia. At the level of the fifth thoracic vertebra, the trachea splits into the **right and left primary bronchi**, supplying the right and left lung, respectively. Within the lung, the primary bronchus divides into secondary and tertiary bronchi, which continue to branch into smaller and smaller passageways with thinner and thinner walls. Airways with a diameter less than 1 mm are called **bronchioles**. Terminal bronchioles open into respiratory bronchioles, which have alveoli bulging from their walls, and which in turn open into clusters of **alveoli**, the airsacs across whose walls gases are exchanged (Fig. 7.2).

The structure of the airway wall changes as the airways branch and become narrower. The largest airways, such as the trachea and the primary and secondary bronchi, have walls rich in cartilage for physical support to ensure airway patency. There is little smooth muscle in these large airways because contraction of the muscle could obstruct the airway and threaten life. Deeper in the respiratory tree, however, cartilage progressively disappears from the airway wall. At the bronchiolar level, all cartilage has disappeared. As the

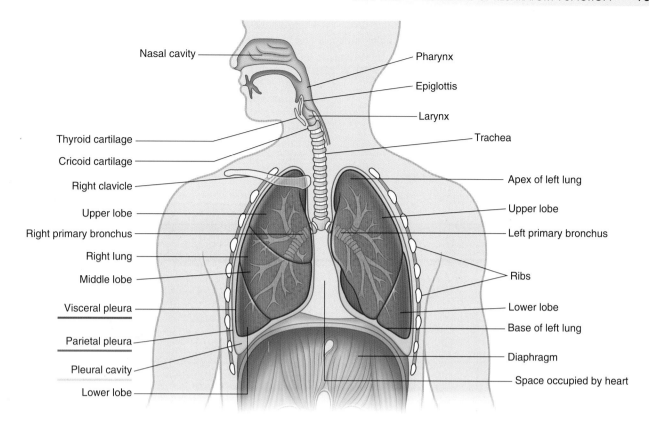

Fig. 7.1 The main structures of the respiratory system. (Modified from Waugh A and Grant A (2018) *Ross & Wilson anatomy and physiology in health and illness*, 13th ed, Fig 10.1. Oxford: Elsevier Ltd.)

cartilage content falls, the proportion of smooth muscle in the airway wall rises. This permits adjustment of airway diameter by bronchodilation and bronchoconstriction to regulate and direct airflow to different areas of the lung.

Anatomy of lung tissue

The lungs occupy most of the space within the thorax and are separated from each other by a region called the **mediastinum** containing the heart, major blood vessels, the trachea, and the oesophagus. The narrow upper section of the lung (the **apex**) projects into the lower neck and the flattened, curved lung **base** sits on the diaphragm. The lungs are subdivided into **lobes**, separated by fissures: the right lung is divided into three lobes and the left lung into two. Each lung lobe is anchored at the **root** (hilum) of the lung and supplied by a secondary (lobar) bronchus. Within each lobe, the lung is subdivided into **segments** by sheets of connective tissue. Each segment is supplied by a tertiary (segmental) bronchus. There are 10 segments in each lung. Each segment is further subdivided into **lobules** by connective tissue sheets called septa. Each lobule is supplied by a respiratory bronchiole, which opens out into clusters of alveoli. The advantage of subdividing each lung into small, separate functional units is that if infection or disease establishes in one area, the physical barriers presented by the connective tissue septa separating it from adjacent areas can limit its spread.

A section of tissue taken from the peripheral lung and examined under the microscope shows an open,

honeycomb-like structure packed with thin-walled alveoli (Fig. 7.3). The alveoli are embedded in elastic tissue, which stretches and recoils with each breath and there are about 150 million alveoli in each lung. The alveolar walls are formed from a single layer of squamous epithelium and so are extremely thin, a feature essential for rapid gas exchange. The total surface area provided by alveoli for gas exchange is over 140m². In addition to the epithelial cells (sometimes called type 1 pneumocytes) are septal cells (type 2 pneumocytes) that secrete **surfactant**, and pulmonary macrophages (dust cells), that patrol the alveolar surface and are part of the innate immune system. Fig. 7.4 shows the structural details of the alveolar wall.

Surfactant

Surfactant is a lipid-rich fluid which reduces alveolar surface tension. Surface tension is the force exerted on the inner surface of any bubble by water molecules (Fig. 7.5A). Water molecules are polar, meaning they have slightly positive regions (their hydrogen atoms) and a slightly positive region (the oxygen atom). Because positive and negative forces have a mutual attraction, the water molecules on the inner surface of the alveoli orientate themselves with their hydrogen atoms pulling towards the oxygen atoms on adjacent molecules. As all the water molecules pull their neighbours towards themselves, this generates a force (surface tension). Because alveoli are basically thin-walled bubbles with no internal support, surface tension tends to collapse them, greatly increasing the respiratory effort required for reinflation (Fig. 7.5B). Surfactant disrupts this water layer, increasing the distances between the water molecules and therefore reducing surface tension and stabilising the alveoli (Fig. 7.5C). Disorders that reduce surfactant or wash it away are associated with collapse of affected alveoli.

Compliance and elasticity

The lung possesses **compliance** and **elasticity**, and it is essential to understand the difference between them because they are opposing forces. Compliance means the stretchability of the lung. Normal healthy lung tissue is very compliant and stretches readily, essential to minimise the work of breathing, which at rest uses only 3% to 5% of basal energy expenditure. Reduced compliance may be a temporary feature of some pulmonary disorders: for instance, in pneumonia,

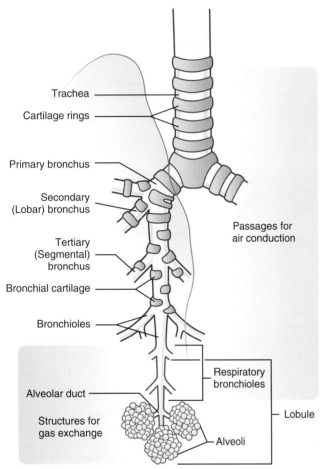

Fig. 7.2 The respiratory passageways. (Modified from Waugh A and Grant A (2018) *Ross & Wilson anatomy and physiology in health and illness*, 13th ed, Fig 10.17. Oxford: Elsevier Ltd.)

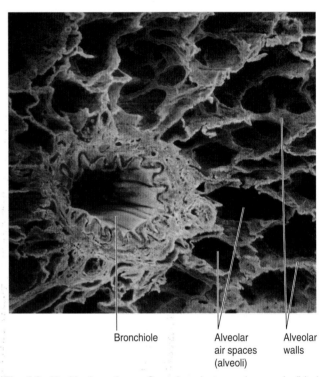

Fig. 7.3 Healthy lung tissue. Scanning electron micrograph. (Modified from Waugh A and Grant A (2018) *Ross & Wilson anatomy and physiology in health and illness*, 13th ed, Fig 10.19. Oxford: Elsevier Ltd.)

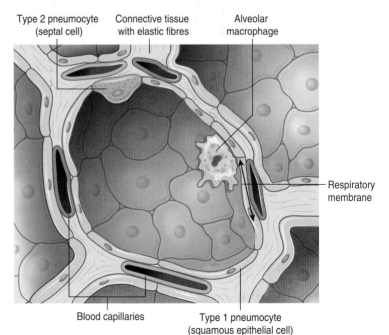

Fig. 7.4 The alveolar wall. (Modified from Waugh A and Grant A (2018) *Ross & Wilson anatomy and physiology in health and illness*, 13th ed, Fig 10.21. Oxford: Elsevier Ltd.)

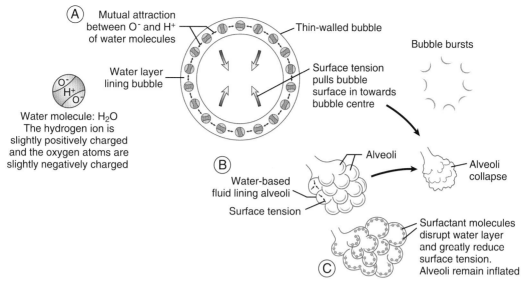

Fig. 7.5 Surface tension and the role of surfactant in alveolar stability. (A) Attraction between water molecules creates surface tension that collapses bubbles. (B) Alveoli without surfactant: surface tension collapses them. (C) Surfactant in the fluid layer lining alveoli disrupts cohesion between water molecules and reduces surface tension.

infected alveoli full of fluid and inflammatory cells consolidate the affected area, greatly reducing compliance. In other conditions, loss of compliance may be permanent (e.g., in tuberculosis, chronic inflammation and lung destruction leads to fibrosis). Fibrotic tissue does not stretch, so lung compliance is reduced and the work of breathing greatly increased.

Elasticity is the ability of a material to return to its original size/shape/length after stretching. The lung is very elastic because the lung tissue in which the alveoli and airways are embedded is rich in elastic fibres. Once an elastic material has been stretched past a certain point, elasticity starts to oppose compliance. For example, think of an elastic band, which can readily be stretched (it is compliant) and returns to its original length when the stretch is released (it is also elastic). It will not stretch indefinitely, however, and the more stretched it is, the more force is required to stretch it further. Eventually, it will stretch no more and breaks. Healthy lung tissue behaves in a similar way: it is compliant, but within limits, and will only stretch so far before its elastic tissues oppose its compliance and cause recoil. The elastic property of lung tissue is as essential to lung function as compliance: having expanded with breathing in, the lung needs to passively recoil to its original size and shape with breathing out. Loss of lung elasticity is as damaging to lung function as loss of compliance. In emphysema, for example, lung tissue, including the elastic matrix, is progressively destroyed. With each breath, the loss of recoil means the lung does not fully expel the inhaled air and air accumulates in the alveoli (air trapping).

The pleura and pleural space

The membranes covering the lungs, the **pleura**, are conventionally described in the plural but in fact are one single, continuous membrane forming a double membrane enclosing the lung. To visualise this, imagine the lung as a fist with the wrist as the primary bronchus, and the pleural membrane as the rubber skin of a partially filled water balloon. The fist can be pushed into the balloon (Fig. 7.6), which then forms a double layer around the fist, with a layer of water in between. This is a reasonable analogy for the relationship between the lung and its pleura, although the fluid between the pleura is not water but a lubricating phospholipid fluid called pleural fluid filtered from blood plasma. On average, about 9 mL of pleural fluid is present around each lung. Its production is continuous and excess is drained away in the lymphatic vessels of the lung. The inner membrane (the **visceral pleura**) sticks firmly to the outer lung surface, including the surfaces of lung tissue forming the fissures between the lung lobes. At the hilum of the lung, it folds back on itself to form the outer layer, the **parietal pleura**, which lines the thoracic cavity, sticking firmly to the inside of the ribcage and the upper surface of the diaphragm. A similar sort of arrangement is found around the heart, with the pericardial membranes; it is designed to allow the organ to expand and recoil/contract within the protective covering of the outer membrane, without being restricted or causing friction against adjacent structures.

The pleural membranes have an additional function in respiratory physiology; they are essential for keeping the lung expanded in the thorax. The lung is physically anchored in the thorax at only one point—the hilum—where the primary bronchi and the major blood vessels enter and leave the lung. Remember that the fundamental framework of the lung is elastic connective tissue. A collapsed lung within the chest cavity is reduced to a much smaller, and more compact mass of tissue attached at the hilum because an elastic material recoils to its point of attachment. There needs to be force applied to the lung tissue to keep it expanded, against the recoil of its own elastic tissue.

The pressure in the pleural space is subatmospheric (about 4 mm Hg less than the atmospheric pressure of air at sea level). This partial vacuum creates a suction that holds the visceral pleura against the parietal pleura, opposing the elastic recoil exerted by the lung tissue. Because the parietal pleura lines the chest cavity, the visceral pleura is held against it and the lung is expanded to fill the thorax (Fig. 7.7). Opening the pleural cavity, by damaging either layer of

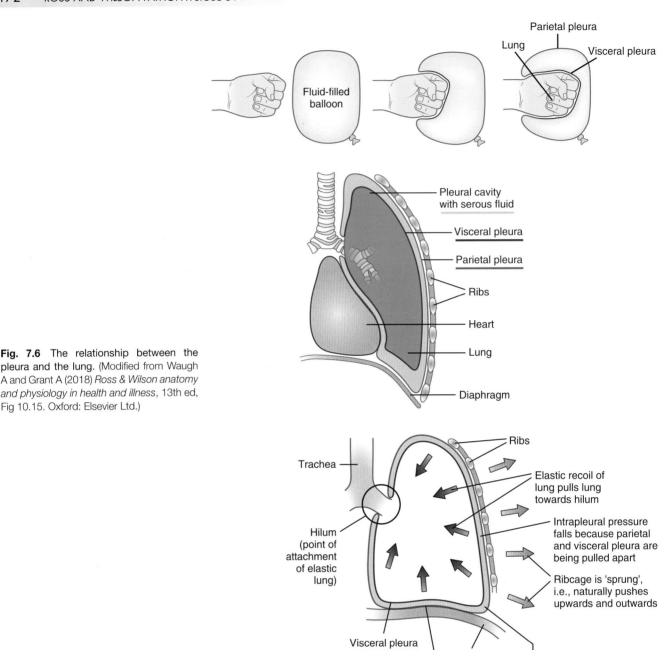

Fig. 7.6 The relationship between the pleura and the lung. (Modified from Waugh A and Grant A (2018) *Ross & Wilson anatomy and physiology in health and illness*, 13th ed, Fig 10.15. Oxford: Elsevier Ltd.)

Fig. 7.7 Generation of negative intrapleural pressure.

the pleural membranes, sucks air into the low-pressure pleural space, and the lung's natural elastic recoil then collapses it towards the hilum (pneumothorax; p.193).

Pulmonary circulation and gas exchange

The right ventricle sends deoxygenated blood to the lungs in the pulmonary arteries. Within the lungs, the pulmonary arteries progressively divide and give rise to the capillary beds that wrap around the alveoli for gas exchange. These capillaries then merge to form pulmonary venules that eventually unite to form the pulmonary veins, which return the now oxygenated blood to the left atrium. Usually, each lung returns two pulmonary veins to the left heart.

Each alveolus is wrapped in a network of pulmonary capillaries. The walls of a capillary and the underlying alveolus are fused together to make the membrane for gas exchange as thin as possible. These fused membranes are called the **respiratory membrane**, which is between 2 and 5 μm thick.

Control of pulmonary blood pressure and flow

The pulmonary vascular system is a high-flow, low-pressure system. Less than 10% of the total blood volume is normally contained within the pulmonary arteries, capillaries and veins and typical pulmonary arterial blood pressure is 25/15 mm Hg. Low pressure is essential to prevent leakage of blood fluid into the alveolar spaces. Control of blood flow through different parts of the lung is essential to direct blood flow towards well-ventilated areas of the lung (see **ventilation/perfusion matching** below). Additional factors specific to the pulmonary circulation can significantly alter blood flow

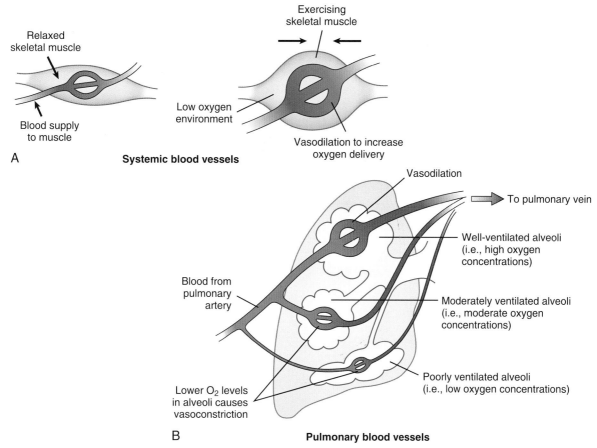

Fig. 7.8   Responses of systemic and pulmonary blood vessels to hypoxia.

and should be considered wherever necessary; for example, because pulmonary blood pressure is so low, changes in body position affect flow much more significantly than in the systemic circulation. Additionally, the pulmonary blood vessels may be passively compressed and expanded by the mechanical processes of breathing. They may also be compressed when surrounding lung tissue becomes inflamed, congested, swollen or fibrotic.

One key difference between systemic blood vessels and pulmonary blood vessels lies in their response to hypoxia. When a systemic blood vessel—for example, in an exercising muscle—is exposed to a hypoxic environment, it responds by dilating to maximise blood flow and oxygen delivery (Fig. 7.8A). However, pulmonary blood vessels constrict when in a hypoxic environment (either the alveolar air is low in oxygen, or oxygen concentrations in the blood are low). This reduces blood flow to poorly oxygenated areas of the lung and diverts it to better oxygenated areas to maximises oxygen uptake (Fig. 7.8B).

GAS EXCHANGE IN THE LUNGS AND TISSUES

Exchange of gases across the respiratory membrane is driven by pressure (P) differences, down a pressure gradient. Oxygen (O_2) diffuses out of the alveolus and into the bloodstream because there is more oxygen in the alveolar air than in the venous blood travelling through the pulmonary capillaries. Likewise, carbon dioxide (CO_2) diffuses out of the tissues and into the bloodstream because there is more CO_2 in the tissues than in the arterial blood entering the

capillary network supplying them. The greater the pressure difference, the faster the diffusion.

The average Po_2 of venous blood is 40 mm Hg (5.3 kPa). It returns to the right side of the heart in the great veins and is pumped to the lungs. In the pulmonary capillaries, it is exposed to much higher O_2 concentrations on the other side of the very thin respiratory membrane: alveolar Po_2 is 100 mm Hg (13.3 kPa) when breathing atmospheric air at sea level. Oxygen diffuses down its concentration gradient from the alveoli into the blood, and equilibration occurs within one-tenth of a second. This means that the blood leaving the pulmonary capillaries and travelling to the left atrium in the pulmonary veins has the same Po_2 (100 mm Hg) as alveolar air. When breathing air with lower O_2 content, for example, at altitude, oxygen levels in pulmonary venous blood reflect this. If alveolar Po_2 is only 70 mm Hg, for example, blood leaving the lungs and returning to the heart would also have a Po_2 of 70 mm Hg. Oxygenated blood travels from the left side of the heart into the systemic circulation, and through the systemic capillary beds, where it is separated from tissues by only the one-cell thick capillary wall. Body tissues continually consume oxygen, and so their O_2 content is low. On average, Po_2 in the tissues is around 40 mm Hg, although it can be much lower (15 mm Hg) in active tissues such as liver or exercising skeletal muscle. Again, this produces a pressure gradient across the capillary wall and oxygen diffuses from high pressure (100 mm Hg in the capillary) to low (40 mm Hg in the tissues).

CO_2 moves in the opposite direction to O_2 in both the pulmonary and the systemic capillaries, but for the same

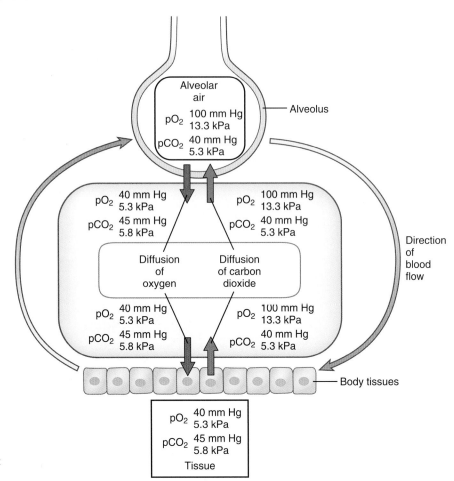

Fig. 7.9 Exchange of gases in the lungs and in the tissues. For simplicity, the heart has not been included in the diagram.

reasons. CO_2 levels in the air we breathe are very low. Average alveolar PCO_2 is about 40 mm Hg. Venous blood arriving at the alveoli in the pulmonary capillaries is, however, rich in CO_2 (45 mm Hg or 5.8 kPa) because it has come from body tissues, which manufacture it as a waste product of metabolism. CO_2 equilibrates across the respiratory membrane even faster than oxygen does, despite the fact that the pressure difference is much smaller than oxygen (only 5 mm Hg compared with 60 mm Hg for O_2) because it is more soluble. Pulmonary venous blood therefore has a PCO_2 of 40 mm Hg, matching the CO_2 level in the alveoli. When it arrives in the tissues, there is another pressure gradient: the PCO_2 of arterial blood is 40 mm Hg, lower than the average tissue PCO_2, on average around 45 mm Hg, although it can be much higher in very active tissues. CO_2 therefore diffuses from the tissues into the blood. Fig. 7.9 illustrates exchange of gases in the lungs and body tissues.

If the respiratory membrane in the lungs is compromised in some way, impaired diffusion of oxygen leads to hypoxaemia and tissue hypoxia, and CO_2 retention leads to hypercapnia and a fall in blood pH (respiratory acidosis).

LUNG VOLUMES AND CAPACITIES

The total amount of air that the lungs can hold is called the **total lung capacity** (TLC). This varies with age, physical build and sex, and for any given individual, it stays fairly constant in health, because it is largely determined by the physical size and characteristics of the thorax. As a convenient example in this discussion a representative figure of 6 L is used (Fig. 7.10A). Of this 6 L, about 1200 mL, called the **residual volume**, remains in the lungs at all times, even after maximal expiration. Residual volume ensures that the lungs cannot be completely emptied by respiratory effort, ensuring that a proportion of alveoli always remains inflated. A completely airless lung permits no gas exchange and cannot be reinflated by normal muscular effort.

The available volume over and above the residual volume is called the **vital capacity** (VC), 4800 mL in our example (6–1.2 L = 4.8L). This is the volume of air that can be moved in and out of the lungs using maximal respiratory effort and, along with residual volume and total lung capacity, is relatively constant because it is determined by the physical characteristics of an individual's thorax. At rest, the amount of air breathed in and out—the **tidal volume**—is much less than this, usually about 500 mL. This shows that healthy lungs possess a great deal of reserve volume, and at rest only about 10% of the available lung volume is being used. The tidal volume can vary enormously and is determined by the body's oxygen requirements. With maximal effort, tidal volume and vital capacity become the same.

The **inspiratory reserve volume** (IRV) is the volume of air that can be inhaled over and above a normal quiet breath in, and the **expiratory reserve volume** (ERV) is the volume of air that can be exhaled over and above a normal quiet breath out. Measurement of lung volumes and capacities are made on a spirometer and shown on a printout called a spirograph or spirogram (Fig. 7.10B). Such measurements are very important in assessing many forms of lung disease, and

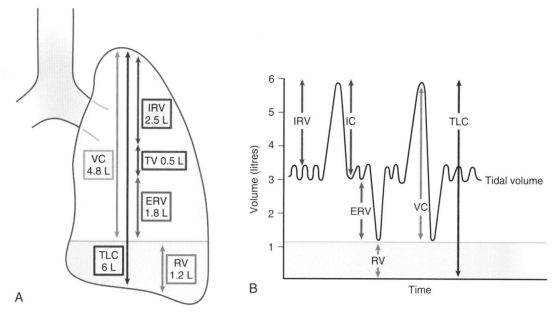

Fig. 7.10   Lung volumes and capacities. (A) The main volumes and capacities. Note that although the diagram shows a single lung, the values shown are for two lungs. (B) A normal spirogram. (B, Modified from Waugh A and Grant A (2018) *Ross & Wilson anatomy and physiology in health and illness*, 13th ed, Fig 10.15. Oxford: Elsevier Ltd.)

interpretation of lung function tests are essential in monitoring disease progression and the efficacy of any treatment.

When interpreting lung function tests, factors such as age, sex, and build must be taken into account because they determine what is normal for an individual. Normal spirometry results from a healthy 10-year-old child, for example, are very different to those from a healthy 30-year-old man. Test results must be compared against reference values calculated from large scale data sets from healthy individuals, which are usually presented as charts, tables, or graphs.

Peak flow

Peak flow (PF) is the maximal speed of airflow achieved by a subject breathing out as hard and fast as possible through a peak flow meter. It is usually expressed as litres per minute (L/min).

FEV₁:FVC ratio

An important tool in assessment of pulmonary function is the ratio of the **forced expiratory volume in one second** (FEV₁) to the **forced vital capacity** (FVC). The FVC is the vital capacity measured with forced exhalation. It is usually measured by asking the subject to take as deep a breath in as possible to reach the total lung capacity, and then to breathe out as hard and as fast as possible through the spirometer until the subject can physically exhale no more air. Measuring the volume of air exhaled gives the vital capacity, and the air left in the subject's lungs is the residual volume. The subject is asked to hold the forced exhalation for 6 seconds, and the curve this generates shows how quickly the subject managed to exhale the full VC. This will clearly vary between individuals and depends on factors such as upper body and abdominal musculature used in forced breathing, and whether the airways are open or narrowed. A young, strong, healthy male, with good upper body strength and clear, unobstructed airways will usually expel his FVC in less time than a middle-aged healthy female whose upper body

strength is likely to be lower. Individuals whose airways are narrowed—for example, in asthma—will take longer to exhale their FVC.

The FEV₁:FVC ratio is a very useful indication of possible airway obstruction. To measure this, the FVC is measured as previously described, and the results are shown on a graph as in Fig. 7.11. Because the test is taken over a fixed period (usually 6 seconds), the rate at which the air is being expelled can be measured. In Fig. 7.11, the FVC is 4 L and is achieved after 2.5 seconds of forced exhalation. This figure also shows that, of that 4 L, 3 L was expelled 1 second into the test. This is the FEV₁ (forced expiratory volume in one second). Expressed as a percentage, this gives us the FEV₁:FVC ratio as 3 L/4 L × 100 = 75%. This means that the subject exhaled three-quarters of their VC in the first second of forced exhalation. Although there is normal variation with age and gender, in general values between 75% and 85% are considered normal. Values lower than this may suggest the presence of obstruction limiting airflow somewhere in the airways.

VENTILATION-PERFUSION MATCHING

Tidal volume at rest is about 500 mL, of which on average 150 mL reaches only the **anatomical dead space** (the upper airways, where no gas exchange takes place). This means that only 350 mL is available to ventilate the alveoli. When the body is upright, this flows mainly into bronchioles in the lung apices because they offer less resistance than those in the lung bases, although this varies with factors such as body position. Therefore, at resting tidal volumes, only a small proportion of total alveoli can receive airflow. The airways supplying these alveoli dilate to encourage ventilation, and the remaining airways constrict. This directs airflow into a limited section of the lung and ensures that as much as possible of the tidal volume actually reaches the alveoli. In addition, pulmonary blood vessels supplying well-ventilated alveoli, where the air is rich in oxygen, dilate to ensure good

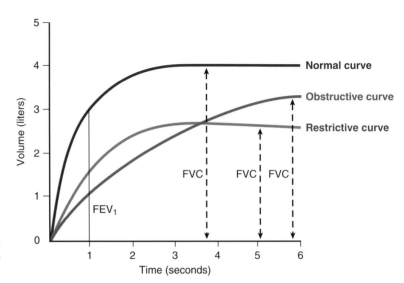

Fig. 7.11 Spirometric measurement of forced vital capacity (FVC) showing forced expiratory volume in one second (FEV$_1$), and the curves obtained in obstructive and restrictive disease. (Modified from Kacmarek RM, Stoller JK, and Heuer AJ (2020) *Egan's fundamentals of respiratory care*, 12th ed, Fig. 20.5. St Louis: Mosby.)

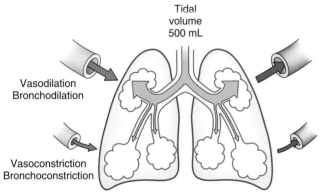

Fig. 7.12 Ventilation/perfusion matching at rest.

blood flow through these capillaries (Fig. 7.8). On the other hand, blood vessels supplying more poorly ventilated parts of the lung, where alveolar air contains less oxygen and more CO_2, constrict. This is called *ventilation/perfusion (V/Q)* matching (Fig. 7.12). The average normal V/Q ratio is 0.8 (because normal alveolar ventilation is 4 L/min and alveolar capillary blood flow is 5 L/min), so they are not equally matched in the healthy lung.

Ventilation-perfusion mismatch

Factors that alter the V/Q ratio of 0.8 cause ventilation/perfusion mismatching. Disorders that reduce airflow into the alveoli reduce ventilation, and the ratio then falls. For example, if ventilation in a group of alveoli falls to 2, the ratio then becomes 2:5 L/min, or 0.4. Examples of such disorders include asthma or pulmonary oedema. Disorders that restrict blood flow increase the ratio; for example, if blood flow to a group of alveoli falls to 1 L/min, the ratio becomes 4:1 L/min, or 4. An example is pulmonary embolism (PE). Altering the V/Q ratio either way, by increasing it or decreasing it, means that pulmonary blood flow is not being targeted to well ventilated alveoli, and leads to compromised gas exchange.

Pulmonary shunting

Pulmonary shunting refers to blood that has travelled from the right ventricle to the left atrium through the pulmonary

capillaries, but that has not passed well-oxygenated alveoli and has therefore been unable to pick up oxygen. This deoxygenated blood mixes with oxygenated blood in the left atrium and dilutes its oxygen content. This can lead to hypoxaemia, and the blood may not have enough oxygen to supply the systemic tissues, leading to hypoxia.

In normal, healthy pulmonary function, V/Q matching ensures that shunted blood makes up only about 3% of the blood returned to the left atrium. This proportion increases in some pulmonary diseases; for example, in obstructive airways disease, where airways are blocked and ventilation is reduced, there are fewer functional, well-ventilated, oxygen-rich alveoli in the lung but the perfusion is just the same; so blood passing through the poorly ventilated areas of the lung pick up little or no oxygen and is unable to excrete its CO_2 load, and returns, still deoxygenated and rich in CO_2, to the left heart, from where it is pumped into the systemic circulation (Fig. 7.13).

INFECTIONS OF THE RESPIRATORY TRACT

Respiratory tract infections are very common. Although the respiratory system has a wide range of very effective defence mechanisms, every inhalation brings a cohort of airborne contaminants and pathogenic organisms into the airways. Most infections are limited to the upper tract and are often viral in origin, relatively mild, and usually self-limiting. Organisms that manage to colonise the deeper airways cause more serious disease, possibly leading to long-term damage and reduced respiratory function.

VIRAL RESPIRATORY TRACT INFECTIONS

Viral upper respiratory tract infections are very common. Most are trivial and short-lived, but if the infection spreads to the lungs themselves, they may cause more serious illness (e.g., viral pneumonia).

COMMON COLD

This common upper respiratory tract infection is usually caused by rhinoviruses, transmitted by aerosol or direct contact. Rhinovirus also causes some lower respiratory tract

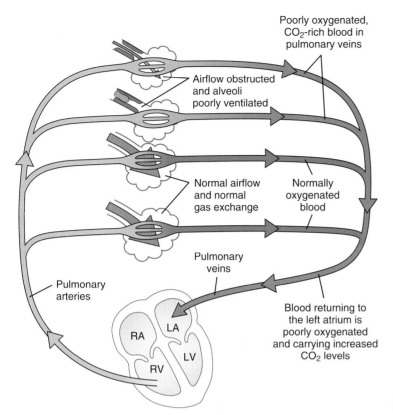

Fig. 7.13 Shunting

infections and bronchiolitis in very young children. Other viruses, including coronavirus, adenovirus, and parainfluenza virus also cause colds. People of all races experience colds; they are commoner in children than adults because adults accumulate immunity to multiple infections over their lifetime. There is a clear seasonal variation, depending on the causative virus: rhinovirus is mainly active in spring and autumn, coronavirus in winter and spring, and adenovirus all year round. The virus attaches to epithelial cells in the upper respiratory tract and triggers a local inflammatory response, releasing cytokines including interleukin 8, which attracts inflammatory cells into the affected area. Commonly, there is sore throat, nasal congestion and discharge, sneezing, and coughing. Generally, symptoms appear 1 to 2 days after exposure and the cold lasts 4 to 5 days. From the early stages of infection, the patient sheds large numbers of viable viral particles into the environment, including before the appearance of symptoms and after symptoms have abated; while this is happening, he may infect others.

CORONAVIRUS INFECTIONS

The coronaviridae family of viruses includes several viruses that cause respiratory and gastrointestinal illness in humans and animals. The first coronavirus to be identified was avian infectious bronchitis virus, reported in 1931 as causing respiratory disease in chicks. In the 1960s, coronaviruses infecting humans were first isolated and identified. At least nine coronaviruses are now known to infect humans, and most cause mild respiratory symptoms characteristic of the common cold; these infections are seasonal and most occur in the winter and spring. However, in recent decades, highly virulent coronaviruses, including SARS-CoV, SARS-CoV-2, and MERS-CoV, have emerged and caused major outbreaks

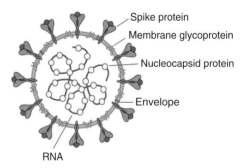

Fig. 7.14 The structure of SARS-CoV-2. (Modified from Rosales-Mendoza S, Comas-García M, and González-Ortega O (2022) *Biomedical innovations to combat COVID-19*, Fig. 12.1. Philadelphia, Academic Press: Elsevier Inc.)

of respiratory disease associated with significant mortality rates. SARS-CoV and MERS-CoV originated in bats; an infection whose original host is non-human but has spread to humans is called a **zoonotic infection**. Wet markets, where live animals are sold, are considered an important contributor to the crossing of these animal viruses into humans. SARS-CoV-2 is also generally considered to be of animal origin, but its main animal host has not been definitively identified.

Coronaviruses are RNA viruses and are so-called because their surface is coated with crown-like projecting spike proteins (corona means *crown*; Fig. 7.14). The virus uses the spike proteins to attach to receptors on the cell membrane of the epithelial cells lining the airways. Once inside the cell, the virus rapidly replicates and generates huge numbers of new viral particles, which infect local tissues and can also spread to other organs including the central nervous system. Risk factors for more severe disease include increasing age, immunocompromise, and co-existing chronic disease, including diabetes, hypertension, respiratory disease, and heart disease.

SARS-CoV

This coronavirus causes **severe acute respiratory syndrome** (SARS) and emerged in 2002 in China, triggering an epidemic that lasted into 2003 and which was associated with a 10% fatality rate. The epidemic was halted by the imposition of strict travel restrictions between countries in which the infection had been identified, including Hong Kong, Taiwan, and China. It is spread mainly by inhalation of infected droplets and initially causes cough, malaise, and fever. The virus binds readily to ACE2 (see Pathophysiology below) on the cell membrane of alveolar cells and lung macrophages in the lower respiratory tract and so causes alveolar inflammation and oedema, lung fibrosis, alveolar collapse, and severe lung injury. In severe cases, there is evidence that the lung damage seen in SARS is associated with abnormal and excessive host immune and inflammatory responses, which worsens the lung injury. There is no specific treatment and no vaccine.

SARS-CoV-2

This coronavirus, closely related to SARS-CoV, causes **COVID-19** (short for coronavirus disease 2019), and first emerged in Wuhan, China, in December 2019. It spread rapidly worldwide; the World Health Organisation declared a pandemic in March 2020. The speed with which the COVID-19 pandemic swept across the world stimulated intensive international efforts to produce a vaccine, of which there are now several. The first to be approved in the UK and the United States was developed jointly by the pharmaceutical firms Pfizer and BioNTech; other important vaccines have also been developed by AstraZeneca in collaboration with Oxford University and by the American company Moderna. As with many viruses, SARS-CoV-2 constantly mutates, producing new strains (variants) with changed surface proteins which may allow vaccine escape: that is, the antibodies generated by existing vaccines may be less effective against a new variant if the virus has changed the protein against which the antibody is effective. Updating vaccines to ensure they are effective against new variants of the virus is likely to be important in ongoing vaccine programmes.

COVID-19 rarely causes severe illness in children and young people unless there are additional risk factors present such as diabetes or asthma, but the risk of severe or critical illness increases in older people, in those with pre-existing chronic conditions including renal, cardiovascular, or lung disease, in obesity, diabetes, sickle cell disease, cancer, or people in who are immunocompromised.

Pathophysiology

In most people, the infection does not spread beyond the upper respiratory tract, but in susceptible or at-risk individuals, it migrates deeper into the respiratory tract and infects the tiny airways and the alveoli, causing pneumonia. In the most severe cases, there is massive lung damage caused by an abnormal and aggressive host immune response to the virus. This involves the release of a range of destructive mediators, including interleukins, interferons, and TNFα, which damage pulmonary blood vessels, destroy alveoli and lead to acute respiratory distress syndrome (ARDS; p.187). This

is a major cause of morbidity and mortality in COVID-19. However, COVID-19 is a multisystem disease, and the virus can affect multiple organs including the heart, kidney, liver, and brain. Severe disease is associated with damage to blood vessel endothelium throughout the cardiovascular system, which in turn increases the coagulability of the blood; thromboembolism is a frequent finding in critically ill patients.

Part of the reason for the widespread pathologies seen in severe COVID-19 disease seems to relate to the receptor site to which the virus binds in the airways. The spike protein on the viral coat binds to **angiotensin converting enzyme 2** (ACE2) on the surface of upper airway epithelial cells, and the cell internalises the virus/ACE2 complex. This gives the virus entry into the cell, where it rapidly divides.

ACE2 is part of the renin-angiotensin-aldosterone system (RAAS; see also p.165 and Fig. 6.43) and is found on the cell surface in nearly all body tissues, including the heart, lungs, kidneys, and central nervous system. It opposes and controls the action of angiotensin II, which is produced when angiotensin converting enzyme (ACE, not to be confused with ACE2) acts on angiotensin I. Angiotensin II is a powerful vasoconstrictor, increases blood pressure, and is implicated in the development of cardiovascular disease. It also triggers salt and water retention and increases the production of a range of inflammatory mediators. ACE2 degrades angiotensin II and, via an indirect pathway, angiotensin I, to angiotensin 1-7. Angiotensin 1-7 antagonises the activity of angiotensin II; it is a vasodilator, reduces blood pressure, and is anti-inflammatory (Fig. 7.15). Its widespread distribution allows ACE2 to protect multiple organ systems from the proinflammatory effects of angiotensin II.

By binding to and neutralising ACE2, SARS-CoV-2 prevents it from degrading angiotensin II. In addition, the virus downregulates ACE2 receptor numbers, further reducing its ability to antagonise angiotensin II. The virally induced loss of the protective action of ACE2 allows the proinflammatory activity of angiotensin II to predominate and, because of the widespread distribution of ACE2, can lead to multiorgan dysfunction and failure.

Signs and symptoms

In most otherwise healthy people, the illness is short-lived and relatively mild. In 2% to 10% of people, however, the

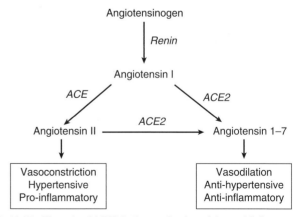

Fig. 7.15 The role of ACE2 in the production of the anti-inflammatory and vasodilator substance angiotensin 1 to 7. (Modified from Plant TM and Zeleznik AJ (2015) *Knobil and Neill's physiology of reproduction*, 4th ed, Fig. 43.17. San Diego: Academic Press, Elsevier Inc.)

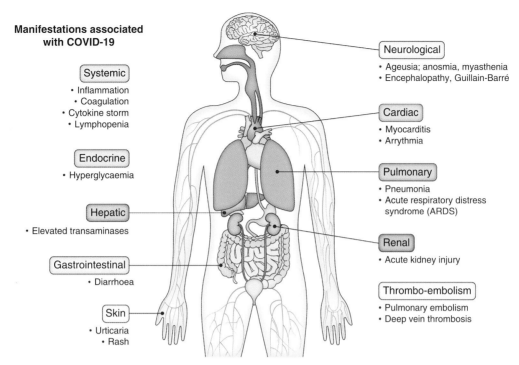

Manifestations associated with COVID-19

Systemic
- Inflammation
- Coagulation
- Cytokine storm
- Lymphopenia

Endocrine
- Hyperglycaemia

Hepatic
- Elevated transaminases

Gastrointestinal
- Diarrhoea

Skin
- Urticaria
- Rash

Neurological
- Ageusia; anosmia, myasthenia
- Encephalopathy, Guillain-Barré

Cardiac
- Myocarditis
- Arrythmia

Pulmonary
- Pneumonia
- Acute respiratory distress syndrome (ARDS)

Renal
- Acute kidney injury

Thrombo-embolism
- Pulmonary embolism
- Deep vein thrombosis

Fig. 7.16 Possible manifestations in COVID-19. (Modified from Asselah T, Durantel D, Pasmant E, et al. (2021) COVID-19: discovery, diagnostics and drug development, *Journal of Hepatology* 74(1): 168–184. https://doi.org/10.1016/j.jhep.2020.09.031.)

infection progresses to cause severe and/or life-threatening disease as described previously. The incubation period is typically 5 to 6 days, although it can be up to 2 weeks, during which time the infected person may infect others. The virus replicates extremely rapidly within airway tissues and is efficiently transmitted in exhaled droplets, especially when talking, coughing, and sneezing. Procedures that generate aerosols, such as in dental work, airway suctioning, endotracheal intubation, or the use of nebulisers, increase the risk of transmission.

Some infected people are asymptomatic, but typical symptoms in mild-to-moderate disease resemble those of a cold, including fever, dry cough, loss of taste (ageusia) and smell, (anosmia) and a sore throat. A range of non-pulmonary signs and symptoms may also be part of the clinical presentation (Fig. 7.16).

A proportion of individuals experience prolonged postviral manifestations, referred to as **long COVID**. It has been estimated that one in seven COVID-19 patients are still experiencing symptoms 12 weeks after diagnosis. Common symptoms include fatigue, poor exercise tolerance, shortness of breath, palpitations, gastrointestinal symptoms, and 'brain fog'. The impact on normal life may be substantial and greatly limit daily activity including an inability to return to work.

Management and prognosis
Antiviral drugs, including remdesivir and molnupiravir, may be useful in some patients. Dexamethasone, an anti-inflammatory and immunomodulatory steroid, improves outcomes for patients who need respiratory support such as oxygen therapy or artificial ventilation. Because severe illness is usually associated with hyperinflammation and the cytokine storm, immunosuppressants and immunomodulators,

such as IL-6 inhibitors, are likely to be increasingly important options in these patients.

MERS-CoV

This coronavirus causes **Middle East Respiratory Syndrome (MERS)** and first appeared in Jordan in 2012, although most cases have occurred in Saudi Arabia. The infection is most commonly acquired from infected dromedary camels, which act as an intermediate host for the virus, although close human-human contact can also spread the virus via infected droplets. The mortality rate may be as high as 35%. There is no specific treatment and no vaccine.

INFLUENZA

The World Health Organisation launched its Global Influenza Strategy 2019–30 with the aim of preventing and controlling global influenza outbreaks, and to improve preparations for future pandemics. It estimates that 290,000 to 650,000 people die every year as a result of the respiratory consequences alone of influenza. The very old and the very young are particularly vulnerable. Influenza viruses are divided into three categories, A, B, and C, and there are several subtypes in each category. Most human influenza is caused by influenza A. Animals are also susceptible to influenza infection; all bird influenza, for example, is caused by influenza A viruses. Other animals susceptible to influenza A infections include pigs, horses, and dogs. Many viral strains are species-specific, but viruses are capable of significant mutation, and the regular appearance of new mutated strains increases the likelihood that a virus may acquire the ability to infect other species. The 1918 Spanish influenza pandemic was caused by an influenza A virus that originated in birds, infected one third of the world's population, and killed 50 million people worldwide (about 1 person in 30).

Box 7.1   Organisms that may cause pneumonia

Organism	Additional information
Streptococcus pneumoniae (pneumococcus)	Gram +ve coccus responsible for other infections, such as pericarditis, meningitis, otitis media. Commonly colonises upper respiratory tract in healthy people and causes pneumonia when spread to the lungs by, for instance, aspiration; the very young, very old, those with chronic disease or the immunocompromised are more susceptible. Commonest cause of community acquired pneumonia.
Staphylococcus aureus	A robust Gram +ve coccus that colonises skin and mucous membranes and survives on environmental surfaces. Heat and salt resistant and a major cause of hospital-acquired infections including pneumonia, bacteraemia, endocarditis, osteomyelitis.
Klebsiella pneumoniae	Gram −ve bacterium; also causes urinary tract infections. Possesses an external protective capsule, so resists body defences. Commonly associated with pneumonia in diabetic and alcohol-dependent people and is common cause of hospital-acquired pneumonia (about 12% of cases). May be normal inhabitant of the nose and throat, or of the gastrointestinal tract.
Pseudomonas aeruginosa	Gram −ve rod-shaped bacterium; also causes skin and soft tissue infections, endocarditis, and colonises wounds and burns; an increasing factor in hospital-acquired infections in general, not just pneumonia. It is an opportunistic pathogen and rarely causes infection in healthy people. It is the commonest cause of lung infection in cystic fibrosis (p.187)
Haemophilus influenzae	Gram +ve bacterium that often possesses a protective capsule and is spread in airborne droplets. Also causes meningitis, especially in children, ear and sinus infections and pericarditis. Common inhabitants of the nose and throat in healthy people.
Fungal species	Relatively uncommon causes of pneumonia but risk increased in immunocompromised people and caused by inhalation of fungal material.
Influenza virus	This is the commonest cause of viral pneumonia.
Respiratory syncytial virus (RSV)	RSV is a very important cause of lower respiratory tract infection in children and the second commonest cause of adult viral pneumonia.

Pathophysiology

The virus enters the respiratory tract and attaches to epithelial cells via a key viral surface protein called **haemagglutinin**. Another key viral protein, an enzyme called **neuraminidase**, releases newly synthesised viral particles from the infected cell surface, allowing the virus to spread. The variants of these proteins define the different subtypes of influenza A. For example, the subtype responsible for Spanish influenza was H1N1 (**h**aemagglutinin type 1 and **n**euraminidase type 1). The virus attaches to and invades respiratory epithelial cells. Once within the epithelial cell, the virus replicates, and multiple new viral particles are released, spreading the infection. The viral infection directly damages and inflames the respiratory epithelium, but in addition to this, systemic signs and symptoms are caused by the host's immune response. Activated T cells and rising levels of circulating inflammatory mediators damage the lungs, increasing the risk of acute respiratory distress syndrome and pneumonia.

Signs and symptoms

The incubation period is between 1 and 4 days. Acute onset of fever, muscle pains, headache, upper respiratory tract congestion, malaise, anorexia, sore throat, and cough are common. There may also be nausea, vomiting, and diarrhoea.

Management and prognosis

In milder cases, rest, fluids, antipyretics, and pain relief are often enough. Antivirals may be used in vulnerable groups. Annually, influenza vaccines are prepared against the strains in circulation at the time and offered to high-risk individuals.

PNEUMONIA

Pneumonia is infection of the lung, including the alveoli and their supporting interstitial tissue. Globally, it is the leading cause of deaths in children under 5 years old, 95% of which occur in the developing world. Risk factors include cigarette smoking, pre-existing chronic disease such as diabetes, alcohol dependency, cardiac disease, chronic obstructive pulmonary disease, childhood and old age, and immunocompromise. A wide range of organisms can cause pneumonia: bacteria, viruses, fungi, and other organisms have all been implicated (Box 7.1). Viral pneumonia is usually less serious than bacterial, but as viruses are immunosuppressive, bacterial pneumonia secondary to an initial viral infection is not uncommon.

In hospitalised patients, especially the seriously ill, people being mechanically ventilated, children, frail elderly, and the immunocompromised, hospital-acquired pneumonia is a significant cause of morbidity and mortality. Up to one third of patients admitted to intensive care units develop pneumonia, and the mortality rate here is high, between one third and half of infected people. The commonest organisms here differ from community-acquired pneumonia (see below); they include *Staphylococcus aureus* and various Gram −ve and anaerobic bacteria, including *Enterobacter, Klebsiella*, and *Pseuodomonas* species.

Community-acquired pneumonia is less common than hospital-acquired pneumonia, with reported rates between 16 and 24 per 10,000 population. The commonest cause is pneumococcus, but in about half of all cases, no causative organism is identified.

Pathophysiology

Infection can be acquired through inhalation or through blood-borne spread. In debilitated people or those with poor immune function, the infection can establish itself throughout the lung and this is called bronchopneumonia (Fig. 7.17A). If the infection is confined to one or more lung lobes, it is called *lobar pneumonia*. This is more common in

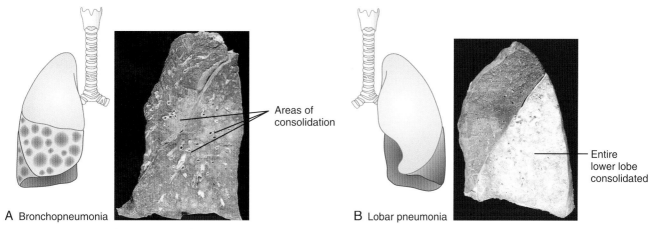

Fig. 7.17 Pneumonia. (A) Bronchopneumonia showing patchy areas of consolidation. (B) Lobar pneumonia showing involvement of one lobe only. (Modified from Kumar V, Singh M, Abbas A, et al. (2022) *Robbins & Cotran pathologic basis of disease*, 10th ed: South Asia Edition, Figs. 15.32, 15.33, and 15.34. New Delhi, RELX India Pvt. Ltd.)

younger, otherwise healthy patients and usually involves the lung bases (Fig. 7.17B).

Whatever the organism of origin, in pneumonia the lung tissue becomes infiltrated with inflammatory and immune cells that migrate in to control the infection. Many of the organisms that cause pneumonia are inherently resistant to pulmonary defence mechanisms. For example, *Streptococcus pneumonia* (pneumococcus), a common cause of community-acquired pneumonia, possesses an external capsule resistant to phagocytosis and other defences, protecting the bacterial cell and allowing it to spread within lung tissue. Activated neutrophils and macrophages release inflammatory mediators, which target the bacteria but also cause lung damage. As inflammation develops, the pulmonary capillaries become congested and fluid leaks into the alveoli, causing pulmonary oedema. Affected areas become consolidated, wet, and firm, with a dense liver-like consistency, and no gas exchange is possible. Lung compliance is greatly reduced and the work of breathing increased.

Aspiration pneumonia is caused by inhalation of stomach contents that have tracked up the oesophagus into the trachea. The pH of gastric juices is very low—usually between pH 1 and 2—and intensely corrosive, and enormous damage can be done to lung tissue. The aspirated material may be vomit, especially in alcohol intoxication, or of gastric contents in anaesthetised people. Aspiration is more likely when abdominal pressure is high—for example, in central obesity or pregnancy—and when lying down.

Signs and symptoms

Pneumonia causes fever, dyspnoea, malaise, productive cough, and pleurisy, which makes breathing very painful. Sputum may be purulent and/or bloodstained. Often, patients report having had a viral respiratory tract infection shortly beforehand.

Management and prognosis

Supportive treatment, including oxygen to reverse hypoxia, is used as appropriate. Antibiotics and other antimicrobial drugs are used according to any culture results identifying the causative organism. Overall mortality is about 5%, but individual outcomes depend largely on the health status of the patient. For example, healthy young adults with community-acquired viral pneumonia almost always recover fully, whereas up to half of intensive care patients with hospital-acquired pneumonia die. Prognosis is poorer in vulnerable groups as described previously.

TUBERCULOSIS

Tuberculosis (TB) causes significant worldwide morbidity and mortality, with an estimated one quarter of the global population infected. Worldwide, incidence is falling, but over 95% of cases are in developing countries, with poorer healthcare and public health education systems. It is an ancient disease and has been identified in human remains as far back in history as the Stone Age. The organisms that cause TB in humans and humans belong to the genus *Mycobacter* and are collectively referred to as the mycobacterium tuberculosis complex (MTI). The organisms that infect humans are *Mycobacterium tuberculosis*, *Mycobacterium bovis*, and *Mycobacterium africanum*.

Initial infection is called **primary TB**. Mycobacteria are highly resistant to immune defences and can remain latent in the tissues for decades. Later (secondary) reactivation is often in response to immunosuppression or other disorders such as malnutrition, diabetes, or alcohol dependence. It may also be a result of reinfection in someone who has recovered from a primary infection at some point in the past. Individuals with primary TB have a 5% to 10% lifetime risk of developing secondary TB, and 80% of cases of TB are reactivation disease, not new infections. Smoking is a major risk factor and causes nearly 8% of all new infections.

Pathophysiology

Mycobacteria are slow-growing, Gram-positive intracellular pathogens, resistant to intracellular killing after phagocytosis by neutrophils or macrophages and very difficult for the body's defence mechanisms to eradicate. Although the infection is transmitted by droplet inhalation, and although the respiratory system is the main body system affected, if viable mycobacteria get into the bloodstream or lymphatic system, they spread to and colonise other organs. The stages of TB are summarised in Fig. 7.18.

After inhalation, the mycobacteria lodge in the lungs and are attacked by pulmonary phagocytes. This triggers an

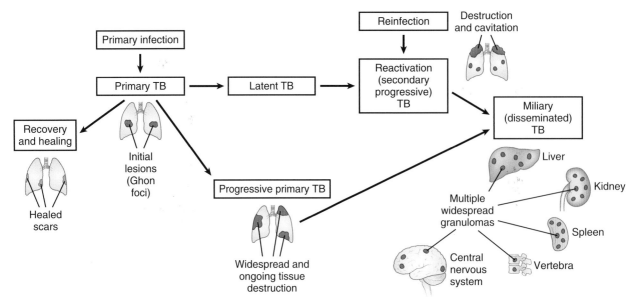

Fig. 7.18   The stages of tuberculosis.

inflammatory response similar to any lung infection, with vasodilation, influx of inflammatory cells, oedema, and consolidation of lung tissue as alveoli fill with fluid rich in inflammatory cells and products of tissue damage. Normally, after engulfing a target, the phagocyte would then empty its lysosomes full of enzymes and other toxic substances around the phagocytosed organism, destroying it. However, mycobacteria actively inhibit this release of lysosomal enzymes and are therefore not destroyed. Living within the phagocyte, they are protected from further attack, and they multiply. Infected macrophages respond by releasing powerful cytokines, including TNFα and interleukins, which activate natural killer cells (p.90) and T-helper cells (p.91), which in turn initiate enhanced cell killing to deal with the infection. One of the body's defensive techniques when dealing with an organism so difficult to eradicate is to seal off areas of infected tissue in discrete masses called **granulomas**, called **Ghon foci** in TB. A granuloma has an outer boundary of fibrotic tissue rich in macrophages and cells derived from macrophages, and its centre is a mass of necrotic tissue (called *caseation tissue*), the result of the body's immune response to the infection site (see Fig. 1.15). If the granuloma is small, it can be cleared completely, and healing may take place. Larger granulomas are much more difficult to resolve and persist for long periods of time. They may calcify (very clearly seen on chest X-rays). Their dense walls prevent spread of the organisms within, but they also protect them from macrophages and other defensive mechanisms, and reactivation many years later causes secondary disease. Over time, TB progressively destroys lung tissue, eliminating alveolar/capillary membranes and the surface area for gas exchange, and creating cavities where functional alveoli should be. The old term for TB, *consumption*, reflects the destructive nature of the infection.

Extrapulmonary (disseminated) TB. TB infection of tissues and organs other than the lungs is called **extrapulmonary TB** and is the consequence of mycobacterial spread from the lungs in the blood or lymph. Individuals who are older, immunocompromised, or vulnerable to infection because of other chronic conditions such as diabetes, HIV infection, alcohol dependence and malnutrition are at greater risk of this. TB can infect any organ, including the heart, genitourinary tract, skin, bone and central nervous system. The spine is a common site of involvement. Infection of the brain and meninges causes cognitive deterioration, blindness, and deafness. Widespread disseminated TB is called **miliary TB** (Fig. 7.18), after millet, which is finely ground oatmeal. Affected organs display large numbers of tiny, scattered granulomas, as though they had been sprinkled with oatmeal. As in the lungs, within these tissues, the mycobacteria proliferate, progressively destroying whichever organ they have seeded.

Signs and symptoms
Pulmonary TB causes a productive cough with bloodstained mucus, chest pain, night sweats, and fever. Because the lung is inflamed and consolidated, and in later stages is fibrosed, it is less compliant than normal and so the work of breathing increases. Cyanosis, hypoxaemia, and hypercapnia are caused by the loss of functional alveolar membranes and impaired gas exchange. In more advanced disease, chronic hypoxaemia leads to increased red blood cell production, which causes a tender, enlarged liver because it is destroying large numbers of red cells. Chronic hypoxaemia increases the workload of the heart, which beats faster and more powerfully to maximise oxygen delivery to the tissues. Ultimately, this can cause heart failure (heart failure secondary to lung disease is called **cor pulmonale**). Destruction of other organs in disseminated TB leads to signs and symptoms associated with their progressive failure; for example, bone pain if bone tissue is involved, and neurological consequences if the nervous system is infected.

Management and prognosis
Aggressive treatment of patients and identified close contacts with prolonged multiple antibiotic therapy is the cornerstone of treatment, but multidrug resistant *Mycobacteria* strains are an increasing global problem. With effective treatment, over 80% of patients can be cured.

MALIGNANCIES OF THE RESPIRATORY TRACT

In non-smokers, primary malignancies of the respiratory tract are relatively rare because lung tissues are fairly stable with low rates of cell turnover. The main cancers of the lung are described on p.82; and the main tumour of the pleura, mesothelioma, is described on p.195.

Metastatic lung cancer
Tumours in the lung are more likely to be secondaries from a primary elsewhere than a primary lung tumour. Thirty percent to 55% of all cancer patients have lung metastases, indicating how common a site the lungs are for secondary neoplastic growth. Certain primary cancers, including renal, bladder, skin, breast, and gastrointestinal cancers metastasise preferentially to the lung. Metastatic growths are usually scattered throughout the lung so surgical removal is not possible. Generally speaking, the discovery of lung secondaries in cancer indicates advanced disease and a poor prognosis.

OBSTRUCTIVE AND RESTRICTIVE LUNG DISEASE

The terms restrictive and obstructive are in common use in the classification of respiratory disorders. Restrictive refers to a reduced ability to expand the lungs and may be caused by lung changes such as fibrosis, which stiffens the lung and reduces its compliance, but it may also be caused by neurological or musculoskeletal problems that impact on the physical process of breathing. Obstructive disease, as the term suggests, is associated with blockage of air flow somewhere in the respiratory tree; so asthma, with the associated bronchoconstriction and inflammatory changes in airway walls, reduces the airway lumen and is classified as an obstructive disorder. Because of reduced airflow, the FEV_1 is reduced, although total lung capacity is normal or near normal; this gives a reduced FEV_1:FVC ratio (Fig. 7.11). In this example, the FVC is 3.3 L and the FEV_1 is 1 L, giving a ratio of 1 L/3.3 L or 30%: less than a third of the vital capacity is exhaled in the first second, well below the normal value of at least 75%. A reduced FEV_1:FVC ratio is characteristic of obstructive disease.

OBSTRUCTIVE AIRWAYS DISEASE

The commonest obstructive disorders are asthma, chronic bronchitis, and emphysema. The latter two frequently occur together as a continuum of respiratory disease, with emphysema developing as end-stage disease in chronic bronchitis, in which case the collective term is chronic obstructive pulmonary disease (COPD).

ASTHMA

The Global Burden of Disease study estimated that worldwide, 262 million people were living with asthma in 2019. It is the commonest cause of chronic disease in children and kills 1000 people every day. Although it is a global disorder, most deaths occur in developing countries. It is almost certainly underdiagnosed and undertreated, so the statistics

do not show the true disease burden. It is primarily associated with childhood but can appear and persist in adults. Although asthma is often considered a single disorder, it is better thought of as a complex group of airway disorders, with varying aetiologies, but all associated with variable and reversible periods of airway inflammation, causing wheeze, cough, shortness of breath, and a tightness in the chest.

The genetics of asthma. Asthma runs in families, indicating a genetic component. However, asthma presents in different ways with different clinical pictures, and is not a single-gene disease. Mutations in multiple asthma-susceptibility genes that potentially contribute to asthma have been identified. The normal healthy genes themselves are involved in inflammatory and immunological responses, so mutations contribute to disordered inflammatory and immunological function. However, research in this area is in its very early stages and exactly what part these genes play in the aetiology of asthma is not known.

Children with one asthmatic parent are twice as likely to have asthma than a child with two non-asthmatic parents, and the risk is increased if the affected parent is the father. However, there is a significant environmental component, with asthma rates higher in urbanised areas compared with rural areas. Although it is found in all racial groups, asthma is more common in some populations than others (e.g., in black Americans than in white Americans).

Atopic (extrinsic) and non-atopic (intrinsic) asthma. Childhood asthma is usually associated with atopy, the tendency to produce large quantities of IgE antibodies to a range of usually harmless allergens (type I hypersensitivity, p.99). There is usually a personal and/or family history of allergic disorders such as eczema. Common potential allergens include house dust, furry animals, fungal spores, and tobacco smoke. Exposure to a triggering allergen initiates the inflammatory response in the airways described below (see Pathophysiology) and the characteristic signs and symptoms of an asthma attack. Adult-onset asthma is generally not associated with atopy or a personal or family history of allergy. The cause of intrinsic asthma is not known, although risk factors and triggers include obesity, male sex, respiratory tract infections, exercise, airborne pollutants, gastro-oesophageal reflux disorder, and some drugs (e.g., aspirin and other non-steroidal anti-inflammatory drugs).

Pathophysiology
Irrespective of the aetiology (i.e., intrinsic or extrinsic), asthma is a chronic inflammatory condition of the airways, associated with episodes of reversible bronchoconstriction, airway oedema, and oversensitivity of the airway smooth muscle to a range of stimuli. The small- to medium-sized bronchioles are worst affected. Mucus production increases, and mucus plugs can block airways, limiting airflow and causing the alveoli distal to the blockage to collapse (atelectasis). Over time, repeated inflammatory episodes lead to permanent changes in the airway wall (remodelling), including thickening of the smooth muscle layer and the epithelial basement membrane, and increased number and activity of goblet cells.

Fig. 7.19 shows the pathological features of an asthmatic bronchiolar wall, compared with that of a healthy one. The wall of the airway is thickened because of generalised oedema and smooth muscle hypertrophy. There is a pronounced

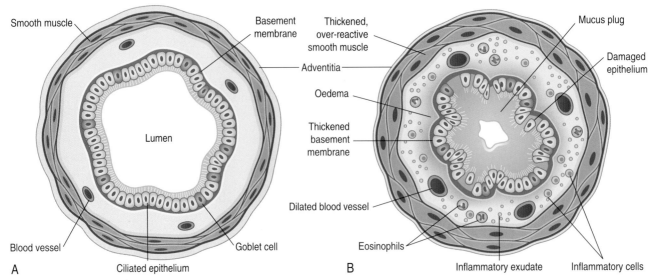

Fig. 7.19 Pathological changes in the asthmatic airway. (Modified from Waugh A and Grant A (2018) *Ross & Wilson anatomy and physiology in health and illness*, 13th ed, Fig 10.30. Oxford: Elsevier Ltd.)

inflammatory cell infiltrate, composed of lymphocytes and eosinophils. Eosinophil accumulation is characteristic of allergic inflammation, so this occurs in atopic asthma but is not seen in intrinsic asthma. The inflammatory cells release mediators that promote the ongoing inflammatory response. The healthy ciliated epithelium is damaged, leading to patchy exposure of the underlying basement membrane, which increases the hypersensitivity of the airways and reduces mucus clearance.

In atopic asthma, the patient produces IgE type antibodies to one or more of a range of allergens as listed previously, which attach themselves to the surface of mast cells in the airways. When the triggering allergen is inhaled into the airways, it is adsorbed onto the airway epithelium, attaches to the IgE antibody, and stimulates degranulation of the mast cell, releasing its range of mediators (see also Fig. 4.14A). Among other mast-cell derived mediators are histamine, prostaglandins, and leukotrienes, responsible for bronchoconstriction, vasodilation, oedema, and recruitment of inflammatory cells into the airway wall.

Signs and symptoms

Wheeze, breathlessness, cough, and tightness of the chest are characteristic of asthma. Exposure to a trigger initiates immediate bronchoconstriction and rapid onset of symptoms, often within minutes. This is called the **early phase response** and is caused by release of preformed mast cell mediators as described previously. It may improve spontaneously or with treatment in the hours after its onset. However, as the inflammatory response develops in the airways, activated inflammatory cells accumulate and produce and release a wide range of inflammatory mediators. This leads to a second phase of bronchoconstriction, called the **late phase response**, which manifests about twelve hours after the original episode.

In severe asthma, with significant obstruction in large numbers of airways, airflow is seriously reduced. The distress of airway obstruction leads to increased respiratory rate and hugely increased respiratory effort. As the frightened person struggles to inhale as much air as possible, not enough time is given for exhalation, and air begins to accumulate in the lungs (air trapping). Trapped air expands the lungs, and air sucked in with each inhalation does not reach the alveoli. Affected alveoli therefore do not participate in gas exchange, leading to **shunting** (Fig. 7.13). As trapped air accumulates, lung tissue becomes progressively more stretched and less and less compliant, and so the work of breathing steadily increases. In addition, as lung volume increases, the ribcage is pushed upwards and outwards, making it harder for the intercostal muscles to lift it further, and restricting inspiration and airflow. The diaphragm's range of movement is also reduced as the expanding lungs compress it from above. This greatly increases the work of breathing and reduces tidal volume. Physical exhaustion in prolonged asthmatic episodes is common and very dangerous, especially in children.

Complete blockage of an airway means the alveoli distal to the blockage receive no inspired air at all. Over time, the air present in these cut-off alveoli is absorbed into the bloodstream, and they collapse (see Lung collapse below).

Management and prognosis

In atopic asthma, allergen avoidance is important. Irrespective of the aetiology, the cornerstones of asthma treatment are the anti-inflammatory glucocorticoids, usually delivered directly into the airways by some sort of inhaler device. β_2 receptor agonists are used to dilate the airways by relaxing the smooth muscle in the airway walls. Asthma is usually a chronic disease; childhood asthma may improve in early adulthood but reappear later in life. Adult-onset asthma, which is usually not allergically mediated, may persist throughout life but may also disappear with time.

Chronic obstructive pulmonary disease

This disease complex involves progressive airflow restriction with or without destruction of lung tissue and is generally associated with chronic bronchitis and its long-term consequence, emphysema. Of all cases of chronic bronchitis, 90% are caused by smoking tobacco, although chronic exposure to other airway irritants—including industrial substances and airborne pollutants—can also cause it. Additionally, a small proportion of cases are caused by an inherited deficiency of α_1-antitrypsin (see α_1-antitrypsin deficiency and emphysema below). Emphysema is the destruction of alveoli when the progressive inflammatory changes in the bronchi extend into the lung tissue itself. The disorder is of global importance. In high-income countries, where tobacco smoking is declining and air purity is monitored and regulated in the environment and in the workplace, its incidence is declining. However, in low- to middle-income countries, it is rising. In 2019 it was the third commonest cause of death worldwide, and more than 90% of those deaths occur in low to middle income countries.

Not all smokers develop COPD: incidence in smokers has been estimated between 20% and 25%. Risk increases with tobacco exposure, which is calculated in **pack-years**. One pack-year is the equivalent of smoking one pack a day for a year. An individual who smokes one pack a day for 25 years has a 25 pack-year smoking history. Alternatively, smoking five packs a day for 5 years also gives a 25 pack-year smoking history and smoking a pack every 2 days takes 50 years to reach a 25 pack-year smoking history. The higher the pack-year history, the higher the risk of developing COPD, as well as other smoking-related disorders, like cardiovascular disease and lung cancer.

Pathophysiology of chronic bronchitis
Changes in the airways, and eventually the lung tissue itself, are characteristic of chronic inflammation secondary to chronic irritation. The airway walls swell and thicken, which limits airflow. Unlike asthma, airflow limitation tends to worsen with time and is not fully reversible, although there may be periods of improved airway function (e.g., associated with warmer, drier summer weather compared with winter weather). Goblet cell numbers increase in the bronchial epithelium, significantly increasing mucus production. Normally, mucus is a beneficial pulmonary defence mechanism; it traps inhaled particles and is then swept by the mucociliary escalator towards the mouth for coughing up or swallowing. Cilia in smokers' airways are shorter and less motile than in non-smokers, impairing their ability to clear mucus (Fig. 7.20). The large quantity of thick, sticky mucus in bronchitis clogs up the airways, blocks airflow, and provides an excellent breeding ground for bacteria, increasing the risk of infection.

When airways become blocked with mucus, the alveoli beyond the blockage receive no air. **Shunting** occurs as blood flowing through the capillaries of these unventilated alveoli is not oxygenated, leading to hypoxaemia and hypercapnia.

With chronic inflammation, the airways become scarred and permanently damaged. The epithelium can ulcerate, and metaplastic changes are seen. **Metaplasia** (p.65) is the replacement of one tissue type with another, in response to a stressor applied to a tissue. In this circumstance, the stressor is the irritation and chronic inflammation in the airways. The pseudostratified ciliated columnar epithelium of the healthy airway is replaced with stratified squamous epithelium to better protect underlying structures. However, the stratified epithelium lacks cilia, and so its protective function is lost (see Fig. 3.7). Because tobacco smoke contains multiple mutagenic chemicals, the epithelium may then become dysplastic and then frankly neoplastic (p.66).

Pulmonary hypertension in COPD. Blocked airways reduce air entry into the alveoli, and so CO_2 levels start to rise in the alveolar air because there is little atmospheric air arriving to flush it out and replenish oxygen levels. The capillaries supplying these alveoli therefore constrict because there is no point in sending blood to alveoli that do not contain oxygen-rich air. This is an important mechanism in V/Q matching during quiet breathing (Fig. 7.12). However, in chronic bronchitis, ventilation throughout the lung is reduced because of extensive airway narrowing. Increasingly large volumes of CO_2-rich air collect in the alveoli, and so pulmonary vasoconstriction is widespread. This leads to pulmonary hypertension, which in turn increases the workload of the right ventricle. A feature of long-standing progressive COPD is therefore right-sided heart failure (p.144), with venous engorgement, liver enlargement, and dependent oedema.

Pathophysiology of emphysema
The airways become progressively fibrotic as a result of the chronic inflammatory changes. Over time, the lung substance itself—including the alveoli and the capillaries that supply them—becomes involved. Loss of the lung tissue includes the elastic tissue in which all the airways and alveoli are embedded. Once this starts to disappear, the lungs become less elastic, meaning that, although they expand readily with inspiration, they lose elastic recoil and progressively expand. Small airways begin to collapse because the elastic tissue they were embedded in helped to hold them open by radial traction (Fig. 7.21). Remember there is no supporting cartilage in the walls of small airways, so they have no internal structural support. As lung tissue is progressively destroyed, the walls of individual alveoli, along with their network of capillaries, are eliminated, merging their airspaces into much larger cavities called **bullae**

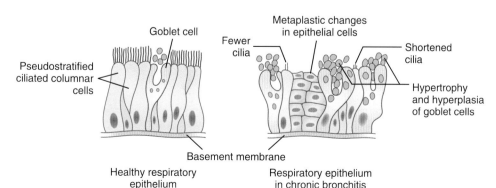

Fig. 7.20 Pathological changes in the respiratory epithelium in chronic bronchitis.

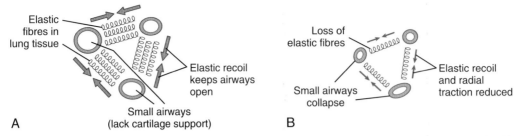

Elastic
fibres in
lung tissue

Elastic recoil
keeps airways
open

Small airways
(lack cartilage support)

A

Loss of
elastic fibres

Elastic recoil
and radial
traction reduced

Small airways
collapse

B

Fig. 7.21 Loss of radial traction in the airways in emphysema. (A) Elastic recoil applies radial traction to airway walls in healthy lung tissue. (B) Loss of elastic tissue in emphysema allows small airways to collapse.

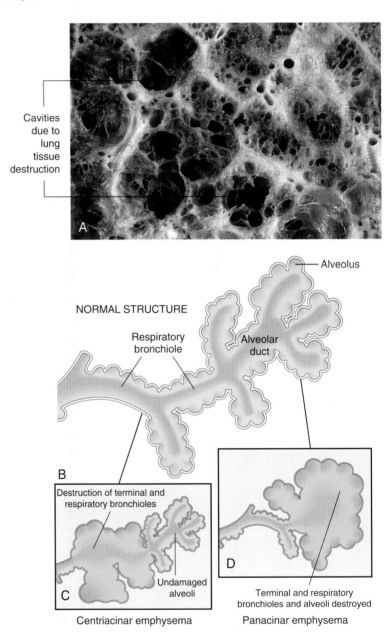

Cavities
due to
lung
tissue
destruction

A

Alveolus

NORMAL STRUCTURE

Respiratory
bronchiole

Alveolar
duct

B

Destruction of terminal and
respiratory bronchioles

Undamaged
alveoli

C

Centriacinar emphysema

D

Terminal and respiratory
bronchioles and alveoli destroyed

Panacinar emphysema

Fig. 7.22 Emphysema. (A) Destruction of lung tissue leaves large cavities non-functional in gas exchange. (B) Normal lung lobule structure. (C) Centriacinar emphysema. (D) Panacinar emphysema. (Modified from (A) Photographs by kind permission of Dr. Yale Rosen under licence of Attribution-ShareAlike 4.0 International (CC BY-SA 4.0) (https://creativecommons.org/licenses/by-sa/4.0/; https://www.flickr.com/people/pulmonary_pathology/); (B) Kumar V, Abbas A, Aster JC, et al. (2021) *Robbins essential pathology*, Fig. 10.13. Philadelphia: Elsevier Inc.)

(Fig. 7.22A). Loss of alveoli and respiratory membrane greatly impairs gas exchange, exacerbating hypoxaemia and hypercapnia. Fig. 7.22B–D shows the normal structure of a lung lobule, and the two main forms of emphysema, which are described according to the anatomical location of the destroyed tissue. In practice, both forms are usually present. Centriacinar emphysema refers to destruction of respiratory bronchioles, and panacinar emphysema is destruction of the respiratory bronchioles and the distal alveoli. If the bullae form around the periphery of the lung, they can breach the pleura, leading to air entry into the pleural space (Fig. 7.23) and pneumothorax.

α₁-Antitrypsin deficiency and emphysema. **Elastase** is an important enzyme released by neutrophils as part of the inflammatory and immune response. As the name suggests, it breaks down elastic fibres. In health, it is tightly controlled by the enzyme inhibitor α_1-antitrypsin. α_1-Antitrypsin deficiency leads to elastase overactivity and destruction of tissues rich in elastic fibres. Because the fundamental lung matrix is elastin-rich, α_1-antitrypsin deficiency causes progressive loss of lung tissue. The faulty gene responsible lies on chromosome 14 and so is inherited as an autosomal trait. It is a rare disorder and affects some populations more than others (e.g., up to 1 in 1500 people in some European populations are affected, whereas it is very rare in Asian people). Symptoms are as for emphysema.

Signs and symptoms

Chronic bronchitis is characterised by a persistent, productive cough with large quantities of thick white mucus. Airway obstruction causes wheeze, breathlessness, and poor exercise tolerance. Repeated respiratory infections are common, in which case the sputum may become green, yellow, and/or bloodstained. Recurrent infections and the associated immune response further damages lung tissue, increasing lung scarring and accelerating the loss of alveoli. Blood gas measurements show chronic hypoxaemia and hypercapnia. Hypoxaemia causes cyanosis, and triggers release of erythropoietin from the kidneys to stimulate red blood cell synthesis in the bone marrow. This increases the oxygen-carrying capacity of the blood, but it also increases blood viscosity, increasing the likelihood of clots and the workload of the heart.

Emphysema is characterised by breathlessness, cough, and poor exercise tolerance. Because there is loss of elastic recoil, the lungs progressively expand as a result of increasing volumes of trapped air in the bullae, giving a characteristic 'barrel' shape to the chest. Hypoxia may affect organ function; for instance, the hypoxic kidney retains sodium and water, causing oedema and increased cardiac workload. The later stages of COPD are associated with respiratory failure, with hypoxaemia (arterial P_{O_2} less than 60 mm Hg) and hypercapnia (arterial P_{CO_2} over 53 mm Hg).

Management and prognosis

Removing the source of the bronchial irritant, which usually involves stopping smoking, may improve or reverse bronchitis, even though some remodelling (e.g., airway scarring) may be irreversible. Destruction of lung tissue is permanent, and obliterated alveoli cannot regenerate.

CYSTIC FIBROSIS

Cystic fibrosis (CF) is a monogenic inherited disorder that disrupts the transport of water and electrolytes across the cell membrane because of faulty membrane chloride channels. It is a multisystem disorder, although lung function is particularly badly affected because pulmonary secretions become thick and viscous, obstructing airflow and causing infections. CF is described in more detail on p.38.

RESTRICTIVE LUNG DISEASE

This general term encompasses a range of disorders that reduce compliance and limit lung expansion. The lung becomes less compliant with fibrosis (e.g., as the result of chronic inflammation and the deposition of scar tissue). Another

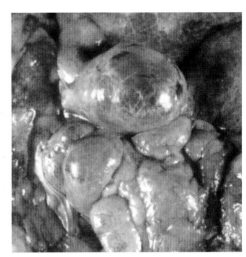

Fig. 7.23 Pleural bullae in emphysema (indicated with white arrows). (From Sens MA, Hughes R (2021) *Diagnostic pathology: forensic autopsy.* Oxford: Elsevier Inc.)

reason for losing compliance is loss of surfactant, which is essential for keeping the alveoli open. The lungs of babies born before the 30th week of gestation are too immature to produce surfactant, leading to the condition respiratory distress of the newborn (RDN). The mature lung may also lose its alveolar film of surfactant if it is washed away by fluid accumulating in the alveoli as a result of, for example, infection or pulmonary hypertension. In addition, conditions that lead to oedema of lung tissue, giving a dense, waterlogged lung, reduce lung compliance and restrict lung expansion.

It is worth noting that not all conditions that restrict lung expansion are caused by pulmonary disease. Damage to the nerves supplying the respiratory muscles (e.g., multiple sclerosis), disease of the respiratory muscles themselves (e.g., muscular dystrophy), or damage or deformity to the thoracic cage (e.g., fractured rib, scoliosis of the spine) are extrinsic causes of restriction.

In restrictive disorders, both lung volume and the capacity for forced exhalation are reduced and so the FEV_1:FVC ratio may be near normal (see Fig. 7.11). In this example, the FVC is 2.5 L and the FEV_1 is 1.5 L, giving a ratio of 60%.

ACUTE RESPIRATORY DISTRESS SYNDROME

ARDS is a form of acute lung injury associated with injury to the respiratory membrane in the lung (i.e., the alveolar-capillary interface at which gas exchange takes place). It is a consequence of many serious illnesses, often not of pulmonary origin, but whose systemic consequences cause acute lung injury. Direct injury includes inhalation of toxic fumes or aspiration of gastric contents. Infection, such as pneumonia or miliary tuberculosis, or from blood-borne organisms, causes a systemic inflammatory response with high circulating levels of inflammatory mediators and cytokines that damage the respiratory membrane. ARDS is a common development after major trauma, especially if significant blood transfusions are needed. In malignant disease, circulating tumour-derived toxins can damage the lung, and in pancreatitis, digestive enzymes released into the bloodstream digest and damage the alveoli (Fig. 7.24). Because ARDS involves loss of functional respiratory membrane, not only is gas exchange impaired leading to hypoxaemia and

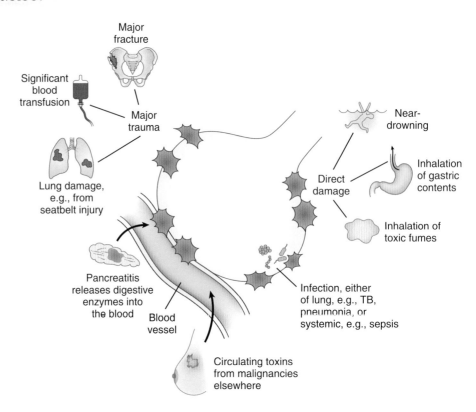

Fig. 7.24 Aetiological agents in ARDS.

hypercapnia, but oxygen therapy also does not improve the situation.

The incidence is higher, and the prognosis is poorer with increasing age, and in smokers.

Pathophysiology

ARDS is associated with diffuse alveolar damage, caused either by direct (inhalational) injury to the alveoli or by circulating infective or inflammatory substances that damage the pulmonary capillaries. Activated neutrophils—and a host of inflammatory cytokines—are closely involved in ARDS development. Whatever the initial inflammatory insult, the key sign in the early stages is pulmonary oedema because pulmonary capillaries become increasingly permeable and fluid leaks into the alveoli. This fluid layer in the alveoli presents a significant barrier to gas exchange, which is badly impaired, leading to hypoxaemia and hypercapnia. Damage to type II alveolar epithelial cells reduces surfactant production, and any surfactant present is diluted and washed away by the fluid in the alveoli; this strongly predisposes to alveolar collapse. Collapsed alveoli are not ventilated, do not contribute to gas exchange, and worsen gas exchange.

Shunting is a significant feature of ARDS, because areas of the lung are lost to gas exchange through alveolar collapse, and blood flowing through these parts of the lung remains deoxygenated and high in CO_2 when it returns to the heart. This is a significant contributing factor to the hypoxaemia seen in ARDS.

Pulmonary hypertension almost always develops, because pulmonary blood vessels constrict in response to the high CO_2 content of the injured lung. This causes V/Q mismatch, worsens alveolar oedema, promotes inflammation, and contributes to the downward spiral of deteriorating respiratory function.

High inhaled oxygen concentrations are always required in the treatment of ARDS, to maximise oxygen transfer across the damaged alveolar membranes.

However, if high-flow oxygen therapy is needed for more than a few days, oxygen toxicity can lead to further lung damage.

If the patient recovers at this point, the inflammatory changes in the lung usually resolve completely and the lung regains normal function. However, in some survivors, a second stage develops, involving lung fibrosis and permanent changes to lung structure.

Management and prognosis

The underlying cause is addressed if possible, and respiratory function supported with high-flow oxygen therapy, mechanical ventilation if required, and fluid restriction to reduce pulmonary oedema. Survival rates in ARDS vary widely. These patients are often already very ill, and the development of this acute lung injury may be a late-stage event. Mortality rates depend on various factors, such as the underlying cause and the age of the patient, but general estimates are in the region of 40%.

Infant respiratory distress syndrome

This is sometimes called **idiopathic respiratory distress syndrome** or hyaline membrane disease. It occurs in babies born very prematurely (before 30 weeks' gestation) who are not yet producing surfactant. In addition to reducing surface tension in the alveoli, surfactant also helps maintain fluid distribution across the alveolar wall and ensures that fluid does not collect in the alveolar air spaces. Therefore, in the absence of surfactant, surface tension increases, compliance falls, and the respiratory effort required to pull air into the lungs is greatly increased. The baby's immature and weak respiratory musculature is not capable of this, and sections of the lung collapse and cannot be inflated. This leads to hypoxia and a developing acidosis because of CO_2 retention. In addition to this, lack of surfactant allows fluid to accumulate in the alveoli, bringing with it protein, including fibrin, which forms a membranous coating (the so-called hyaline membrane) inside the alveoli that blocks gas exchange. Because of this physical obstruction at the alveolar membrane, even high-flow oxygen therapy may not be effective in reversing the hypoxia. The baby is in clear respiratory distress, with shallow breathing, sunken chest, and possibly cyanosis. There is often hypotension and bradycardia.

Management and prognosis

Prevention wherever possible is important. If premature delivery is anticipated, the mother can be given steroids to accelerate the baby's lung development. Once delivered, mechanical ventilation, oxygen therapy, administration of artificial surfactant and supportive measures are used. Care must

be taken when using high-flow oxygen for extended periods, because it inhibits normal development in the retina, leading to blindness, and damages the alveoli and their blood supply.

INTERSTITIAL LUNG DISEASE

Interstitial lung disease (ILD) is an umbrella term encompassing over 180 disorders, affecting mainly the alveolar walls and the lung tissue in which the alveoli are embedded. There is a range of known causes, including systemic connective tissue disorders (Table 7.1) and inhalation of irritant materials (Table 7.2). Certain drugs are also associated with ILD (Box 7.2). The risk of developing ILD after drug exposure usually increases with dose and length of treatment time but sometimes develops rapidly after relatively low dose treatment. If

Table 7.1   Connective tissue disorders associated with interstitial lung disease

Disorder	Key information
Sarcoidosis (p.105)	This chronic inflammatory disorder affects multiple body systems, especially the lung and the mediastinal lymph nodes. The cause is not known, although there is evidence of excessive T-cell activity. In the lung, there is granuloma (p.16) formation and cavitation. Many patients are asymptomatic and may even improve but in others progressive fibrosis and declining lung function occur.
Systemic sclerosis (scleroderma, p.104)	This autoimmune inflammatory disorder affects multiple body systems. In the lung, it causes progressive collagen deposition, causing fibrosis, thickening of the pleura, damage to pulmonary blood vessels, pulmonary hypertension and right-sided heart failure as the right ventricle struggles to pump blood through the narrowed and damaged pulmonary vasculature.
Rheumatoid arthritis (p.338)	The commonest pulmonary manifestation of rheumatoid arthritis is Interstitial lung disease (ILD), with or without pleural involvement. Risk factors include male sex, smoking, increased age, and high levels of circulating autoantibodies, including rheumatoid factor. The mechanism of lung damage is not understood but may be secondary to deposition of autoantibodies in lung tissue, which triggers a chronic inflammatory response. A range of studies have shown clinically silent ILD is present in large proportions of RA patients.
Systemic lupus erythematosus (SLE) (p.105)	Pulmonary involvement occurs in 50%–70% of SLE cases. Autoantibodies circulating in SLE deposit in lung tissue and trigger a chronic inflammatory response. The pleura are frequently involved, leading to pleural effusion.
Sjogren's syndrome (p.105)	This autoimmune, chronic inflammatory disorder mainly affects the eyes and salivary glands, and frequently the lungs, which become infiltrated with lymphocytes, chronically inflamed and fibrotic.

Table 7.2   Inhaled irritants associated with interstitial lung disease

Irritant	Key information
Asbestos	Asbestos is fibrous and comes in two forms (amphiboles and chrysotile). One type of amphibole, called crocidolite, is most commonly involved in human disease. Its tiny fibres (4μm long by 1.3 μm diameter) make it all the way to the alveoli, where they deposit and are toxic to alveolar macrophages, which cannot clear them. The inflammation and fibrosis they trigger lead to destruction of lung tissue and greatly increase the risk of the highly malignant pleural tumour, mesothelioma.
Silicates	Silica is a very common mineral found in rock, so stoneworkers, quarriers, glassmakers, and sandblasters (among others) are exposed to high levels of airborne silicate dust. When deposited in the lungs it triggers inflammatory and fibrotic changes seen as small nodules on X-ray. Mild cases may be symptom free but more severe disease is progressive.
Fungal spores	Farmer's lung is caused by inhalation of *Aspergillus* fungal spores in mouldy hay, which trigger a type III hypersensitivity response (p.101). Avoidance of the allergen usually resolves the problem, but chronic exposure leads to permanent inflammatory and fibrotic changes
Coal dust	Coal workers' lung (coal workers' pneumoconiosis, black lung) is caused by deposition of anthracite dust in the lung. Not all miners develop this disorder but the risk is increased in smokers. Pulmonary macrophages ingest the dust but cannot destroy it and a progressive inflammatory response is initiated, with formation of fibrous nodules. The most severe form, progressive massive fibrosis, leads to cavitation, emphysema, lung destruction, raised pressure in the pulmonary arteries because of massive destruction of the pulmonary blood vessels, and right-sided heart failure.
Organic dusts	Inhalation of certain organic dusts can trigger hypersensitivity reactions in the lung (e.g., cotton fibres) and cause byssinosis, and bird faeces causes bird fancier's lung (seen, e.g., in people who keep pigeons or other birds).

Box 7.2 Drugs associated with interstitial lung disease

Drug	Examples
Chemotherapeutic agents	Bleomycin, cyclophosphamide, methotrexate
Anti-inflammatory drugs	NSAIDs, penicillamine, gold, methotrexate
Some antibiotics	Nitrofurantoin, sulphonamides
Oxygen	Risk increases with oxygen concentration, and extended period of therapy
Drugs of abuse	For example, heroin, especially in overdose, and talc, used as a bulking agent in preparations of illicit drugs for intravenous use

there is no identifiable cause, the condition is referred to as **idiopathic pulmonary fibrosis**. Whatever the cause, all interstitial lung diseases involve inflammation and fibrosis, reduce lung compliance, destroy alveoli, and reduce lung volumes.

Although ILD is often associated with chronic, progressive disease, acute ILD can follow trauma or injury, in which case it is often associated with ARDS and secondary to a similar range of insults.

Pathophysiology

ILD is associated with lung inflammation, which may be chronic, acute, or somewhere in between. Many cases are progressive, leading to permanent lung fibrosis. In the acute stage, the lung is infiltrated with inflammatory cells, becomes oedematous, haemorrhagic, and congested, and if the airways are involved, there may be bronchoconstriction and production of large quantities of mucus. The lung becomes less compliant, and the work of breathing is increased. Gas exchange is impaired because the alveoli fill with fluid. This inflammatory fluid is rich in protein, which precipitates out of solution and lines the alveoli with a so-called *hyaline membrane*, further obstructing gas exchange.

Chronic ILD is characterised by low-grade, ongoing inflammation, and deposition of fibrous tissue in the lung. Granulomas can form, and the chronic inflammation can destroy alveoli, generating cavities and honeycombing the lung. The fibrous tissue makes the lung stiff and non-compliant, so lung volumes fall.

Signs and symptoms

Patients experience breathlessness and reduced exercise tolerance. Lung function tests show reduced total lung capacity, vital capacity, and FEV_1. FEV_1:FVC ratio can be relatively normal because both of these measures are reduced. Fibrotic changes/cavitation show on X-rays. As the lungs stiffen and become less compliant, pulmonary hypertension develops, which in turn increases pressure in the pulmonary arteries and leads eventually to rising pressures in the right side of the heart. This results in heart failure.

Management and prognosis

Acute ILD, usually seen with ARDS after acute lung injury, carries a high mortality. Healing involves resorption of the alveolar fluid and clearing of cell debris, inflammatory matter, and the hyaline membranes by macrophages. Full lung function may be restored in some survivors, but in others there may be permanent scarring in the lung after healing.

Chronic disorders tend to progress over a period of years, with a steady deterioration in lung function, even after withdrawal of an identified causative agent (e.g., an affected coal miner giving up work does not halt disease progression). Stopping smoking is essential because smoking accelerates the inflammatory and fibrotic changes.

NON-PULMONARY CAUSES OF RESTRICTIVE LUNG DISEASE

Impaired lung function after a restrictive pattern (i.e., reduced lung volumes, reduced FEV_1, and a normal or close to normal FEV_1:FVC ratio) is seen in conditions that restrict normal lung expansion, even when the lung itself may be healthy. Conditions that increase intra-abdominal pressure, including pregnancy and central obesity, limit the downward movement of the diaphragm.

Musculoskeletal conditions

Bruised or fractured ribs make breathing painful, reducing lung expansion. Deformities of the vertebral column/thoracic cage Fig 13.17, such as scoliosis, kyphosis, or lordosis, deform the thoracic cage, compress the lungs, and limit the degree to which the lungs can expand on inspiration. In myasthenia gravis, both respiratory nerve and respiratory muscle function are normal, and the problem lies with the acetylcholine receptors of the neuromuscular junction (p.328), which are destroyed by autoantibodies. This means that the muscle cannot respond to the acetylcholine neurotransmitter released by the motor nerve. Muscular dystrophies, a group of muscle wasting disorders, frequently involve the respiratory muscles.

Neurological conditions

Disorders that damage or impair conduction in the nerves supplying the muscles of respiration reduce their ability to stimulate contraction, causing muscle weakness and possible paralysis. Disorders in this group include multiple sclerosis and Guillain-Barré syndrome, in which autoantibodies to peripheral nerves cause progressive paralysis of skeletal muscles, including the respiratory muscles.

PULMONARY VASCULAR DISEASE

As described previously, the pulmonary circulation is physiologically different from systemic blood vessels.

PULMONARY HYPERTENSION

This is defined as mean pulmonary arterial pressure greater than 25 mm Hg. It is usually caused by heart or lung disease (i.e., is secondary pulmonary hypertension). Primary pulmonary hypertension is much rarer, usually manifests in young adulthood, is commoner in women than men, and has a low survival rate.

SECONDARY PULMONARY HYPERTENSION

Whatever the cause (some of the main ones are explained below), the changes found in the pulmonary vasculature associated with secondary pulmonary hypertension follow a common development.

Pathophysiology

In the development of secondary pulmonary hypertension, progress is self-perpetuating; hypertension accelerates the changes, which in turn worsen the hypertension. Initially, the smooth muscle layer in the pulmonary blood vessel wall thickens, so the vessel's capacity to constrict is enhanced and its ability to dilate is reduced. As the condition progresses, the wall becomes thicker and thicker, less and less compliant, and fibrotic tissue appears. As with any blood vessel, the hypertension predisposes to atherosclerosis, which worsens the hypertension.

Causes of secondary pulmonary hypertension

These are numerous.

Hypoxia. As described previously (see Fig. 7.8), hypoxia in the lung, either because of low oxygen levels in the alveoli or low oxygen levels in the blood, causes pulmonary vasoconstriction. When the hypoxia is chronic, vasoconstriction is prolonged, and blood pressure rises. Blood vessels throughout the body respond to sustained increases in blood pressure with changes in the structure of their walls, which thicken and become less compliant. This makes them stronger and more able to withstand extended periods of high pressure, but it further increases blood pressure, promotes wall thickening and reduces the capacity of the blood vessel to dilate when required. Situations associated with chronic hypoxia include obstructive disease (bronchitis, emphysema), high altitude, obesity (because of impairment of respiratory muscles), sleep apnoea, kyphoscoliosis, or degenerative neuromuscular diseases affecting the respiratory system (e.g., multiple sclerosis, muscular dystrophy, myasthenia gravis).

Increased pulmonary blood flow/blood viscosity. If increased volumes of blood flow into the pulmonary circulation, or blood flow is sluggish and slow because the blood is thicker than normal, pulmonary blood pressure rises. This triggers the chain of events described previously, leading to wall thickening and steady worsening of the hypertension. Predisposing conditions include polycythaemia, in which high red cell numbers increase blood viscosity, and sickle cell disease, in which sickled red blood cells generate turbulence and slow blood flow. Failure of the ductus arteriosus or the foramen ovale to close completely after birth (p.152) also causes pulmonary hypertension in the newborn, because although they divert blood away from the lungs in the unborn child, after birth they divert large volumes of blood from the systemic circulation into the pulmonary artery.

Destruction or obstruction of pulmonary blood vessels. Destruction of alveoli—along with their associated blood vessels, reduces the total capacity of the pulmonary vasculature—increasing pressure because blood flow through the lungs is forced through fewer vessels. Compression or obstruction of pulmonary blood vessels, by fibrosis, blood clots, expanding tumours or infection all increase pressure, triggering changes in pulmonary vascular structure.

Left-sided heart failure. The pulmonary veins return blood to the left atrium, from where it passes into the left ventricle and is pumped into the systemic circulation. If there is any obstruction or the pumping action of the left ventricle is impaired, then blood backs up from the left heart, through the pulmonary veins and into the pulmonary capillaries, causing long-term changes as described previously. This may be caused by disease of the myocardium, mitral valve incompetence, or pericarditis restricting the normal pumping action of the heart.

PULMONARY EMBOLISM

An **embolism**, an abnormal mass travelling in the blood, can be trapped in a pulmonary artery or one of its branches, preventing blood flow to the areas of the lung beyond the blockage. Usually, the embolus is a thrombus or a fragment of a thrombus, often detached from a deep venous thrombosis formed in the leg, pelvis, or abdomen, but air, fat, amniotic fluid, or tumour masses travelling in the blood are other causes of PE. In this text, the abbreviation PE will be used to mean thromboembolism unless otherwise specified.

PULMONARY THROMBOEMBOLISM

Postmortems in people who have died of other causes frequently reveal PE, often in the form of multiple microemboli, which has been asymptomatic in life. It is thought that small emboli are naturally lysed by the fibrinolytic processes of the bloodstream, and that this is an ongoing process in otherwise healthy people. The true incidence of thromboembolism, and PE, is probably much higher than reported, because many cases are asymptomatic. Globally, however, larger pulmonary emboli are a major cause of death in hospitalised patients. It has been estimated that PE is the third commonest cause of death in people who die in hospital. Risk increases with age, in smokers, in those with central venous lines in place and with periods of immobility and is higher in black people than in whites. 10% of symptomatic PE cases are fatal.

Pathophysiology

Blockade of a pulmonary blood vessel usually causes ischaemia and infarction of the lung tissue supplied by that vessel. At the site of blockage, an inflammatory response is initiated, releasing inflammatory and other mediators including serotonin and thromboxane A_2 into the circulation, which cause vasoconstriction and increase pulmonary blood pressure. This further impedes blood flow through the lungs. A so-called *saddle embolus* (Fig. 7.25A) is a large blood clot that travels through the right ventricle and lodges in the pulmonary trunk, blocking both the right and left pulmonary arteries. Such massive obstruction is immediately fatal. If the embolism is major but does not cause immediate death, pressure builds up behind it, through the pulmonary artery, and into the right side of the heart, increasing its workload and potentially causing right-sided heart failure. In addition, less blood passes through the lung into the pulmonary vein, so return to the left side of the heart falls, leading to low left sided output and systemic hypotension. Fig. 7.25B shows the main consequences of a PE.

The non-perfused section of the lung stops producing surfactant after several hours of blood deprivation, leading to collapse of the alveoli involved, which worsens hypoxaemia. These areas are ventilated but not perfused, leading to a higher-than-normal V/Q ratio, which also contributes to hypoxaemia.

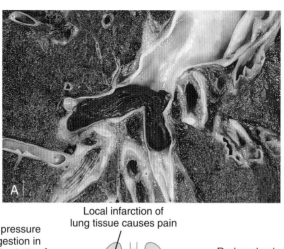

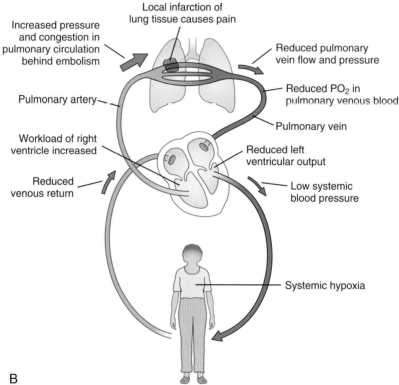

Fig. 7.25 Pulmonary embolism. (A) A saddle embolism blocking both pulmonary arteries. (B) The main consequences of a pulmonary embolism. (Source: A, From Gould B, Dyer R (2011) *Pathophysiology for the health professions*, 4th ed. Philadelphia: Saunders.)

Signs and symptoms

The consequences for the affected individual depend on the size of the pulmonary artery affected and the health status of the person. Small emboli may be completely asymptomatic. Clearly, if the embolism is large and it blocks a major vessel, more lung tissue is deprived of oxygen and the consequences are greater. Assuming the embolism does not cause instant death, the symptoms usually reflect the degree to which pulmonary blood flow is impeded. The person is breathless and frightened. If there has been infarction, then pleuritic pain on breathing and a cough with bloodstained sputum may occur. A non-fatal massive embolism causes signs and symptoms of heart failure and shock caused by inadequate return of blood to the left side of the heart: there is hypotension, tachycardia, pallor, and tachypnoea. There may be angina if blood supply to the myocardium via the coronary arteries is reduced. There may be venous congestion, as blood backs up in the right heart and the large veins because its path through the lungs is blocked. Blood oxygen levels fall and blood CO_2 levels rise because of lung collapse and impaired gas exchange.

Management and prognosis

Oxygen therapy is used to reverse hypoxaemia. Anticoagulants are used to prevent further clot development and fibrinolytics dissolve existing clots. Support for a failing heart, in the form of inotropic agents to strengthen the force of myocardial contraction, can be useful in the short term.

PLEURAL DISORDERS

Damage to the pleura is associated with collapse of all or part of the lung because it opens the sealed intrapleural space and allows air to enter. Pleural disorders may be painful because the parietal pleura (but not the visceral pleura) contains a rich population of free sensory nerve endings, which transmit pain sensation via somatic nerves to the brain.

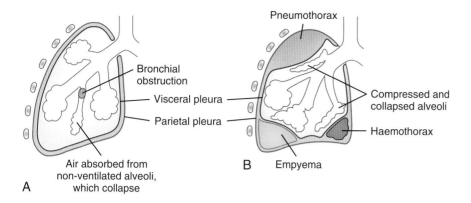

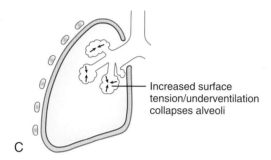

Fig. 7.26 The three types of atelectasis. (A) Obstruction collapse. (B) Compression collapse. (C) Expansion collapse.

Pleurisy

Pleurisy is a general term meaning inflammation of the pleura and occurs with a range of disorders, including lung infections and tumours, PE, rheumatoid arthritis, connective tissue disorders including systemic lupus erythematosus, scleroderma and sarcoidosis, and certain drugs (e.g., methotrexate). It causes sharp, localised pain with breathing because of the friction generated when the inflamed membranes rub against one another, and the friction rub can be heard with a stethoscope (**pleural rub**). Pleurisy may resolve completely, but occasionally the healing process produces fibrotic adhesions between the pleura, which can restrict lung expansion and cause residual pain.

LUNG COLLAPSE (ATELECTASIS)

The term *atelectasis* means collapse or partial collapse of all or part of a lung. The healthy lung is kept inflated because of the equilibrium between two opposing forces: the elastic recoil of the lung tissue, constantly pulling the lung towards the hilum, and the negative pressure in the intrapleural space, holding the visceral pleura and the parietal pleura together (Fig. 7.7). Any factor that disturbs this equilibrium can lead to atelectasis, and a number of conditions and events may be involved (Fig. 7.26).

Obstruction collapse

When an airway is blocked, whether by secretions, a tumour, or a foreign body, the alveoli it supplies receive no more air. Over a period of time, the air already in the alveoli is slowly absorbed into the bloodstream and is not replaced, and so the alveoli collapse (Fig. 7.26A). Airway obstruction is the commonest reason for lung collapse.

Compression collapse

Inflammation and/or infection in the lung lead to collection of a protein-rich inflammatory fluid, blood, and/or pus in the tissues. If this involves the pleura, these materials collect in the pleural space and compress the soft lung tissue, preventing alveolar expansion with breathing, and leading to collapse (Fig. 7.26B). Blood in the pleural space is called **haemothorax**, and pus in the pleural space is called **empyema**. Increased volume of pleural fluid is called **pleural effusion** (see Pleural effusion below). Damage to either the visceral or parietal pleura opens the sealed pleural space, and air enters (**pneumothorax**; see below). Any expanding lesion in the chest (e.g., a lung tumour) compresses the lung tissue, prevents alveolar expansion, and leads to lung collapse.

Expansion collapse

Inadequate surfactant in the alveoli increases surface tension and predisposes to collapse (Fig. 7.26C). This may be caused by prematurity or acute lung injury. The risk of atelectasis is increased in post-operative patients, especially after general anaesthetics and opioid analgesia because both depress respiratory effort. The pain, drowsiness, and reduced mobility after surgery can reduce the depth and rate of respiration, such that large areas of the lung may not be adequately ventilated and end up partially collapsed.

PNEUMOTHORAX

Pneumothorax is the presence of air in the pleural space. Normally, the intrapleural space contains a few milliliters of pleural fluid, and the intrapleural pressure is subatmospheric. This generates the suction responsible for holding the visceral and parietal pleura together. If one or other of the pleural membranes is ruptured, air rushes in to equalise pressure between atmospheric air and the pleural space. The visceral pleura can be breached by a tumour growing in the lung periphery, or by an expanding lung cavity created by, for example, emphysema or interstitial lung disease. In this case, the air enters the pleural space from the alveoli. If the chest wall and parietal pleura are damaged—for example, by a broken rib or stab wound—air is sucked in from

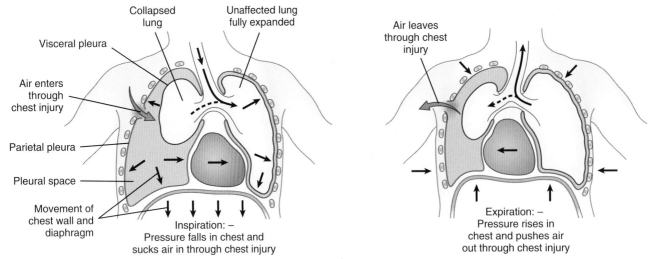

Fig. 7.27   Open pneumothorax. (Modified from Des Jardins T and Burton G (2020) *Clinical manifestations and assessment of respiratory disease,* 8th ed, Fig. 23.2. St Louis: Elsevier Inc.)

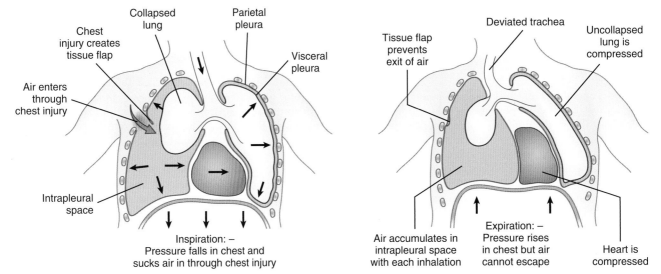

Fig. 7.28   Closed (tension) pneumothorax. (Modified from modified from Des Jardins T and Burton G (2020) *Clinical manifestations and assessment of respiratory disease,* 8th ed, Fig. 23.3. St Louis: Elsevier Inc.)

the exterior. The pleural space is now in direct communication with the external atmosphere, and once the intrapleural pressure is equal to atmospheric pressure, air moves in and out of the chest according to the pressure changes of breathing. When the respiratory muscles contract and the chest expands, the pressure in the chest falls and sucks air in through the breach in the chest wall. During expiration, the chest volume falls, pressure rises, and air is expelled again. This is called an **open pneumothorax** (Fig. 7.27).

Closed (tension) pneumothorax. In tension pneumothorax, the injury does not leave an open hole in the damaged pleura but creates a partially attached flap of tissue that acts as a valve (Fig. 7.28). When pressure falls in the chest during inspiration, the flap is pulled away from the breach and allows air to enter. However, when pressure rises in the chest during expiration, the flap is pushed against the breach and prevents air from leaving. In this way, air rapidly accumulates in the pleural space with each breath in and cannot escape. This compresses the lung on the affected side and collapses

it. In addition, the expanding air space compresses other structures in the chest, most notably the heart, which is displaced away from the affected lung, restricting its pumping action. Total lung capacity rapidly falls, gas exchange is reduced, and hypoxaemia follows. Compression of the aorta and the great veins impedes cardiac output and venous return. Tension pneumothorax is a medical emergency.

Primary pneumothorax. In primary pneumothorax, there is no clearly identified underlying cause. It is most common in tall young people, in whom the lung is subject to greater stretch because of their longer than average chest. There is an association with the presence of lung blebs (cavities less than 2 cm in diameter within lung tissue) or bullae (spaces over 2 cm in diameter within lung tissue) that are otherwise asymptomatic.

Signs and symptoms

Acute pneumothorax presents with dyspnoea, cyanosis, tachycardia, tachypnoea, and distress. Shunting develops because of the non-ventilated alveoli, leading to hypoxaemia,

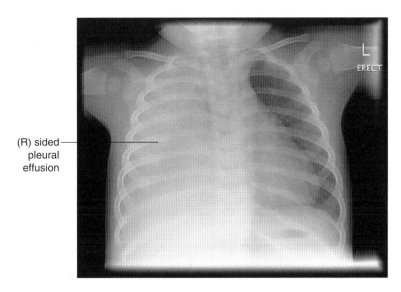

(R) sided pleural effusion

Fig. 7.29 Right-sided pleural effusion on chest X-ray. (Collection of Prof. Adam Jaffe.)

and the V/Q ratio is decreased. The chest on the affected side may expand because of accumulation of air, especially in a tension pneumothorax. X-ray shows the extent of lung collapse and any changes in position of thoracic structures.

Management and prognosis

If only a small proportion of the lung has collapsed (15%–20% of lung capacity), it may reinflate itself over time without treatment. In these circumstances, healing of the lesion and reabsorption of the gases in the pleural space takes about a month. Larger pneumothoraces may be relieved by insertion of a chest drain, allowing air to leave but not re-enter the pleural space.

PLEURAL EFFUSION

This is fluid accumulation in the pleural cavity caused by production exceeding drainage (Fig. 7.29). There are two types, depending on the underlying cause.

Pressure effusion. When blood pressure rises in the pulmonary capillaries, fluid is pushed into lung tissues. This can cause pulmonary oedema, as described previously, and if the capillaries are close to the lung surface, fluid is pushed into and accumulates in the intrapleural space. This effusion fluid is low in protein and has normal white cell numbers because it is generated by rising pressure rather than an inflammatory condition. Pulmonary hypertension of any aetiology can cause pleural effusion. Kidney disease and liver failure may also cause this type of effusion, not because of rising blood pressure but because of falling plasma osmotic pressure. In liver failure, plasma protein production is low, so plasma protein levels fall, which reduces plasma osmotic pressure and allows fluid to leak out of capillaries and into tissues, including the lungs. Abnormal protein excretion in the urine is a feature of some kidney disorders, leading to reduced plasma protein levels and reduced plasma osmotic pressure. Pleural effusions secondary to pressure changes in the blood affect both lungs equally.

Inflammatory effusion. These effusions are likely to be localised and affect only one lung or part of one lung because they are caused by inflammation, trauma, or impaired lymphatic drainage. The inflammatory fluid is protein rich and may contain significant numbers of white blood cells because the pulmonary blood vessels are more permeable than normal. Malignancy is a common cause of pleural effusion. An expanding tumour may block drainage channels, and its local inflammatory environment causes vasodilation and other inflammatory changes, leading to exudation into the pleural space. Infections may also cause pleural effusions, not only because they block lymphatic drainage, but also because of the inflammation associated with them. Empyema (pus in the pleural fluid) may also be a feature in infection.

Pathophysiology

Large volumes of effusion fluid compress the lungs and prevent efficient expansion. If fluid continues to accumulate, especially if both lungs are affected, there may be atelectasis and compression of the heart and great vessels in the mediastinum. This may impede cardiac pumping and the flow of blood in and out of the heart.

Signs and symptoms

These vary depending on the size of the effusion and the underlying cause. There may be dyspnoea, tachycardia, pain, and distress. If there is significant atelectasis, gas exchange is impaired and hypoxaemia develops. There may be cough and a pleural rub heard on auscultation with a stethoscope. X-ray shows any area of atelectasis and displacement and compression of thoracic organs.

Management and prognosis

This depends on the extent of the effusion and the underlying cause. The effusion may resolve naturally with time or with treatment. Occasionally, drainage of the excess fluid is indicated.

MESOTHELIOMA

This aggressive malignancy of the pleura is rare, with a global incidence of fewer than 1 in 100,000 people per year, but there are significant differences from country to country. The male:female ratio is 3:1. There is a strong link with asbestos exposure, and other risk factors include smoking and increasing age.

Pathophysiology

Although 87% of mesotheliomas arise in the pleura, this malignancy is not exclusive to the lung. Mesothelial cells, the cells of origin in mesothelioma, are simple squamous epithelial cells, and form the membranes lining the pleural, peritoneal, and pericardial cavities, among others. Of all pleural mesotheliomas, 80% develop in individuals in the age range 60 to 80 years and who had been exposed to asbestos up to 40 years earlier. The tumour begins as small nodules scattered on the pleura, which expand and merge, forming a thick sheet of neoplastic tissue that envelopes the lung. It frequently invades other thoracic structures but is generally slow to metastasise to distant sites.

Signs and symptoms

Breathlessness, fatigue, weight loss, night sweats, and chest wall pain are common. There is often pleural effusion.

Management and prognosis

Without treatment, survival time is on average about 6 months after presentation. Even with treatment, survival rates are dismal, and often measured in months rather than years. Treatment includes chemotherapy and radiotherapy, and if the disease is confined to the chest, lung removal may be considered.

BIBLIOGRAPHY AND REFERENCES

Cloutier, M. M. (2018). *Respiratory physiology* (2nd ed). Elsevier.

Duffy, S. P., & Criner, G. J. (2019). Chronic obstructive pulmonary disease: Evaluation and management. *Medical Clinics of North America, 103*(3), 453–461.

Papi, A., Brightling, C., Pedersen, S. E., & Reddel, H. K. (2018). Asthma. *The Lancet, 391*(10122), 783–800.

Useful websites

British Lung Foundation: https://www.blf.org.uk

Global Asthma Report 2018: http://www.globalasthmareport.org

Influenza statistics: https://www.thelancet.com/journals/lancet/article/PIIS0140-6736(17)33293-2/fulltext

The pathophysiology of pneumonia: https://emedicine.medscape.com/article/234753-overview

Disorders of Neurological Function

8

CHAPTER OUTLINE

INTRODUCTION
   The cells of the nervous system
   The action potential
   The synapse and nerve–nerve communication
The central nervous system
   Functional anatomy of the brain
   The spinal cord
The peripheral nervous system
   The cranial nerves
   The spinal nerves
   The autonomic nervous system
   The somatic (voluntary) nervous system
CENTRAL NERVOUS SYSTEM
PATHOPHYSIOLOGY
CNS infections
   Meningitis
   Encephalitis
   Rabies
   Poliomyelitis (polio)
Inflammatory and immune mediated CNS
   disorders
   Multiple sclerosis
Neurodegenerative disorders
   Alzheimer disease
   Vascular dementia
   Frontotemporal dementia
   Motor neurone disease (MND)
Mental health disorders
   Bipolar disorder
   Anxiety and panic disorders
   Schizophrenia
   Autism

Seizures and epilepsy
Central nervous system tumours
   Gliomas
   Medulloblastoma
   Meningioma
   Schwannoma
   Primary CNS lymphoma
Disorders of motor control
   Parkinson disease
Cerebrovascular disorders
   Stroke
   Intracranial haemorrhage
Congenital and developmental disorders
   Neural tube defect (NTD)
   Cerebral Palsy (CP)
Headache syndromes
   Tension headache
   Cluster headache
   Migraine
PERIPHERAL NERVOUS SYSTEM
PATHOPHYSIOLOGY
Peripheral neuropathy
   Carpal tunnel syndrome
   Guillain-barré syndrome
   Myasthenia gravis
Cranial nerve syndromes
   Trigeminal neuralgia
   Bell palsy
PAIN
   Classification of pain
   Pain transmission

INTRODUCTION

Working in tandem with the endocrine system, the nervous system provides key communication, integration, and response systems essential to the function of all body organs. It is conventionally divided into two parts: the **central nervous system** (CNS), comprising the brain and spinal cord, and the **peripheral nervous system** (PNS), comprising all neural tissue outwith the CNS.

THE CELLS OF THE NERVOUS SYSTEM

Neurones generate and transmit electrical signals in the form of **action potentials**. The general structure of a neurone is shown in Fig. 8.1. Although not all nerve cells are anatomically identical, they all possess a **cell body** that houses

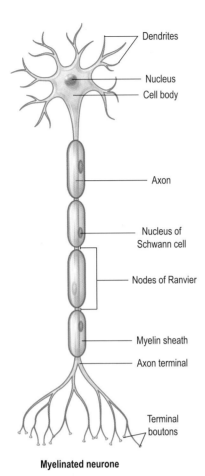

Dendrites

Nucleus

Cell body

Axon

Nucleus of
Schwann cell

Nodes of Ranvier

Myelin sheath

Axon terminal

Terminal
boutons

Myelinated neurone

Fig. 8.1 General structure of a neurone. (Modified from Waugh A, Grant A (2018) *Ross & Wilson anatomy and physiology in health and illness* 13th ed, Fig. 7.2. Oxford: Elsevier Ltd.)

the nucleus, a long slender fibre called the **axon** along which the action potential travels, and multiple **dendrites**, fine filamentous extensions that receive input from adjacent nerve cells. The axon conducts action potentials away from the neuronal cell body towards the target tissue. In the central nervous system, the target cells are other neurones, and in the peripheral nervous system the axon innervates muscle, glands, and other body tissues. Within the CNS, the axons are usually very short, but PNS axons may extend from the spinal cord to their target tissue: nerves running from the spinal cord to the toes can be up to a metre in length. At the **axon terminal**, where the nerve ending is close to its target tissue, it breaks up into a sheaf of fine threadlike filaments, each of which forms a tiny **terminal bouton** responsible for communicating with a dendrite of the target cell. A neurone may receive input from hundreds of adjacent nerves via its receiving dendrites. Many nerve axons are coated in a myelin sheath, which improves the speed and efficiency of impulse conduction.

Glial cells: neuronal support cells

There are about as many glial cells as neurones in the brain. Glial cells—originally believed to be passive 'glue' cells simply holding neurones together—are now known to be essential for controlling the microenvironment in the brain and regulating key neuronal functions, including synaptic

transmission. The glia are important in the brain's response to injury and their numbers expand significantly when brain tissue is damaged. In addition, they control the chemical composition of the brain environment through their uptake of a range of substances including neurotransmitters, ions, and toxins.

There are several types of glial cells. Some produce the myelin sheath associated with many nerves: in the CNS this function is performed by **oligodendrocytes** and in the PNS, myelin is produced by **Schwann cells**. Another type, **microglia**, are phagocytes, and clear debris and infecting organisms from the CNS. **Ependymal cells** are glial cells lining the spinal cord and the ventricles in the brain and produce cerebrospinal fluid. **Astrocytes**, star-shaped glial cells with multiple processes, provide physical support for nerves and help form the blood-brain barrier (see below).

THE ACTION POTENTIAL

Action potentials are produced by the movement of sodium and potassium ions across the nerve cell membrane. Sodium concentrations are higher in extracellular fluid and potassium concentrations are higher in the intracellular fluid because of the action of the sodium-potassium pump (Na^+/K^+ pump) in the nerve cell membrane, which pumps sodium out and potassium in against their concentration gradients and prevents the ions from equilibrating on either side of the cell membrane. The Na^+/K^+ pump requires energy, in the form of ATP, to operate. The gradients created by the Na^+/K^+ pump are essential for the electrical excitability of the nerve cell. Nerve cells receive continuous input from communicating nerve cells, via their dendrites. When the level of input reaches threshold, it triggers an action potential in the nerve. The action potential is generated by a rapid and short-lived change in the permeability of the nerve cell membrane to sodium and potassium, allowing these electrically charged ions to flood through the membrane down their concentration gradients and generating an electrical current. Initially, sodium channels along the nerve axon open, and sodium ions flood into the nerve, **depolarising** it. A millisecond later, potassium channels open, and potassium ions flood out of the nerve. Locally, the concentrations of sodium and potassium ions are now the same on both sides of the nerve cell membrane, and for the nerve to fire again, the gradients must be restored. The sodium and potassium channels therefore close, and the Na^+/K^+ pump rapidly pumps sodium back out of the nerve and potassium back in, regenerating the ionic differences essential to allow the nerve to conduct another action potential. This is called **repolarisation**.

THE SYNAPSE AND NERVE–NERVE COMMUNICATION

Nerve cells communicate with one another via the release of neurotransmitters at the synapse. These chemical messengers diffuse across the tiny gap between the terminal boutons of the presynaptic nerve and bind to receptors on the dendrites of the post-synaptic nerve (Fig. 8.2). This binding may either stimulate or inhibit the post-synaptic nerve membrane; controlled, integrated brain activity depends on the continued and regulated adjustment of the balance between excitatory and inhibitory signals.

The CNS uses a large number of neurotransmitters, some of which are found exclusively in the brain and spinal cord and some of which are also found in peripheral tissues,

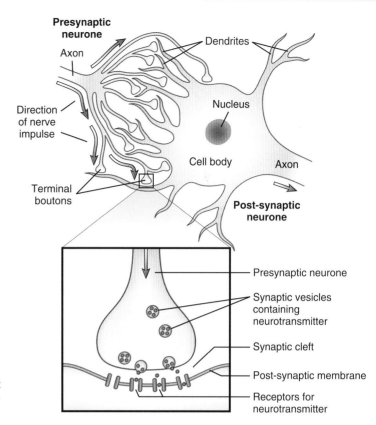

Fig. 8.2 Synaptic transmission. (Modified from Waugh A, Grant A (2018) *Ross & Wilson anatomy and physiology in health and illness* 13th ed, Fig. 7.7. Oxford: Elsevier Ltd.)

not necessarily as neurotransmitters. Some important neurotransmitters are presented in Box 8.1. Abnormalities of synaptic transmission can cause significant neurological dysfunction and are found in a range of neurological disorders, including epilepsy and depression.

THE CENTRAL NERVOUS SYSTEM

Conventional description of the CNS separates it into two structures—the brain and the spinal cord—protected within the bony shelter of the cranium and vertebral column and cushioned and nourished by the constant circulation of cerebrospinal fluid (CSF).

Blood supply to the brain

About 15% of the left ventricular cardiac output at rest goes to the brain. The brain is supplied with blood by the internal carotid and vertebral arteries, which feed blood into a circular arrangement of arteries called the **circulus arteriosus** (circle of Willis) lying on the base of the brain (Fig. 8.3). The vertebral arteries unite at the back of the brain to form the basilar artery, which delivers blood into the posterior part of the circle, and the right and left internal carotids supply blood from the right and left sides respectively. From the circle arise the arteries that supply the majority of the brain tissue: the anterior cerebral artery, the middle cerebral artery, and the posterior cerebral artery. The brainstem and cerebellum are supplied by arteries branching directly from the basilar and vertebral arteries (i.e., not from the circulus arteriosus).

Anterior cerebral artery

This supplies most of the frontal lobes, including some of the motor cortex.

BOX 8.1 Some important CNS transmitters and their function

Neurotransmitter	Comments
Acetylcholine	Widespread; excitatory; controls memory, alertness, learning and motor functions
Noradrenaline	Regulates pathways concerned with emotion, alertness, motivation, sleep, mood, learning and cardiovascular control
Endorphins	Found in pain pathways in the brain and spinal cord; endorphin release deactivates synapses that transmit pain signals
Histamine	Stimulates vomiting; maintains daytime alertness as part of the body's diurnal rhythm
Dopamine	Found mainly in the nigrostriatal pathways that control voluntary motor activity; stimulates vomiting; important in reward, reinforcement and pleasure pathways; inhibits lactation
Serotonin	Contributes to control of mood, arousal, sexual activity, sleep and appetite
GABA (gamma amino butyric acid)	Widespread inhibitory transmitter in brain
Glycine	Inhibitory transmitter in brainstem and spinal cord
Glutamate	Widespread in CNS; principal excitatory transmitter

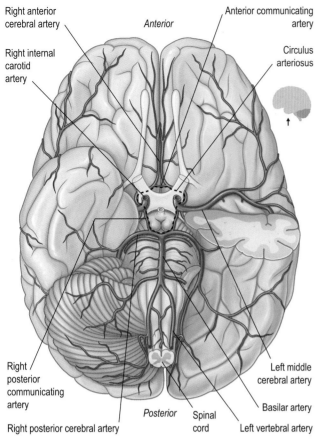

Fig. 8.3 The circulus arteriosus, viewed from below. (Modified from Waugh A, Grant A (2018) *Ross & Wilson anatomy and physiology in health and illness* 13th ed, Fig. 7.31. Oxford: Elsevier Ltd.)

Middle cerebral artery

This supplies a portion of the frontal, temporal, and parietal lobes, including the sensory and motor supply to the face, throat, hand, arm, and speech area. The lenticulostriate arteries arise from the middle cerebral artery to supply the basal ganglia and brainstem. The middle cerebral artery is the largest of the cerebral arteries and the most likely to be involved in ischaemic stroke.

Posterior cerebral artery

This supplies the occipital and temporal lobes.

Venous drainage of the brain

Venous blood drains from the brain through a complex system of channels called **dural venous sinuses**, which lie within the dura mater, the fibrous lining of the skull and the outermost of the three meninges covering the brain.

The meninges

The brain and spinal cord are wrapped in three membranes, the meninges: the **pia mater**, the **arachnoid mater**, and the **dura mater** (Fig. 8.4A). The dura mater, formed of two layers, is a tough, fibrous coat lining the inside of the skull and extending down the vertebral canal, enclosing the spinal cord and the filum terminale to the level of the second sacral vertebra. The space between the skull and the dura mater is called the **epidural space** and is filled with fat and blood vessels. The space between the dura mater and the middle meningeal membrane, the arachnoid mater, is called the **subdural space** and contains a network of blood vessels. The arachnoid mater is thin with no blood vessels, and is separated from the innermost membrane, the pia mater, by the **subarachnoid space**, which is filled with cerebrospinal fluid (Fig. 8.4B).

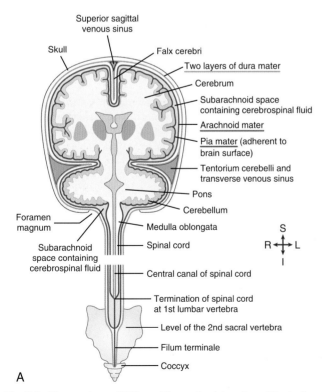

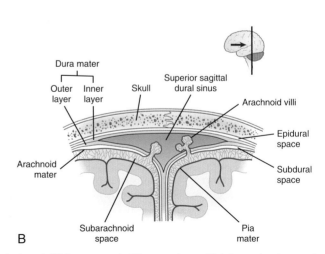

Fig. 8.4 The meninges. (A) Viewed from a frontal section of the brain and spinal cord. (B) Arrangement at the superior sagittal sinus, showing arachnoid villi. (Modified from Waugh A, Grant A (2018) *Ross & Wilson anatomy and physiology in health and illness* 13th ed, Fig. 7.14. Oxford: Elsevier Ltd.)

CSF and raised intracranial pressure

Lying within the brain is an interconnected system of chambers called the *cerebral ventricles* (Fig. 8.5A), lined with ependymal cells. CSF is filtered from the bloodstream by specialised tufts of capillaries called **choroid plexuses** in the ventricular lining. It is produced at a rate of about 650 mL/ day and circulates through the ventricular system and into the subarachnoid space (Fig. 8.5B), extending down into the vertebral column to the level of the 2nd sacral vertebra (S2; Fig. 8.4A). It is reabsorbed into the bloodstream through the **arachnoid villi (arachnoid granulations)**, small outpouchings of the arachnoid mater through the dura

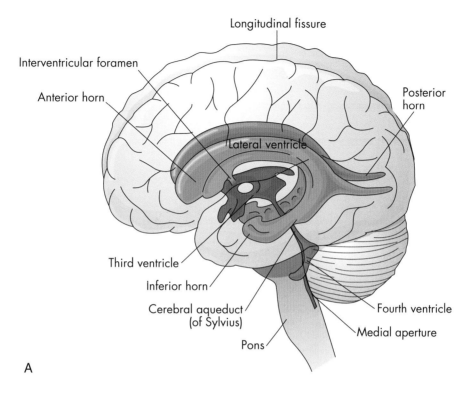

Longitudinal fissure

Interventricular foramen

Anterior horn

Posterior horn

Lateral ventricle

Third ventricle

Inferior horn

Cerebral aqueduct (of Sylvius)

Pons

Fourth ventricle

Medial aperture

A

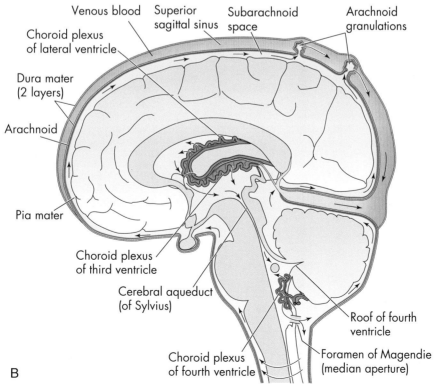

Venous blood   Superior sagittal sinus   Subarachnoid space   Arachnoid granulations

Choroid plexus of lateral ventricle

Dura mater (2 layers)

Arachnoid

Pia mater

Choroid plexus of third ventricle

Cerebral aqueduct (of Sylvius)

Choroid plexus of fourth ventricle

Roof of fourth ventricle

Foramen of Magendie (median aperture)

B

Fig. 8.5   The production, circulation, and reabsorption of CSF. (A) The cerebral ventricles. (B) Circulation of CSF in the subarachnoid space.

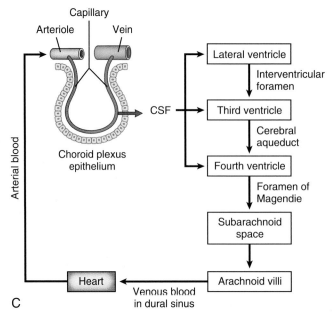

Fig. 8.5 cont'd   (C) Summary of the formation and circulation of CSF. (Modified from (A) and (B) J Craft, C Gordon, S Huether, et al. (2015) *Understanding Pathophysiology ANZ,* 2nd ed, Fig. 6.21. Sydney: Elsevier Australia.)

mater into the blood filling the dural sinuses (Fig. 8.4B). Fig. 8.4C summarises the route of formation and circulation of CSF. Normal intracranial pressure (ICP) is maintained between 10 to 15 mm Hg because CSF reabsorption into the blood through the arachnoid villi matches the rate of production. Raised ICP may occur because of obstruction of the circulation of CSF by a tumour, serious head injury, or a cerebral haemorrhage. Other causes include cerebral oedema, perhaps because of water overload or meningitis.

Consequences of raised ICP. Raised ICP compresses and damages delicate brain tissue. Seizures are common. There may be headache, vomiting, reduced level of consciousness, visual disturbances including diplopia, and papilloedema (swelling of the optic disc). Sustained raised pressure displaces the brain and can force parts of the brainstem and/or cerebellum through the foramen magnum at the base of the skull. This is called **coning**, which causes significant damage to brainstem structures and usually leads to coma and death unless treated. Hydrocephalus, the accumulation of CSF circulating within the CNS in babies or children, enlarges the head because the skull bones have not fully fused together and is very likely to cause compressive injury to the brain.

FUNCTIONAL ANATOMY OF THE BRAIN

The brain contains around 86 billion neurones and is described in four major regions: the **brainstem**, the **diencephalon**, the **cerebral hemispheres** (the telencephalon), and the **cerebellum** (Fig. 8.6).

Brainstem

The brainstem is composed of the **medulla oblongata**, the **pons**, and the **midbrain** and connects the spinal cord to brain structures above. It contains the respiratory and cardiovascular control centres and is the bridge that allows higher centres in the brain to communicate with the body and sensory input from the body to reach the higher centres. Key protective reflexes—such as the swallowing, gag, corneal, cough, and sneeze reflexes—are generated here.

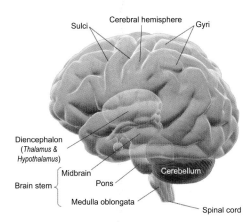

Fig. 8.6   The main regions of the brain. (Modified from Blausen gallery 2014. Wikiversity J. Med., https://doi.org/10.15347/wjm/2014.010. ISSN 20018762)

For these reasons, brainstem damage is often catastrophic and may endanger life. An important group of dopamine-releasing neurones, originating in the substantia nigra of the midbrain and projecting to the striatum (the **nigrostriatal pathway**), are essential to voluntary motor control and will be further discussed in the section on Parkinson disease. Also located in the midbrain is the **ventral tegmental area**, which sends dopamine-releasing neurones involved in the pathogenesis of schizophrenia to areas of the cortex, the limbic system and the striatum.

Ten of the twelve cranial nerves (nerves III–XII) exit the brain from the brainstem.

Diencephalon

This region of the brain—sitting superiorly to the brainstem and connecting it to the cerebral hemispheres—contains key regulatory brain areas including the **thalamus** and the **hypothalamus**. The thalamus, an important integratory structure, receives and integrates sensory information from the body and sends it to the cerebral cortex. The thalamus

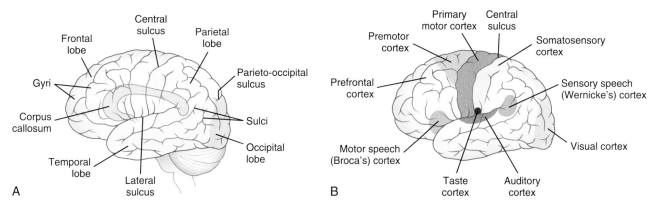

Fig. 8.7 The anatomy of the brain. (A) The lobes, sulci, and gyri of the brain. (B) Functional areas of the cerebral cortex. (Modified from (A) Waugh A, Grant A (2018) *Ross & Wilson anatomy and physiology in health and illness* 13th ed, Oxford, Elsevier Ltd; Fig. 7.18; (B) modified from Waugh A, Grant A (2018) *Ross & Wilson anatomy and physiology in health and illness* 13th ed, Oxford, Elsevier Ltd; Fig. 7.20.)

also has connections with the cerebellum and other brain areas important in voluntary motor control.

The hypothalamus represents only 0.3% of the total brain mass, but it is a key integrator of a wide range of essential physiological functions, including temperature regulation, some emotional responses, appetite, and reproduction. It is also the main controller of autonomic nervous system function and communicates directly with autonomic nerves in the brainstem and spinal cord to regulate essential autonomic functions such as cardiovascular control. Additionally, it has endocrine functions, playing a critically important role in the hypothalamic-pituitary axis and control of key endocrine organs (p. 251).

Cerebral hemispheres

The paired cerebral hemispheres (the telencephalon) make up the majority of the total volume of the brain and are divided into four main lobes (Fig. 8.7A). They are composed of mostly white matter—the axons that connect neuronal cell bodies with one another—and are joined by a thick bridge of axons called the **corpus callosum**. The surface layer, a thin coating of grey matter only about 2 to 3mm thick and formed by neuronal cell bodies, is called the **cerebral cortex** and houses sophisticated higher functions including memory, judgement, reasoning, intellectual capacity, consciousness, thinking, and learning. The surface of the cerebral hemispheres show folds, called **gyri** (singular = gyrus), separated by narrow fissures and dips called **sulci** (singular = sulcus), and allow more grey matter to be packed into a smaller volume. Distinct areas of cerebral cortex are devoted to discrete functions (Fig. 8.7B). Deep in the cerebral hemispheres lie the **basal ganglia**, collections of cell bodies involved primarily in voluntary motor control, which will be discussed in more detail in the section on Parkinson disease. Two parts of the basal ganglia—the caudate nucleus and the putamen—form a structure called the **striatum**, which is important as an integrator, receiving input from, and feeding output to, multiple areas of the brain including the cerebral cortex, the limbic system and the midbrain. In addition to its role in voluntary muscle control, the striatum is important in learning, planning, motivation, and reward processing. Its extensive connectivity seems to be impaired in schizophrenia.

Cranial nerves I and II (olfactory and optic) leave the brain from the cerebrum.

The limbic system

This group of structures is associated functionally rather than anatomically: that is, they are not collected in the same location but are considered together because they have the common functions of memory, emotion, motivational behaviours, and learning. They are heavily interconnected, allowing them to operate as an integrated unit despite being dispersed in the brain. Some limbic structures are found deep in the cerebral hemispheres, including the **hippocampus**, involved in memory, and the **amygdala**, involved in the processing of emotion. The system also includes the **periaqueductal grey matter** of the midbrain, involved in transmission of pain signals, and some groups of nerves from the thalamus and hypothalamus.

Cerebellum

'Cerebellum' means 'little brain', and this structure, lying posterior to the main body of the brain, with its ridged and folded surface, does resemble a scaled-down version of the main organ. As with the brain itself, the cerebellum is composed mainly of axons (white matter) with the neuronal cell bodies lying on the surface, forming a thin external layer of grey matter. It contains a disproportionately high number of neurones compared with its size and receives sensory input from nearly all sense organs of the body, including visual input, auditory, and balance information from the ears and proprioceptor information from skeletal muscles and joints. With this information, the cerebellum maintains rapid, integrated and finely tuned control of balance, equilibrium, and voluntary muscle movement.

THE SPINAL CORD

The spinal cord, a rope of nerves extending from the brainstem down the bony tube formed by the stacked vertebrae of the vertebral column, is enclosed by the dura, arachnoid and pia maters and extends as far as the first lumbar vertebra (Fig. 8.8A). The cord tip (the **conus medullaris**) is anchored at the base of the vertebral canal by the **filum terminale**, a filament of connective tissue. The spinal cord is the vital link between brain and body. From the gaps between the stacked vertebrae, the 31 spinal nerves exit from the spinal column to supply body tissues (Fig. 8.8B). Every spinal nerve is a mixed nerve (i.e., it carries both motor and sensory fibres and therefore carries two-way information: incoming

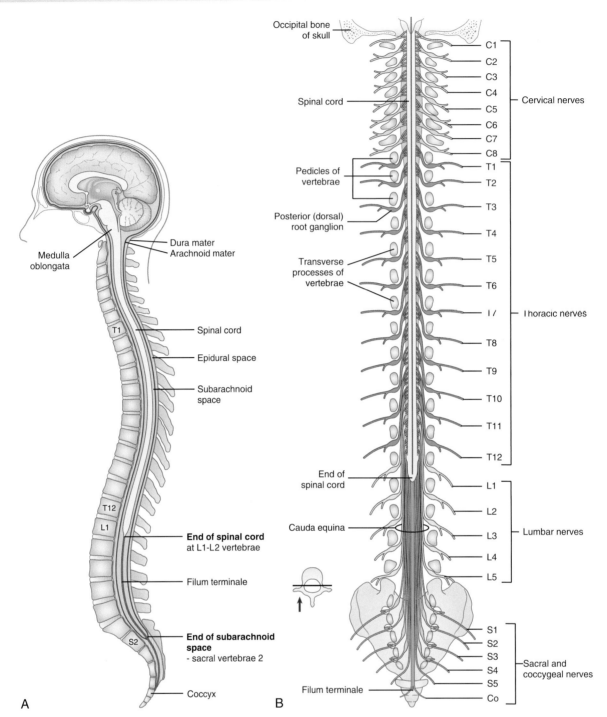

Fig. 8.8 The spinal cord. (A) The spinal cord and its meninges. (B) The spinal nerves. (Modified from (A) Waugh A, Grant A (2018) *Ross & Wilson anatomy and physiology in health and illness* 13th ed, Fig. 7.26. Oxford: Elsevier Ltd.; (B) modified from Waugh A, Grant A (2018) *Ross & Wilson anatomy and physiology in health and illness* 13th ed, Fig. 7.27. Oxford: Elsevier Ltd.)

sensory data from the body streams into the brain), and instructions are transmitted from the brain to the body.

A cross-section of the spinal cord shows a central butterfly-shaped area of grey matter, containing the cell bodies and their synapses with the spinal neurones. It forms two 'horns' anteriorly and two posteriorly. The dorsal (posterior) horns are formed from the cell bodies of sensory nerves, bringing information from the body to the spinal cord to be transmitted to the brain. The ventral (anterior) horns carry motor nerves, supplying skeletal muscle and other body organs

such as glandular tissue. The outer region of the cord is made of white matter and is composed of the neuronal axons running up and down the spinal cord (Fig. 8.9).

Spinal tracts

Nerves going to, or coming from, the same place, or that are carrying out similar functions (e.g., skeletal muscle control) are bundled together into **tracts**. For example, the spinothalamic tracts contain nerves transmitting ascending sensory information on pain, temperature, pressure, and touch

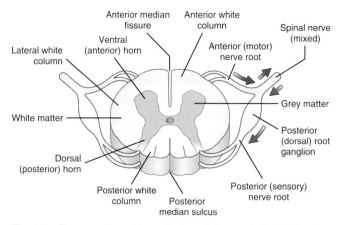

Fig. 8.9 Cross-section of the spinal cord. Arrows indicate direction of nerve impulse traffic. (Modified from Waugh A, Grant A (2018) *Ross & Wilson anatomy and physiology in health and illness* 13th ed, Fig. 7.28. Oxford, Elsevier Ltd.)

from the body to the thalamus from where the information is passed to relevant brain areas. Damage to the spinothalamic tract therefore interferes with the individual's ability to perceive these sensations.

Motor control: the pyramidal tract

The motor cortex controls voluntary movement. The corticospinal tract and the corticobulbar tract, collectively called the **pyramidal tract** because they pass through the pyramids of the medulla, transmit instructions from the motor cortex to the brainstem and down the spinal cord to skeletal muscles, maintaining tone, posture and permitting voluntary movement. Damage to the nerves in the pyramidal tract causes loss of motor control and paralysis. Motor pathways of the pyramidal tract contain two nerves: **the upper motor neurone** (UMN) and the **lower motor neurone** (LMN). The UMN has its cell body in the primary motor cortex in the frontal lobe of the brain, and its axon travels through the internal capsule, the midbrain, and the medulla, and down the spinal cord to the level of the muscle that it innervates. Here it synapses with the second motor nerve in the chain, the LMN, which exits from the anterior root of the spinal cord and runs to the skeletal muscle that it innervates (Fig. 8.10). Damage to either the UMN or LMN interferes with skeletal muscle control.

Motor control: extrapyramidal tracts

Although the pyramidal tract is the main mechanism of voluntary muscle control, other pathways exert significant influence over its activity. These are called **extrapyramidal pathways**, and their nerves link the basal ganglia and cerebellum to the motor cortex. The basal ganglia and cerebellum are not under voluntary control, but their constant input into the motor cortex is essential for smooth, co-ordinated voluntary muscle action, and they allow the motor cortex to constantly adjust its instructions to muscles to suit changes in body posture or mechanical requirements. The cerebellum constantly feeds information into the brain regarding the position of the body in space, essential for maintaining balance and posture during activity. The basal ganglia, collections of nerve bodies deep in the brain, are essential for smooth, practiced voluntary movement.

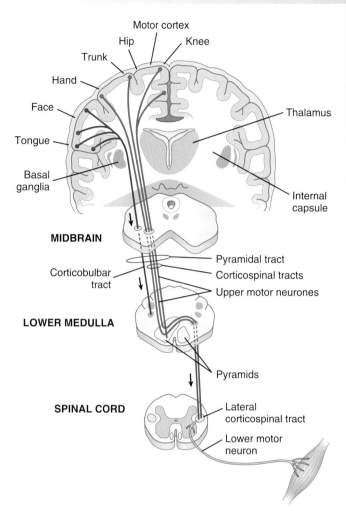

Fig. 8.10 Motor pathways. The upper motor neurone of the pyramidal pathway originates in the motor cortex, travels down the spinal cord, and synapses with the lower motor neurone.

THE PERIPHERAL NERVOUS SYSTEM

Nerves outside the brain and spinal cord are considered part of the peripheral nervous system.

THE CRANIAL NERVES

The 12 cranial nerves arise from the base of the brain and are numbered (using Roman numerals) I through XII. Their names and functions are summarised in Table 8.1.

THE SPINAL NERVES

The 31 pairs of spinal nerves exit the spinal cord from the intervertebral foramina formed between the interlocking vertebrae of the spine (Fig. 8.8B). Each spinal nerve passes from the spinal column as two roots. The **anterior root** emerges from the spinal cord at the front and the **posterior root** emerges from the spinal cord at the back. The anterior root carries descending fibres transmitting motor signals from the brain to the skeletal muscles; the posterior root carries ascending fibres, transmitting sensory information from the body to the brain. The two roots merge into the spinal nerve itself, and because the spinal nerves carry both sensory and motor fibres, they are called **mixed nerves** (Fig. 8.9).

Table 8.1   The cranial nerves

Number	Name	Motor function	Sensory function
I	Olfactory	None	Sense of smell
II	Optic	None	Vision
III	Oculomotor	Controls eyeball movement, the iris muscle and the muscles of the eyelid	None
IV	Trochlear	Controls eyeball movement	None
V	Trigeminal	Controls the muscles of chewing	Sensation from face; taste
VI	Abducent	Controls eyeball movement	None
VII	Facial	Controls muscles of facial expression	Sense of taste
VIII	Auditory	None	Senses of balance, posture and hearing
IX	Glossopharyngeal	Controls muscles of pharynx and the tongue, and salivary secretion	Sensation from tongue and throat
X	Vagus	Motor control of multiple body organs including respiratory, renal and gastrointestinal tract, blood vessels, spleen	Sensation from multiple body organs including respiratory, renal and gastrointestinal systems, blood vessels, spleen
XI	Accessory	Controls muscles of neck and shoulder	None
XII	Hypoglossal	Controls the tongue	None

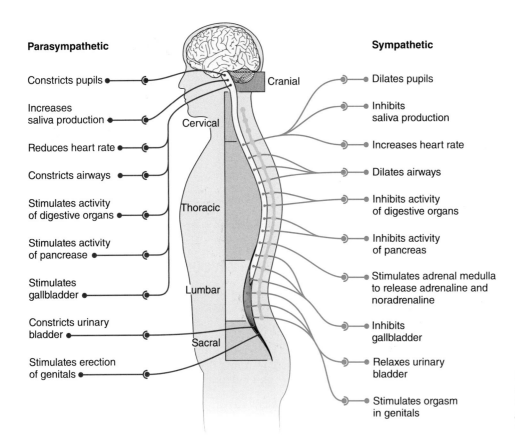

Fig. 8.11 The autonomic nervous system. (From Hines RL and Jones SB (2022) *Stoelting's anesthesia and co-existing disease*, 8th ed, Fig. 15.71. Philadelphia: Elsevier Inc.)

THE AUTONOMIC NERVOUS SYSTEM

The autonomic nervous system (ANS) manages body functions not under conscious control. Its fibres travel in and out of the brain within spinal nerves and in some of the cranial nerves. Conventionally, the ANS is divided into two branches, the **sympathetic** and the **parasympathetic** branches, whose nerves flow from different areas of the vertebral column, as shown in Fig. 8.11. Between them, the sympathetic and parasympathetic nervous systems generate the homeostatic balance required for moment-to-moment physiological control of body functions, adjusting according to the situation. Sympathetic activity predominates at times of activity or stress and is associated with fight or flight responses. Parasympathetic activity predominates when at rest. So, for example, during a period of exercise, sympathetic activity increases heart rate and cardiac contractility, respiratory rate, and depth, generates hyperglycaemia and increases blood flow to the myocardium and skeletal muscle, whereas at rest the parasympathetic nervous system reverses these changes and promotes gastrointestinal blood flow and the production of digestive enzymes.

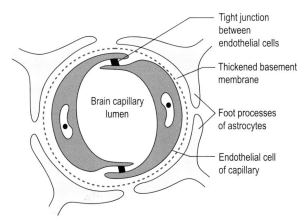

Fig. 8.12 The blood-brain barrier. (Modified from Singh V (2020) *Textbook of clinical neuroanatomy,* 4th ed, Fig. 15.23. New Delhi: RELX India Pvt Ltd.)

THE SOMATIC (VOLUNTARY) NERVOUS SYSTEM

The voluntary nervous system innervates skeletal muscle, producing movement of the whole body or part of the body. Information from the eyes, ears, skin, and other sensory receptors is also relayed into the voluntary nervous system so that the motor centres of the brain have all the information needed to maintain posture and balance and initiate appropriate voluntary responses. This includes protective reflex actions, which do not actually involve the brain because the incoming sensory information arriving at the dorsal horn of the spinal cord along sensory nerves is transmitted directly to motor nerves exiting the anterior horn of the spinal cord to activate appropriate skeletal muscles. For example, placing the hand accidentally on a hot surface leads to rapid reflex withdrawal, with the brain only being informed of the event a fraction of a second later.

The neuromuscular junction

The synapse between a motor nerve and a skeletal muscle cell is called the **neuromuscular junction**, and the neurotransmitter is acetylcholine. Disorders and drugs blocking neuromuscular transmission paralyse skeletal muscle, including the diaphragm (e.g., myasthenia gravis; p. 328).

CENTRAL NERVOUS SYSTEM PATHOPHYSIOLOGY

The CNS is well protected within the bones of the skull and the vertebral column but is subject to a wide range of disorders. Additional specialist defence mechanisms isolate it from the rest of the body and provide additional protection.

The blood-brain barrier (BBB)

This is a specialised interface between the blood passing through blood vessels in the brain, and the brain tissue on the other side of the blood vessel wall. It is designed to control the brain's internal environment as tightly as possible: it limits the movement of substances between the blood and the brain; it protects the organ from blood borne toxins, infections, and other unwanted substances; and it shields it from fluctuations in the composition of blood plasma. The anatomy of the BBB is shown in Fig. 8.12. The capillary

endothelial cells form tight junctions with adjacent cells, greatly reducing the permeability of the capillary wall, and they sit on a thicker basement membrane than non-brain capillaries. In addition, foot processes extended from astrocytes wrap around the capillary, providing an additional barrier.

Immunological defence in the CNS

The microglia of the brain are its only resident immune cells and are responsible for protecting it from infection. In health, the blood-brain barrier excludes peripheral immune cells and immune and inflammatory proteins such as complement and antibodies from entering the brain, shielding its delicate tissues from the aggressive and potentially damaging effects of immune and inflammatory activation. The systemic defence response, involving activation of multiple inflammatory and immune cell types and the release of a wide range of inflammatory mediators, can cause significant tissue injury, which in most tissues would usually be repaired as part of the healing process. Because neurones are generally not capable of division and renewal, such healing does not occur, and injury leads instead to cell death and scarring. In addition, the astroglia maintain an anti-inflammatory environment through release of anti-inflammatory and immunosuppressant cytokines, suppressing the initiation and progression of inflammation. In brain injury or infection, the blood-brain barrier admits large numbers of peripheral immune cells for protection and repair, but this process is carefully regulated so that there is not excessive inflammation or damage. The disadvantage to this immunological dampening is that infection of the CNS may not be adequately dealt with.

CNS INFECTIONS

Microbial invasion of the CNS is relatively common, usually bacterial or viral, but sometimes fungal or amoeboid infections are found. Infective meningitis involves the membranes covering the brain, infective encephalitis refers to infection of the brain tissue itself and infective myelitis is infection of the spinal cord. Some infections are secondary to primary infections elsewhere, with CNS involvement only part of the clinical picture (e.g., neurosyphilis and tuberculosis).

MENINGITIS

Most accurately, meningitis means inflammation of the meninges, not infection, but although sterile meningitis can occur, the term has come to imply infection. The arachnoid and pia maters are involved, and once the infection has accessed the subarachnoid space, it is quickly carried in the CSF throughout the brain and down the spinal cord. Meningitis may be fatal unless treated, although viral meningitis is significantly less dangerous than other forms. Box 8.2 lists some important organisms associated with infective meningitis. The infection usually spreads to the CNS from elsewhere in the body (e.g., respiratory, genitourinary, or gastrointestinal infections), and the organisms usually arrive in the bloodstream. Sometimes infection occurs because of cranial fracture or contamination caused by an invasive procedure or neurosurgery.

There is significant variation between countries regarding the main infecting organism because different organisms

BOX 8.2 Causative organisms in meningitis

Bacteria	*Neisseria meningitidis* (meningococcus)
	Streptococci
	Haemophilus influenzae
	Escherichia coli
Viruses	Enteroviruses
	Influenza virus
	Herpes viruses: varicella zoster (chickenpox), herpes simplex, Epstein-Barr virus
	Human immunodeficiency virus
	Mumps
Fungi	Cryptococcus
	Candida
Parasites	Amoeba
	Cysticerci

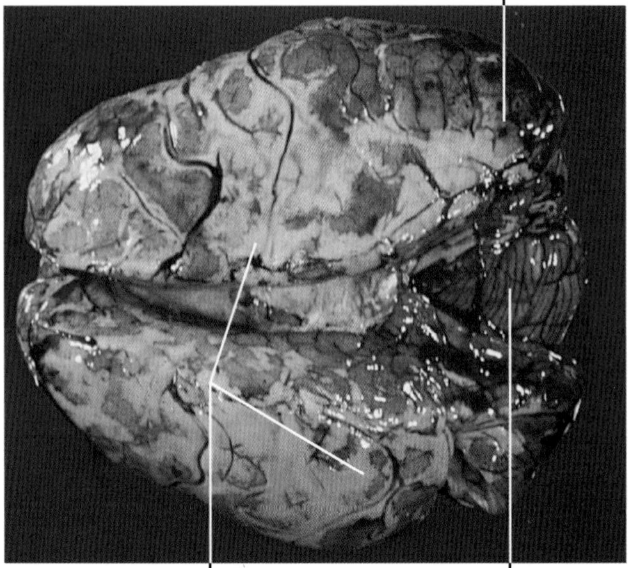

Fig. 8.13 Bacterial meningitis. (Modified from Elsevier Inc. (2021) *ICD-10-CM/PCS coding: theory and practice,* 2021/2022 ed, Fig. 10.3. St Louis: Saunders.)

are endemic in different areas of the world. As with many infections, overall rates are higher in developing countries with less comprehensive healthcare systems and poor living conditions. Where vaccination programmes are available, they have reduced the incidence of specific forms of meningitis.

Risk factors include immunocompromise (e.g., corticosteroid treatment or immunodeficiency), poor general health, crowded or cramped living conditions, chronic illness such as diabetes, alcohol dependency, malnutrition, splenectomy and liver and renal impairment. The very young and the very old are also at increased risk compared with the general population.

Non-infective meningitis is sometimes seen in autoimmune disorders, such as systemic lupus erythematosus, in which brain tissues are attacked by the autoimmune processes, or because of meningeal irritation caused by tumour invasion.

Pathophysiology

Viral meningitis is usually self-limiting, and although it causes severe headache, malaise, and fever, the condition almost always resolves within a few days without specific treatment. However, there is evidence that some viral infections may increase the risk of subsequent bacterial meningitis, probably by damaging the blood-brain barrier. Bacterial meningitis is very different to the viral form and untreated cases carry an 80% mortality. If the infection is contained within the subarachnoid space, the prognosis is better, but if organisms cross the pia mater and invade the brain tissue itself, the consequences are significantly worse. As the bacteria proliferate, they trigger an immune and inflammatory response in the brain that causes swelling, which obstructs CSF circulation, and can increase intracranial pressure. In addition, the swelling can compromise blood flow and areas of the brain may become hypoxic and ischaemic. Sluggish blood flow and rising levels of inflammatory mediators trigger clotting, forming microthrombi that further interfere with perfusion. Increased pressure and inflammatory exudate compress brain tissue and cranial nerves, causing nerve injury that may be permanent even after recovery: for example, hearing loss follows damage to cranial nerve VIII (auditory nerve). Pus formation

(Fig. 8.13) causes obstruction and adhesions, worsening the damage. Inflammatory cells, including neutrophils (which are normally completely excluded from the brain) infiltrate the brain and release damaging free radicals and other cytotoxic agents that cause further injury. Because the CNS is relatively isolated from peripheral immune defences, its ability to clear infection is compromised, contributing to the overwhelming speed with which invading bacteria can colonise here.

Fungal meningitis usually affects immunocompromised people and is usually caused by *Cryptococcus.*

Signs and symptoms

The classic triad of bacterial meningitis is headache, fever, and neck stiffness. There may also be drowsiness, photophobia, nausea, vomiting, and rash (Fig. 8.14). It usually presents acutely and evolves rapidly, with the possible development of sepsis and neurological abnormalities, including seizures.

Prognosis and management

Rapid intervention is important. Identifying the causative organism is essential for appropriate antimicrobial treatment. Aggressive management of sepsis and any indication of rising intracranial pressure, and supporting renal function are also important. Prognosis is poorer in older people, those with risk factors as outlined previously, and in patients who present with indications of sepsis and/or a low Glasgow Coma Scale score. Even if the patient recovers, there can be permanent residual damage including cranial nerve damage (e.g., hearing or vision loss), the onset of seizures, ataxia and other motor issues, or paralysis.

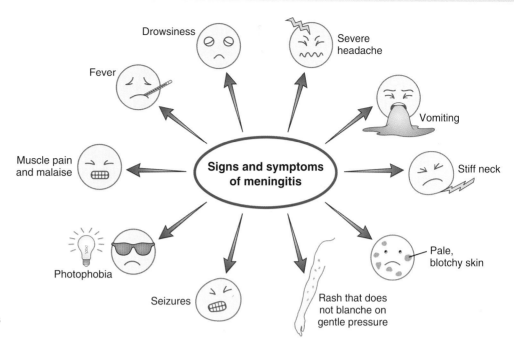

Fig. 8.14 Signs and symptoms of meningitis.

ENCEPHALITIS

This is infection of the brain itself, usually of viral origin. The commonest culprits are herpes simplex and mosquito-borne viruses. It is likely that many mild cases are asymptomatic and so are not counted in epidemiological statistics. The commonest forms of mosquito-borne encephalitis include St. Louis encephalitis (found across the United States) and Japanese virus encephalitis, endemic to Japan, southeast Asia, China, and India. Measles virus may cause encephalitis. Incidence tends to be highest in the very young and the very old.

Pathophysiology

Generally, the virus enters the CNS via the bloodstream from a primary site of infection elsewhere. In the case of mosquito-borne disease, the virus enters the bloodstream as the result of a bite. Humans are a dead-end host for the virus and are not part of the normal viral life cycle, which is lived between mosquitos and another host, often birds or small mammals. Herpes simplex exists in two forms, HSV1 and HSV2, and both can cause herpes encephalitis. The virus is ubiquitous, and most people carry one or both forms. It is easily transmitted from person to person by close personal contact including sexual activity and mother to child at birth. The virus invades and establishes itself in the nervous system and causes encephalitis when it travels into the brain along nerve tracts. Once in the brain, the virus invades neurones and triggers an inflammatory response, which affects the cell bodies to a much greater degree than white matter (the nerve axons). There may be bleeding, oedema and necrosis of brain tissue, and the swelling can increase intracranial pressure. Signs and symptoms depend on which areas of the brain are infected and the extent of injury. The meninges are often involved too.

Signs and symptoms

The condition may follow a benign and self-limiting course or it may be fatal, and the clinical presentation can be very variable. The viral infection itself as it develops in the body before invading the brain causes typical viral signs and symptoms: fever, headache, malaise, perhaps nausea and vomiting, lethargy, and myalgia. Specific viruses are also associated with specific symptoms (e.g., measles, rash). Indications of encephalitis include photophobia, neck pain and stiffness, seizures, paralysis, confusion, and altered consciousness. Intracranial pressure may rise because of brain inflammation and swelling.

Management and prognosis

The very old and the very young and those with pre-existing neurological conditions or immunocompromise have a poorer prognosis. Depending on the virus involved, untreated encephalitis can carry a significant mortality, and the incidence of permanent deficits after recovery is even higher, but the picture is very variable and the disease can be mild and self-limiting. The mainstay of treatment is anti-viral therapy.

RABIES

This viral infection, caused by a rhabdovirus, is carried in the salivary glands of a variety of mammals including canines, felines, bats, and raccoons. A bite from an infected animal is the usual route of transmission to humans, but there are documented cases of person-to-person infection via contaminated blood or tissues. It has a global distribution but has been eliminated from many countries and large areas of others by animal vaccination. However, the virus is adaptable and develops new strains to ensure its survival in new hosts and in changing climatic conditions. The story of rabies and the insight of Louis Pasteur, a French chemist working on early vaccines in the late 19th century, are inseparably linked. In

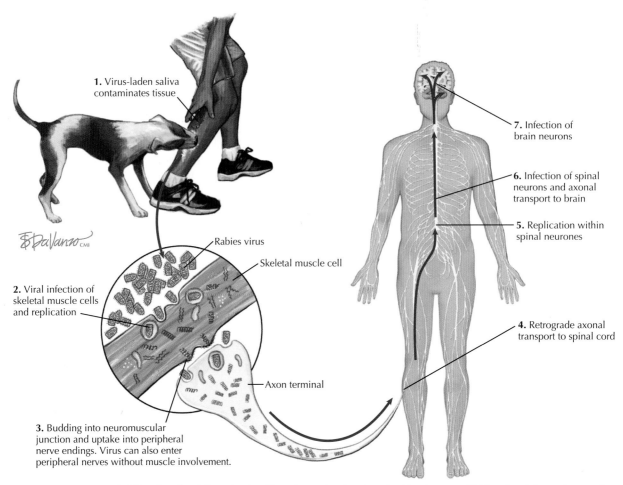

1. Virus-laden saliva contaminates tissue

7. Infection of brain neurons

6. Infection of spinal neurons and axonal transport to brain

5. Replication within spinal neurones

Rabies virus

Skeletal muscle cell

2. Viral infection of skeletal muscle cells and replication

4. Retrograde axonal transport to spinal cord

Axon terminal

3. Budding into neuromuscular junction and uptake into peripheral nerve endings. Virus can also enter peripheral nerves without muscle involvement.

Fig. 8.15   Rabies infection. (1) The bite of an infected animal introduces the virus into the bloodstream. (2) The virus infects damaged muscle. (3) The virus infects local nerves. (4) Viral particles travel along nerve axons towards the spinal cord. (5) The virus establishes itself in the spinal cord. (6) The virus travels up the spinal cord to the brain. (7) The virus establishes itself and proliferates in the brain. (Courtesy of Center for Disease Control and Prevention.)

1885 a 9-year-old boy called Joseph Meister was brought to doctors at the University of Paris because he had been badly bitten by a rabid dog. Over the course of a week, Pasteur gave Joseph a series of injections containing dried spinal cord from rabbits that had died of rabies. The treatment worked: Joseph did not develop rabies.

Pathophysiology
After infection, the virus replicates at the site (e.g., muscle tissue deep to a bite). It then invades local nerves by binding to acetylcholine receptors at the neuromuscular junction (p. 323). The nerve internalises the receptor for recycling, bringing the virus with it (Fig. 8.15). Once in the nerve, the virus is now protected from immune attack and spreads back up the axon towards the spinal cord. Unusually, the infection triggers little inflammatory response in the host, so there are no symptoms at this stage and motor function is unaffected. Once the virus reaches the CNS, however, the consequences are devastating.

Signs and symptoms
The incubation period between exposure and the appearance of symptoms is usually between 1 and 3 months, but it can be significantly shorter or longer. Once the virus invades the CNS, non-specific signs and symptoms such as

malaise, fever, headache, and anorexia are reported. Within a few days, neurological dysfunction appears, with seizures, muscle twitching, and progressive paralysis. Some patients become very agitated, hyperactive, and violent, with hallucinations and profound disorientation ('furious' rabies), whereas others remain quiet, calm, and apathetic ('dumb' rabies). The final outcome, however, does not vary: the patient slips into coma, and death is usually secondary to respiratory arrest.

Management and prognosis
The wound must be carefully and thoroughly cleaned. If rabies infection is likely, and the individual has not been immunised against rabies, treatment involves infiltration of ant-irabies antibodies around the wound site, and anti-rabies vaccine. The vaccine (it was an early version of this that Pasteur gave to Joseph Meister) stimulates an active immune response to the infection which should clear the infecting virus before it has time to infect the nervous system, but it takes around 2 weeks before this gives an adequate antibody response, and the anti-rabies antibodies produce short-term cover in the meantime. Provided this is done before the virus reaches the shelter of the nervous system, it is almost always effective in preventing the disease. Once the virus invades the CNS, the chances of survival are negligible.

POLIOMYELITIS (POLIO)

This viral condition, which affects children far more severely than adults, is caused by poliovirus, a subgroup within the enterovirus genus. It is a crippling condition that sometimes kills and can cause permanent and severe disability in surviving children. Globally, vaccination programmes have eradicated polio from the developed world, cutting cases by 99% between 1988 and 2019. The World Health Organisation's (WHO's) Global Polio Eradication Initiative reported in 2019 that it had eliminated two of the three types of poliovirus across the world. As of 2022, only wild poliovirus type 1 remains endemic, and in only two countries: Pakistan and Afghanistan.

Pathophysiology

Infection usually occurs by the faeco-oral route and the virus incubates in the mucosal lining of the oropharynx and lower gastrointestinal tract over a period of 1 to 3 weeks. The virus enters the nervous system either by crossing the blood-brain barrier from circulating blood, or by entering peripheral nerves and travelling up the axon towards the CNS. It establishes itself in the anterior motor horn of the spinal cord and can progressively destroy the lower motor neurones responsible for supplying skeletal muscles. As a result of their loss of innervation, affected muscles become paralysed and atrophied. After resolution of the infection, surviving nerves and their associated muscles may recover either completely or partially, with complete or partial regain of function.

Signs and symptoms

Polio infection is usually a mild febrile illness, and fewer than 1 in 20 infected children develop neurological symptoms. However, in these children, the disease can cause catastrophic paralysis, including of the respiratory musculature, which can kill. Initially, the affected muscles go into painful, extended spasms that give way to complete loss of tone and paralysis. There may also be sensory abnormalities (paraesthesias). Muscles may recover over a period of months, or the paralysis may be permanent. If the medulla, pons, and cerebellum are affected (so-called *bulbar involvement*), then key life support functions such as respiration are compromised, and speech, swallowing, and cardiovascular control are impaired.

Management and prognosis

Management is supportive, with bed rest and respiratory/cardiovascular support as required. Physiotherapy is an essential part of recovery to maximise regain of function. One in 200 children is left with irreversible paralysis, and up to 10% of these children die because of respiratory paralysis.

INFLAMMATORY AND IMMUNE MEDIATED CNS DISORDERS

As described previously, the CNS is an immunologically protected environment, with limited capacity to mount inflammatory and immunological responses. Inflammation of the brain, its meninges, or the spinal cord is usually, but not always, caused by infection. Non-infective neurological conditions that cause inflammation include multiple sclerosis.

Sometimes the CNS is involved as a consequence of a systemic inflammatory or immune disorder: for example, 40% of systemic lupus erythematosus sufferers experience CNS symptoms.

MULTIPLE SCLEROSIS

Multiple sclerosis (MS) is found globally and occurs in all racial groups, but its geographical distribution varies significantly with latitude. In general, the disease occurs more frequently in countries further from the equator, with the incidence highest in North America and Europe. Some population groups show lower than average rates (e.g., people of Japanese and Chinese extraction, the Inuit, New Zealand Maoris) and some show higher than average rates (e.g., Sardinian and Palestinian people), indicating a genetic component in addition to geographical factors. MS is an autoimmune disorder, so in common with autoimmunity in general, there is a higher female:male ratio. It is usually diagnosed in younger adults (20–40 years), although up to 5% of diagnoses are made in childhood.

MS is not an inherited disease, although there is a heritable component: having a parent or sibling with the disease does slightly increase the risk of developing the disorder. Several genes have been linked to MS, including genes that code for the stimulation and proliferation of immune cells, and genes belonging to the HLA complex (p. 91), which underpin the ability of immune cells to differentiate between 'self' proteins that belong to the body and foreign proteins that do not (e.g., bacterial or viral proteins). If genes in these key areas of body defence are abnormal, it can lead to failure of self-tolerance and contribute to autoimmune processes. It is generally believed that the disease arises in genetically susceptible people after exposure to a specific trigger: a viral infection (e.g., with Epstein-Barr virus), or vitamin D deficiency (associated with low sunlight exposure).

Pathophysiology

In MS, the myelin sheath of nerves in the brain and spinal cord is destroyed, usually in a series of inflammatory episodes interspersed with periods in which the disease is quiescent (remission), allowing some repair and healing. With repeated episodes, however, the neural tissue becomes permanently scarred and damaged, leading to significant and progressive neurological deficits and disability. Affected areas, called **plaques** (Fig. 8.16), usually develop close to a blood vessel and become infiltrated with inflammatory cells, including T cells and macrophages, which release a range of cytokines and mediators, including interleukins and tumour necrosis factor. This initiates a destructive and progressive inflammatory cycle that degrades myelin and destroys oligodendrocytes, exposing nerve axons to the local environment rich in inflammatory mediators and cytokines released by the inflammatory cells. This interrupts nerve conduction in the affected axons and with time destroys the axons themselves.

The immune cells thought to be central to myelin destruction are autoreactive T cells that target myelin. They are activated in peripheral tissues, perhaps by a precipitating infection, and cross the blood-brain barrier into the CNS, where they initiate myelin injury. B cells are also involved, and individuals with MS have elevated levels of antibodies in active

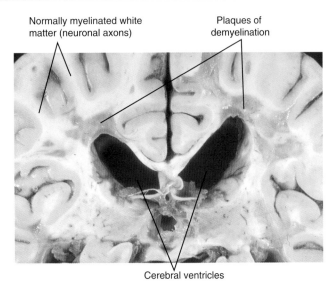

Normally myelinated white matter (neuronal axons)

Plaques of demyelination

Cerebral ventricles

Fig. 8.16 Frontal section through a brain affected with multiple sclerosis. Multiple areas of demyelination ("plaques") are visible. (From Klatt E (2015) *Robbins and Cotran atlas of pathology*, 3rd ed, Fig. 19-109. St. Louis: Elsevier Inc.)

plaques, in the CSF, and circulating in the bloodstream. In addition, B cells are believed to be important activators of the autoimmune T-cell response. Although MS has traditionally been considered an autoimmune disorder, the specific protein that acts as the autoantigen has not yet been identified.

Signs and symptoms

These depend on the location of the plaques, and so presentation can be variable. Involvement of the optic nerve is very common: about 40% of MS patients experience optic neuritis at some stage of their disease, and it is the presenting symptom in one in five patients. Visual signs and symptoms indicating optic neuritis include blurred vision, changed perception of colours, and reduced visual fields including loss of central vision. A wide range of motor and sensory symptoms of the trunk and limbs, including paraesthesia and spasticity may occur, leading to progressive loss of motor control and mobility. Depression, fatigue, pain, trigeminal neuralgia, and facial twitching may be seen. Intellectual impairment, including memory loss and concentration difficulties, occurs. Cerebellar involvement causes ataxia and weakness, with an inability to perform fine co-ordinated voluntary muscle movement. If nerves of the autonomic nervous system are affected, there may be issues with bladder and bowel control and loss of sexual function.

Management and prognosis

Most people (up to 90%) follow a **relapsing/remitting pattern** of disease, with episodes becoming closer together and more severe with time and recovery between attacks less and less complete. Disability therefore becomes steadily worse, and eventually the remissions disappear altogether, and the disease becomes progressive. A small number of patients experience a single attack and have no further symptomatic episodes, even though patches of demyelination are demonstrable on scans. Occasionally, the disease follows a rapid, malignant, and aggressive course, leading to an early death (**fulminant** MS). Some patients experience a progressive course from diagnosis, with no remissions; their prognosis is worse than relapsing/remitting patients. Life expectancy in MS is slightly less than normal, although the quality of life, especially in advanced disease, can be significantly reduced because of disability. There is currently no cure for MS. Until the early 1990s, treatment centred around symptom management and control of acute attacks, and although these remain keystones of care today, in 1993 the introduction of interferon-β opened the era of disease-modifying treatment. Anti-inflammatory steroids are given in exacerbations to subdue the acute response, and this shortens the acute episode and reduces the degree of damage done by the inflammatory flare. Muscle spasticity is managed with physiotherapy and drugs such as dantrolene, and dysaesthesias (abnormal sensations) are treated with drugs such as gabapentin and carbamazepine. Newer immunotherapies, including interferons and cytokine inhibitors and drugs that inhibit T- and B-cell activity, have shown considerable promise in slowing disease progression and this area of medicine is actively developing.

NEURODEGENERATIVE DISORDERS

Neurodegenerative disorders are generally more common in older people. The signs and symptoms depend on the area of the brain affected; for example, in Parkinson disease, nerves between the basal ganglia and the substantia nigra degenerate, progressively destroying the capacity for voluntary muscle control.

Dementia

Dementia describes a set of symptoms including progressive impairment of intellectual function and loss of memory, often with personality changes, and is associated with a number of neurological disorders including multiple sclerosis, Huntington disease, Parkinson disease, alcohol dependence, repeated trauma, diabetes, infections and cerebrovascular disease, which impairs blood flow to the brain. The incidence of dementia increases with age: the number of people worldwide living with dementia more than doubled between 1990 and 2016, mainly caused by ageing populations.

ALZHEIMER DISEASE

Alzheimer disease (AD) is the most common cause of dementia. It is named after Alois Alzheimer, a German psychiatrist who, in 1906, presented a detailed case report of a 50-year-old woman who had died after a 5-year period of progressive memory loss, behavioural changes, and confusion. The disease is more common in older age groups: in 2016, an estimated 10% of Americans over the age of 65 were reported to be suffering from the disease, with up to one third of over 85s given an AD diagnosis. Globally, the disease is becoming more common, probably because of increasing lifespans, and rates are increasing fastest in developing countries because this is where average lifespans are currently increasing most significantly. However, there is evidence that in high-income countries, the incidence is stabilising, likely because increasing numbers of people are becoming health-conscious, eating healthily, stopping smoking, remaining active into their retirement years and managing chronic conditions like hypertension and diabetes better.

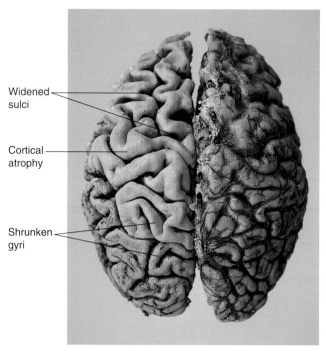

Widened sulci

Cortical atrophy

Shrunken gyri

Fig. 8.17   The superior surface of the brain of an individual with Alzheimer's disease. Widened sulci, cortical atrophy and shrunken gyri are seen. (Modified from Prayson RA (2012) *Neuropathology*, 2nd ed, Fig. 6.1. Philadelphia: Elsevier Inc.)

Factors that increase the risk of cardiovascular disease (e.g., smoking, physical inactivity, diabetes, high blood cholesterol, and hypertension) also increase the risk of dementia in general, including AD. Genetics play a part; having a first-degree relative with AD doubles an individual's risk, but the actual chance of developing the disease is also influenced by other factors, including lifestyle, low educational attainment and environmental influences. A rare familial form of AD exists, accounting for only about 1% of cases, caused by one or more specific gene mutations. Children of people with one of these mutations have a 50:50 chance of inheriting the faulty gene, in which case they will certainly develop AD, often at a young age.

Pathophysiology

The affected brain shows clear atrophy of the cerebral cortex and neuronal loss (Fig. 8.17). Insoluble plaques of **beta-amyloid protein** develop in the cortex, affecting intellectual functions, and in the hippocampus, which participates in memory formation. These plaques are also seen in the brains of healthy older people and are not always found in postmortem examination of brain tissue from confirmed AD patients, so they are not in themselves diagnostic for AD. The function of beta-amyloid in health is not known, although it may help neurones attach to one another. The plaques cause local neuronal damage and trigger an inflammatory response, causing local destruction of brain tissue. Beta-amyloid protein is produced from a larger precursor, amyloid precursor protein (APP). One of the genes that mutate in the rare, familial form of AD, *APP*, codes for APP, and the mutated gene produces abnormally high levels of

amyloid protein. *APP* is carried on chromosome 21; people with Down syndrome have three copies of this gene, which explains their high risk of dementia.

Another protein believed to participate in the pathology of AD is **tau protein**, a thread-like protein found inside neurones and which holds the intracellular network of microtubules together. The microtubules direct and guide movement of substances inside nerve axons. In AD, the tau threads become tangled, the microtubule system falls apart, and the ability of the neurone to regulate its internal traffic and to communicate with other neurones is lost. The knots of tau protein are visible in the neurones as **neurofibrillary tangles**, another finding in AD. However, as with amyloid plaques, these tangles are found in healthy ageing brains and in other neurodegenerative diseases, so are not diagnostic for AD. It may be that the development of AD relates to the extent of plaque and tangle formation: the more plaques and tangles, the greater the risk of symptomatic brain damage

Other pathological processes have been suggested to contribute to AD aetiology; for example, levels of damaging free radicals in the brain are higher in AD than in age-matched controls, so inflammation may contribute to the pathology. Oestrogen may be protective because pre-menopausal women are at lower risk than age-matched men for AD.

Signs and symptoms

Physical changes in the brain as described previously precede the onset of signs and symptoms, sometimes by decades. The initial indication is usually loss of short-term memory, although failure of longer-term memory normally occurs early in the disease as well. There may be behavioural changes and difficulty with language because the person loses the ability to locate specific words for something they want to talk about. They lose visuospatial skills, depth perception, and the ability to keep track of moving objects, making driving hazardous and leading to clumsiness and increased risk of falls. The ability to make judgements and decisions fails, and concentration becomes poor.

Management and prognosis

There is no cure. Treatment is supportive and has no effect on the progression of the disease. There is a great deal of research ongoing, including in the areas of reducing amyloid production or reducing amyloid levels, or stabilising tau protein.

VASCULAR DEMENTIA

This form of dementia is caused by damage and obstruction to blood vessels supplying the brain and is the second commonest cause of dementia. Vascular dementia is associated with Alzheimer disease; the risk of developing the latter is increased in people with known vascular dementia.

Pathophysiology

Degeneration of nervous tissue is secondary to an inadequate blood supply. The vascular changes can be widespread, affecting multiple brain areas (diffuse vascular dementia), but sometimes focal, if only certain blood vessels are affected, leading to a more restricted pattern of signs and symptoms reflecting the specific brain areas involved. Multi-infarct dementia is caused by obstruction of blood supply in the tiny blood vessels in the brain. Blood vessels can be obstructed by microthrombi, atherosclerotic changes in their walls, or sometimes inflammatory/immune vasculitis, as in systemic lupus erythematosus.

FRONTOTEMPORAL DEMENTIA

This term includes a number of disorders in which the frontal and temporal lobes of the brain atrophy. Frontal lobe involvement presents primarily with personality changes, disinhibition, apathy, and emotional blunting. Temporal lobe involvement is characterised mainly by speech problems because this is the location of the sensory speech area of the cortex. Unlike AD, memory loss is not an early event in the disorder.

Pathophysiology

Tau protein is seen inside the affected neurones, sometimes in tangles like AD, but sometimes as smooth, rounded pebble-like structures called *Pick bodies*. Abnormal collections of other proteins, most notably one called *TDP-43*, may also be present. It is not known why these proteins aggregate and accumulate inside nerves, but they severely disrupt neuronal function.

MOTOR NEURONE DISEASE (MND)

These disorders cause progressive and catastrophic degeneration of upper motor neurones (UMN) and/or lower motor neurones (LMN) and other nerves involved in voluntary muscle control. There are four main conditions, and the initial clinical presentation varies depending on which group of motor nerves is affected, but as the disease progresses the distinction between them blurs (Fig. 8.18).

Amyotrophic lateral sclerosis (ALS)

This is the commonest form of MND. Risk increases with age and in smokers. It is found in all races and countries; it is slightly commoner in white people than black people and in men than women. U.S. and European statistics show an incidence of 2 to 3 per 100,000 people; 5% to 10% of cases have a family history (familial ALS), and their disease manifests earlier than in people with no family history (sporadic ALS).

Pathophysiology

Both upper and lower motor neurones of motor pathways are destroyed, leading to progressive atrophy and paralysis of skeletal muscle. Initially, one limb tends to be affected, but with time the disease spreads relentlessly to involve all limbs. There is a strong association with other disorders of the cerebral cortex, especially frontotemporal dementia. The cause of ALS is not known, but a range of genetic abnormalities have been found in affected nerves in both familial and sporadic ALS. One gene frequently mutated in ALS is *SOD1*, which produces the enzyme **superoxide dismutase**. This enzyme is responsible for clearing toxic and inflammatory free radicals from the cellular environment, so if it is not functioning correctly, neuronal damage may result. Additionally, the faulty superoxide dismutase produced by the gene is incorrectly folded and can precipitate out in large aggregates inside the neurone, triggering apoptosis, which may be one of the factors in the progressive neuronal death seen in this disease. Although specific genetic mutations have been identified in many of the familial forms, it is likely that sporadic ALS is caused by a combination of environmental and genetic factors.

Signs and symptoms

The disorder generally begins with weakness in one part of the body, usually a limb. There are no sensory signs and symptoms because sensory nerves are unaffected. There may be foot drop, or problems picking up and holding items. Gait may become clumsy and stumbling, and fine movements are difficult. There may be rigidity, spasticity, and painful cramping of skeletal muscles, and as muscle denervation proceeds, the muscles atrophy and become weaker and weaker. Muscle spasm, combined with immobility, can lead to painful contractures.

Management and prognosis

ALS is incurable and the outcome is inevitable. Death is usually caused by respiratory failure. Younger people live longer after onset of symptoms than older people, and male sex is associated with longer survival. However, about 50%

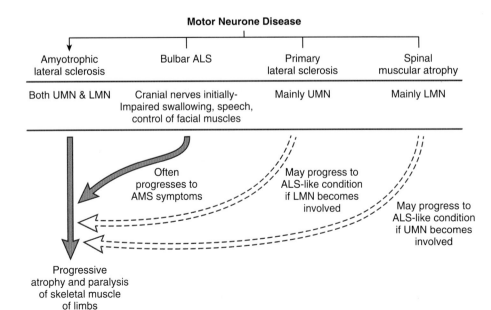

Fig. 8.18 The classification of motor neurone disease.

of people die within 3 years. The only drug known to extend life is riluxole, a glutamate antagonist, although its exact mechanism of action in this disease is unknown. Other treatments offered are symptomatic and include muscle relaxants, physiotherapy and serotonin selective reuptake inhibitors (SSRIs) for depression.

Progressive bulbar palsy (bulbar ALS)

In this disorder, the motor nerves in the medulla oblongata degenerate. This affects the glossopharyngeal (cranial nerve IV), the vagal (cranial nerve X), and the hypoglossal (cranial nerve XII) nerves. Speech and swallowing problems appear early. This form carries a worse prognosis than ALS itself. As the disease progresses, limb involvement develops, and the clinical picture follows that of ALS.

Primary lateral sclerosis

This is the least common form and primarily affects the UMN. It may be that it represents an early stage of ALS because sometimes it evolves to affect lower motor neurones as well. Initial indications of the disease usually begin in the legs with stiffness and spasticity, which is often painful. With progression, the back and the arms become involved and balance, gait, and physical activity become steadily more compromised. It tends to progress more slowly than the other forms of motor neurone disease, but eventually it causes paralysis of all four limbs, and when it affects the brainstem and cerebellum (usually late in the disease), swallowing, speech, and breathing are impaired. Average survival time after the onset of symptoms is about 20 years.

Spinal muscular atrophy

This group of inherited disorders is characterised by LMN degeneration. It causes muscle weakness and atrophy and is considered by some experts to be a precursor of ALS, partly because the clinical course is very similar to ALS and many patients develop UMN disease as well.

MENTAL HEALTH DISORDERS

Mental health disorders represent a wide spectrum of conditions in which thought, perception, emotion, or behaviour change from the individual's norm and affect their ability to function in daily life, interact with others and maintain normal, healthy relationships. Dementia (described previously) represents one form of mental illness.

Psychosis

The term *psychosis* describes psychiatric episodes or illness in which reality is not perceived or interpreted normally. **Hallucinations** are psychotic events in which an individual experiences (sees, hears, feels, or smells) people or things that are not actually there; for example, the person may believe there are spiders crawling all over their body, or the person may see a dead relative sitting at the table. They may hear disembodied voices threatening them or giving them instructions or advice. **Delusions** are beliefs or ideas that do not fit with reality; for example, an individual may believe that he or she has special powers or was brought up on a different planet. Another feature of psychosis is disordered thinking, in which thoughts and ideas may race through someone's head; the person may be unable to articulate

thoughts in speech and consequently may be incoherent and nonsensical.

Depressive illness

Depression is a common disorder, and the incidence is rising globally. It is commoner in women than in men; the lifetime risk in females is 20% to 25% compared with 7% to 12% in males, and the WHO's 2023 statistics estimated that at any one time 5% of the world's population has depression. The condition represents a spectrum, ranging from mild illness that may occur only once in an individual's lifetime, to severely disabling depression that can lead to suicide. The link between depression and suicide is very clear. Depression increases the risk of suicide tenfold, and suicide is the second commonest cause of death in young adults.

Risk factors include female sex and genetics. Stressful life events, such as childbirth, bereavement, loss of employment, childhood abuse or neglect, chronic illness, or being the victim of violence may trigger depressive episodes at the time or increase risk later in life. Other cases of depressive illness show a clear tendency to run in families and having a first-degree relative with the disorder increases an individual's chances of becoming a sufferer. In identical twins, for example, concordance rates can be over 60%.

Pathophysiology

The onset of depression is likely to be the result of genetic, environmental, endocrine, and neurological factors; that is, it has a complex, multifactorial origin. One of the most long-standing theories in the cause of depressive illness, the monoamine hypothesis, dates from the 1950s and was based on observations suggesting that the levels of monoamine neurotransmitters, in particular **noradrenaline** and **serotonin**, were reduced in depression (Fig. 8.19). The idea that receptors for these transmitters might be malfunctional in depression has also been suggested. The monoamine hypothesis has the advantage of being simple and is supported by some experimental and clinical evidence; for example, some drugs that increase monoamine levels in the brain are effective in the treatment of depression, and some drugs that deplete the brain of monoamines can induce depression. However, significant contradictory findings that have not been explained reduce the credibility of the monoamine hypothesis and strongly suggest that, at best, it can only be part of the story. One of the most important is the time lag, sometimes of weeks, between initiation of treatment with drugs that increase brain monoamine levels and improvement of symptoms, even though imaging demonstrates that transmitter levels rise immediately. Another is that one third to one half of patients do not improve on these drugs. Other neurotransmitters increasingly considered important in the regulation of mood include **dopamine**, which is important in reward and pleasure-seeking behaviours, **GABA**, and **glutamate**.

Signs and symptoms

The presentation can be very variable, but key signs and symptoms include low mood, loss of interest and enjoyment in favourite activities and pastimes, feelings of worthlessness and guilt, suicidal ideas and thoughts, tiredness, insomnia or sleeping more than usual, decrease or increase in appetite and body weight, poor concentration, poor judgement

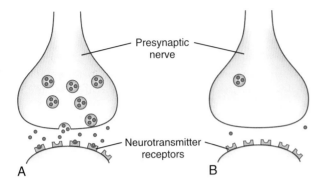

Fig. 8.19 The monoamine hypothesis. (A) Normal levels of monoamines (adrenaline, serotonin, dopamine) in nerve pathways regulating mood. (B) Deficient monoamines reduce synaptic transmission and depress mood.

and decision-making, anxiety and apathy, or agitation. Severe depression may cause psychotic episodes.

Prognosis and management

Depression may be treated with both psychological and pharmacological approaches. Antidepressant drugs generally increase the levels of monoamine neurotransmitters (mainly noradrenaline and serotonin) in the brain and are generally most effective in moderate to severe depression. It has recently been shown that ketamine, a drug conventionally used in anaesthesia, rapidly improves depressive symptoms in people for whom traditional antidepressants have not worked, perhaps through improving synaptic connections in the brain and/or by enhancing the effect of the neurotransmitter glutamate. A range of psychological interventions, including cognitive behavioural therapy, are used. Physical exercise and alternative treatments—for example, art therapies and mindfulness—have also been successfully used to manage depression; they are likely to increase the brain's release of endorphins, endogenous substances that improve mood and the sense of well-being. Having one depressive episode increases the risk of further episodes.

BIPOLAR DISORDER

In this condition, periods of good mental health are interspersed with episodes of altered mood, either depression or abnormally elevated mood (mania). There is no difference in incidence between the sexes, and there is a strong heritable component; having an affected first-degree relative increases an individual's risk sevenfold. The disorder usually manifests itself in young adulthood.

Pathophysiology

Although genetics play a significant part in this disorder, no single mutated gene is responsible; rather, the interaction of over 20 different susceptibility genes, each of which individually contributes a slight increase in risk, is believed to underpin the condition. Some of these genetic mutations are associated with abnormal nerve function and identification of the function of these genes might therefore help in finding new treatments. For example, one gene associated with bipolar disorder, *CACNA1C*, is found on chromosome 12 and codes for a subunit on a calcium channel found in the brain. Mutations in this gene may therefore lead to abnormal calcium movement across neuronal membranes,

and there is evidence that some drugs used to treat bipolar disorder work by modulating calcium channel function. Mutations in this gene are also associated with schizophrenia (see Schizophrenia below); in fact, several genes associated with bipolar disorder are also associated with schizophrenia, suggesting a degree of commonality in the underlying pathophysiology of the two conditions.

There is evidence for neuronal loss or dysfunction in the hippocampus in patients with bipolar disorder. The hippocampus is important in the regulation of memory and emotion, and abnormalities in this part of the brain have also been documented in other psychiatric disorders such as severe depression.

Signs and symptoms

Extreme mood swings characterise this disorder, often with periods of normal mood in between. The signs and symptoms of depression are described previously and may include psychotic symptoms such as hallucinations and delusions. Manic phases are characterised by hyperactivity, rapid and incessant speech, extreme euphoria, irritability and distractability, grandiose ideas and unrealistic plans and expectations, risk-taking behaviours and decisions, and poor sleep patterns.

Management and prognosis

The disease is lifelong and the more extreme forms, in which the patient rapidly cycles between mood extremes, can be incapacitating. A range of drugs may be used in its management. One of the key agents, lithium, is thought to exert at least part of its effect through blocking the increased neuronal calcium signalling associated with bipolar disorder. Antidepressants are used in depressive phases but must be used with care to prevent tipping the patient into a manic phase. Anticonvulsant drugs, which reduce neuronal excitability, are also used.

ANXIETY AND PANIC DISORDERS

Anxiety is a normal emotional and physiological response to an unfamiliar or potentially threatening situation. Activation of the sympathetic nervous system increases alertness and cerebral blood flow to optimise a response to possible dangers, and increases heart rate, blood glucose and lipid levels, respiratory rate, and blood pressure. These all represent protective mechanisms and, provided they are activated at appropriate times and deactivated when not required, contribute usefully to helping people cope with stressful events. Anxiety disorder, in which inappropriate fears, troublesome thoughts, and sometimes phobias towards harmless agents, is one of the commonest psychiatric conditions. There is a 3:2 female:male ratio, and indications usually appear fairly early in life. Anxiety disorders often occur with other mental health conditions, including depression and drug or alcohol dependence, and can cause significant social withdrawal, reduced day-to-day functionality, and decreased quality of life.

Pathophysiology

Activation of the sympathetic nervous system and adrenaline release produce many of the symptoms. The underlying cause of the disorder is not understood. There is increased activity of sympathetic and serotonergic neurones in the brain, and serotonin receptor activity in some parts of the brain associated with levels of arousal has been shown to be abnormal in some studies, but the actual causative changes have not been identified.

Signs and symptoms
Sympathetic activation causes systemic signs and symptoms, such as sweating, tachycardia, hyperventilation, palpitations, and tremor. There may be diarrhoea, nausea, abdominal pain, headache, and insomnia. The patient may report a fear of impending doom, a sensation of impending death, or a sense of becoming detached from reality and losing control. There may be episodes of complete panic, in which the anxiety becomes overwhelming and the patient may be incapacitated.

Management and prognosis
It is important to identify co-existing psychiatric issues such as depression so that appropriate treatment can be offered to manage these elements of the disorder. The anxiety can be treated with psychological approaches including relaxation techniques, desensitisation programmes for phobias and cognitive behavioural therapy.

SCHIZOPHRENIA

This major psychiatric disorder is associated with psychotic episodes, including hallucinations, delusions, and disordered thinking. Incidence is higher in developed and developing countries than in the least developed countries and has been estimated at up to 1% of the population. Immigrants from a low-risk area to a higher-risk area acquire the increased risk of their new environment. The disorder usually manifests before the age of 30, and although it occurs equally in males and females, it tends to be more severe in males. The cause is not known, although there is a genetic predisposition (e.g., identical twins can have up to 50% concordance, even if separated at birth), and environmental factors seem to play a part. Children of older fathers have an increased risk, and other risk factors include obstetric difficulties either before or at the time of birth and living in cities. It is thought the underlying cause is some abnormality of brain development associated with increased genetic susceptibility that is triggered by some later environmental influence.

Pathophysiology
The changes in the schizophrenic brain are complex and include both changes in neurotransmitter levels, activity, and structural alterations. Changes in neurotransmitter levels, including **glutamate**, **serotonin**, and **GABA**, have been implicated in schizophrenia, but the best established abnormality is increased **dopamine** activity. Most of the brain's dopamine-synthesising nerves originate in the midbrain and are organised into four main groups projecting to different areas and with different functions. One pathway links the substantia nigra in the midbrain to the corpus striatum. This is called the **nigrostriatal pathway** and regulates voluntary muscle control (see Parkinson disease). The **tuberoinfundibular pathway** regulates prolactin release from the pituitary gland. The other two pathways project from the ventral tegmental area (VTA) in the midbrain. The **mesocortical pathway** links the VTA to the cortex and is important in cognitive functions. The **mesolimbic pathway** links the VTA to the

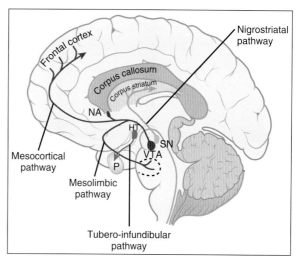

Fig. 8.20 Dopamine pathways in the brain. (1) The nigrostriatal pathway. This is deficient in Parkinson disease. (2) The mesocortical pathway. Underactivity in this pathway is linked to the negative symptoms of schizophrenia. (3) The mesolimbic pathway. Overactivity in this pathway is linked to the positive symptoms of schizophrenia. (4) The tuberoinfundibular pathway. This regulates lactation. NA: nucleus accumbens; SN: substantia nigra; VTA: ventral tegmental area; HT: hypothalamus; P: pituitary gland. (From Satoskar RS, Rege N, and Bhandarkar SD (2021) *Pharmacology and pharmacotherapeutics*, 26th ed, Fig. 5.1. New Delhi: RELX India Pvt Ltd.)

nucleus accumbens, the hippocampus, and other structures of the limbic system and is important in reward, motivation, and addiction (Fig. 8.20). Both pathways are dysfunctional in schizophrenia. Although the link between schizophrenia and dopamine was made in the early 1960s, dopamine's role in schizophrenia and the precise pathways involved are not fully understood. It seems that dopamine hyperactivity in the mesocortical pathway causes the negative symptoms of schizophrenia and hyperactivity in the mesolimbic pathway causes the positive symptoms (Box 8.3; and see Signs and symptoms below). The main drugs currently available to treat schizophrenia are all dopamine receptor blockers. Recent work has also suggested that neural responses to the stimulatory neurotransmitter glutamate may be deficient in schizophrenia. Glutamate operates through the NMDA receptor, and NMDA receptor antagonists such as ketamine can initiate psychotic states similar to schizophrenia. Some studies have shown that drugs that activate NMDA receptors may be neuroprotective and beneficial in schizophrenia, although the evidence compared with that for dopamine receptor blockers is modest.

There are clear physical changes in the size and composition of the brain in schizophrenic people compared with non-schizophrenics. Brain volume is reduced, the ventricles are enlarged, the cerebral cortex becomes progressively thinner, the sulci are wider, and the gyri are flatter. Fig. 8.21 shows MRI scans of the brains of two identical 44-year-old male twins, one of whom (right image) has schizophrenia. Compared with his healthy twin, the schizophrenic brain has enlarged ventricles and reduced brain volume. In particular, the pre-frontal cortex and the grey matter of the temporal lobes are affected. The amygdala, hippocampus, and hypothalamus reduce in size, and their connectivity (i.e., their capacity to communicate with other brain areas) is also reduced. These changes lead to impaired short- and long-term memory, abnormal emotional processing and responses, and declining cognitive capacity and decision-making ability.

Signs and symptoms

Schizophrenia is associated with significant psychotic signs and symptoms and a lack of insight (a person's inability to recognise that they are ill). Positive symptoms are characterised by experiences and behaviours (e.g., abnormal hallucinations, delusions, and disorganised speech and behaviours). Hallucinations, usually of the auditory type, are very common. People may have delusions that they are being controlled, watched, persecuted, or having their mind read, and they may develop aggressive or agitated behaviour. Negative symptoms reflect a reduction or loss of normal emotional responses and behaviours, including poverty of speech, emotional flattening, and a loss of interest in people, places, and activities that would normally be enjoyed. Patients may stop washing and eating, cease to take any interest in their appearance, and withdraw from social contact. Cognitive symptoms include loss of intellectual capacity, poor memory, slow or poor decision-making, and a deterioration in the ability to read social and interpersonal cues. People may have difficulty paying attention, planning and organising even mundane daily activities, and limited comprehension. They have no insight into their condition and become suspicious, angry, and impatient with others.

BOX 8.3 Positive and negative symptoms of schizophrenia

Positive symptoms	Negative symptoms
Hallucinations (visual, auditory, olfactory)	Social withdrawal
Delusions	Poverty of speech
Disorganised speech	Emotional flattening
Bizarre behaviours	Loss of interest
Disordered thoughts	Failure of self-care
Inaccurate and inappropriate beliefs	Poor concentration and memory
	Poor comprehension and judgement

Management and prognosis

Schizophrenia often follows an initially unpredictable and fluctuating course over the first few years after diagnosis. Sometimes symptoms may disappear for long periods of time, but there is no cure and complete recovery is highly unlikely. Most people find they have to manage their condition all their lives. Anti-psychotic drugs block D2 dopamine receptors in the brain, and although they are particularly effective in controlling the positive symptoms and thought disorder of schizophrenia, they have significant side effects, not least the onset of drug-induced parkinsonism because dopamine in the nigrostriatal pathway controls voluntary motor activity. Lifelong drug treatment may be required. Psychosocial interventions, such as cognitive behavioural therapy and social skills training, can help maintain the person in their community, hold down a job, live independently,

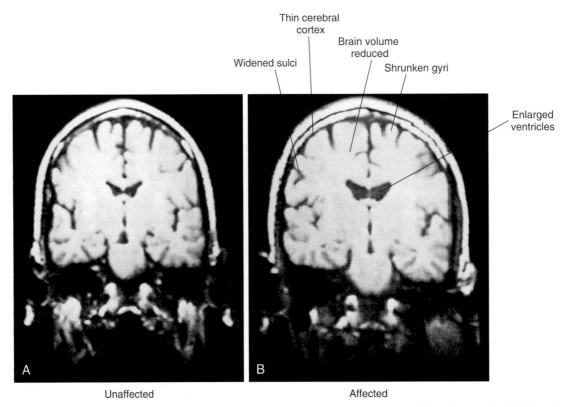

Fig. 8.21 MRI brain scans of identical twins showing enlarged ventricles in the schizophrenic twin. (A) unaffected twin. (B)Affected twin. (From Fortinash KM and Worret PA (2004) *Psychiatric mental health nursing*, 3rd ed. St Louis: Mosby, p. 240. Courtesy Daniel Weinberger, MD, Clinical Brain Disorders Branch, Division of Intramural Research Program, NIMH, 1990.)

and minimise hospitalisations. It is also important to manage co-morbidities, such as diabetes and cardiovascular disease. The risk of suicide in people with schizophrenia is higher than average and highest in young males with depressive symptoms, active hallucinations and delusions, and co-existing drug or alcohol problems.

AUTISM

Autism is a spectrum of neurodevelopmental disorders associated with altered perceptions of the environment, communication difficulties, learning difficulties and difficulty forming and maintaining interpersonal relationships. It includes conditions such as Asperger syndrome, which is usually associated with normal to high intellectual function and good language skills. Autism is usually diagnosed by the age of three, and the range of signs and symptoms is wide. Globally, its incidence is rising, although this may reflect changing diagnostic criteria and/or rising awareness; and although data collection is not performed consistently in all countries, it is estimated that about 1 in 130 people is affected by some form of the condition. Risk factors include prematurity, older parents, family history and male sex. Genetics play a part: some genetic disorders (e.g., fragile X syndrome and Rett syndrome) are strongly associated with autism. Several other gene defects are also regularly found in autism.

Pathophysiology

Although the underlying abnormality is not fully understood, there is evidence of impaired neural connectivity and synaptogenesis (synapse formation) in the brains of autistic people, although there are actually more neurones present than normal. Current evidence suggests that there is a failure of neuronal migration and neuronal pruning, essential processes in the development and maturation of the brain during normal embryonic development, childhood, and adolescence. It has been estimated that the total number of neurones produced during embryonic brain development is reduced by half at the time of birth. During normal brain development, newly formed neurones migrate along predetermined pathways as part of the complex organogenesis of the brain, but many more are formed than are needed, so they do not all survive. This is called **neuronal pruning**. In early childhood, synaptic connections between brain neurones proliferate hugely, and then rapidly diminish as those that are not required or used are eliminated by phagocytic glial cells. This is called **synaptic pruning** and streamlines the connectivity between brain areas and establishes efficient and effective communication pathways. Autism is associated with excessive neuronal numbers and excessive synaptic connections, which interferes with efficient neural connectivity and communication.

Signs and symptoms

The typical triad of symptoms is composed of poor social interaction, difficulties with language and communication, and the presence of restricted and repetitive interests, activities, and patterns of behaviour. There may be behavioural abnormalities such as abnormal responses to pain and environmental and physical stimulation. Not all disorders on the spectrum exhibit the typical triad, however; for example, people with Asperger syndrome usually have no language difficulties. Autism is associated with gastrointestinal symptoms, including diarrhoea and constipation; the more severe the autism, the more severe the symptoms.

Management and prognosis

The condition is permanent and how well the child does usually depends strongly on their intellectual capacity. High-functioning autistic people may live close to normal lives, whereas those at the other end of the spectrum may need lifetime care. Support with speech therapy, occupational therapy, and psychosocial education helps each individual reach personal potential.

SEIZURES AND EPILEPSY

A seizure (sometimes called a *convulsion* or *fit*) is caused by an abnormal or excessive episode of electrical activity in the brain. The signs and symptoms depend on where in the brain this arises, how far it spreads, and how long it lasts. Epilepsy is the condition of being prone to seizures, and epileptic people can experience more than one type of seizure.

Seizures can cause motor and/or sensory disturbances, with or without loss or impairment of consciousness. Seizures are described according to where they start in the brain, the degree of awareness during the seizure and the nature of the signs and symptoms associated with the event. Recent changes in the classification of seizures have led to the discontinuation of some older terms; some key terminology associated with seizures is listed in Table 8.2. The group or groups of neurones in which the disordered electrical activity begin is called the **epileptogenic focus**.

Aura

An aura is a brief sensory disturbance that may take the form of an emotional, sensory, or thought change. It is itself a form of seizure, and it precedes the main clinical event, giving a characteristic warning that a seizure is imminent. It is not the same as a **prodromal event**, which may precede the seizure by up to several days. Prodromal awareness may be experienced as changes in feeling or behaviour, and although this is not actually part of the seizure, it may give the individual enough warning to take rescue steps: avoid triggers, take medication, warn friends and family, or avoid potentially dangerous activities (e.g., climbing ladders or going swimming).

Not everyone has either a prodromal syndrome or an aura; many seizures occur with no prior warning.

Focal seizures

This is the commonest form of seizure in epilepsy, and the epileptogenic focus is localised in one part of one cerebral hemisphere of the brain. The signs and symptoms are determined by the area of the brain in which the abnormal activity originates. If the individual remains aware during the event with full memory afterwards, it is called a **focal aware seizure**. In some such seizures, there are no motor symptoms, and the individual can talk to others around them, but others may be 'frozen' for the duration of the seizure and unable to communicate, although they are fully awake. In a **focal impaired awareness seizure**, the epileptogenic focus is usually in the temporal or frontal lobe, which are the areas of the brain most important in awareness (Fig. 8.22).

Table 8.2 Key terminology associated with seizures

Term	Comment	Older/alternative terminology
Myoclonic	Brief, jerking contractions of a muscle or groups of muscles	
Tonic	Sudden stiffening of a muscle or a group of muscles (e.g., of the arm or the leg), causing rigidity in the affected part	
Clonic	Sustained, rhythmical contraction of a muscle or group of muscles giving a period of repeated jerking of the affected part	
Tonic/clonic	Both features of tonic and clonic seizures are seen; the tonic phase comes first followed by clonic jerking movements	Grand mal
Motor	Skeletal muscle is involved	
Non-motor	May involve a range of symptoms: autonomic changes e.g. increased heart rate; emotional changes, e.g. dread, anxiety, pleasure; confusion; visual, taste or auditory disturbances	
Atonic	Muscle tone is suddenly lost and the affected part becomes limp	
Focal	The epileptogenic focus arises in one area of one hemisphere of the brain	Partial
Focal aware	As focal, but with no loss of consciousness	Simple partial
Focal impaired awareness	As focal, but the individual loses awareness of their surroundings	Complex partial
Evolving	The seizure begins as a focal event, but spreads to both hemispheres; consciousness is always impaired or lost	Secondary generalised
Generalised	Areas in both brain hemispheres are involved in the seizure	
Absence	A (usually brief) period of loss of awareness of and responsiveness to local environment	Petit mal

(International League against Epilepsy, 2017)

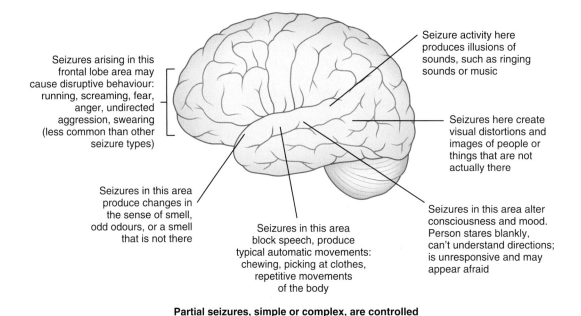

Partial seizures, simple or complex, are controlled by the function of the brain area in which they occur

Seizures arising in this frontal lobe area may cause disruptive behaviour: running, screaming, fear, anger, undirected aggression, swearing (less common than other seizure types)

Seizures in this area produce changes in the sense of smell, odd odours, or a smell that is not there

Seizures in this area block speech, produce typical automatic movements: chewing, picking at clothes, repetitive movements of the body

Seizure activity here produces illusions of sounds, such as ringing sounds or music

Seizures here create visual distortions and images of people or things that are not actually there

Seizures in this area alter consciousness and mood. Person stares blankly, can't understand directions; is unresponsive and may appear afraid

Fig. 8.22 Focal impaired awareness (partial) seizures and their origins in the brain.

Individuals are unable to respond to others around them. They stare blankly and may exhibit repetitive behaviours and movements called *automatisms*, including hand rubbing, lip smacking, chewing, bicycling of the legs, or picking at their clothes. Although some people lose all awareness, others may still be aware of their surroundings.

In some people, the epileptogenic focus that initiates the focal seizure spreads to other areas of the brain, involving both cerebral hemispheres, tonic-clonic activity, and loss of consciousness. This is called an **evolving seizure** and leads to a **generalised convulsion**.

Generalised seizures

By definition, these involve both cerebral hemispheres and awareness and/or consciousness is usually impaired or lost.

Tonic-clonic seizures. The tonic phase comes first, and the patient experiences sudden and widespread muscle rigidity. A fall at this point can lead to serious injury. The clonic phase follows, with alternating cycles of muscle contraction and relaxation of the limb muscles and violent, rhythmical, spasmodic jerking. The patient may bite their tongue, lose continence, and if respiration is impaired, become cyanosed. The seizure usually lasts less than 3 minutes, and afterwards the patient is generally sleepy, irritable, and disorientated. They may have no memory of events immediately preceding the seizure and may take several hours to fully recover. If the tonic-clonic seizure began as a focal event, it is referred to as a **focal to bilateral tonic-clonic seizure**, to distinguish it from a seizure that began in both hemispheres, in which case it is called a **generalised onset tonic-clonic seizure**.

Absence seizures. These are generalised seizures usually seen in children. When mild, they may be misinterpreted as periods of daydreaming, and they are generally short, lasting about 10 to 20 seconds, with the individual carrying on at the end of the seizure as though nothing had happened. Sometimes, however, a train of absence seizures may occur in fairly close succession, leading to confusion and disorientation at their conclusion. They may occur frequently, perhaps 20 or 30 times a day, interfering considerably with function. Even when single and brief, the attacks can cause significant disruption; for example, a child may miss a teacher's instructions or the thread of a conversation.

Status epilepticus. This means prolonged seizure activity lasting 5 minutes or more, with no intervening periods of recovery and is a medical emergency. In known epileptic people, it is usually caused by failure to take prescribed medication, but it can arise secondary to a range of injuries and diseases such as meningitis, an undiagnosed brain tumour or a metabolic disturbance such as hypoglycaemia. It is not known why the seizure does not self-terminate, but it induces a massive sympathetic response that increases heart rate, induces cardiac arrhythmias and (initially) hypertension. There may be hyperthermia resulting from the prolonged and excessive muscle activity, and acidosis resulting from muscle metabolism and impaired respiratory function. With continued seizure activity, blood pressure drops, cerebral perfusion falls, blood oxygen levels fall and acidosis gets progressively worse. Status epilepticus carries a 10% to 15% mortality.

Causes and triggers of seizures and epilepsy

In a significant number of people diagnosed with epilepsy, an underlying cause is never found. However, a wide range of diseases and conditions cause seizures. In children, common causes include fever, birth-related hypoxia, infection, head trauma, and congenital malformations. In young adults, head trauma is the commonest cause. In older age, cerebrovascular disease, stroke, tumours, and degenerative disorders become increasingly prevalent. Other causes include electrolyte deficiencies, including low levels of sodium, calcium and magnesium, hypoglycaemia, and circulating toxins (e.g., from renal or liver failure), and additionally, many drugs may trigger seizures. Epilepsy may be genetic: a range of inherited disorders, including inborn errors of metabolism and some mitochondrial diseases feature epilepsy in their clinical picture.

A number of trigger factors can initiate seizure in susceptible individuals (e.g., sleep deprivation, flashing lights, stress, menstruation, loud music, or strong emotions). Alcohol and hangovers are also common triggers.

Pathophysiology of seizures

The epileptogenic focus determines the nature and severity of the seizure, but the underlying event is an excessive electrical discharge in the brain. Recording brain electrical activity on an electroencephalograph (EEG) can be diagnostic. Fig. 8.23 shows abnormal EEG activity during an absence seizure lasting 7 seconds in a teenage boy. Normal brain function requires both excitatory and inhibitory discharge in neural circuits, and seizures can arise if activity in either of these two balancing elements is increased or decreased. The

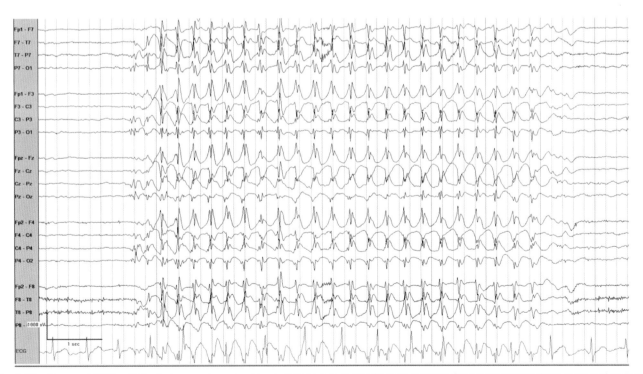

Fig. 8.23 Abnormal EEG activity during an absence seizure. (From Levin K and Chauvel P (2019) *Clinical neurophysiology: basis and technical aspects,* Fig. 7.6. Netherlands: Elsevier BV.)

range of possible abnormalities that may disturb this balance is very wide, and there is a correspondingly wide range of possible aetiologies in seizures and epilepsy. For example, changes in the brain that enhance excitatory nerve activity increase the likelihood of seizures and may underpin some forms of epilepsy. The brain's main excitatory neurotransmitter, glutamate, acts on NMDA receptors. In some forms of inherited epilepsy, these receptors are more sensitive and remain activated for longer than normal. Drugs that increase the levels of stimulatory neurotransmitters may trigger seizures as a side effect (e.g., the tricyclic antidepressants, which increase levels of excitatory noradrenaline and serotonin in the brain). Alternatively, reducing activity in inhibitory pathways may also reduce the seizure threshold and increase their risk and incidence. Gamma aminobutyric acid (GABA) is an important inhibitory neurotransmitter, and reduction in GABA receptors, GABA levels, or GABA activity have all been associated with increased risk of seizures.

Management and prognosis

Identifying and correcting any underlying issues (e.g., treating infections or rectifying electrolyte imbalances) is essential. If the risk of further seizures is high, anti-epileptic drug treatment can be offered. A range of anticonvulsant drugs are available, and the choice of drug is determined largely by the type of epilepsy present because not all anticonvulsant drugs are equally effective in all types of seizure disorder; indeed, some drugs may make certain types worse.

CENTRAL NERVOUS SYSTEM TUMOURS

Because neuronal cell turnover is very low, primary tumours of nerve cells themselves are relatively rare, and the commonest tumours arise from glial cells and other support cells in the CNS. Nearly all occur in the brain: only about 3% of CNS tumours arise in the spinal cord. The International Agency for Research on Cancer data (2020) place brain and other CNS cancers as the 20th commonest cancers worldwide but the 12th leading cause of cancer-related death, reflecting the gravity of the disease and the limitations of current treatment options. The Global Burden of Disease Study (2016) reported that CNS cancer rates increased by over 17% between 1990 and 2016. For most CNS cancers, the main risk factor is age, although some occur mainly in children. Paediatric brain cancers generally have a very poor prognosis. Most brain tumours arise spontaneously, although some have a familial tendency,

As with other cancers, identifying the cell of origin, the genetic mutations present, and the molecular characteristics of the tumour are important for treatment decisions and for prognosis. The most recent WHO classification of primary CNS tumours was made in 2016, and only the most common will be discussed here. Most brain tumours are benign, but even a benign tumour can be life threatening in the closed cranial cavity if it compresses key brain areas, causes bleeding, or compromises blood flow and cannot be removed or reduced by surgery or other treatments. Most malignant tumours are metastatic growths that have seeded from a primary elsewhere. About 80% of cancers can metastasise to the brain; the commonest sources of brain secondaries are melanomas and lung, breast, renal, and colorectal malignancies.

Primary CNS malignancies vary enormously in their behaviours and growth patterns. They are generally described in terms of their malignant potential or grade and are ranked from low grade (grade I) to high grade (grade IV). Low-grade tumours can carry a mean survival time of over 5 years, but eventually, at higher grade, more aggressive tumour cell types self-select and predominate, the patient's condition deteriorates. High-grade tumours are aggressive and can cause death in weeks or months.

Consequences of CNS tumours

Irrespective of the nature of the tumour, the expanding mass can erode blood vessels and cause bleeding into the brain or compress blood vessels and impair blood flow to an area of tissue. Compression or obstruction of the ventricles or interconnecting ducts can block CSF circulation and increase intracranial pressure, compressing and injuring delicate neural tissue. The brain tissue becomes oedematous, increasing pressure damage. There may be seizures, headaches, and personality changes. In addition to these general effects, there may be signs and symptoms associated with the direct damage done locally by the expanding or infiltrating tumour; for example, a cerebellar tumour causes balance and co-ordination difficulties, and a tumour growing in the visual cortex causes visual impairment.

GLIOMAS

A range of cancers can arise from the CNS glial cell population or from their stem cell precursors. Gliomas are the commonest type of malignant brain tumour and range from high-grade aggressive tumours to slower growing low-grade cancers.

Astrocytoma

This is the commonest form of glioma in both adults and children and may be high- or low-grade. Tumour growth patterns vary: some are infiltrative and diffuse, and others are more compact. Their clinical effects depend on where the tumour originates and how quickly it grows, and they can arise anywhere in the brain.

Glioblastoma

This type of astrocytoma (Fig. 8.24) is always high grade and is the commonest form of glioma. Its clinical course is short and aggressive, and median survival time even with optimal treatment is less than 12 months. Common gene mutations occur in the *LOH*, *p53*, and *EGF* genes, but a number of additional genetic mutations have also been identified, showing that there are a number of different disease entities within this group of cancers. Most occur in the cerebral hemispheres. Treatment is palliative; surgery, radiotherapy, and chemotherapy may all be options, but the condition is currently incurable. Younger patients tend to survive longer than older patients, but the overall 5-year survival rate is less than 10%.

Oligodendroglioma

This type of glioma is generally fairly slow growing and may respond well to chemotherapy. It usually arises in the cerebral hemispheres, most frequently in the frontal lobes, and occurs more often in men than women, usually in middle age. Survival time in the slowest growing forms can be up to 10 years.

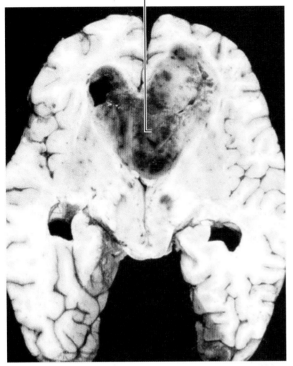

Glioblastoma showing
haemorrhage and necrosis

Fig. 8.24 Glioblastoma. (From Moini J, Avgeropoulos N and Samsam M (2021) *Epidemiology of brain and spinal tumors*, Fig. 7.7. Philadelphia: Elsevier Inc.)

MEDULLOBLASTOMA

This is the commonest malignant brain tumour in children, accounting for up to 20% of all paediatric brain malignancies. It arises from undifferentiated, embryonic cells in the cerebellum, and is usually fast growing and invasive. Unlike most primary brain tumours, which tend not to metastasise because the brain has no lymphatic system, medulloblastomas can spread throughout the brain and spinal cord and even outside the CNS. The growing tumour causes hydrocephalus and cerebellar dysfunction (motor and co-ordination abnormalities).

MENINGIOMA

This is the commonest benign brain tumour and occurs more frequently in women than men. Of all meningioma tumours, 90% are benign, although some are highly malignant. They arise from the arachnoid mater and can appear anywhere on the brain surface or within the ventricular system; sometimes they grow on the spinal meninges. They generally attach to the dura and can grow into the skull bone itself, and although they compress the underlying brain tissue, they do not invade it and are easily separated from it at surgery. After treatment, recurrence can occur, but the risk is relatively low. Known risk factors include prior exposure to radiation and neurofibromatosis type 2, a rare genetic disorder also associated with schwannoma formation.

SCHWANNOMA

This benign tumour arises from the Schwann cells forming part of the nerve coverings of the cranial and spinal nerve roots within the cranial cavity and spinal column. Schwann cells are not found within the brain itself: the function of myelin production in the brain is performed by oligodendrocytes. The commonest site for schwannoma formation is along the vestibular branch of the eighth (auditory) cranial nerve, causing gait, balance, and hearing problems. They can also cause facial numbness and paralysis because the facial nerve (CN VII) lies immediately beside the auditory nerve and can be compressed by the growing tumour (Fig. 8.25). Sometimes called **acoustic neuromas**, schwannomas are more common in women and with increasing age and are associated with certain genetic disorders including neurofibromatosis type 2 (NF2). In NF2, the gene coding for production of a protein called **merlin** is mutated. Merlin is a tumour suppressor protein (p. 75); it ensures that in growing tissues, cell-cell contact inhibits cell proliferation, an important regulatory mechanism in preventing excessive cell division. In NF2, merlin is non-functional and cell growth continues, causing tumours. NF2 is also associated with other CNS tumours, including meningioma.

PRIMARY CNS LYMPHOMA

Risk factors for this cancer include immunosuppression, for example, in long-term steroid treatment or in HIV infection and increasing age. Globally, its incidence is rising, and it is more common in males than females. It is considered a form of non-Hodgkin lymphoma, originating from a B cell in the brain, pia or arachnoid mater, spinal cord, or the eyes. It rarely spreads outside the CNS, but it is usually aggressive, and although it can sometimes be cured, survival rates are low, especially in older people and in those with comorbidities. As the malignant cells proliferate, they infiltrate and injure brain tissue, causing inflammation and necrotic changes. There are frequently multiple tumours present, and the signs and symptoms depend on their location and which areas of the brain are involved. Raised intracranial pressure is common, as are seizures and changes in personality and behaviour.

DISORDERS OF MOTOR CONTROL

When all processes and components controlling skeletal muscle function are healthy and operating normally, they produce smooth, controlled, and integrated movement to ensure balance, locomotion, and maintenance of posture. Although seemingly straightforward, even simple movements require a complex and integrated collaboration of neural input from the motor cortex, the premotor cortex, the cerebellum, and other key subcortical areas, including the basal ganglia. Injury, disease, or degeneration of any of the multiple pathways involved in the complex process of motor control can disrupt or abolish this. Motor neurone disease is discussed previously. Huntington disease is discussed in Chapter 2.

PARKINSON DISEASE

Parkinson disease (PD) was first described in 1817 in an article entitled 'Essay on the Shaking Palsy', written by James Parkinson, a surgeon-apothecary in London. Its incidence increases with age, and it affects 1 in 100 people aged over 60 years. It is commoner in men than women and occurs in all racial groups, and its incidence is rising worldwide. The cause is not known, although some cases are directly linked

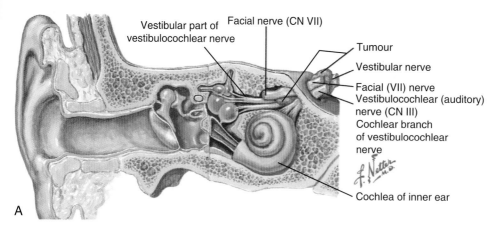

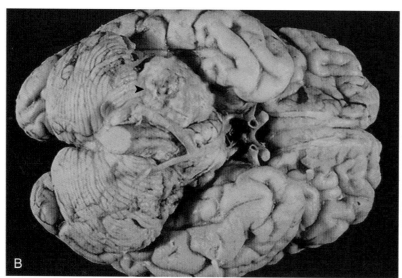

Fig. 8.25 Acoustic neuroma. (A) Anatomical location of the tumour. (B) Acoustic neuroma (black arrow) clearly visible on the base of the brain. (Modified from (A) Srinivasan J, Chaves C, Scott B, Small J (2020) *Netter's neurology*, 3rd ed, Philadelphia, Elsevier Inc; Fig. 49.18; and (B) Klatt E, Robbins and Cotran (2020) *Atlas of pathology*, 4th ed, Fig. 19.145. Philadelphia: Elsevier Inc.)

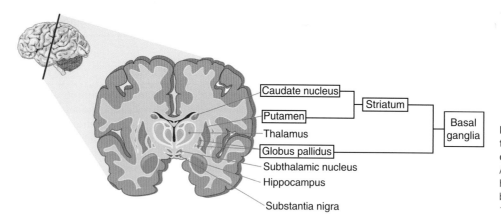

Fig. 8.26 The principal brain structures involved in voluntary motor control. (From Draoui A, El Hiba O, Aimrane A, El Khiat A, and Gamrani H (2020) Parkinson's disease: from bench to bedside, *Revue Neurologique* 176(7–8), 543–559.)

to certain drugs or CNS infection. The underlying aetiology is progressive loss of the dopamine-releasing neurones of the nigrostriatal pathway (Fig. 8.21), leading to severe depletion of dopamine levels in the striatum. Most cases are thought to result from a combination of a genetic predisposition and a contributory environmental factor. For example, exposure to pesticides increases risk. Caffeine and cigarette smoking have both been shown to reduce risk. Associations between melanoma and diabetes and PD have also been demonstrated. Heredity does play a part but is more likely to be a contributing factor in young people who develop the disorder before 50 years of age.

Motor control and the nigrostriatal pathway

The main brain structures involved in the initiation and regulation of voluntary muscle movements are shown in Fig. 8.26. Decisions about voluntary muscle movement (e.g., picking up a cup of coffee or changing from walking to running) are made in the motor cortex, which sends instructions to the skeletal muscles. Excitatory input from the thalamus stimulates the motor cortex and therefore initiates and increases muscle movement, but this input must be constantly regulated to ensure only muscle groups needed for the desired movement are activated, and that the degree of activation is appropriate for the desired movement. For example, more muscle groups and more overall movement are needed to bend and pick a pile of heavy books off the floor than to lift a coffee cup off a nearby table. In addition, muscle groups that oppose a desired action must be relaxed to allow the movement to take place. For example, when the biceps contract to lift the cup, the triceps must relax to allow the arm to bend at the elbow. The excitatory activity of the thalamus is regulated by the **basal ganglia**—the **caudate nucleus** and the **putamen** of the striatum—and the **globus pallidus**. Nervous input from the basal ganglia inhibits the thalamus, and prevents muscle overactivity and allows muscle relaxation.

The striatum is supplied with dopaminergic nerves from the substantia nigra in the midbrain- the nigrostriatal pathway. When the nigrostriatal pathway is activated, and dopamine is released in the striatum, the striatum increases its inhibition of the thalamus and input to the motor cortex is reduced. This in turn reduces skeletal muscle activity (Fig. 8.27A).

Pathophysiology

PD is caused by degeneration of the nigrostriatal pathway, which reduces the ability of the basal ganglia to inhibit the excitatory action of the thalamus on the motor cortex (Fig. 8.27B). The nigrostriatal nerves release dopamine at their nerve endings in the striatum, so dopamine levels in the striatum fall; this can be demonstrated in PD sufferers by neuroimaging scans. In addition, a characteristic neurological finding is the presence of Lewy bodies in the neurones of the substantia nigra, although this is not diagnostic for PD, because they are found in other neurological disorders, including dementia.

Signs and symptoms

Because the underlying pathological changes in PD decrease the ability of the brain to reduce skeletal muscle tone, the initial indications of the disease are usually muscle rigidity, a resting tremor and bradykinesia (slow and delayed movement). The earliest symptom is usually a resting tremor, which may begin unilaterally but becomes bilateral with time. The patient becomes stooped and develops a shuffling gait. He may report a loss of the sense of smell, clumsiness, and reduced manual dexterity, and may have reduced facial expression. There may be dystonia (increased or abnormal muscle tone) leading to abnormal position or posture; for example, a foot may turn in, or an arm may be pulled in across the chest or abdomen. There may be autonomic signs and symptoms, including constipation, excessive salivation, and urinary urgency. Depression is common, and the incidence of dementia is increased, usually as a late development in advanced PD.

Management and prognosis

Dopamine cannot be used for replacement therapy because it does not cross the blood-brain barrier, but the precursor in its biosynthetic pathway, L-DOPA, does and was first used in the 1960s with startling effect: up till that time, the few drugs licensed to treat PD had very limited efficacy and none reversed the progressive nature of the disease. L-DOPA crosses the blood-brain-barrier and is converted into dopamine, restoring dopamine levels in the striatum. However, PD is a progressive disorder, and although L-DOPA can manage symptoms, often giving complete remission that might last

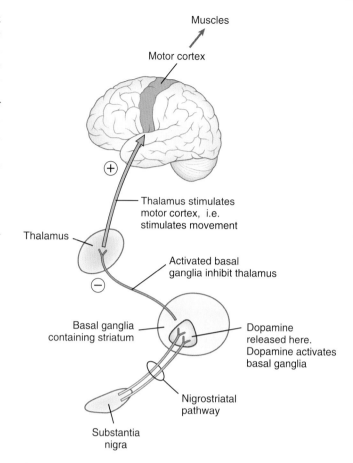

A

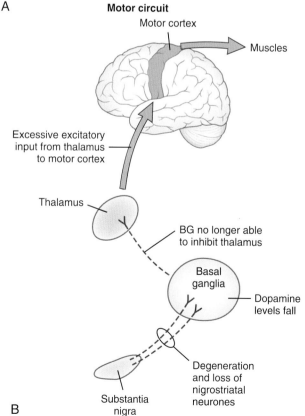

B

Fig. 8.27 The relationship between the nigrostriatal pathway, the thalamus and the motor cortex. (A) In health. (B) Nigrostriatal degeneration in Parkinson disease.

for years, it does not halt or reverse the neurological degeneration that causes it, and most patients eventually develop severe disability.

CEREBROVASCULAR DISORDERS

The central nervous system has a high metabolic rate and high oxygen demands. Despite representing only 2% of total body weight, the brain receives 15% of the resting cardiac output and uses 20% of the body's oxygen and 60% of resting glucose requirements. Neurones are highly sensitive to reduced oxygen and glucose supply because their capacity to generate energy from anaerobic and other metabolic sources is very limited and brain tissue has no glucose stores. Disruption to brain blood supply can significantly threaten function, and because neurones do not regenerate, damage from hypoxia or haemorrhage is frequently permanent.

Disruption of blood supply to brain tissue may occur either by reduction in the oxygen supply to the area (ischaemic injury) or by the rupture of an artery, causing bleeding into brain tissue (haemorrhagic injury). In either event, the effect on the brain depends on the location and extent of the injury, and also on how long the affected area is subject to reduced blood flow. Multiple small infarctions may not individually cause neurological symptoms but are associated with the development of dementia.

Ischaemic injury

If the brain does not receive enough oxygen and glucose, it cannot generate ATP for energy, and its ability to maintain the electrical potential across neuronal cell membranes is rapidly impaired (the Na^+/K^+ pump requires energy to operate). As a result, neurones cannot generate or conduct action potentials and they fail. If hypoxia continues, the cells swell (because sodium is accumulating in the cell because of failure of the Na^+/K^+ pump), damaging its internal structure; calcium floods into the cell and apoptosis is activated.

Hypoxia in the brain can be caused by obstruction of a blood vessel, usually by atherosclerosis, thrombosis, or embolism. It may also occur because of low perfusion pressures (e.g., hypotension secondary to developing shock or haemorrhage). It can also be caused by anaemia, when the blood flow may be normal but oxygen levels in the blood are low.

Haemorrhagic injury

Bleeding into the brain disrupts blood flow to distal tissue, triggers an inflammatory response and causes mechanical injury caused by the mass of the clotting blood (the haematoma) at the site of the bleed. The breakdown of erythrocytes and release of their contents into the brain triggers an inflammatory response that injures neurones and increases the permeability of local blood vessels. This reduces the efficiency of the blood-brain barrier and causes oedema and the entry of bloodborne substances and cells normally excluded from the brain, worsening the inflammatory response. Peripheral immune cells, especially neutrophils, infiltrate the site of damage and release their inflammatory mediators, which worsens the brain injury. Haem and iron, released from haemoglobin breakdown, are themselves directly neurotoxic. The developing haematoma causes mechanical injury, compressing adjacent brain tissue and compromising blood supply. It may displace brain tissue (herniation) and increase intracranial pressure.

Risk factors for cerebrovascular disease

Many risk factors for cerebrovascular disease are the same as for vascular disease in general (see Chapter 7). They include hypertension, diabetes, hyperlipidaemia, atherosclerosis, obesity, smoking, and increasing age. Hypertension is particularly important because it predisposes to atheroma of the cerebral arteries, which weakens, roughens, and narrows them, increasing the likelihood of thrombosis and rupture. Intracerebral haemorrhage is more common in people on anticoagulant medication. Vascular abnormalities within the brain (e.g., berry aneurysms) also increase the risk of an intracranial bleed. Head injury and trauma may interfere with blood supply to the brain, causing ischaemia. Conditions that predispose to thrombus formation (e.g., mitral valve disease or atrial fibrillation) can generate travelling emboli that may partially or completely block cerebral blood vessels. Myocardial infarction increases the risk of thromboembolic stroke because it increases the risk of clot formation within the heart.

STROKE

The term *stroke*, or *cerebrovascular accident* (CVA), means death of brain tissue after disruption of its blood supply. World Stroke Organisation statistics (2022) indicate that, worldwide, stroke is the second commonest cause of death and the third commonest cause of disability, and that the incidence of stroke is declining in high-income countries, presumably as a result of improved health education and the adoption of healthier lifestyles, whereas in low- and middle-income countries the rates are steadily rising.

The pathogenesis of stroke may be ischaemic or haemorrhagic. About 80% of strokes are caused by cerebral infarction because brain tissue dies as a result of gradually developing cerebrovascular disease or a sudden blockage of a cerebral vessel because of thrombosis or embolism. The remaining 20% are caused by haemorrhage, either subarachnoid or intracerebral (within the brain itself). The signs and symptoms of stroke depend on the area of brain damaged, which in turn depends on the blood vessel affected (Fig. 8.28 and Fig. 8.3).

Ischaemic stroke

Most ischaemic strokes occur because of disease of the **middle cerebral artery**. Middle cerebral artery strokes affect motor and sensory areas of the frontal, temporal, and parietal lobes including the motor speech area (which is found in the dominant hemisphere only). The next most commonly affected is the anterior cerebral artery. Anterior cerebral artery strokes affect the frontal lobes, the regions of the brain controlling rational and logical thought, personality, and other higher functions. The motor cortex is also found in the frontal lobes, and a stroke affecting this area causes weakness or paralysis in the limbs of the side opposite to the affected lobe. The posterior cerebral artery supplies the occipital and parietal lobes, including the visual cortex and stroke affecting this artery can involve significant visual defects.

About 20% of ischaemic strokes affect the **lenticulostriate arteries**, branches of the anterior and middle cerebral arteries that are very susceptible to developing atherosclerosis as a consequence of hypertension. These vessels supply deep structures in the brain, including the basal ganglia, and strokes here can cause facial drooping, sensory and motor loss, confusion and memory loss and problems with producing and understanding speech.

Transient ischaemic attack (TIA)
These episodes are caused by temporary reductions in blood flow to part of the brain. The symptoms are similar to those of a stroke but resolve quickly. TIAs indicate cerebrovascular disease and are highly predictive of stroke.

Signs and symptoms
The signs and symptoms depend on the location and extent of the injury but commonly include paralysis, usually of body parts on one side only (hemiparesis), and sensory deficits, again usually on one side only. There may be loss of speech, visual disturbances, facial asymmetry, and reduced level of consciousness.

Management and prognosis
If the stroke is not immediately fatal, some recovery of function may be possible, but this depends partly on how quickly the stroke is diagnosed and appropriate treatment e.g., thrombolytic therapy is commenced. Generally, the more extensive the area of brain affected, the poorer the prognosis, although this does not always hold true; for example, although brainstem strokes are rare, even small infarctions can be fatal because of the key life-support function of this part of the brain. Other factors predisposing to a poorer outcome include increased age and pre-existing chronic

conditions such as diabetes and heart disease. Most people post-stroke are left with some residual deficits, which may be relatively minor, but that may also be so severe as to require constant care and support. Onset of seizures occurs in a significant number of post-stroke patients.

INTRACRANIAL HAEMORRHAGE
Brain haemorrhage may occur within the brain itself, or between the surface of the brain and the skull. It can be spontaneous, or secondary to trauma, and if it causes death of neurones it can cause stroke. Bleeding between the dura mater and the internal surface of the skull (epidural haemorrhage) or between the dura mater and the arachnoid mater (subdural haemorrhage) are usually caused by head trauma. Subarachnoid haemorrhage is bleeding into the subarachnoid space between the arachnoid and pia maters (Fig. 8.29).

Subarachnoid haemorrhage
This may be caused by blood forcing its way through from a bleeding area deeper in the brain into the subarachnoid space, or from skull trauma, but it is usually caused by rupture of a cerebral artery aneurysm (see Fig. 6.35). Most aneurysms arise in the internal carotid artery close to its junction with the circulus arteriosus, and at points where the large anterior cerebral arteries branch into smaller arteries. At branching points, blood turbulence and the risk of arterial wall damage are highest. Risk factors for aneurysm rupture include increasing age, hypertension (including hypertension of pregnancy), family history of cerebrovascular disease, and the presence of atherosclerosis. Half of patients present with sudden, agonising ('thunderclap') headache

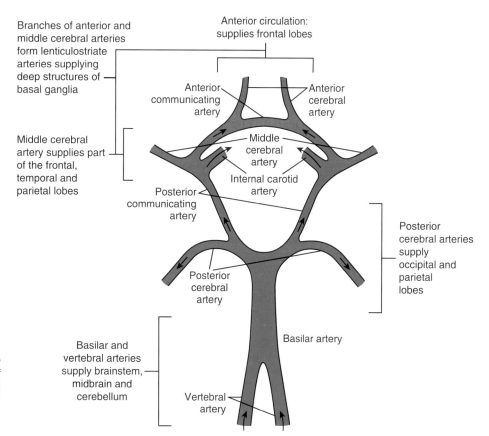

Fig. 8.28 The arterial blood supply to the brain. Arrows indicate direction of blood flow. (Modified from Hines RL and Jones SB (2022) *Stoelting's anesthesia and co-existing disease*, 8th ed, Fig. 12.8. Philadelphia: Elsevier Inc.)

Branches of anterior and middle cerebral arteries form lenticulostriate arteries supplying deep structures of basal ganglia

Anterior circulation: supplies frontal lobes

Anterior communicating artery

Anterior cerebral artery

Middle cerebral artery

Internal carotid artery

Middle cerebral artery supplies part of the frontal, temporal and parietal lobes

Posterior communicating artery

Posterior cerebral arteries supply occipital and parietal lobes

Posterior cerebral artery

Basilar artery

Basilar and vertebral arteries supply brainstem, midbrain and cerebellum

Vertebral artery

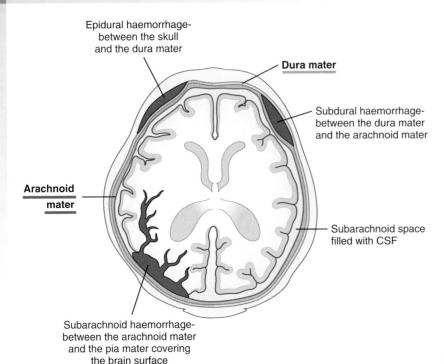

Epidural haemorrhage-
between the skull
and the dura mater

Dura mater

Subdural haemorrhage-
between the dura mater
and the arachnoid mater

Arachnoid
mater

Subarachnoid space
filled with CSF

Subarachnoid haemorrhage-
between the arachnoid mater
and the pia mater covering
the brain surface

Fig. 8.29   Sites of cerebral haemorrhage.

because blood in the CSF irritates the meninges, and up to 45% may lose consciousness at the time of the bleed. The accumulating blood increases intracranial pressure. Meningeal irritation causes neck and back pain, and there may be loss of or impaired vision, seizures, and photophobia. With hindsight, many patients report having experienced what are called *prodromal signs and symptoms*; that is, they may have had headaches, visual disturbances, dizziness, and other events preceding the actual haemorrhage, possibly caused by the aneurysm leaking a little or, as it expanded, pressure on adjacent nerve tissue. Prognosis is variable: many patients die almost immediately after the haemorrhage, and up to 40% may die in the 4 weeks post-haemorrhage. Long-term neurological deficit is extremely common in survivors.

CONGENITAL AND DEVELOPMENTAL DISORDERS

Abnormalities of brain and spinal cord development during intrauterine life are often incompatible with life, and others cause irreversible neurological deficits in surviving children.

NEURAL TUBE DEFECT (NTD)

This group of congenital abnormalities occurs during embryogenesis and can affect the spine or brain. By about 18 days after conception, the developing embryo is made up of three so-called *germ layers*: the **ectoderm**, the **mesoderm**, and the **endoderm**, and each germ layer progresses through embryogenesis and fetal development to produce specific cells and tissues of the growing baby. The nervous system develops from a flattened plate of cells in the ectoderm called the **neural plate** (Fig. 8.30). At about 26 to 29 days of gestation, the neural plate folds down into the mesoderm below, forming a tube called the *neural tube*. This process is called **neurulation**. Within this tube, the brain and spinal cord and the bones of the skull and cranium will differentiate and develop under the tight control of a complex and integrated sequence of growth factors and developmental

processes. If sealing of the tube is not complete somewhere along its length, it leaves a gap in the coverings of the brain or the spinal cord, a defect called a *neural tube defect* (NTD). This disrupts the tightly controlled developmental environment necessary for correct neurological development, usually with permanent consequences in surviving children. In some forms of NTD, the neural tissue and its membranes are exposed; in others, skin has developed over the defect. The most significant defects are lethal, and most babies born with any degree of NTD will have permanent disability. Globally, NTDs are the commonest form of congenital CNS malformations, and mainly involve the spinal cord. In some countries (e.g., the United States), the incidence is falling, but it is higher in other countries, including northern China and the UK. NTDs are usually discovered during prenatal screening.

Risk factors for NTD
The main maternal risk factors for having a baby with an NTD are folate and vitamin B_{12} deficiency, smoking, diabetes, obesity, and some anti-epileptic drugs. Additionally, a pregnancy history of previous NTD babies increases risk, suggesting a genetic contribution. Dietary supplementation with folic acid has reduced the incidence of NTD in many countries. Body cells need folic acid and vitamin B_{12} to synthesise proteins and purines, essential building blocks of DNA and production of proteins, myelin, and lipids. Deficiency of either vitamin significantly disrupts cell function. These key biochemical roles are presumed to be at least part of the explanation as to why their deficiency in pregnancy increases the risk of NTD. However, many women who have babies affected by an NTD have normal serum folate and/or B_{12} levels, so there must be other contributory factors. It is believed that in women whose serum vitamin levels are normal, there are faults in the metabolic pathways that process them, so that even with adequate vitamins available, the cell cannot use them properly. Deficiencies in genes that

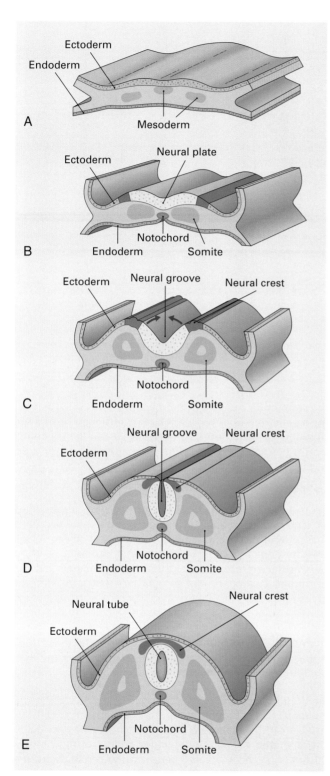

Fig. 8.30 Development of the neural tube. (From Ellison D, Love S, Chimelli LMC, Harding B, Lowe J, and Vinters HV (2004) *Neuropathology*, 2nd ed. Oxford: Elsevier Ltd.)

code for enzymes important in folate/vitamin B_{12} metabolism have been linked to NTD, supporting this idea.

Anencephaly

In this form of NTD, the cranium and much of the brain fail to form, with devastating effects; the baby dies in the womb or shortly after birth (Fig. 8.31). Because the neural tube at the cranial end has not fused properly, the developing brain is not safely enclosed in the neural tube but is instead bathed in the amniotic fluid filling the uterus and cannot develop properly.

Encephalocele

This is a defect in the skull bones, allowing the meninges with or without brain tissue to herniate through it. It usually occurs in the midline, and usually involves the occipital bone, but it can occur anywhere between the occiput and the nose.

Spina bifida

This condition results from failure of the neural tube to fuse somewhere along the spinal column. If the defect is minor and not apparent on inspection, it is called **spina bifida occulta** or *closed spina bifida*; it may be that neurological development of the spinal cord has proceeded adequately, and there are no symptoms. If there is a gap in the vertebral column, and only the meninges are protruding through, it is called a *meningocele*; if there is spinal cord (neural) tissue in there as well, it is called a *myelomeningocele* (Fig. 8.32). Neural tissue in a myelomeningocele is dysfunctional because it did not develop within the closed neural tube, and the neurological difficulties suffered by the child relates to the level of the spinal cord where the defect is located. Most children will be unable to develop bowel or bladder control, and the bladder becomes contracted because of lack of neural control. This in turn increases the pressure inside the bladder, which is transmitted up the ureters to the kidneys and may cause infection, hydronephrosis, and renal failure. Control and sensation in the lower limbs may be abnormal, so the child may develop contractures and need to use a wheelchair. Hydrocephalus is relatively common, because of obstruction in the flow of CSF. Provided this is treated, most people with spina bifida are of normal intelligence.

CEREBRAL PALSY (CP)

This is a collection of disabilities featuring motor and movement impairments. It is the commonest cause of childhood disability and occurs in all races and all countries. CP is caused by injury to the developing brain, either during uterine development or in early childhood, and a wide range of insults can interfere with brain development and lead to CP (Box 8.4). Because neuronal development is an extended process and is still ongoing in early childhood, the timing of the causative insult determines the nature of the disability, and the clinical presentation can be very varied. If the corticospinal motor tracts are affected, there is impaired motor control, increased motor tone, scoliosis (Fig. 13.17), and contractures. If the basal ganglia, thalamus, or cerebellum are involved, there are problems with voluntary muscle movement and increased muscle tone, fine motor control, balance, and walking. Other common features of CP include seizures, visual and hearing impairment, impaired intellectual development and function, and difficulties with speech and language.

The degree of disability varies hugely. Some people attain independent living and have life expectancy approaching normal. As the degree of disability increases, support requirements increase, mobility decreases, and life expectancy tends to reduce.

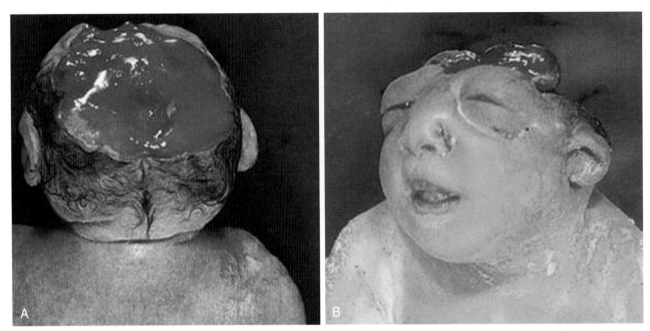

Fig. 8.31   Anencephaly. The brain and cranial vault have failed to develop; the cranial cavity is completely open because the cranial bones are absent. **(A) Posterior view. (B) Anterior view.** (From Volpe J, Inder T, Darras B, de V L, du Plessis A, Neil J, and Perlman J (2018) *Volpe's neurology of the newborn*, 6th ed, Fig. 1.3. Philadelphia: Elsevier Inc.)

HEADACHE SYNDROMES

Headache is a common experience in the general population; everyone has headaches now and again. Some conditions are associated with repeated headache, often severe, that may be incapacitating.

TENSION HEADACHE

This is the commonest cause of recurring headache. The pain is mild to moderate in intensity, usually bilateral, described as squeezing or tightening in the head and does not worsen with exercise. It can be associated with increased tension in the neck and scalp muscles, generating continuous nervous input into the brain from these tissues. With time, the brain begins to misinterpret this constant stream of signals as pain: this is an example of central sensitisation (p. 236) and increases the frequency and intensity of the headaches. A link has also been made between chronic stress and chronic tension headache. Excess cortisol release in chronic stress causes permanent changes in areas of the brain, including the hippocampus, which may sensitise the brain to incoming sensory information and lead to increased perception of pain.

CLUSTER HEADACHE

Cluster headaches, as the name suggests, occur repeatedly over a period of time, sometimes several weeks, with long periods of headache-free remission in between. The headaches are severe, occur on one side of the head, tend to last between 15 minutes to two to 3 hours, and can be as frequent as eight times a day. Along with the headache, other signs and symptoms on the affected side only include eyelid swelling or drooping, sweating, nasal congestion and runny nose, miosis and watering of the eye. The disorder appears to be caused by a fault in the posterior hypothalamus, and the regularity of the attacks suggests some dysfunction of one of the circadian clock systems of the body, controlled by the supraoptic chiasma in the hypothalamus. The underlying mechanism however is not known, although central sensitisation involving input from the facial and the trigeminal nerves has been reported. For most sufferers, the disorder persists throughout life.

MIGRAINE

Globally, this common headache disorder has a prevalence of 10%. White people have higher rates than people of African and Asian extraction and there is a strong female preponderance, except in prepubertal children, in whom boys are more often affected than girls. It is believed that hormonal factors account for the fact that most sufferers are females of reproductive age. There is a strong genetic predisposition, and a wide range of triggers, including fatigue, hormonal changes (including the normal fluctuations of the menstrual cycle), stress, and some drugs (e.g., nitrates, ranitidine, histamine). An individual susceptible to migraine is called an **migraineur**.

Signs and symptoms

In about 60% of sufferers, the headache is preceded by a **prodromal (premonitory) phase**, which may be days before the migraine begins; they include food cravings, anorexia, lethargy, and increased sensitivity to smells, light, and sounds. About a third of patients then experience an **aura**, a collection of symptoms immediately preceding the headache. Auras are usually visual because they are generated by altered neurological activity in the visual cortex. They include **scotoma**, which is loss of part of the visual field, either as large chunks of peripheral vision or areas within the visual field. Sometimes the areas of vision loss are bordered by a shimmering, glittering, flashing, brightly coloured border. Not all migraineurs experience aura, and aura is not always followed by headache, so it is not likely that aura initiates headache. The headache is severe, unilateral, pulsatile, and

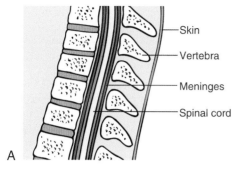

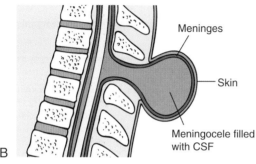

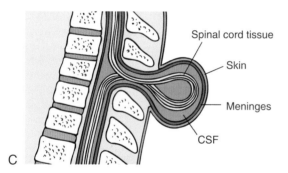

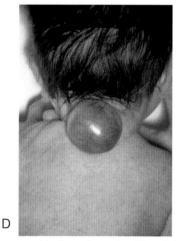

Myelomeningocele with an intact sac

Fig. 8.32 Spinal defects. (A) Normal spinal structure. (B) Meningocele. (C) Myelomeningocele. (D) Spina bifida. (Modified from (A–C) McCance K, and Huether S (2015) *Pathophysiology*, 7th ed, Fig. 20.6. St. Louis: Mosby; and (D) St Bartholomew Hospital/Science Photo Library.)

BOX 8.4 Causes of cerebral palsy

Maternal factors in pregnancy	Poor nutrition
	Anaemia that reduces oxygen levels in maternal blood
	Maternal illness or infection (e.g., rubella, cytomegalovirus)
	Placental bleeding or placental failure that restricts oxygen supply to the fetus
	Twin/multiple pregnancy
	Metabolic abnormalities (e.g., hypoglycaemia, electrolyte imbalances)
	Hypothyroidism
	Seizures
	Hypertension
Birth factors	Fetal hypoxia
	Mechanical injury to the baby during birth
	The use of drugs (e.g., analgesics, anaesthetics, during birth)
Factors in early childhood	Infection (e.g., meningitis)
	Head injury
	Exposure to neurotoxins (e.g., lead or mercury)

---

post-dromal phase, with fatigue and reduced ability to concentrate follows (Fig. 8.33).

Pathophysiology
The disorder is complex and the underlying abnormalities incompletely understood. Various theories have been proposed. It has been shown that the cerebral cortex of migraineurs is hyperexcitable compared with non-migraineurs, even between attacks, contributing to the increased susceptibility to migraine. Currently, it is thought that the primary causative abnormality is neurological, and that this causes changes in cerebral blood flow that cause the headache.

In the prodromal phase, and during the headache itself, there are changes in activity in the neuronal circuits of the hypothalamus and pathways linking the thalamus and the cortex. This is linked to the abnormal sensory processing associated with migraine. However, migraine involves changes in neuronal connectivity between multiple brain areas, reflecting the wide range of neurological abnormalities experienced before and during a migraine attack. Aura is associated with a phenomenon called cortical spreading depolarisation (formerly called cortical spreading depression), a wave of depolarisation that spreads steadily at a rate of 2 to 3 mm/min across the cerebral cortex in response to some neurological injury (Fig. 8.34). The advancing wavefront is associated with significant increase in blood flow and massive disruption of ion balance across nerve cell membranes. Unable to control sodium and potassium movement across their membranes, nerves lose function and their activity is depressed. Neurones behind the spreading wavefront swell because of accumulation of intracellular sodium and ischaemic because blood vessels constrict. This may also contribute to migraine pain. Cortical spreading depolarisation is not exclusive to migraine; this phenomenon is also seen in other brain disorders, including epilepsy and traumatic brain injury. The headache phase of migraine has been linked to increased activity in the pons.

---

worsened by physical activity. There is often photophobia and phonophobia (noise intolerance), nausea and vomiting, and sometimes aphasia, confusion, sensory changes such as numbness or tingling, or even temporary paralysis. A

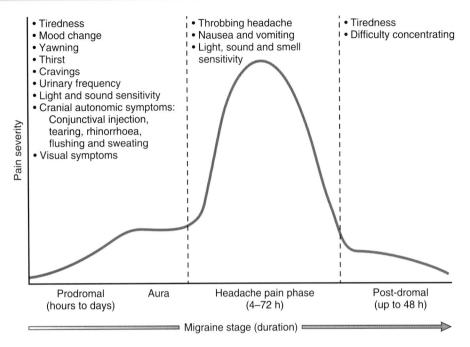

• Tiredness
• Mood change
• Yawning
• Thirst
• Cravings
• Urinary frequency
• Light and sound sensitivity
• Cranial autonomic symptoms:
  Conjunctival injection,
  tearing, rhinorrhoea,
  flushing and sweating
• Visual symptoms

• Throbbing headache
• Nausea and vomiting
• Light, sound and smell
  sensitivity

• Tiredness
• Difficulty concentrating

Pain severity

Prodromal
(hours to days)   Aura   Headache pain phase
                               (4–72 h)

Post-dromal
(up to 48 h)

Migraine stage (duration)

Fig. 8.33 The stages of a migraine episode. (Modified from Karsan N and Goadsby PJ (2018) Biological insights from the premonitory symptoms of migraine, *Nat Rev Neurol* 14(12): 699–710.)

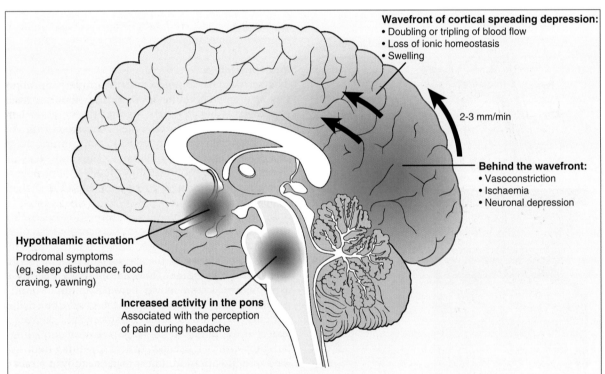

Wavefront of cortical spreading depression:
• Doubling or tripling of blood flow
• Loss of ionic homeostasis
• Swelling

2-3 mm/min

Behind the wavefront:
• Vasoconstriction
• Ischaemia
• Neuronal depression

Hypothalamic activation
Prodromal symptoms
(eg, sleep disturbance, food
craving, yawning)

Increased activity in the pons
Associated with the perception
of pain during headache

Fig. 8.34 Changes in the brain associated with migraine. Reprinted with permission from Elsevier (Ashina M, Terwindt GM, Al-Karagholi MAI-M et al. Migraine: disease characterisation, biomarkers, and precision medicine. *The Lancet.* 2021; 397(10283):1496-1504).

The pain of migraine may be caused by a combination of factors. Central sensitisation leads to misinterpretation of incoming sensory information as painful stimuli (recall the cerebral cortex is hypersensitive in migraine sufferers) and in addition the processing of sensory signals in key areas of the brain associated with pain, including the thalamus, is abnormal. The soup of neuropeptides released as a result of neuronal dysfunction triggers inflammation and vasodilation in the meninges, which also causes pain. One such neuropeptide, calcitonin gene-related peptide (CGRP),

has recently been widely studied because administration of CGRP in migraine-susceptible people induces migraine, and drugs that block its action show promise as anti-migraine treatments.

Management and prognosis

Avoidance of known triggers is an important part of management. Rest and sleep in a dark room can help a sufferer through an attack. Drug treatment is of variable efficacy and varies between individuals. Anti-emetics can relieve vomiting and non-steroidal anti-inflammatories can reduce pain. Serotonin receptor agonists, the triptans, are useful in some people; serotonin causes vasoconstriction, reducing meningeal inflammation. However, regular use of anti-migraine medications can make the migraines worse and more frequent. Migraine sufferers are at increased risk of stroke, seizures, and depression.

PERIPHERAL NERVOUS SYSTEM PATHOPHYSIOLOGY

The main pathologies of the peripheral nervous system (PNS) are caused by damage to any of the functional parts of peripheral nerves—the axon and its myelin sheath and the cell body—and of the neuromuscular junction.

PERIPHERAL NEUROPATHY

The umbrella term **peripheral neuropathy** refers to dysfunction or disease of peripheral nerves and can affect motor nerves, sensory nerves, or both. The commonest cause of peripheral neuropathy is diabetes mellitus. Peripheral neuropathy may affect a specific nerve (**mononeuropathy**) or multiple nerves (**polyneuropathy**). A range of insults and disorders can cause polyneuropathy, including alcohol dependence (which mainly affects sensory nerves), toxins such as lead, some drugs (e.g., phenytoin), and vitamin B_1, B_6, and B_{12} deficiencies. Polyneuropathy may occur in cancer because of infiltration of nervous tissue by cancer cells, the toxic effects of tumour-released factors, and the cytotoxic effects of radiation and drug therapies.

CARPAL TUNNEL SYNDROME

The carpal tunnel is formed by the ligament called the *flexor retinaculum*, which crosses the anterior aspect of the wrist, attaching the pisiform and the hamate bones on the medial side to the trapezium and scaphoid bones on the lateral side (Fig. 8.35A). The median nerve and nine flexor tendons that operate the hand pass through the narrow bony channel formed by this arrangement. Narrowing of the channel can compress and damage the median nerve. It has both sensory and motor functions, so symptoms include numbness, tingling, pain, loss of strength, and reduced motor control in the thumb and first four fingers (Fig. 8.35B). Subjecting the hand and wrist to long-term repetitive movements, or regular vibration or excessive force, as in hammering, is an important risk factor. Others include increasing age, female sex, hand/wrist deformity, hypothyroidism, arthritis, fracture or dislocation of the wrist, diabetes, and pregnancy.

GUILLAIN-BARRÉ SYNDROME

This inflammatory polyneuropathy involves loss of the myelin sheath of affected nerves with progressive loss of function. It is present in all racial groups and seen at all ages, although there is a peak in youth and a second peak in older age. Its incidence is between 1 and 3 in every 100,000 people, with males being at slightly higher risk than females.

Pathophysiology
Guillain-Barré syndrome usually occurs after an infection, and the inflammatory process causing the polyneuropathy

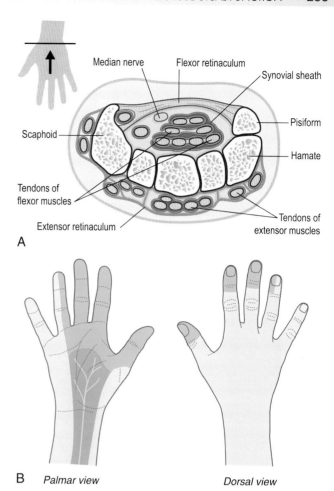

Fig. 8.35 The carpal tunnel. (A) Transverse section showing the median nerve and flexor tendons in the wrist. (B) The areas of the hand served by the median nerve. (From (A) Waugh A and Grant A (2018) *Ross & Wilson anatomy and physiology in health and illness*, 13th ed, Fig. 16.52. Oxford: Elsevier Ltd.; and (B) Drake R, Vogl AW, Mitchell A (2020) *Gray's anatomy for students*, 4th ed, Fig. 7.114. Philadelphia: Elsevier Inc.)

is immunologically mediated. The preceding infection is usually respiratory or gastrointestinal. Causative organisms include *Campylobacter jejuni*, cytomegalovirus, Epstein-Barr virus, *Mycoplasma pneumoniae*, and varicella zoster, but a wide range of pathogens can trigger it. It is thought that these organisms possess lipopolysaccharide antigens that resemble a component of myelin closely enough that the immune cells and antibodies produced to combat the infection also attack the myelin of nerve cells. This is called **molecular mimicry** and is seen in other post-infective immunological disorders, for example, rheumatic heart disease after streptococcal infection. In the process, autoreactive T- and B-lymphocytes infiltrate peripheral nerve tissues, macrophages are activated and myelin is stripped from peripheral axons. This impedes or completely eliminates conduction of action potentials, leading to reduced or abolished nerve function.

Signs and symptoms
The main manifestations are symmetrical weakness or paralysis of skeletal muscle, which generally spreads from the lower extremities upwards. If it involves the respiratory muscles, it can be life threatening and may require ventilatory

support. The onset of weakness is sudden and develops over a period of 2 to 4 weeks. If there is cranial nerve involvement (seen in up to three-quarters of people), there may be facial droop, paralysis of the oculomotor muscles, diplopia, and a loss of normal pupillary function. There are usually sensory changes, including numbness and paraesthesia, which may actually precede the onset of muscle weakness.

Prognosis and management

Most people recover fully within a few weeks or months. The condition can kill, if the respiratory muscles are compromised, and the most seriously affected survivors can take years to recover and may be left with some residual deficit. Supportive treatments including physiotherapy, speech therapy, and occupational therapy aid recovery. During the acute phase of the illness, glucocorticoids are used to reduce the inflammation, and immunotherapy, for example plasma exchange to remove autoantibodies, can also be used.

MYASTHENIA GRAVIS

In this autoimmune condition, autoantibodies destroy the ability of skeletal muscle to respond to motor nerve activity at the neuromuscular junction (p. 328).

CRANIAL NERVE SYNDROMES

Damage to individual cranial nerves as part of wider syndromes (e.g., Guillain-Barré syndrome), leads to specific motor and/or sensory signs and symptoms associated with the distribution of that nerve. Some conditions affect individual cranial nerves, giving well-defined disease entities.

TRIGEMINAL NEURALGIA

This condition is characterised by attacks of severe, knife-like pain in the structures supplied by the trigeminal nerve (cranial nerve V): the upper and lower jaw— and sometimes the eye. It is usually one-sided because the cause is usually compression of the nerve root where it enters the pons. The usual cause of compression is an abnormal, expanded blood vessel loop. This compression irritates and inflames the nerve and causes demyelination. Hypertension, which damages blood vessels, is therefore an important risk factor. Other causes of trigeminal neuralgia include multiple sclerosis and sarcoidosis affecting the trigeminal nerve, and tumours compressing the nerve. Some cases are idiopathic. Pain is provoked by multiple, often trivial, triggers such as chewing, shaving or cold air. The condition tends to become more severe with time, with attacks becoming more severe and remission periods between attacks shorter. The condition is treated with anticonvulsant drugs, which carry significant risk of side effects.

BELL PALSY

This condition is caused by damage to the facial nerve (cranial nerve VII). The precise reason for this is unknown, but it may be caused by compression of the nerve in the facial canal, a very narrow (0.66 mm) tunnel in the temporal bone of the skull through which the facial nerve travels on its way to supply the tissues of the face. The nerve becomes swollen, probably secondary to a viral infection (e.g., herpes simplex), which compresses it within the narrow confines of the facial canal. This further irritates and inflames the nerve, leading to demyelination and nerve injury. It causes sudden, unilateral facial paralysis, with facial drooping, visual impairment, reduced tear production, pain in the eye and ear area and taste disturbances. Most people, especially younger people, recover fully but some experience deeper and more prolonged paralysis and do not regain full neurological function. The disorder occurs in all populations, with an average incidence of 15 to 30 cases per 100,000 population, but risk is higher in diabetic and immunocompromised people, in young women, and in older age. It usually resolves completely within 3 to 6 months.

PAIN

The International Association for the Study of Pain defines pain as 'an unpleasant sensory and emotional experience associated with actual or potential tissue damage, or described in terms of such damage'. It is a subjective experience, influenced significantly by emotional states, psychological factors, social conditioning, and cultural expectations, and can be very difficult to assess accurately. Pain is usually an important protective mechanism; it alerts the individual to actual or possible tissue damage and encourages behaviours that protect injured body parts and promote healing.

CLASSIFICATION OF PAIN

Pain can be described in terms of its origin (neuropathic or nociceptive) or its duration (acute or chronic).

Neuropathic and nociceptive pain

Neuropathic (neurogenic) pain originates from damaged or dysfunctional nervous tissue (e.g., diabetic neuropathy, phantom limb pain, or nerve entrapment). **Nociceptive pain** is caused by stimulation of pain receptors (nociceptors) in tissues and so is usually associated with tissue injury (e.g., osteoarthritis, myocardial infarction, or bone fracture). Some conditions are associated with both (mixed pain, e.g., in malignancy, when the expanding tumour invades local nerves and local tissues).

Neuropathic pain

Neuropathic pain is one of the so-called *positive symptoms* in neuropathy, that is, those symptoms resulting from abnormal nerve signalling because of the neuropathic condition. Others include **paraesthesias** (abnormal unprovoked sensation) and **dysaesthesias** (unpleasant but not painful abnormal sensations). Neuropathic pain is characteristically constant and spontaneous (i.e., not triggered by a specific stimulus) and may be described as shooting, electric, burning, stabbing, or gnawing.

Phantom limb pain. Removal of a body part (e.g., a hand or the lower leg) may be followed by the person reporting continual, often excruciating, pain from the missing region despite its absence. This is called *phantom limb pain* and is associated with increased excitability and spontaneous firing in the severed sensory nerves that had supplied the absent tissues.

Referred pain. This is pain perceived as originating from a particular area, when in fact its origin is elsewhere. A common example is the pain from a myocardial infarction, which can be referred to the left shoulder, jaw, and left arm, when

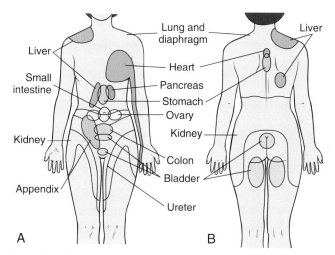

Fig. 8.36 Sites of referred pain. (A) Anterior view. (B) Posterior view. (From Huether S and McCance K (2020) *Understanding pathophysiology*, 7th ed, Fig. 15.3. St Louis: Elsevier Inc.)

in fact the injured tissue is in the heart. The reason pain is referred is that the sensory input from the injured tissue travels along nerve pathways that merge with sensory nerves from other body regions on their route into the central nervous system, and the brain cannot distinguish with complete accuracy the precise origin of the pain signal. Fig. 8.36 shows the areas to which pain from some body organs is referred.

Nociceptive pain

Nociceptors are unmyelinated free nerve endings that respond to stimuli strong enough to cause tissue damage, including trauma, extremes of temperature, and corrosive chemicals. Most are polymodal, meaning they respond to different kinds of potentially damaging stimuli. They also respond to endogenous agents, including inflammatory mediators such as bradykinin and prostaglandins. Nociceptor density varies greatly in different body areas. The skin is particularly rich in nociceptors, as are the cornea, musculature, joint capsules, and the periosteum covering bone. Most body organs also possess nociceptors. **Visceral pain** originates in body organs and the linings and coverings of organs and cavities and is less well localised than **somatic pain**, which originates mainly in skin, connective tissues, and the musculoskeletal system. The two main types of sensory nerves transmitting pain signals (and also thermal information) to the brain after nociceptor activation are **Aδ fibres** and **C fibres**. Aδ fibres are large diameter (2–5 μm), myelinated nerves that conduct action potentials at speeds between 12 to 30 m/sec. They transmit sharp, fast, well-localised pain information and are important in the withdrawal reflex when a body part is quickly pulled away from a painful stimulus. C fibres are smaller diameter (0.4–1.3 μm), non-myelinated fibres that conduct more slowly (0.5–3 m/sec) and are associated with poorly localised, diffuse, often chronic pain.

Acute and chronic pain

Acute pain is usually associated with tissue damage and resolves with healing. It is generally accepted to be a useful, if unpleasant, aspect of healing, signalling the need to protect a vulnerable body part. It is usually well localised,

proportional to the degree of injury, and often described as stabbing, aching, sharp, or twisting.

Chronic pain, on the other hand, persists beyond normal healing time and has no apparent biologic value. It is common and can have drastic psychological consequences, with significant distress and disruption of quality of life. It is usually poorly localised and notoriously difficult to manage with conventional pain management approaches. It is associated with physiological changes, including long-term sensitisation of pain pathways, abnormal processing of pain signals in the brain, and a loss of pain inhibition mechanisms. It can cause major physical, social, and psychological disruption; it tends to reduce physical activity, interfere with sleep, and cause significant stress, fear, anxiety, depression, and anger. Many of these are self-perpetuating and the individual may enter a cycle of negative behaviours and a downwardly spiralling loss of confidence, social withdrawal, and deteriorating mental and physical health.

PAIN TRANSMISSION

Activated nociceptors transmit pain signals to the spinal cord via Aδ and C fibres, from where the signal is sent up to the brain, where it activates a number of key centres important in processing the signal and determining the body's response. The chain of nerves that carry pain messages from the periphery to the brain is shown in Fig. 8.37.

Sensory (afferent) pain pathways

Aδ and C fibres carrying signals from tissues to the spinal cord are called **primary afferents** or **first order neurones**. The first order neurone enters the spinal cord via the dorsal horn, and synapses with the **second order neurone**, the second nerve in the chain, which crosses to the other side of the spinal cord and from the dorsal horn to the ventral horn, and ascends to the thalamus, located just above the brainstem. The thalamus is an important integrating station that receives incoming information from spinal cord tracts and relays it to higher centres in the brain. From here, **third-order neurones** transmit the pain signal to a range of higher structures, all of which contribute to the experience of pain, the behavioural and emotional responses to the pain, and to modulation of the pain signal. For example, the cerebral cortex is responsible for putting the pain into context e.g., whether or not the pain has been experienced before and making rational decisions about actions or behaviours to be undertaken in response. The amygdala is important in the emotional response to pain, and the hypothalamus is important in autonomic pain responses (e.g., sweating, increased heart rate). The network of pain nerves in the brain, linking the key centres processing and integrating pain information, is extensive and uses a number of neurotransmitters. Substance P, cholecystokinin and glutamate are excitatory neurotransmitters that activate pain-transmitting synapses, whereas endogenous opioids and GABA (gamma-amino butyric acid) are inhibitory neurotransmitters that shut down transmission at pain synapses.

Modulation of pain signals

Pain signals are modulated at multiple sites in the brain and spinal cord, either decreasing or increasing the sensation of pain.

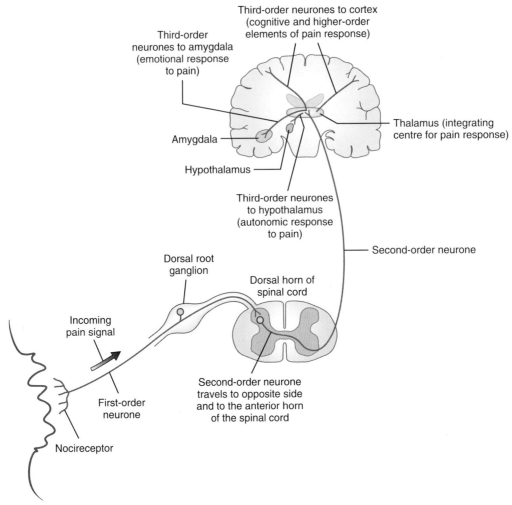

Fig. 8.37 Ascending pain pathways.

Inhibition of pain signals

Pain signals can be blocked at various sites in the brain and spinal cord. These gating mechanisms allow the brain to influence the experience and perception of pain. This can have a significant survival advantage. The American anaesthetist, Henry Beecher, working in the European battlefields of World War II, recorded his observations that severely injured soldiers frequently required significantly less analgesia than would normally be expected, allowing them to function at least temporarily while they withdrew from the battle front and indicating the presence of some sort of internal pain suppression mechanism. In 1965 Melzack and Wall published a paper entitled "Pain Mechanisms: A New Theory", which proposed a mechanism by which transmission of pain signals between the first and second order neurones in the spinal cord may be blocked. They likened this mechanism to a gate, a very user-friendly simile, and the gate control theory remains today a cornerstone in pain research. When the blocking mechanism is operating, synaptic transmission is inhibited and pain signals are not transmitted up the spinal cord: the gate, in other words, is closed. The gate can be closed in a number of ways, including by the brain itself, via a process called **descending inhibition**. In response to ascending pain signals, a region of the midbrain called the periaqueductal grey matter (PAG) activates descending neurones in the spinal cord that send

inhibitory impulses back down the spinal cord to the dorsal horn synapse between the first order and second order neurones bringing the pain signal in from the injured tissues. Here, they release inhibitory neurotransmitters, switch the synapse off, and reduce the ascending neuronal pain traffic (Fig. 8.38). Similar 'gates' also appear to operate in other sites in pain pathways within the brain itself, using a range of inhibitory transmitters to provide significant capacity for internal analgesia. These internal pain inhibition mechanisms may be deactivated in some chronic pain conditions.

Sensitisation

Sensitisation is increased responsiveness of neurones transmitting pain signals either in the central nervous system (**central sensitisation**) or in peripheral nerves (**peripheral sensitisation**). Nerve injury leads to inflammation of the nerve, an important factor in the development of sensitisation, and the glial cells supporting the neurones release inflammatory and immune factors that decrease the stimulus threshold needed to activate the nerve and increase the excitability of the nerve membrane. Sensitisation leads to **hyperalgesia**, in which stimuli trigger disproportionately intense pain, and to **allodynia**, in which non-painful stimuli such as gentle stroking elicit pain. These are both common experiences in damaged or inflamed tissues and are an important part of body defences: the supersensitivity of injured

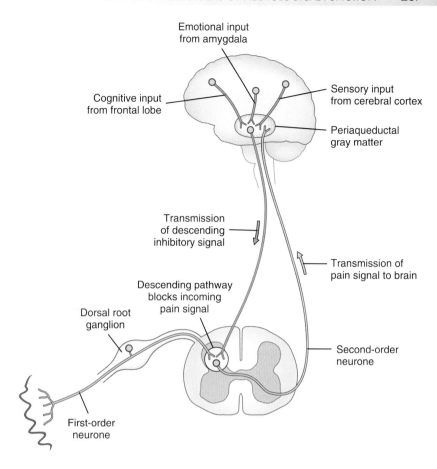

Fig. 8.38   Descending inhibition of pain.

tissue increases the incentive to protect and care for affected body parts. However, long-term abnormally increased sensitivity of central and peripheral nociceptive nerve pathways is a feature of chronic and neuropathic pain, leading to pain amplification and prolongation even when the original painful stimulus has been removed.

BIBLIOGRAPHY AND REFERENCES

Baron, R., Binder, A., & Wasner, G. (2010). Neuropathic pain: Diagnosis, pathophysiological mechanism and treatment. *The Lancet Neurology, 9*, 807–819.

Draoui, E., Hiba, O., Aimrane, A., et al. (2019). Parkinson's disease: From bench to bedside. *Revue Neurologique.* https://doi.org/10.1016/j.neurol.2019.11.002.

Harrison, P. J., Geddes, J. R., & Tunbridge, E. M. (2018). The emerging neurobiology of bipolar disorder. *Trends in Neurosciences, 41*(1). https://doi.org/10.1016/j.tins.2017.10.006.

Kesby, J. P., Eyles, D. W., McGrath, J. J., & Scott, J. G. (2018). Dopamine, psychosis and schizophrenia: The widening gap between basic and clinical neuroscience. *Translational Psychiatry, 8*(3).

Louis, D. N., Perry, A., Reifenberger, G., et al. (2016). The 2016 world health organisation classification of tumours of the central nervous system: A summary. *Acta Neuropathologica, 131*(6), 803–820.

Malhi, G. S., & Mann, J. J. (2018). Depression. *Lancet, 392*, 2299–2312.

Melzack, R., & Wall, P. D. (1965). Pain mechanisms: A new theory. *Science, 150*, 971–979.

Ransohoff, R. M., & Brown, M. A. (2012). Innate immunity in the central nervous system. *Journal of Clinical Investigation, 122*(4), 1164–1171.

Riegelhaupt, P. M., & Angst, M. S. (2019). (2019) Nociceptive physiology. In H. C. Hemmings, & T. D. Egan (Eds.), *Pharmacology and physiology for anesthesia* (2nd ed.) (pp. 311–331). Elsevier.

Stafstrom, C. E., & Carmant, L. (2015). Seizures and epilepsy: An overview for neuroscientists. *Cold Spring Harbor Perspective in Medicine.* https://www.ncbi.nlm.nih.gov/pmc/articles/PMC4448698/pdf/cshperspectmed-BEP-a022426.pdf.

Wallin, M. T., Culpepper, W. J., Nichols, & (GBD 2016 Multiple Sclerosis Collaborators)., et al. (2019). Global, regional and national burden of multiple sclerosis 1990-2016: A systematic analysis for the global burden of disease study 2016. *The Lancet Neurology, 18*(3), 269–285.

Wang, J., Wu, X., Lai, W., et al. (2017). Prevalence of depression and depressive symptoms among outpatients: A systematic review and meta-analysis. *BMJ Open.* https://doi.org/10.1136/bmjopen-2017-017173.

Yenkoyan, K., Grigoryan, A., Fereshetyan, K., & Yepremayan, D. (2017). Advances in understanding the pathophysiology of autism spectrum disorders. *Behavioural Brain Research, 331*, 92–d101.

Useful Websites

Alzheimer's Disease International: https://www.alz.co.uk/

Global, regional and national burden of brain and other CNS cancer, 1990–2016: a systematic analysis for the Global Burden of Disease study 2016 (2019) GBD Brain and Other CNS cancer collaborators, *Lancet Neurol* 18: 379–393. https://doi.org/10.1016/S1474-4422(18)30468-X.

Global , regional and national burden of Alzheimer disease and other dementias, 1990–2106: a systematic analysis for the Global Burden of Disease Study (2016) GBD 2016 Dementia Collaborators *Lancet Neurol* 18(1). https://doi.org/10.1016/S1474-4422(18)30403-4.

Epilepsy Foundation: https://www.epilepsy.com

Parkinson's disease: a great explanation of the neural circuitry and the role of the nigrostriatal pathway: https://www.khanacademy.org/science/health-and-medicine/nervous-system-diseases#parkinsons-disease

Useful website describing sensory and motor pathways: https://open.oregonstate.education/aandp/chapter/14-5-sensory-and-motor-pathways/

Relating signs and symptoms of stroke to the causative blocked vessel: https://www.americannursetoday.com/identify-the-vessel-recognize-the-stroke/

WHO information on stroke: https://www.who.int/bulletin/volumes/94/9/16-181636/en/

WHO information on poliomyelitis: https://www.who.int/news-room/fact-sheets/detail/poliomyelitis

WHO information on Alzheimer disease: https://www.alz.co.uk/research/WorldAlzheimerReport2018.pdf

9

Disorders of the Special Senses

CHAPTER OUTLINE

THE EYE
The normal eye
Glaucoma
Refractive errors of the eye
Disorders of the anterior eye
 Infection and inflammatory conditions
 Cataract
Retinal disorders
 Age-related macular degeneration (AMD)
 Retinal detachment
 Retinoblastoma
 Ocular malignant melanoma

THE EAR
The normal ear
Deafness
 Conductive deafness
 Sensorineural deafness
Ear infections
 Otitis externa
 Otitis media
Inner ear disorders
 Ménière's disease
 Labyrinthitis

The eyes (the organs of sight) and the ears (the organs of hearing and balance) are frequently affected by systemic disorders as well as the organ-specific conditions discussed here, and their function may also be reduced as part of the normal ageing process. Impairment or loss of vision or hearing of any aetiology are life-changing developments.

THE EYE

Vision is the most significant sense. Damage to the eye, or the optic nerve that carries visual input from the eye to the visual cortex in the brain, may be caused by infection, trauma, inflammatory or immunologically mediated processes, chemical injury, neoplastic change, or the ageing process. In addition, a wide range of systemic disorders (e.g., neurofibromatosis, rheumatoid arthritis, migraine, and diabetes) can cause ocular and visual complications.

THE NORMAL EYE

The eyeball sits within a bony orbit, a cavity formed by the bones of the face, which holds the eye and its associated muscles, blood vessels, nerves, and supporting connective tissue. The main structures of the interior of the eye are shown in Fig. 9.1. The outer layer of the eyeball, the **sclera**, is a tough, fibrous coating that supports the eyeball and is continuous with the perineurium (the outer coat) of the optic nerve. Anteriorly, the sclera is seen as the white of the eye, and at the front becomes the clear **cornea**, which allows light to enter the eye. The middle layer, the **uvea**, forms the iris and ciliary body at the front of the eye, and forms the choroid along the lateral and posterior eyeball wall, responsible for nourishing the retina. The inner layer, the **retina**, contains the light-sensitive rods and cones (photoreceptors) that absorb light entering the eye and convert the energy of the light waves into action potentials, to be transmitted to the visual cortex of the brain along the optic nerve (cranial nerve II).

The retina

The healthy retina, seen through an ophthalmoscope, is shown in Fig. 9.2. The area where the optic nerve leaves the eye is clearly visible as the pale optic disc. The network of retinal blood vessels is clearly visible, and evidence of systemic vascular disease (e.g., in hypertension) is often picked up on routine eye examination. Additionally, the macula lutea, containing a cup-shaped depression called the fovea, shows as a more deeply pigmented region on the retina.

The retina contains several types of specialised nerve cells dedicated to receiving light signals, converting them to action potentials, initial processing of the signals and transmitting them to the brain. There are three main layers of nerve cells, collectively called the **neural retina**, lying against a layer of deeply pigmented retinal epithelial cells, whose function is to absorb any photons of light that pass through the photoreceptor layer without being absorbed there (Fig. 9.3A and B). The deepest layer of nerve cells, lying immediately adjacent to the retinal pigmented epithelium, consists of the photoreceptors themselves, the **rods**, and **cones** (Fig. 9.3C). The photoreceptors convert light photons to action potentials, and transmit them to a layer of **bipolar cells**, which in turn activate a layer of **ganglion cells**. Transmission of the signal here is modulated by a layer of interneurons

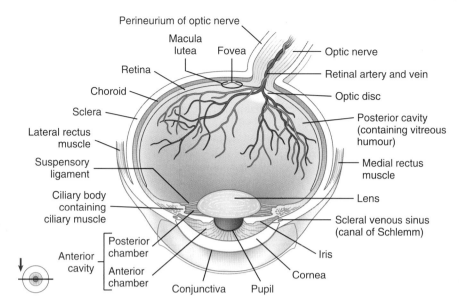

Fig. 9.1 The interior of the eyeball. (Modified from Waugh A and Grant A (2018) *Ross & Wilson anatomy and physiology in health and illness*, 13th ed, Fig. 8.8. Oxford: Elsevier Ltd.)

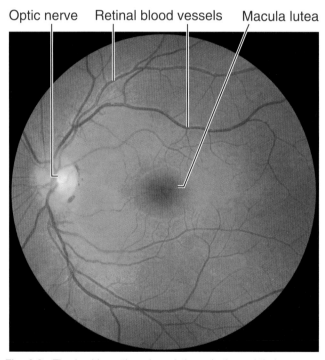

Fig. 9.2 The healthy retina viewed through the ophthalmoscope. (Modified from http://commons.wikimedia.org/wiki/File:Fundus_ photograph_of_normal_right_eye.jpg.)

called **amacrine cells**. The ganglion cells possess long axons that travel across the retinal surface towards the optic disc, where they merge to form the optic nerve.

Rods and cones. Rods are highly sensitive photoreceptors that can function in extremely low light levels, but they do not detect colour. Cones are much less sensitive than rods, so need higher light levels, but give clear, detailed vision and colour discrimination. The distribution of rods and cones around the retina is not even. Cones are concentrated in the fovea (Figs. 9.1 and 9.2), where light from a directly viewed object strikes the retina. This gives sharp, bright colour vision. Light from objects in the field of vision but not being directly looked at strikes the peripheral retina, where rods are more abundant, so their detail and sometimes colour are less distinct. At the optic disc, there are no rods or cones at all because this is where the ganglion cells running along the surface of the retina merge to form the optic nerve.

The lens
This is a flattened, elastic disc made of fibre-shaped cells containing specialised, transparent proteins called **crystallins**, which align themselves within the lens to allow light to pass through the cell without impediment and are also essential for lens elasticity. The lens has no blood vessels, again to prevent obstruction of light. The lens focuses light on the retina. In adults, the lens has an average diameter of about 9 mm and is enclosed in a capsule. Suspensory ligaments attach around the perimeter of the lens capsule like spokes radiating out from the hub of a wheel and anchor the lens behind the iris in the circular space formed by the ring-shaped ciliary body. The ciliary muscle fibres lie circularly in the ciliary body so that the ciliary muscle acts as a sphincter; when it relaxes, the circular space in its centre opens up, pulling on the ligaments and stretching and thinning the lens. When the ciliary muscle contracts, the sphincter closes down, the pull on the ligaments and on the lens is reduced, and the lens bulges. The ability of the lens to bend (refract) light, to ensure sharp and accurate focussing on the retina, is determined by its thickness. Focussing light from close objects requires maximal refraction of light, and the lens must be as thick as possible. For near vision, therefore, the ciliary muscle needs to contract (Fig. 9.4A), explaining why prolonged periods of close work can lead to eye strain and headache. Distance vision is much easier on the eye because the ciliary muscle is relaxed (Fig. 9.4B) The ability of the lens to adjust its focussing power is called **accommodation**.

Intraocular pressure
The shape of the eyeball is maintained by the pressure of the fluids it contains. **Aqueous humour**, an ultrafiltrate of plasma, is continuously produced by the ciliary body and circulates mainly through the anterior cavity of the eye, nourishing the lens and cornea, neither of which have their own blood

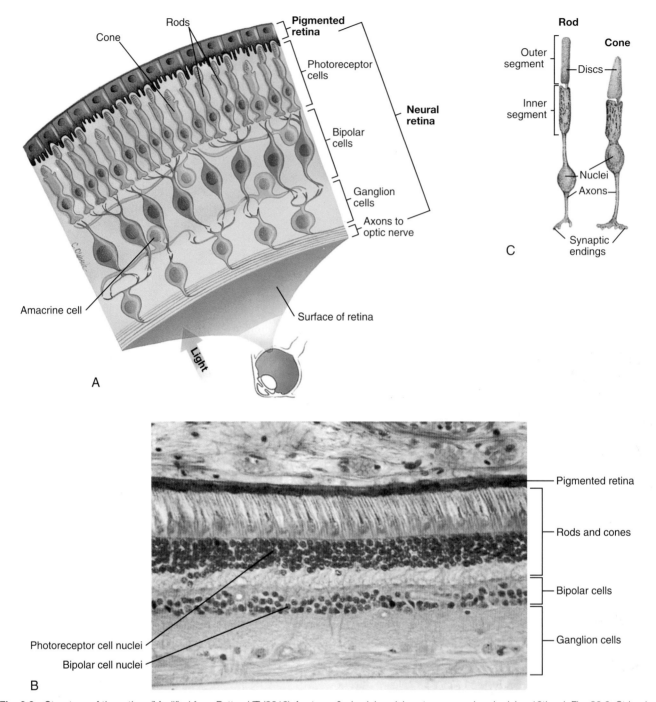

Fig. 9.3 Structure of the retina. (Modified from Patton KT (2019) *Anatomy & physiology laboratory manual and e-labs,* 10th ed, Fig. 30.2. St Louis: Elsevier Inc.)

supply. It drains away through a meshwork of tissue in the angle between the cornea and the iris (the scleral venous sinus or canal of Schlemm; Fig. 9.5A). The posterior cavity is full of a jelly-like substance called **vitreous humour**. Intraocular pressure (IOP) is maintained between 12 and 15 mm Hg. This is an important factor in holding the neural retina against its underlying pigmented epithelium because the cellular attachments between the two layers are weak and they are easily separated (retinal detachment). Rising intraocular pressure is also dangerous and a key contributor to glaucoma.

Floaters. Floaters are specks, ribbons, or patches that move across the field of vision. They are more common in older people because they are usually caused by degenerative changes in the consistency of the vitreous humour, which tends to become more fluid with age. Any particles floating in this more fluid centre cast a shadow on the retina and are perceived as floaters. They are not usually a sign of disease, although if they appear suddenly they may indicate that the vitreous has separated from the retina, or that there is a retinal detachment.

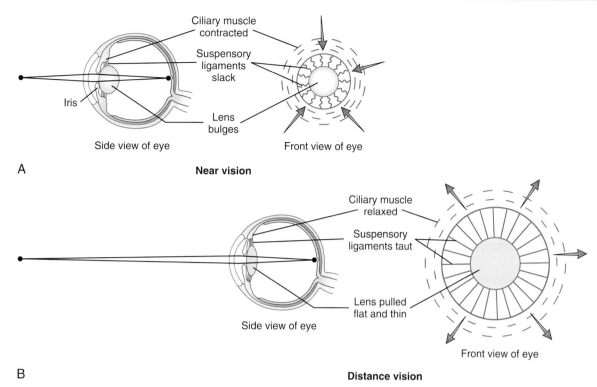

Fig. 9.4 Accommodation of the eye. (A) Distant vision. Light rays from a distant object are parallel as they pass through the pupil and require less refraction to focus on the retina. (B) Near vision. Light rays from a near object are still diverging when they travel through the pupil and require maximal refraction from the lens to focus them on the retina. (Modified from Waugh A and Grant A (2018) *Ross & Wilson anatomy and physiology in health and illness*, 13th ed, Fig. 8.18. Oxford: Elsevier Ltd.)

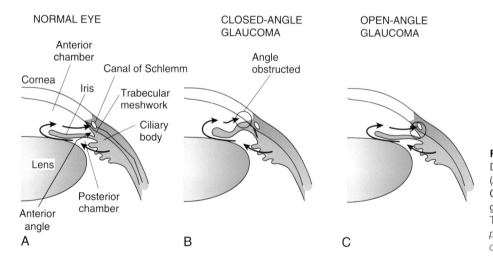

Fig. 9.5 Circulation of aqueous humour. Direction of flow is indicated by arrows. (A) Normal circulation and drainage. (B) Closed-angle glaucoma. (C) Open-angle glaucoma. (Modified from McKenry LM, Tessier E, and Hogan MA (2006) *Mosby's pharmacology in nursing: revised and updated*, 22nd ed, St Louis: Mosby.)

GLAUCOMA

The characteristic event in glaucoma is optic nerve damage. It is usually caused by raised intraocular pressure (IOP), which damages the delicate retinal ganglion cells and the optic nerve, causing blindness. Depending on the aetiology, it may affect one or both eyes. Risk increases with age and in some racial groups (e.g., people of African origin). There are many reasons why IOP may rise.

Closed-angle glaucoma. This refers to obstruction of the angle of the eye, the junction between the iris and the cornea, where aqueous humour drains from the anterior chamber (Fig. 9.5B). The angle can be naturally acute be-cause of the anatomy of the eye; in long-sighted people, for example, the eyeball is relatively short, so the space between the iris and the cornea is more compact than in a longer eyeball. This predisposes one to closed-angle glaucoma. Some racial groups have genetically determined narrower angles than others; for example, people of American Indian origin are at higher risk than American whites. When the pupil is dilated, the iris muscle is thicker around its junction with the cornea, which can cause angle obstruction, especially in older people. Disease processes can also thicken tissues around the iris-corneal junction, narrowing the angle and causing glaucoma; these include infection or haemorrhage.

Open-angle glaucoma. This arises from a raised IOP, even when the iris-corneal angle is open and unobstructed (Fig. 9.5C) and accounts for 90% of glaucoma cases. It can be caused by age-related fibrotic changes in the drainage meshwork of the iris-corneal angle, reducing its permeability and outflow. Obstruction at any point within the aqueous humour circulatory system can also increase IOP: inflammation, infection, or an expanding tumour can all be responsible.

Glaucoma of normal IOP. Although most cases of glaucoma are caused by raised IOP, some people with the condition have normal intraocular pressure. The pathophysiology of normal-tension glaucoma is unclear, but one suggestion is that the optic nerve damage is caused by atherosclerotic changes in the tiny blood vessels supplying the optic nerve, reducing its blood supply.

Pathophysiology

Rising IOP stretches the eyeball wall, including the retina. This pulls on the axons of the ganglion cells, which converge on the optic disc from all areas of the retina and damages them. The higher the pressure, the greater the stretch tension and the more likely the damage will be irreversible. The shape and size of the eyeball are also important; in short-sighted people, whose eyeballs are slightly bigger than normal, the eyeball wall is often slightly thinner, and stretches more easily than smaller, thicker-walled eyeballs. Short-sighted people are therefore at increased risk of glaucoma.

Signs and symptoms

These depend on how rapidly the condition develops. Acute closure of the angle between the iris and cornea and a rapid rise in IOP causes eye pain, headache, nausea, and vomiting. The cornea becomes oedematous because of the build-up of fluid behind it, causing blurred vision and haloes around lights. Chronic glaucoma is painless and permanent neurological damage can be done before diagnosis, reinforcing the importance of regular eye checks, especially in older people.

Management and prognosis

Raised IOP must be reduced immediately, usually using drugs to increase outflow of aqueous humour or reduce its production. Even with prompt treatment, about 10% of sufferers experience some degree of permanent visual impairment.

REFRACTIVE ERRORS OF THE EYE

When light from a viewed object is not focussed accurately on the retina, it gives a blurred and indistinct picture. Errors of refraction, in which light rays are not bent precisely enough by the cornea and the lens, are very common. Normal vision, in which light rays from a viewed object are brought to sharp focus on the retina, is called **emmetropia** (Fig. 9.6A). If the focal point of light falls behind the retina, the condition is called *long sight* (**hyperopia**), and if the focal point is in front of the retina, the condition is called *short sight* (**myopia**). Both can usually be corrected easily with appropriate lenses (Fig. 9.6).

Myopia

Myopic people generally have good close vision but cannot see objects at a distance. The condition is usually the result of the eyeball being slightly longer than normal (Fig. 9.6B), which also predisposes to other conditions, including retinal detachment. It is corrected with a divergent lens that spreads the light rays out slightly before they reach the lens so that the focal point falls on the retina (Fig. 9.6C).

Hyperopia

In long sightedness, the eyeball is usually a little shorter than normal (Fig. 9.6D), which also predisposes to other conditions, including glaucoma. In hyperopia, distance vision is often good but close vision is poor. It is corrected with a convergent lens that brings the light rays closer together before they hit the lens so that the focal point falls on the retina (Fig. 9.6E).

Presbyopia

This is loss of near vision due mainly to a loss of elasticity of the lens with age. An inelastic lens does not bulge as much as an elastic lens, and its refractive power and range of accommodation are therefore reduced. All individuals over the age of 50 are affected to some degree by lens stiffening that progressively increases the near point (the closest distance at which an object can be brought into focus) and accounts for the observation that older people have to hold their reading material farther away than they did in their youth!

DISORDERS OF THE ANTERIOR EYE

The anterior eye is composed of the cornea, the iris, the lens, the ciliary body, and the aqueous humour that circulates through the pupil and bathes the anterior structures.

INFECTION AND INFLAMMATORY CONDITIONS

A range of microbes, including bacteria, fungi, and viruses, can cause eye infections. The eye represents a breach in the continuity of the skin of the face, increasing the likelihood of infection. Its defence mechanisms include the lubricating and washing action of the tear film and the antibacterial action of lysozyme and antibodies in tears, but eye infections are still relatively common.

Conjunctivitis

The conjunctiva is the membrane lining the inner surface of the eyelid and covering the sclera of the eye. Inflammation or infection of the conjunctiva is common. It is usually self-limiting, although it can cause corneal scarring. The eye becomes red, and the eyelids may be swollen if their conjunctival lining is involved. There is irritation, pain, and sometimes photophobia, and bacterial conjunctivitis causes purulent discharge. The commonest causes of bacterial conjunctivitis are streptococcal and staphylococcal species. Conjunctivitis can also be viral or fungal in origin.

Trachoma

This eye infection is the global leading cause of blindness caused by infection. The causative organism is *Chlamydia trachomatis*. It is spread by flies that pick up the bacteria when

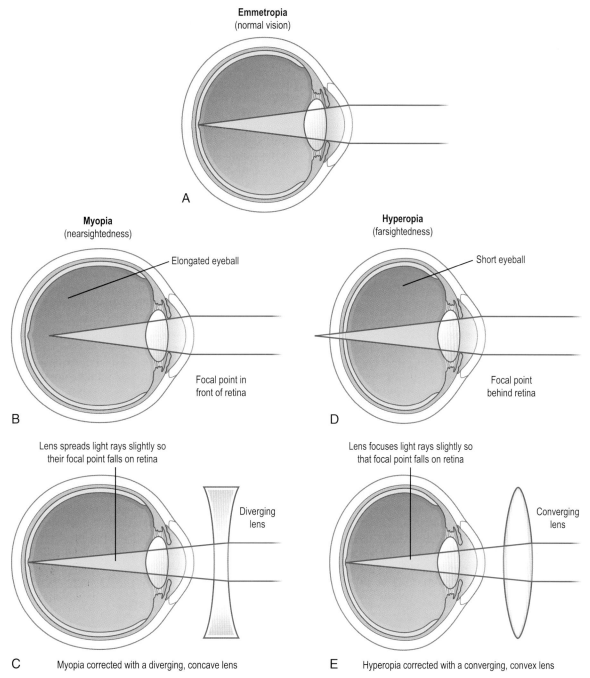

Fig. 9.6 Correction of short and long sight with appropriate lenses. (A) Emmetropia. (B) Myopia. (C) Corrected myopia. (D) Hyperopia. (E) Corrected hyperopia. (Modified from Waugh A and Grant A (2018) *Ross & Wilson anatomy and physiology in health and illness*, 13th ed, Fig. 8.29. Oxford: Elsevier Ltd.)

landing on the eyes or noses of infected people and carry the infection to others. It is also spread by direct person-to-person contact and via contaminated clothing or bedding. The disease is endemic in some parts of Africa, Asia, the Middle East, Central and South America, and aboriginal communities in Australia; WHO data (2021) estimates the global number of people living at risk of trachoma blindness as 136 million. It flourishes in impoverished communities living in conditions of poor sanitation and hygiene. Women are more likely to be blinded than men, possibly because they are more likely to be caring for children and dealing with contaminated household linens.

Pathophysiology

Chlamydia are obligate intracellular bacteria; some members of the species infect the genitalia and cause sexually transmitted disease. The bacteria invade the conjunctival epithelial cells, causing infiltration with immune cells and triggering intense inflammation (Fig. 9.7). Follicles, collections of lymphoid cells that appear as small pale lumps on the inner eyelids, may appear. A single infective episode heals without complication, but repeated reinfection occurs in populations where the disease is endemic, with serious consequences. The prolonged, intense inflammation caused by recurrent infection causes corneal clouding and

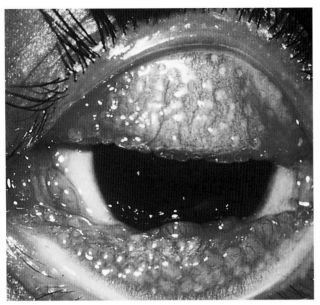

Fig. 9.7 Trachoma conjunctivitis. Conjunctival follicles clearly seen. (From Kanski J and Bowling B (2009) *Clinical ophthalmology: a synopsis*, 2nd ed, Fig. 8.9. London: Elsevier Ltd.)

scarring, drying, degeneration and loss of the conjunctiva, and fibrous changes in the eyelids, which tighten across the eye and turn inwards. This brings the eyelashes into contact with the conjunctiva, causing intense pain, further inflammation and corneal scarring and eventually leading to blindness.

Management and prognosis
A global programme driven by the World Health Assembly aiming to eliminate trachoma worldwide is achieving significant success, with 14 countries previously plagued with trachoma declared trachoma-free by the WHO in January 2022. There is currently no vaccine, although work is ongoing in that area. Antibiotics and surgery are keystones of treatment, as are eliminating the overcrowding, poor sanitation, and lack of hygiene practices that allow the disease to persist.

CATARACT

In cataract, the lens becomes clouded, usually as the result of ageing (senile cataract), but other factors that can trigger it include alcohol consumption, diabetes, some drugs (e.g., corticosteroids), and irradiation, including sun exposure. Sometimes cataracts are congenital.

Pathophysiology
Opacification (clouding) of the lens usually results from age-related changes in the central portion of the lens (**nuclear sclerosis**). This is a complex process. With age, the central part of the lens is slowly compressed as new lens fibres are laid down on the outer lens surfaces, which stiffens it and reduces its transparency. The cellular processes that transport water, nutrients, and antioxidants begin to fail in the ageing lens, further injuring its central portion. The sclerosing fibres become stiffer and discoloured because the crystallin proteins degenerate, contributing to the progressive lens clouding. The increased risk of cataract in

diabetes is linked to the production of advanced glycation end products (p.261).

Signs and symptoms
The cloudy lens decreases the sharpness of vision (this is usually the presenting symptom) and can make certain colours, particularly blues, less bright. Vision in reduced light may be very poor because not enough light penetrates the opaque lens to give a clear image on the retina. Existing short sight, in which light rays are already focused in front of the retina instead of on it, can be significantly increased (myopic shift) because cataract thickens the lens and brings light rays to focus even farther from the retina.

Management and prognosis
Lens replacement, in which the damaged lens is liquefied and extracted from its capsule and replaced with an artificial lens, is one of medicine's success stories. The procedure takes about twenty minutes, carries a very low risk of complications when performed by experienced and well-trained operators and can completely reverse blindness brought on by the cataract.

RETINAL DISORDERS

Systemic disorders that damage retinal blood vessels and cause retinal disease include hypertension, diabetes, and arterial embolism. Retinal disease or damage leads to loss of the visual signal from the affected area, giving an area in the visual field with poor or no vision (scotoma).

AGE-RELATED MACULAR DEGENERATION (AMD)
Globally, AMD is the leading cause of irreversible vision loss in moderate- to high-income countries and is commoner in whites than people of other races. Degeneration of the macula lutea, usually age-related, leads to loss of central vision because the macula lutea is the area on the retina where light falls from a directly viewed object. Of all patients with AMD, 90% have dry AMD, and the remaining 10% have wet AMD, although up to one fifth of patients diagnosed with dry AMD progress to the wet form. The main risk factor is increasing age: most patients are over 50 years old. Other risk factors include family history, hypertension, ultraviolet light exposure, smoking, and hypercholesterolaemia. The condition may be bilateral or affect only one eye. Because AMD destroys the macula but spares the peripheral retina, it causes progressive visual impairment and eventual loss of the centre of the visual field, but peripheral vision is unaffected.

Dry AMD: pathophysiology
This condition develops over years and is associated with atrophy and detachment of the retina from the choroid in the region of the macula. The affected tissue is the basement membrane separating the retinal pigmented epithelium from the choroid below. This membrane is called *Bruch's membrane* (Fig. 9.8A) and with age it accumulates fatty deposits of degraded extracellular materials called drusen (Fig. 9.8B). Drusen are not diagnostic for AMD, but they are characteristic of the disease. Over time, the retinal pigmented epithelium and choroid degenerate, disrupting the blood supply to the overlying retina, which atrophies and

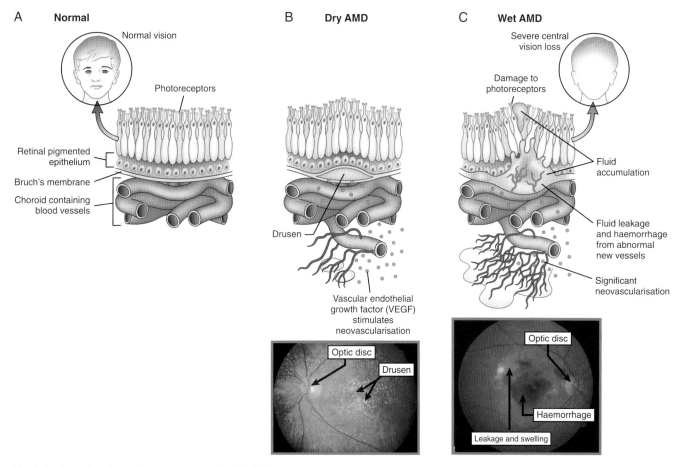

Fig. 9.8 Age-related macular degeneration (AMD). (A) The normal retina with intact Bruch's membrane. (B) Dry AMD showing drusen separating the retinal pigmented epithelium and Bruch's membrane, and the initiation of neovascularisation. (C) Wet AMD showing leakage, haemorrhage, and swelling. (Modified from (B) ISM/Science Photo Library. Reproduced with permission and (C) El-Baz AS, Suri J (2021) *State of the art in neural networks and their applications*, Fig. 2.9A. Philadelphia: Academic Press.)

dies with irreversible vision loss. Inflammation caused by drusen formation releases growth factors, including vascular endothelial growth factor (VEGF), which trigger the growth of new blood vessels (neovascularisation). This is normally an essential part of tissue healing but in this situation may lead to the development of wet AMD. The most advanced form of dry AMD is associated with a phenomenon called **geographical atrophy**, so called because the outline of the atrophic central portion of the retina is sharply defined like the border of a country on a map (Fig. 9.9).

Wet (exudative) AMD: pathophysiology

Wet AMD (also called *neovascular* or *exudative AMD*) is characterised by significant neovascularisation (Fig. 9.8C). The structure of these new blood vessels is abnormal, and their walls are more permeable than usual, so they leak exudate into the tissue around them (hence 'wet' AMD), causing subretinal oedema. Sometimes they bleed, causing subretinal haemorrhage, and this can cause a sudden onset of symptoms. Any swelling or bleeding here can cause the retina to detach from the pigmented epithelium. This disrupts the delicate architecture of the retina, leading to vision loss.

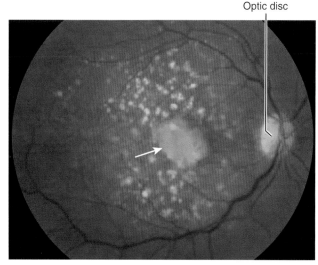

Fig. 9.9 Geographical atrophy (arrowed) in the region of the macula lutea in dry AMD. (Courtesy Alan Bird, Moorfields Eye Hospital, London.)

Signs and symptoms

As AMD of either aetiology progresses, central vision is lost. In addition, other visual difficulties occur, including poor night vision and problems adapting when light levels change (e.g., walking from sunshine into a darkened room). Reading, recognising faces, and coping with work requiring sharp central vision, e.g., chopping vegetables and sewing become increasingly difficult. Peripheral vision is always preserved.

Management and prognosis

There is no cure for AMD. There is an association between AMD and Alzheimer disease, and wet AMD sufferers are at increased risk of cardiovascular disease and stroke. Dry AMD usually progresses much more slowly than wet AMD. Recent evidence from the Age-Related Eye Disease Study strongly suggests that vitamin, zinc, and antioxidant supplements delay the onset of dry AMD and slows the progress of established disease.

There are no drugs available to treat dry AMD. Small-scale studies using stem cell therapy have shown major improvements in wet AMD, and VEGF inhibitors (e.g., ranibizumab) can be very effective in curbing the growth of new blood vessels and slowing vision loss.

RETINAL DETACHMENT

Separation of the neural retina from the underlying pigmented epithelium is called *retinal detachment*. It can be caused by several factors, including older age, ocular surgery or trauma, loss of intraocular pressure, AMD, or as an unpredicted event with no apparent initiating factors.

Pathophysiology

Fig. 9.10 shows some causes of retinal detachment. The neural retina can be detached from its underlying epithelium if fluid or other materials is introduced between the two layers or if it is pulled away by the vitreous. Risk factors include severe short-sightedness because this is associated with a long,

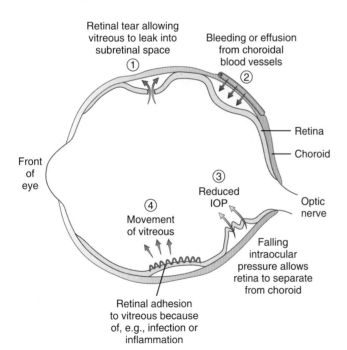

Fig. 9.10 The pathophysiology of retinal detachment.

stretched eyeball, stretching the retina and increasing the chance that it will separate from its underlying epithelium. Factors that reduce intraocular pressure (e.g., eye trauma or removal of the lens without replacing it) also predispose to retinal detachment.

Signs and symptoms

Patients report flashing lights, the sudden appearance of floaters, and a shadow over their field of vision. If the retina around the macula is involved, central vision will be poor.

Management and prognosis

Depending on the aetiology, the prognosis can be very good provided the detachment is diagnosed and treated quickly. Treatment is usually surgical, to repair the damaged retina, but underlying causes must also be addressed. There is increased risk of cataract in the affected eye.

RETINOBLASTOMA

This cancer of childhood is discussed on p.48.

OCULAR MALIGNANT MELANOMA

This is the commonest malignant eye tumour but is not in itself a common cancer and arises in **melanocytes**. Melanocytes are rich in the pigment **melanin** and are found in the skin, the choroid, ciliary body, iris of the eye, and in some other pigmented tissues (e.g., neurones of the substantia nigra pathway in the brain; see Fig. 8.20). Cutaneous malignant melanoma is much more common than ocular melanoma; fewer than 1 in 20 cases of malignant melanoma arise in the eye. Men are at greater risk than women, and the incidence is higher in lighter-skinned races.

Pathophysiology

Ocular melanoma usually develops in the choroid at the back of the eye and is generally aggressive and fast growing. It is occasionally found in the iris or the sclera. It frequently metastasises early, mainly to the liver, lung, and skin. Occasionally, a choroid tumour may be a secondary growth from a primary somewhere else.

Signs and symptoms

The growing tumour causes retinal detachment with vision loss and increased intraocular pressure. The patient may report floaters and eye pain. There may be systemic issues (e.g., weight loss, cough, or change in bladder or bowel habits) that may indicate that the tumour has metastasised or is itself a metastatic growth.

Management and prognosis

The 10-year mortality rate for treated ocular malignant melanoma is up to 50%, usually caused by the cancer spreading to distant organs. It is usually not possible to preserve good sight in the affected eye, and vision is usually poor or lost. The treatments themselves (radiotherapy, surgery, chemotherapy, and immunotherapy) can themselves injure the eye.

THE EAR

The ear contains the organs of hearing, balance, and receptors for proprioception that detect the position and

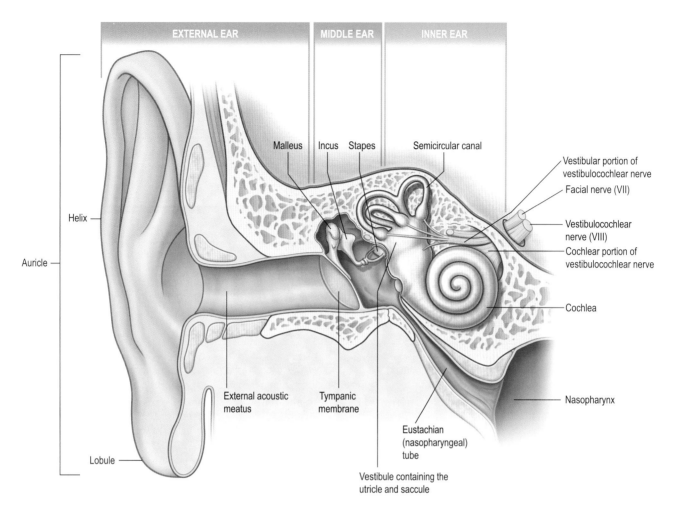

Fig. 9.11   The anatomy of the outer, middle, and inner ear. (Modified from Waugh A and Grant A (2018) *Ross & Wilson anatomy and physiology in health and illness*, 13th ed, Fig. 8.1. Oxford: Elsevier Ltd.)

movement of the body and body parts in space. The main structures of the ear are shown in Fig. 9.11.

THE NORMAL EAR

The ear is conventionally described in three areas: the external, middle, and inner ear. The external ear (auricle) is a folded flap of cartilage covered with skin, which contains specialised secretory glands producing **cerumen** (earwax) to protect and lubricate the external ear canal. The external ear channels sound waves through the external ear canal towards the **tympanic membrane** (eardrum), which marks the boundary between the outer and middle ear. Incoming sound waves vibrate the tympanic membrane.

The middle ear

This air-filled bony chamber hollowed out of the temporal bone is linked directly to the throat via the Eustachian (nasopharyngeal) tube. Vibrations from the tympanic membrane are amplified and transmitted into the inner ear by a bridge of three tiny bones, the hammer (**malleus**), anvil (**incus**), and stirrup (**stapes**), the tiniest bones in the body. The malleus is fastened firmly to the inner surface of the tympanic membrane and forms a synovial joint with the incus, which in turn forms a synovial joint with the stapes, which in turn

is fastened firmly to the **oval window**, a membranous plate leading into the inner ear.

The inner ear

The sensory organs of the inner ear are contained within a network of tunnels built into the temporal bone. These tunnels are lined with membranes and filled with fluid called **endolymph**. The specialised sensory receptors of hearing, balance, and proprioception, found in the inner ear, are designed to detect movement in endolymph, convert these signals into action potentials, and transmit them to the brain.

The oval window opens into the vestibule, which in turn opens into the semicircular canals (the organs of balance) and the cochlea (the organ of hearing). The vestibule, cochlea, and semicircular canals are collectively referred to as the **labyrinth**, and the vestibule and the semicircular canals together are called the *vestibular apparatus*.

The vestibular apparatus

The vestibule itself contains two important sensory structures, the **utricle** and the **saccule**, which detect changes in the position of the head with respect to gravity. The specialised nerve cells that detect head movement in the utricle and saccule are hair cells, the tips of which are embedded in a heavy gelatinous membrane above them. Movement of the

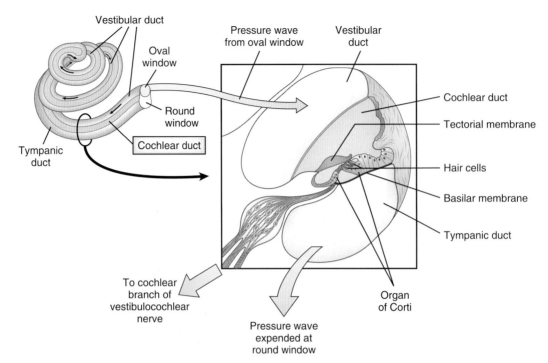

Fig. 9.12   The cochlea. (Modified from Standring S (2021) *Gray's anatomy,* 42nd ed, Fig. 43.9. Oxford: Elsevier Ltd.)

head results in movement of the membrane as gravity pulls on it, stimulating the hair cells. Nerve fibres from the hair cells run to the vestibular portion of the vestibulocochlear nerve (auditory nerve, cranial nerve VIII), and carry this information to the brainstem and cerebellum, informing them about head movement and position. This governs balance and posture and allows the eyes to remain fixed on an object even when the body is moving relative to that object.

The semicircular canals. There are three of these arch-shaped tunnels, sitting at right angles to each other, and all are filled with endolymph. They detect rotational movement of the head. One end of each tunnel is expanded and contains a collection of specialised hair cells, embedded in a jelly-like blob of proteins and polysaccharides called the *cupula.* Head rotation sets up waves in the endolymph, which distorts the soft cupula and stimulates the hair cells. Nerve fibres from the hair cells travel in the vestibular portion of the vestibulocochlear nerve to the brain.

The cochlea. The cochlea is a curled tunnel ('cochlea' means shell) containing the **organ of Corti,** the organ of hearing. The cochlea contains three fluid-filled membranous tubes lying alongside one another within the coiled cochlea (Fig. 9.12). The vibrations of the stapes are transmitted through the oval window into the **vestibular duct**. The floor of the vestibular duct forms the ceiling of the middle duct, the **cochlear duct**, which contains the organ of Corti. The floor of the cochlear duct is also the roof of the third tube, the **tympanic duct**, and is called the **basilar membrane**. The organ of Corti sits on the basilar membrane. Vibration of the stapes against the oval window generates pressure waves in the fluid in the vestibular and tympanic ducts, which in turn distorts the basilar membrane and stimulates the organ of Corti. As with the semicircular canals, the specialised sensory receptors in the organ of Corti are delicate hair cells sitting on the basilar membrane (Fig. 9.13). Their tips lie against a membrane that overlies them, the **tectori-**

al membrane. When the basilar membrane is disturbed by fluid waves in the vestibular and tympanic ducts, the tips of the hair cells are pushed against the tectorial membrane, which bends the hair cells and stimulates them. Nerve fibres running from the hair cells unite to form the cochlear portion of the vestibulocochlear nerve, carrying impulses to the auditory cortex, where they are perceived as sound.

DEAFNESS

Hearing loss (deafness) is generally divided into two categories depending on the aetiology: **conductive deafness**, in which the transmission of sound waves to the inner ear is blocked in some way, and **sensorineural deafness**, in which the organ of Corti itself or the auditory nerve transmitting information from the inner ear to the brain is damaged.

CONDUCTIVE DEAFNESS

A wide range of factors can reduce the transmission of sound waves from the exterior to the cochlea. One of the commonest causes of conductive deafness is the build-up and impaction of earwax in the external ear canal, often worsened by attempts to clean the ear with cotton buds or other items. If the eardrum is perforated, its ability to vibrate in response to arriving sound waves is reduced or lost. The presence of fluid (e.g., in otitis media) in the middle ear dampens the vibration of the auditory ossicles and reduces the transmission of sound waves through the oval window.

Otosclerosis

This usually leads to hearing loss in young adulthood and is caused by malformation of the auditory ossicles because of abnormal bone growth, usually around the stapes, which fuses it in place and prevents it from vibrating normally. This blocks sound wave transmission to the cochlea through the oval window. There is a strong hereditable component,

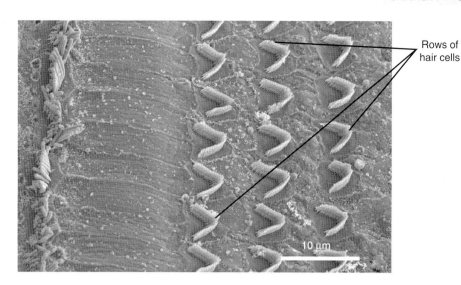

Rows of
hair cells

Fig. 9.13 Cochlear hair cells. In life, the tips would be in contact with the tectorial membrane above them. (From Paxinos G (2015) *The rat nervous system*, 4th ed, Fig. 1. San Diego: Academic Press.)

and it is more common in females than males. Sometimes surgery can release the stapes, but this carries the risk of permanent deafness.

SENSORINEURAL DEAFNESS

Exposure to excessive noise at any age can permanently damage cochlear hair cells. Other causes include tumours, infections, or trauma affecting the vestibulocochlear nerve. Some drugs (e.g., gentamicin and furosemide) are directly ototoxic. These drugs accumulate in the endolymph of the cochlea and cause irreversible damage to the hair cells in the organ of Corti.

Presbycusis

This is sensorineural age-related hearing loss. It usually affects both ears and is progressive. Males and females are equally affected, and estimates suggest up to a third of people in the 65 to 74 age range have some degree of age-related hearing loss; the proportion of people affected rises with increasing age. With age, cumulative noise injury to the cochlear hair cells causes them to atrophy, beginning at the proximal end of the cochlea, responsible for detection of high-pitched tones, which are therefore lost first. In addition, the number of nerve fibres involved in carrying auditory signals to the brain fall with advancing age, leading to loss of hearing across all frequencies, not just high-pitched sounds. The ability to hear speech clearly is therefore reduced. Additionally, the basilar membrane tends to become thicker and less flexible with age, reducing its sensitivity to movement of the cochlear fluid.

EAR INFECTIONS

Infections of any part of the ear can cause pain and impair hearing.

OTITIS EXTERNA

Infections of the outer ear (**otitis externa**) are relatively common because it is exposed to the external environment. Some common skin conditions e.g., eczema and psoriasis can involve the external ear. Acute otitis externa is usually associated with swimmers because chronic exposure to water washes the natural cerumen of the ear out of the ear canal and the underlying skin can break down, increasing the risk of infection. Foreign objects lodged in the external ear canal increase the risk of infection if the skin is broken or inflamed as a result. Otitis externa is usually easily treated and does not cause long-term problems, although in immunocompromised people an established otitis externa infection may spread deeper in the ear or to the face or neck. If the inflammation leads to perforation of the eardrum, hearing is likely to be impaired.

OTITIS MEDIA

This is inflammation of the middle ear, usually as a result of infection, usually by microbes ascending to the middle ear from the throat along the Eustachian tube. It is most common in children, whose Eustachian tubes are shorter than in adults: up to 90% of cases occur in children under 6 years of age. It is more common in developing countries than wealthier countries, and boys and girls are equally affected. It is the second commonest childhood disorder after upper respiratory tract infection and may present acutely or develop into a chronic disorder.

Pathophysiology

In infective otitis media, the commonest causative organisms are those associated with respiratory infections because the middle ear infection almost always ascends from the throat via the Eustachian tube. Otitis media is therefore often viral in origin. The inflammatory response to infection produces exudate that collects in the middle ear cavity, which is filled with air in the healthy ear, preventing normal vibration of the auditory ossicles and causing deafness. Accumulating pus and inflammatory fluid can cause the eardrum to bulge into the external ear canal or to perforate. Otitis media can also spread to the inner ear, and cause labyrinthitis.

'Glue ear' is a non-infective otitis media with effusion into the middle ear that occurs in children, whose Eustachian tubes are narrow and short and easily blocked. As a result, air cannot reach the middle ear cavity from the throat and the pressure within falls. This pulls fluid from the mucosal lining of the cavity, producing an effusion fluid that is sterile initially but may become infected because it is an excellent medium for bacterial growth. It usually improves as the child grows and the Eustachian tube lengthens and widens but may persist as a chronic disorder for some time until this happens, and, untreated, cause permanent damage. Cleft palate causes glue ear, because the anatomical deformities associated with cleft palate affect the structure of the Eustachian tube and the muscles that keep it open.

Signs and symptoms

Otitis media causes pain and deafness. If there is infection, there may be fever, malaise, and discharge from the ear if the eardrum perforates.

Management and prognosis

Acute otitis media usually settles within 2 or 3 days and pain relief and fever reduction are generally enough; antibiotics are only used if there is evidence of bacterial involvement. Glue ear frequently recurs and the hearing loss it causes can interfere with the development of speech and language in children. A tiny grommet can be inserted through the eardrum to keep the pressure in the middle ear equal to atmospheric pressure, preventing the development of the negative pressure that generates the effusion.

INNER EAR DISORDERS

Inner ear disorders can affect balance and hearing. Vertigo, the sensation that either the person or their surroundings are moving (often rotating) even when they are stationary, is a common presenting symptom. It usually means that the vestibule and semicircular canals are involved, although vertigo can also result if central pathways involved in the processing of the signals from the inner ear are damaged (e.g., in brainstem injury).

MÉNIÈRE'S DISEASE

This condition can appear at any age and many cases have a significant family history. Most diagnoses are made in the 40 to 60 years age range, more commonly in women than men. There is an association with migraine.

Pathophysiology

This disorder is associated with increased endolymph in the inner ear. This increases inner ear pressures and applies mechanical stress to the sensitive structures here, including the hair cells of the cochlea and semicircular canals. The cause of the accumulation of endolymph is not known.

Signs and symptoms

There is a sensation of pressure in the ear, accompanied by dizziness, vertigo, nausea, vomiting, and deafness.

Management and prognosis

Initially, symptoms appear in recurring episodes but as the disease progresses the periods of remission in between episodes can disappear and the person experiences constant hearing loss and imbalance. For most people, the disorder reaches a stable state and stops progressing, although there may be permanently impaired balance and hearing.

LABYRINTHITIS

This is inflammation of the structures of the inner ear. It therefore interferes with balance or hearing, and sometimes both. Inflammation may be infective or non-infective. Non-infective labyrinthitis is usually associated with a systemic autoimmune disease, in which the inappropriate immune activation damages the inner ear.

Infective labyrinthitis

This may be bacterial or viral. Viral labyrinthitis is commoner than bacterial. The infection can arrive in the inner ear via the bloodstream or from the middle ear. In addition, there are bony tunnels through the temporal bone that directly link the vestibule and the cochlea with the subarachnoid space, and in this way infecting organisms in the CSF may travel into the inner ear.

Viral labyrinthitis in otherwise healthy adults usually follows an upper respiratory tract infection and resolves after a few weeks, during which time the main signs and symptoms include vertigo, deafness, nausea, and vomiting. Viral labyrinthitis can cause childhood deafness from either pre- or post-natal infection. Congenital deafness is usually caused by maternal infection with rubella or cytomegalovirus (CMV). Rubella causes German measles, and although it usually causes a mild febrile illness in children, it can be catastrophic for the unborn child if the mother becomes infected during the early stages of pregnancy, during which time organogenesis is ongoing. Rubella infection can cause miscarriage or stillbirth. Surviving babies can have significant disability including deafness, because by mechanisms not yet understood the virus is directly toxic to the organ of Corti in the cochlea. The introduction of immunisation to rubella has slashed the incidence of congenital rubella in all countries with an immunisation programme. CMV, a herpesvirus, is carried by nearly everyone, although it usually does not cause disease in healthy people. Transmission from mother to baby in utero is associated with a range of congenital disabilities, including deafness. The virus causes cochlear inflammation and damage, although the mechanism is not known. Measles (caused by the rubeola virus) and mumps (caused by the paramyxovirus) cause labyrinthitis and permanent deafness in infected children.

Bacterial labyrinthitis is usually a consequence of otitis media or bacterial meningitis and so is associated with the same organisms that cause these infections.

BIBLIOGRAPHY AND REFERENCES

Fleckenstein, M., Mitchell, P., Freund, K. B., et al. (2018). The progression of geographic atrophy secondary to age-related macular degeneration. *Ophthalmology*, *125*, 369–390.

Forrester, J. V., Dick, A. D., McMenamin, P. G., Roberts, F., & Pearlman, E. (2016). *The eye: Basic sciences in practice* (4th ed.). Elsevier.

Gul, A., Rahman, M. A., Salim, A., et al. (2009). Advanced glycation end products in senile diabetic and nondiabetic patients with cataract. *Journal of Diabetes and Its Complications*, *23*, 343–348.

Useful websites

Age-Related Eye Disease Studies: National Eye Institute research on age-related eye diseases: https://www.nei.nih.gov/research/clinical-trials/age-related-eye-disease-study-areds.

Ocular manifestations of systemic disease: American Academy of Ophthalmology.: https://med.virginia.edu/ophthalmology/wp-content/uploads/sites/295/2015/12/Systemic.pdf.

Useful resource on glaucoma: https://www.hopkinsmedicine.org/wilmer/services/glaucoma/book/chapter_what_is_glaucoma.html.

WHO factsheet on trachoma: https://www.who.int/news-room/fact-sheets/detail/trachoma

Disorders of Endocrine Function

10

CHAPTER OUTLINE

INTRODUCTION
    Principles of endocrine control
THE PITUITARY GLAND AND ITS DISORDERS
    Pituitary tumours
Disorders of anterior pituitary hormones
    ACTH oversecretion and Cushing disease
    Growth hormone disorders
    Hyperprolactinaemia
Disorders of the posterior pituitary
    Diabetes insipidus
THE ENDOCRINE PANCREAS AND DIABETES
MELLITUS
    Insulin and glucagon
    Glucose and energy metabolism
Diabetes mellitus
    The main features of diabetes mellitus

Complications of diabetes mellitus
Types of diabetes mellitus
    Type 1 diabetes mellitus
    Type 2 diabetes mellitus
    Hyperglycaemia of pregnancy
    Diabetes of other specific types
THE THYROID GLAND AND ITS DISORDERS
    Hyperthyroidism
    Hypothyroidism
THE PARATHYROID GLANDS
    Hyperparathyroidism
    Hypoparathyroidism
THE ADRENAL GLAND AND ITS DISORDERS
    The adrenal medulla
    The adrenal cortex

INTRODUCTION

Endocrinology is the study of the production and function of chemical messengers, **hormones**, synthesised and secreted by a range of glands and tissues. Many hormones are released into the bloodstream and, once in the circulation, act on distant tissues. Other hormones, generally referred to as **local hormones**, regulate the activity of cells in the vicinity of their release. Fig. 10.1 shows the body's main endocrine glands. Effective body function relies on a wide range of hormones, which regulate fundamental processes including growth and repair, metabolism, reproduction, response to stress, and water and electrolyte balance. In general, endocrine disorders can be categorised as either reduced or excessive secretion of a hormone, or an abnormal body response to a specific hormone. Endocrine glands can develop tumours, become infected, or be destroyed by autoimmune mechanisms. In addition, because there is a close functional relationship between many of the body's key glands, abnormalities in one gland can have significant knock-on effects on the function of others.

PRINCIPLES OF ENDOCRINE CONTROL

In complex multicellular organisms, sophisticated control and regulatory mechanisms are needed for precise coordination of internal functions and rapid, accurate, and controlled internal communication. The nervous system and the endocrine system, acting together, fulfil these roles. Although both operate via the interaction of specific substances with specific cellular receptors to initiate or inhibit specific cellular processes, there are important differences in the nature of their action. Neurotransmitters released by activated nerves generally initiate finely controlled and rapid changes that can usually be immediately reversed when the nerve stimulation, and neurotransmitter release, stop. Hormones, on the other hand, once released into the bloodstream or into local tissues, persist until they are cleared by enzymatic degradation, either in the blood or in the tissues. Body functions controlled by hormones are therefore generally of slower onset but are sustained and long lasting.

THE PITUITARY GLAND AND ITS DISORDERS

The pituitary gland is sometimes called the *master gland* because it controls the activity of so many other endocrine glands, but it is itself under the control of the hypothalamus.

The hypothalamic-pituitary axis

The relationship between the hypothalamus and the pituitary gland is fundamental to the regulation of certain key endocrine glands, most notably the thyroid gland, the

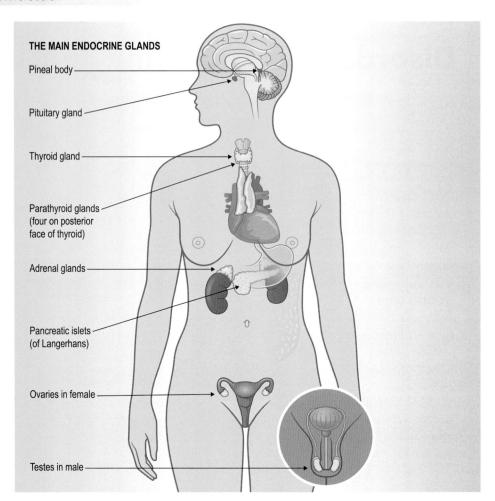

THE MAIN ENDOCRINE GLANDS

Pineal body

Pituitary gland

Thyroid gland

Parathyroid glands
(four on posterior
face of thyroid)

Adrenal glands

Pancreatic islets
(of Langerhans)

Ovaries in female

Testes in male

Fig. 10.1 The main endocrine glands. (Modified from Waugh A and Grant A (2018) *Ross & Wilson anatomy and physiology in health and illness*, 13th ed, Fig. 9.1. Oxford: Elsevier Ltd.)

adrenal glands, and the gonads. Understanding this relationship, also referred to as the **hypothalamic-pituitary axis (HPA)**, is essential to understanding the consequences of disease or disorder in any of the glands involved. The pituitary gland sits immediately below the hypothalamus and is linked to it by a short stalk called the infundibulum (Fig. 10.2). It sits in the sella turcica, a bony hollow in the sphenoid bone, and has two lobes, made of different types of tissue. The anterior pituitary is made of **glandular tissue**, and it produces and secretes its own hormones, but it does this in response to instructions from the hypothalamus. The posterior pituitary is very different: it is essentially a finger of brain tissue extending down from the hypothalamus and so consists of **nerve tissue**. The hypothalamus communicates with the pituitary gland in two ways: a network of blood vessels connects the hypothalamus and anterior pituitary, and the connection between the hypothalamus and posterior pituitary is via nerve axons.

Vascular connection: anterior pituitary. Running through the infundibulum and linking the hypothalamus to the anterior pituitary is a network of blood capillaries (Fig. 10.2). Glandular cells in the hypothalamus produce hormones that travel in these connecting capillaries to the anterior pituitary and control its hormone production. Some hypothalamic hormones stimulate anterior pituitary secretion, and these are called **releasing hormones**. Others, called **inhibiting hormones**, downregulate it.

The anterior pituitary secretes six key hormones, from five different types of glandular cells, which between them have wide-ranging effects on body function (Fig. 10.3). The secretion and function of these hormones are summarised in Box 10.1. These hormones will be discussed in more detail in the sections describing relevant pathophysiology.

Neural connection: posterior pituitary. The part of the infundibulum that forms the posterior pituitary is a downgrowth of nerves from the hypothalamus. The cell bodies of these neurones lie in the hypothalamus, and their axons run down the infundibulum and terminate in the posterior pituitary (Fig. 10.3). These neurones are specialised to secrete and transport hormones. Two hormones, **oxytocin** and **antidiuretic hormone (ADH)** are produced in the hypothalamus and transferred to the axon terminals in the posterior pituitary below via axonal transport. The posterior pituitary therefore acts as an endocrine gland because it releases oxytocin and ADH although it does not actually synthesise these hormones itself.

Feedback inhibition and regulation of the HPA

Levels of hormones released by the target endocrine glands controlled by the HPA (e.g., tri-iodothyronine (T_3) and thyroxine (T_4) from the thyroid gland) are constantly measured by the pituitary gland and/or the hypothalamus. When thyroid hormone levels fall in the blood, the hypothalamus increases its secretion of thyrotrophin releasing hormone

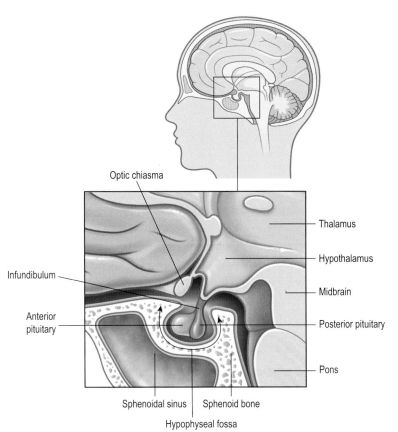

Optic chiasma

Infundibulum

Anterior pituitary

Thalamus

Hypothalamus

Midbrain

Posterior pituitary

Pons

Sphenoidal sinus Sphenoid bone

Hypophyseal fossa

Fig. 10.2 The pituitary gland, showing its relationship to the hypothalamus and other brain structures. (Modified from Waugh A and Grant A (2018) *Ross & Wilson anatomy and physiology in health and illness*, 13th ed, Fig. 9.2. Oxford: Elsevier Ltd.)

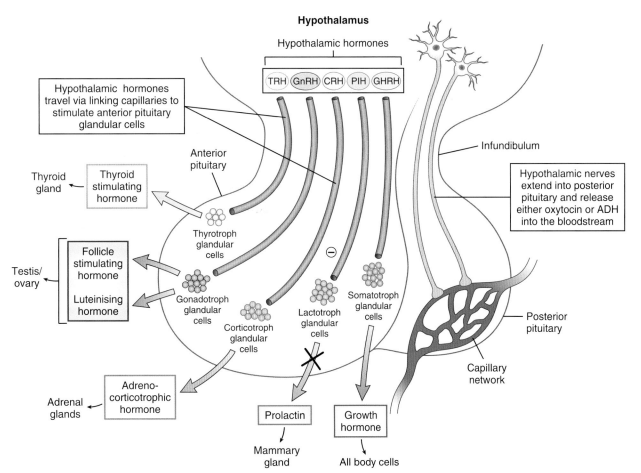

Hypothalamus

Hypothalamic hormones

TRH GnRH CRH PIH GHRH

Hypothalamic hormones travel via linking capillaries to stimulate anterior pituitary glandular cells

Anterior pituitary

Infundibulum

Hypothalamic nerves extend into posterior pituitary and release either oxytocin or ADH into the bloodstream

Thyroid gland

Thyroid stimulating hormone

Thyrotroph glandular cells

Follicle stimulating hormone

Luteinising hormone

Testis/ ovary

Gonadotroph glandular cells

Corticotroph glandular cells

Lactotroph glandular cells

Somatotroph glandular cells

Posterior pituitary

Capillary network

Adreno-corticotrophic hormone

Adrenal glands

Prolactin

Mammary gland

Growth hormone

All body cells

Fig. 10.3 Hormones of the hypothalamus and the glandular cells and hormones of the anterior pituitary gland. *CRH*, Corticotrophin releasing hormone; *GHRH*, growth hormone releasing hormone; *GnRH*, gonadotrophin releasing hormone; *PIH*, prolactin inhibiting hormone; *TRH*, thyrotrophin releasing hormone.

BOX 10.1 Anterior pituitary hormones, their functions, and the hypothalamic hormones that regulate their production

Anterior pituitary hormone	Anterior pituitary glandular cell	Released by (hypothalamic hormone)	Inhibited by (hypothalamic hormone)	Target gland/ tissue of anterior pituitary hormone	Response of target gland/tissue
Adrenocorticotrophic hormone (ACTH)	Corticotrophs	Corticotrophin releasing hormone (CRH)	—	Adrenal cortex	Stimulates glucocorticoid (e.g., hydrocortisone) secretion
Follicle stimulating hormone (FSH)	Gonadotrophs	Gonadotrophin releasing hormone (GnRH)	—	Gonads	Stimulates follicle development in the ovary and sperm production in the testis
Luteinising hormone (LH)	Gonadotrophs	Gonadotrophin releasing hormone (GnRH)	—	Gonads	Maintains the corpus luteum in the ovary and stimulates testosterone production in the testis
Growth hormone (GH)	Somatotrophs	Growth hormone releasing hormone (GHRH)	Somatostatin	Body tissues in general	Stimulates growth and development
Prolactin	Lactotrophs	-	Dopamine	Mammary gland	Stimulates lactation
Thyroid stimulating hormone (TSH)	Thyrotrophs	Thyrotrophin releasing hormone (TRH)	-	Thyroid gland	Stimulates release of T_3 and T_4

(TRH), stimulating the anterior pituitary to increase secretion of thyroid stimulating hormone (TSH). The result is increased stimulation of the thyroid gland and an elevation in T_3 and T_4 blood levels. The opposite happens when T_3 and T_4 blood levels rise: TRH and TSH levels drop, and thyroid secretion falls. This control mechanism responds to exogenous hormone as well: therefore, thyroxine treatment in hypothyroidism suppresses secretion of thyroid hormones by the thyroid gland.

PITUITARY TUMOURS

There are no known risk factors specifically for pituitary tumours, except for a few rare inherited syndromes (only about 5% of pituitary tumours have an identified family history). Pituitary tumours are associated with a range of genetic abnormalities, including loss of the tumour suppressor gene *p53* (p.75) and mutations of the tumour promotor gene *ras* (p.76). Most pituitary tumours arise from a single cell; and if the expanding tumour cell population continues to secrete the hormone made by its cell of origin, it is called a *functioning tumour*. Tumour cells that lose the capacity to secrete their hormone produce a non-functioning tumour.

Pituitary adenoma

The commonest pituitary neoplasm is a benign adenoma (Fig. 10.4). This neoplasm is more frequent in females than males and usually arises in young to early middle adulthood. They almost always develop in the anterior pituitary and are thought to be commonly present without causing signs and symptoms because they are often discovered incidentally at postmortem. The cell of origin can be any of the five different glandular cell types, and in functioning tumours, hormone secretion increases as the tumour enlarges. Hypersecretory syndromes are a common reason for the patient to seek medical help, and oversecretion of anterior pituitary hormones is considered under the relevant headings below. Usually, functioning adenomas arise from ACTH, GH or prolactin-secreting cells (**corticotrophs, somatotrophs,** or

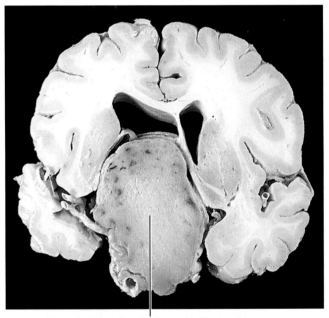

Large non-functional adenoma with massive displacement of overlying brain tissue

Fig. 10.4 Pituitary adenoma. (Modified from Kumar V, Abbas A, Aster JC, et al. (2021) *Robbins essential pathology*, Fig. 16.1. Philadelphia: Elsevier Inc.)

lactotrophs). It is not common for thyrotrophs or gonadotrophs to undergo neoplastic change and produce tumours. A further issue with this form of neoplasm is compression of adjacent brain tissue as the tumour grows. Because it is benign, it is generally capsulated and does not invade local tissue, but its expansion in the limited space of the sella turcica can cause pressure effects on the hypothalamus above, or on the nearby optic nerve, causing visual disturbances. Non-functioning tumours can lead to hypopituitarism by compressing and damaging adjacent, otherwise healthy, pituitary tissue.

Malignant pituitary tumours

Primary malignancies of the pituitary gland are rare, although metastatic growths from primaries elsewhere can establish here. The origin of malignant pituitary neoplasms is not clear; they may arise spontaneously in a glandular cell (giving rise to a carcinoma) or may be caused by malignant transformation of an existing benign adenoma. A range of genetic mutations has been identified but for much of them little research has been done and has not yet provided information on possible diagnostic markers or drug targets.

DISORDERS OF ANTERIOR PITUITARY HORMONES

Anterior pituitary conditions may be associated with under- or oversecretion of hormones and may be caused by an abnormality in the pituitary itself or of the hypothalamus. **Hypopituitarism** means deficiency of any one or any combination of the pituitary hormones and may be congenital or acquired.

Causes of congenital hypopituitarism

Failure of the pituitary gland to develop in utero (which may occur along with developmental abnormalities of other tissues in the area, such as the optic nerve) can affect any of the five different types of hormone-secreting cells, and therefore give deficiencies in one or more pituitary hormones. Rarely, pituitary failure may be part of an inherited endocrine syndrome.

Causes of acquired hypopituitarism

Injury (for example head trauma or surgery) to the pituitary can cause failure. Irradiation, for example for a cranial tumour, can also cause necrosis and failure, especially of somatotrophs (GH secretion), which are particularly susceptible to radiation damage. Infection (e.g., meningitis or disseminated tuberculosis) are other causes. Primary or secondary tumours of the pituitary can cause hyposecretion by compressing and damaging normal pituitary tissue.

ACTH OVERSECRETION AND CUSHING DISEASE

Adrenocorticotrophic hormone (ACTH) stimulates growth and activity of the adrenal cortex, which responds by increasing secretion of cortisol, the principal glucocorticoid hormone in humans. Pituitary release of ACTH can increase because of a functioning tumour of corticotroph cells, resulting in a condition called **Cushing disease**. This produces a wide range of signs and symptoms associated with excessive levels of cortisol. Because essentially the same syndrome is caused if a disorder of the adrenal cortex itself leads to hypercortisolism, Cushing syndrome is discussed below under disorders of the adrenal cortex.

GROWTH HORMONE DISORDERS

GH stimulates growth in all body tissues and is the main endocrine factor controlling normal growth and development. Inadequate or excessive secretion of GH has different consequences in children compared with adults because children are actively growing and laying down increased body mass. GH exerts at least part of its growth-stimulating action by releasing proteins, called *insulin growth factors* (IGFs), which as the name suggests, act like insulin on body cells. Insulin and IGFs promote cell proliferation and maturation in almost every tissue in the body, and regulate carbohydrate, protein, and fat metabolism.

GH deficiency in children: Pituitary dwarfism

In children, untreated failure of the pituitary to secrete adequate GH causes reduced growth rate and short stature, although body proportions remain normal. The child may have facial features characteristic of a younger child, with slow hair growth and delayed dental development. The average height of an adult with dwarfism is 4 feet.

Pathophysiology

The cause of GH deficiency may be congenital (e.g., failure of the pituitary gland to develop in utero), or there may be an inherited endocrine disorder that affects pituitary function. If the problem lies with disrupted pituitary development, other pituitary hormones may also be affected, including LH and FSH. If this is the case, the child may experience delayed puberty or may not go through puberty at all. Blood lipid levels are higher than normal, which can lead to cardiovascular disease in later life. Acquired causes include factors described previously, the commonest being pituitary adenoma. The problem may alternatively lie with the hypothalamus, which may not be secreting adequate GHRH. In some cases, the underlying cause of the pituitary failure may not be identified.

Management and prognosis

Babies born with GH deficiency are usually not diagnosed until later in childhood, when a parent or carer notices the child is smaller than its peers. Sometimes it is not picked up till puberty, when the expected growth spurt and/or pubertal changes do not happen. There is an increased risk of cardiovascular-related death in adulthood because of increased blood lipid levels, but in general, life expectancy is near normal unless there are additional problems. Treatment with GH is generally considered safe and may be extended into adulthood if this is of benefit.

GH deficiency in adults

Although there is no clearly defined syndrome associated with low GH levels in adults, in healthy people GH and IGF levels remain high even after puberty. They do decline steadily with age, but the fact that they are still produced in adult life suggests a role for them in the control of body mass and tissue growth. Adults with low GH levels may experience fatigue, intolerance of heat or cold, and poor concentration and memory. Bone density and muscle mass fall, and the skin can become dry and thin. Weight gain is common, and there is loss of sex drive. Treatment with GH may be beneficial.

GH excess: Gigantism in children and acromegaly in adults

Gigantism, the result of GH excess before the epiphyseal growth plates of bone have closed, and **acromegaly**, the effects of GH excess after closure of the epiphyseal plates, represent two ends of a disease continuum rather than two separate disorders. Both are rare, with up to 11 new cases a year per million people.

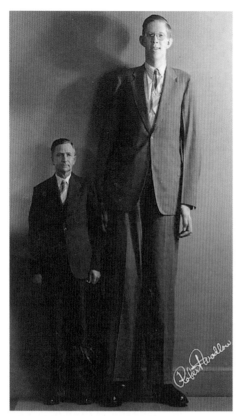

Fig. 10.5 Robert Wadlow, the Alton Giant. (From Iacovazzo D and Korbonits M (2016) Gigantism: X-linked acrogigantism and GPR101 mutations, *Growth Hormone & IGF Research*, 30–31: 64–69. https://doi.org/10.1016/j.ghir.2016.09.007.)

The tallest recorded individual was Robert Pershing Wadlow, born in 1918 (Fig. 10.5). Despite a normal birth weight of 9 lb, he achieved a final adult height of 8 ft 11.1 in (2.72 m), and is better known as the *Alton Giant*, after his place of birth. His gigantism, as is the case in 95% of gigantism and acromegaly, was the result of a functioning pituitary adenoma.

Pathophysiology

Most cases of gigantism and acromegaly are caused by a pituitary adenoma of somatotrophs, which in turn maintains very high levels of IGF and promotes excess growth. Very occasionally, a tumour of the hypothalamus, or ectopic secretion of GH by a primary tumour in another tissue (usually lung or pancreatic cancers), can be the source of the excess GH. A number of genetic mutations have been found, and although most cases are sporadic (i.e., caused by random mutation), several uncommon familial syndromes predispose to gigantism and acromegaly.

Gigantism is characterised by abnormal height resulting from excessive levels of GH on the growth plates of the skeleton. It can occur at any age before puberty, after which rising levels of sex steroids close the epiphyseal plates of long bones and prevent further linear growth. Excess GH after puberty produces the signs and symptoms of acromegaly, in which the stimulant effect of GH cannot increase bone length, but it thickens and coarsens soft tissues, and enlarges bone. This gives characteristically broad and thickened facial bones, protrusion of the jaw, large hands and feet, and large

ears. Almost all tissues and organs are affected; the viscera enlarge, including the heart, predisposing to heart failure, and overgrowth of bone and joint tissues causes joint disorders and skeletal degeneration and deformity. There may be nerve entrapment (e.g., carpal tunnel syndrome) as bony channels become overgrown and narrowed. There are also metabolic changes because raised GH increases blood lipid levels, insulin resistance, and hyperglycaemia. Diabetes mellitus is common in acromegaly and gigantism. High blood lipid levels contribute to atherosclerosis, which, along with heart enlargement, worsens cardiovascular function. Enlargement of upper respiratory structures increases the risk of obstruction, and sleep apnoea is very common (90%).

Management and prognosis

If untreated, progressive acromegaly is significantly life limiting. Not only does it strongly predispose to cardiovascular disease, but persistently high levels of GH and IGF expose tissues to a strong and constant growth stimulus, which in turn increases the risk of malignancy, especially of the colon. Treatment options include surgery and/or radiotherapy to remove or reduce the pituitary adenoma, and growth hormone antagonists such as pegvisomant. In addition, drugs that enhance the effects of somatostatin (Box 10.1), which inhibits pituitary release of GH, can bring GH and IGF blood levels into the normal range.

HYPERPROLACTINAEMIA

This is the commonest pituitary hypersecretion abnormality in both males and females. In the non-pregnant woman, constant release of **dopamine** (referred to as **prolactin inhibitory hormone, PIH**, in this context) from the hypothalamus inhibits prolactin production by the anterior pituitary (Fig. 10.6A). During pregnancy, dopamine release here stops, allowing prolactin levels to rise in the blood. After the birth, prolactin is the main hormone maintaining milk production. Prolactin in males stimulates testosterone production and spermatogenesis.

Pathophysiology

Some of the main causes of prolactin hypersecretion are shown in Fig. 10.6B. Because dopamine from the hypothalamus inhibits prolactin release from the anterior pituitary, drugs that block dopamine activity here switch this control mechanism off and allow prolactin levels to rise. Antipsychotic drugs used in psychiatry (e.g., clozapine, risperidone) antagonise dopamine and can cause galactorrhoea (milk production not associated with pregnancy). A significant number of drugs in other categories (e.g., opioids, oestrogens, some anti-emetics, and some anti-depressants) also block dopamine and cause hyperprolactinaemia. Other known causes of hyperprolactinaemia include stress because prolactin is believed to play an important part in the stress response. Rising prolactin levels in stress increase cortisol secretion from the adrenal glands, a key event in the stress response. Primary hypothyroidism is another recognised cause. In primary hypothyroidism, the thyroid gland fails to produce adequate thyroid hormone, and the anterior pituitary and hypothalamus respond by increasing the levels of TSH and TRH in an attempt to bring thyroid hormone levels up to normal. However, TRH is also a potent stimulator of prolactin release.

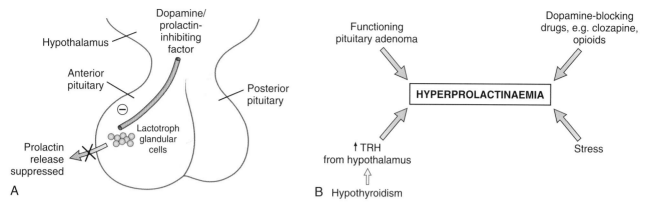

Fig. 10.6   (A) Dopamine (prolactin inhibiting factor) suppresses anterior pituitary secretion of prolactin. (B) Some causes of hypersecretion of prolactin.

Prolactinomas, functioning pituitary adenomas arising from lactotroph (prolactin-secreting) cells, comprise about 40% of pituitary adenomas and are another cause of hyperprolactinaemia.

Signs and symptoms

Prolactin inhibits the release of FSH and LH from the anterior pituitary. These hormones promote the reproductive cycle in women and spermatogenesis in men. During breastfeeding, this suppression of fertility reduces the mother's chances of becoming pregnant, usually advantageous for both mother and baby, but if prolactin levels are abnormally high over extended periods as a result of drugs or any of the conditions described above, then normal reproductive function is suppressed. Women usually present with infertility, galactorrhoea, and menstrual irregularities. Men may experience reduced libido and gynaecomastia (abnormal breast development).

Management and prognosis

Identifying the cause of the elevated prolactin levels determines the treatment; for example, medication-induced hyperprolactinaemia should be reversible when the drug responsible is withdrawn, and pituitary adenomas can be treated. Dopamine agonists, which switch the inhibition of prolactin secretion back on, can also be used. Hyperprolactinaemia itself is not usually considered to have a significant effect on life expectancy.

DISORDERS OF THE POSTERIOR PITUITARY

These are less common than disorders of the anterior pituitary, but a variety of conditions, including head injury and inflammatory and infectious conditions involving the hypothalamus can affect secretion of the two posterior pituitary hormones, ADH and oxytocin. Oxytocin is responsible for triggering and maintaining uterine contractions during childbirth and so has a very specific and limited function, whereas ADH has a key role in maintaining water balance.

DIABETES INSIPIDUS

This condition is caused by hyposecretion of ADH. ADH acts on the distal convoluted tubules and collecting ducts of the kidney, opening water channels in the wall of the nephron, and increasing water reabsorption from the filtrate. It therefore reduces the volume of urine excreted. Deficiency of ADH prevents the kidney from reabsorbing water, leading to the production of large volumes of dilute urine.

THE ENDOCRINE PANCREAS AND DIABETES MELLITUS

Diabetes mellitus (DM) is a group of metabolic disorders associated with insulin deficiency or an abnormal response to insulin, both of which seriously disrupt the cellular pathways responsible for energy production and fuel storage, most significantly related to glucose metabolism. The underlying cause, pathophysiology, and treatment of the different types of DM differ, but DM of any aetiology is associated with hyperglycaemia; a fasting blood glucose level over 7 mmol/L (126 mg/dL) is diagnostic for diabetes. The disorder may appear suddenly, or have a slow and insidious onset, depending on the underlying aetiology. The term *diabetes* derives from the Greek word *diabetes*, which means to pass through and refers to the large volume of urine associated with the disorder (as in diabetes insipidus described previously). Mellitus derives from the Latin for 'honey' and refers to the sweet taste of the urine produced by affected people because of its high glucose content. The earliest recorded mention of DM is found in ancient Egyptian writings dating from 1550 BC. They recorded a disorder in which people were extremely thirsty, lost weight, and produced large volumes of urine. Since then, the disease has been described in medical literature from cultures across the world, but before the mid-20th century there was no cure, and people generally did not survive for long after diagnosis. It was a grim and painful death because sufferers, often children, permanently exhausted and underweight, progressively wasted away in slow starvation despite eating calorie and nutrient-rich foods. In fact, high-calorie diets accelerated the patient's decline, and the only intervention known to extend life was a very low-calorie, low-carbohydrate diet, which few people tolerated for long. In 1889 von Mering and Minkowski induced diabetes in dogs by removing the pancreas. It was concluded that the pancreas produced a substance that prevented diabetes, and this was confirmed when, in 1921, Banting and Best injected pancreatic extract into diabetic dogs, reversing the animals' disease. Shortly afterwards, in conjunction with other workers, they purified this substance, which we know as insulin, and gave the world the cure for diabetes.

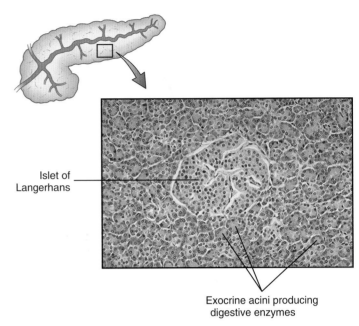

Fig. 10.7   Pancreatic tissue, showing an islet of Langerhans surrounded by exocrine tissue which produces digestive enzymes. (Modified from Klatt E (2015) *Robbins and Cotran atlas of pathology,* 3rd ed, Fig. 9.13. Philadelphia: Elsevier Inc.)

INSULIN AND GLUCAGON

Insulin is a small protein, composed of 51 amino acids, and is produced and released by **β-cells** of the islets of Langerhans in the pancreas (Fig. 10.7). **α-cells** in the islets release **glucagon**, also a small protein hormone. Insulin and glucagon are the major hormones regulating body fuel metabolism. Their actions are usually antagonistic: that is, they act in opposition to each other to maintain the metabolic balance between packaging nutrients away in storage forms for future use while still keeping an adequate supply of essential fuel molecules in the bloodstream and immediately available for body cells.

Insulin

When digested nutrients—glucose, fatty acids, and amino acids—enter the blood after a meal, insulin levels rise very quickly in response. Insulin stimulates body cells to extract these nutrients from the circulation and to deposit them in fuel storage sites; in other words, it is an **anabolic** hormone. Its principal effects are on liver, adipose tissue, and skeletal muscle (Fig. 10.8), but all body cells rely on insulin to be able to extract nutrients from the bloodstream to fuel their activities. Glucose is stored as glycogen (the conversion of glucose to glycogen is called glycogenesis), mainly in liver and muscle, and when glycogen storage sites are full, insulin converts glucose to fat (triacylglycerol) and stores it in adipose tissue. Insulin stimulates the conversion of amino acids to protein, which are laid down into body protein stores, usually muscle, and stimulates the conversion of fatty acids into triacylglycerol, which is laid down in adipose tissue. Between meals, insulin levels fall, and these stored nutrients are then released into the blood to maintain fuel supplies to body cells.

Insulin, like its closely related cousin IGF, is also an important stimulator of cellular proliferation in both pre- and post-natal growth and development.

Insulin receptors

All body cells express insulin receptors on their cell membranes because all body cells need glucose for fuel. When

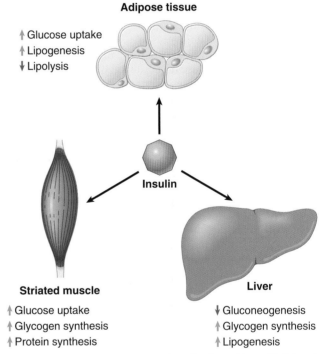

Fig. 10.8   The metabolic actions of insulin. (From Kumar V, Abbas A, and Aster J (2014) *Robbins & Cotran pathologic basis of disease: South Asia edition*, Fig. 24.29. India: Elsevier India.)

insulin binds to its receptor, it initiates a range of metabolic changes as described above, depending on the cell type involved. In particular, insulin-receptor binding leads to the production of specialised glucose transport channels called GLUT-4 transporters, which are inserted into the cell membrane and import glucose into the cell.

Insulin release

Insulin is synthesised as a pro-peptide, that is, a larger precursor molecule, called *pro-insulin*. This is enzymatically broken down in the β-cell to release insulin (Fig. 10.9). The

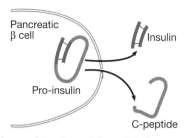

Fig. 10.9 Release of insulin and C-peptide from pro-insulin. (From Ralston S, Penman I, Strachan M, et al. (2018) *Davidson's principles and practice of medicine*, 23rd ed, Fig. 20.4. Edinburgh: Elsevier Ltd.)

remainder of the pro-insulin molecule after insulin has been cut out is called *C-peptide* (because of its shape), and measuring C-peptide levels is a useful indicator of how much natural insulin an individual is producing. Injected insulin gives high blood insulin levels, but no C-peptide, whereas blood insulin that has been endogenously synthesised is accompanied by high C-peptide levels.

The main stimulus for insulin release is rising blood glucose, which is detected directly by pancreatic β-cells. Rising levels of fatty acids and amino acids also stimulate β-cells and increase insulin release. If the nutrients are eaten and absorbed via the gastrointestinal tract, the effect on insulin release is more powerful than if the nutrients are injected directly into the bloodstream. The explanation for this lies in the fact that when foodstuffs enter the gastrointestinal tract, digestive organs release hormones into the blood that enhance pancreatic insulin release. These hormones, collectively called **incretins**, include cholecystokinin and glucagon-like peptide.

Insulin is secreted continuously into the bloodstream between meals, to allow body cells to extract glucose for energy. This is called **basal secretion**. Within 2 minutes of glucose arriving in the bloodstream after a meal, insulin levels rise, and peak after 5 or 6 minutes before falling again. This represents release of preformed, stored insulin from the pancreas and prevents the hyperglycaemia that would otherwise follow the commencement of a meal. A second, slower, more sustained rise in insulin levels begins almost immediately, leading to a prolonged rise in blood insulin levels that lasts until blood glucose levels are stabilised (Fig. 10.10). The second phase is caused by release of newly synthesised insulin. This biphasic response is abnormal in some forms of DM.

Glucagon

In contrast to insulin, glucagon mobilises stored nutrients, releasing glucose from glycogen, amino acids from protein, and fatty acids from fats. It therefore increases blood glucose levels.

GLUCOSE AND ENERGY METABOLISM

Glucose is often referred to as the preferred fuel molecule for body cells, but the biochemistry is not quite as straightforward as that. Glucose is not used directly for energy, but rather to produce ATP, a high-energy molecule used by all body cells to fuel all types of chemical reactions. In the presence of oxygen, one molecule of glucose can be metabolised to produce 38 molecules of ATP. The initial step is to split the glucose molecule into two pyruvate molecules in a

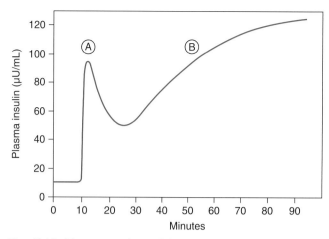

Fig. 10.10 The pancreatic β-cell biphasic response to glucose ingestion (at time 0). (A) Plasma insulin levels rise rapidly as the pancreas releases its stored insulin. (B) Prolonged raised plasma levels caused by release of newly synthesised insulin. (Modified from Seifter J, Walsh E, and Sloane D (2022) *Integrated physiology and pathophysiology*, Fig. 28.7. Philadelphia: Elsevier Inc.)

process called **glycolysis**, which takes place in the anaerobic environment of the cell cytosol. Glycolysis does not use oxygen and produces only two molecules of ATP. In healthy cells with a good oxygen supply, the pyruvate molecules enter the mitochondria and are converted into acetyl-CoA, which is then processed in two aerobic ATP-producing metabolic pathways, the citric acid cycle and oxidative phosphorylation, to produce a further 36 molecules of ATP. In the absence of oxygen, the pyruvate released from glycolysis is converted to lactate, which accumulates (Fig. 10.11).

DIABETES MELLITUS

WHO data reports that between 1990 and 2017 the number of people worldwide with DM increased fourfold, and around 1 in 10 people now has diabetes. It is the ninth commonest cause of death globally, and the economic burden it imposes on healthcare systems is enormous.

THE MAIN FEATURES OF DIABETES MELLITUS

The main types of diabetes are described below, but the following pathophysiological changes are characteristic of DM, irrespective of the aetiology.

Hyperglycaemia

High blood sugar levels are a diagnostic feature of DM because in the absence of insulin cells cannot extract glucose from the bloodstream. In addition, because cells are literally starved of glucose, the liver converts other substances—amino acids, lactic acid, and glycerol—into glucose, a process called *gluconeogenesis*. This additional glucose is released into the bloodstream in a futile attempt to supply the tissues; of course, in the absence of insulin, the additional glucose merely worsens the hyperglycaemia. It is important to be aware of what the person has eaten recently, as blood sugar levels can exceed normal values for a short time after a high carbohydrate meal, but the body's glucose regulatory mechanisms are so effective that this is rapidly brought back into the normal range in non-diabetic people. A fasting plasma glucose level below 100 mg/L (5.6 mmol/L) is considered normal.

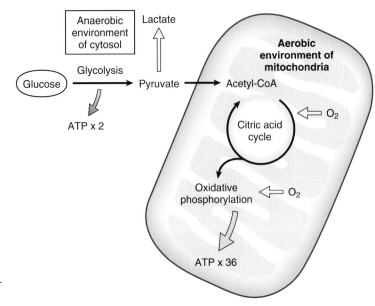

Fig. 10.11 The metabolic fate of glucose in aerobic and anaerobic conditions.

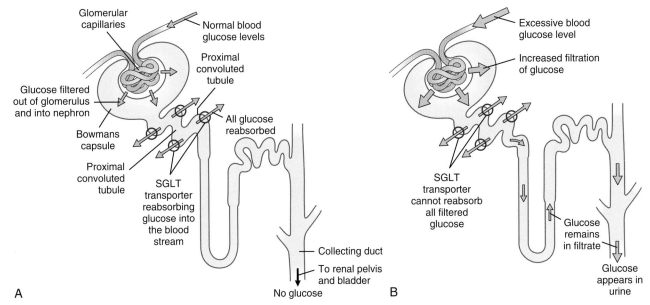

Fig. 10.12 Glucose handling in the nephron. (A) In health. (B) In diabetes mellitus.

Glycosuria

In the kidney, glucose is freely filtered from the blood across the glomerular membrane into the filtrate, because its molecular weight is low enough to permit it to pass through the filtration pores. The proximal convoluted tubule of the nephron then reabsorbs it into the blood using specialised carriers, **SGLT transporters**, related to the GLUT4 transporter used by body cells to import glucose (Fig. 10.12). As long as blood glucose levels are within the normal range, the amount of glucose appearing in the filtrate should not exceed the capacity of the SGLT carriers in the nephron wall to reabsorb it all, and none should appear in the urine (Fig. 10.12A). The maximum amount of glucose that can be reabsorbed per minute is called the *transport maximum* and is generally reached when plasma glucose levels reach about 11 mmol/L. When blood levels exceed this, as in uncontrolled DM, the glucose load in the filtrate exceeds the capacity of the nephron to reabsorb it, and glycosuria results (Fig. 10.12B).

Polyuria

Increased urine output is characteristic of DM because glucose in the urine increases its osmolarity and reduces water reabsorption. Daily urine volumes therefore rise. The excess water loss causes thirst, a characteristic symptom in uncontrolled DM. It also causes dehydration and increases the osmolarity of body fluids. One key consequence of this is that the acid products of impaired glucose metabolism, ketone bodies and lactic acid, are therefore more concentrated in body fluids, worsening the acidosis characteristic of diabetes.

COMPLICATIONS OF DIABETES MELLITUS

Although the natural course of DM of the different aetiologies is not identical, many of the pathophysiological changes that develop as a consequence of the metabolic abnormalities of the disease are associated with all of them to a lesser or greater extent.

Microvascular complications of diabetes mellitus

These are the major cause of mortality and morbidity in DM of any aetiology.

The most common sites of microvascular damage are the blood vessels of the retina, the kidney and the tiny blood vessels supplying the nerves of the peripheral nervous system, the vasa nervorum. Diabetic retinopathy, diabetic nephropathy, and diabetic neuropathy are the result. The main predisposing factor here is hyperglycaemia, which causes thickening of the basement membrane of the blood vessel endothelium, induces a chronic inflammatory state in the blood vessel wall, and impairs oxygen diffusion into the tissues. Persistently high glucose levels lead to glucose binding irreversibly to proteins in the blood vessel wall, forming **advanced glycation endproducts (AGEs)**. AGEs contribute to the ongoing vascular injury and accelerate the evolution of the abnormal insulin response in type 2 DM. Evidence from the United Kingdom Prospective Diabetes Study showed clearly that controlling hyperglycaemia delays the development of diabetes-associated vascular disease.

Diabetic retinopathy. Diabetic retinopathy is a leading cause of blindness worldwide. Retinal blood vessels, damaged by persistent hyperglycaemia, become leaky, leading to retinal oedema, which distorts and blurs vision. As the retinopathy progresses, new blood vessels begin to develop in the retina (retinal neovascularisation), but these are fragile and bleed easily, causing haemorrhage, hypoxia and death of the specialised retinal tissue, and blindness. Examined through the ophthalmoscope, the diabetic retina exhibits characteristic changes: narrowed, distorted or blocked vessels, tiny aneurysms where the weakened, damaged wall bulge, fatty deposits and haemorrhages (Fig. 10.13).

Diabetic neuropathy. This affects nerves (both sensory and motor) of the peripheral nervous system and is probably the most common complication of diabetes. It is mainly caused by microvascular damage in the vasa nervorum, but there is also evidence that hyperglycaemia directly injures the nerves themselves, initiating a chronic inflammatory response that causes demyelination and reduces conduction speeds, and causes degeneration of nerve axons.

Peripheral neuropathy shows what is called a 'stocking and glove' distribution (i.e., it affects the hands, feet, and lower leg), with the most distal areas (toes and fingers) affected first. Sensory nerve destruction causes paraesthesias (including tingling, pricking, aching, and hypersensitivity to touch) and numbness, increasing the risk that injury, often to the feet, may go unnoticed. Pain in diabetic neuropathy is common, tends to worsen with time, and because it is neuropathic in origin (i.e., is caused by direct damage to nervous tissue) does not respond to conventional analgesics. It can therefore have a substantial, negative impact on an individual's quality of life and be difficult to manage.

Lack of proprioceptive fibres means that the individual's balance and muscle co-ordination may be poor, increasing the risk of falls. If motor nerves are involved, the muscles they supply develop weakness and may atrophy. There may also be autonomic nerve damage, impairing the function of important body systems, including the cardiovascular, genitourinary and gastrointestinal organs, and producing a wide range of signs and symptoms, including erectile dysfunction, diarrhoea or constipation, arrhythmias, poor baroreceptor function leading to poor regulation of blood pressure, urinary retention, and sweating.

Diabetic nephropathy. The glomerular capillaries are progressively destroyed, leading ultimately to renal failure. Diabetic nephropathy is the commonest cause of chronic renal failure in the Western world and develops in about 40% of diabetic people. In addition to the vascular damage, the extracellular matrix in which the glomerular capillaries are embedded proliferates, which along with the vascular damage injures the filtration membrane, allowing proteinuria and reducing the glomerular filtration rate.

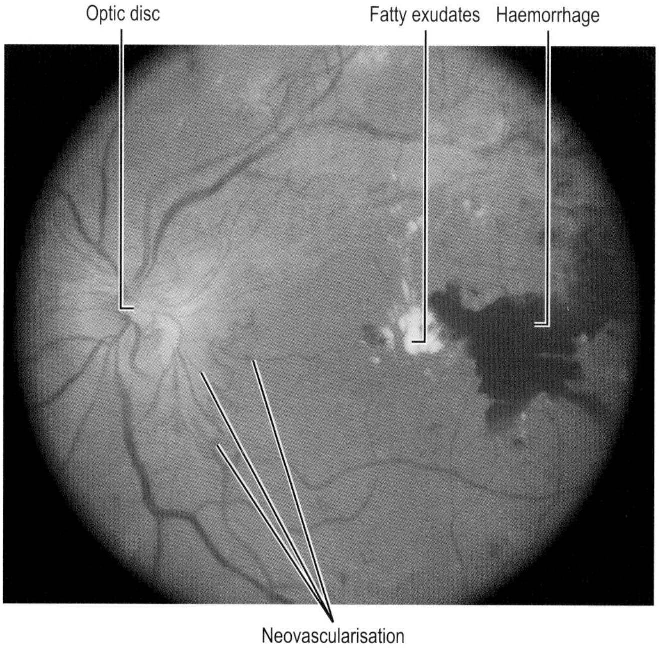

Fig. 10.13 The diabetic retina, showing neovascularisation of the optic disc, fatty exudates, and haemorrhage. (Modified from Swartz M (2021) *Textbook of physical diagnosis,* 8th ed, Fig. 10.103. Philadelphia: Elsevier Inc.)

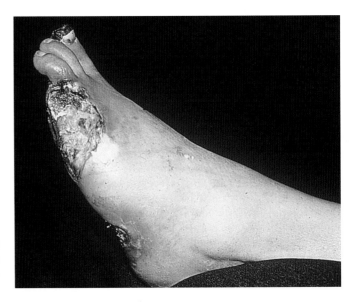

Fig. 10.14 Diabetic foot, showing two large gangrenous ulcers. The two smallest toes have been amputated. (From Johnson R, Feehally J, and Floege J (2015) *Comprehensive clinical nephrology*, Fig. 32.3. Philadelphia: Elsevier Inc.)

Macrovascular complications of diabetes mellitus

DM also injures larger blood vessels, leading to atherosclerosis, calcification, and chronic inflammation. This form of vascular injury is more common in type 2 DM than type 1. Hyperglycaemia is a known trigger, but in addition to this, the hyperlipidaemia of DM (caused by the increased breakdown of fats in the disease) is a major contributing factor. In addition, the blood lipid profile is usually unfavourable, with high levels of 'bad' low density lipoprotein and low levels of 'good' high density lipoprotein. The pathophysiology of atherosclerosis is described on p.158. Developing atherosclerotic plaques can cause stroke, myocardial infarction, or peripheral vascular disease, depending which blood vessels are affected. In addition, atherosclerosis increases the incidence of hypertension in diabetes.

Diabetic foot

This is very common in diabetes and accounts for nearly half of all diabetes-related hospital admissions. Because of poor circulation, increased incidence of infection, and poor sensation, diabetic people are predisposed to developing foot ulcers, which heal poorly and frequently lead to gangrenous changes, necrosis, and the necessity of amputation (Fig. 10.14). Scrupulous foot care and good glycaemic control greatly reduce the likelihood of diabetic foot developing.

Ketoacidosis

This is associated mainly with type 1 DM. In the absence of insulin, cells cannot take up glucose from the bloodstream, and hyperglycaemia ensues. Without glucose, the cell's main ATP-producing pathways are therefore unavailable. Body cells require a constant source of ATP, and the main alternative fuel source to glucose is the triacylglycerols, the body's stored fats. The body cells convert triacylglycerols to acetyl-CoA, which the liver then converts to ketone bodies-acetoacetate and 3-hydroxybutyrate. Acetoacetate is then converted to acetone. This is called **ketogenesis**, and the ketone bodies can be used by body cells, including the brain, for energy. In starvation, when the body is breaking down its reserves to produce energy for survival, ketones are an important source of fuel for body cells. Rising levels of ketones in the blood can spill into the urine (ketonuria) and cause metabolic acidosis (ketoacidosis). They are excreted in the breath, giving it a distinctive odour of acetone.

Diabetic ketoacidosis (DKA) is a medical emergency. It requires immediate treatment with insulin to restore glucose supply to body cells, and fluid and electrolyte replacement. Monitoring blood potassium levels is particularly important because DKA induces a profound reduction in total body potassium. This happens because, to restore acid-base balance, cells take up hydrogen ions from the acidic extracellular fluid, but in exchange, they release potassium. This potassium is then lost from the body in the osmotic diuresis caused by the hyperglycaemia. Because a high intracellular potassium concentration, maintained by the Na^+/K^+ pump, is essential to keep nerve and muscle cells electrically active, hypokalaemia can cause life-threatening cardiac arrhythmias and cardiac arrest.

DKA can be triggered by failure to adhere to treatment, allowing hyperglycaemia and a metabolic shift to ketone production to follow, or by a physiological stressor such as infection or injury. When this happens, the adrenal glands release cortisol as part of the stress response, and one of cortisol's actions is to induce insulin resistance, reduce tissue uptake of glucose, and cause hyperglycaemia. Additional insulin is normally required to compensate for this and prevent DKA.

Other complications of diabetes mellitus

Diabetic people are at elevated risk of cataract, caused by deposition of AGE and denaturation of the proteins in the lens. The risk of certain cancers, including uterine and pancreatic malignancies, is increased. Infections are more common in diabetes than in the general population.

TYPES OF DIABETES MELLITUS

The WHO (2019) classification of diabetes mellitus lists five main types: type 1 diabetes, type 2 diabetes, hyperglycaemia first detected during pregnancy, diabetes of other specific types, and hybrid forms of diabetes. Only the first four will be considered here. Identifying the type of DM present is important for determining treatment.

TYPE 1 DIABETES MELLITUS

Globally, type 1 diabetes mellitus (T1DM) accounts for 5% to 10% of DM cases. It is usually diagnosed in childhood, and so is sometimes referred to as juvenile-onset diabetes, although a significant number of cases are diagnosed in adulthood. Globally, its incidence is rising, and there is significant geographical variation in its distribution. Diabetes UK (2013) listed Finland (incidence 57.6 per 100 000 children aged under 15) as the country with the highest rate of T1DM in the world. Other countries high on the list include the United Kingdom (24.5 per 100 000) and Kuwait and Denmark (both about 22 per 100 000). The lowest rates in this age group are found in Venezuela and Papua New Guinea, with 0.1 per 100 000 children. This illustrates the huge global variation, which has not been adequately explained, although it is likely that genetic variation between populations plays a significant part. Girls and boys are equally affected, and white populations have higher rates than non-white populations. Although there is a clear genetic predisposition, there is no single 'diabetes' gene: multiple genes are involved. In identical twins, if one is type 1 diabetic, the risk to the other is only 30% to 50%, and the risk to a child if the mother has T1DM is less than 4%.

Pathophysiology

T1DM is characterised by destruction of the β-cells of the pancreatic islets and leads to an absolute deficiency of insulin. β-cell destruction can occur very quickly, or take a slower, more protracted course. In up to 90% of affected people it is an autoimmune disorder, and autoantibodies to key enzymes of the pancreatic islets and sometimes to insulin itself are found. Autoreactive T-cells directed against β-cells also contribute to their destruction. These people have a higher incidence of other autoimmune disorders, for example, coeliac disease and rheumatoid arthritis. As well as the genetic predisposition, it is also thought that some cases develop after a triggering event, such as a viral infection, which initiates the autoimmune response. Histological examination of the pancreas shows infiltration with a range of inflammatory and immune cells, including macrophages, T cells, and B cells.

It is not clear what the underlying pathological changes are that cause β-cell destruction in those people without an obvious autoimmune mechanism.

Signs and symptoms

The biphasic insulin secretion response to rising blood glucose levels (Fig. 10.10) is completely abolished because the pancreas is producing no insulin. The individual presents with weight loss, fatigue, a raging thirst, polyuria, and (in children) failure to thrive. There may also be a history of urinary tract infections because the high glucose content of the urine favours microbial growth. In the total absence of insulin, the risk of ketoacidosis is high. It has been estimated that about 50% of hospital admissions in young diabetics are caused by poor control and consequential ketoacidosis.

Prognosis and management

Because the pancreatic islets are usually completely destroyed, the patient produces no insulin of their own and requires lifelong insulin treatment. Even in developed countries with advanced healthcare, T1DM reduces the expected lifespan by 13 years. However, how well patients do in the long term is strongly influenced by how well controlled their blood glucose levels are. Good glycaemic control delays the onset of complications and can reduce their severity when they do develop.

TYPE 2 DIABETES MELLITUS

Type 2 diabetes mellitus (T2DM) accounts for up to 95% of all cases of DM. Risk factors include increasing age, smoking, obesity, a family history, a sedentary lifestyle, and a diet high in processed foods, red meat, fat, and carbohydrates. Body fat distribution is also important. People who carry a higher proportion of their body fat around their abdominal organs are at higher risk, even when their body weight falls in the normal range. T2DM is traditionally more common in older adults, but because the numbers of overweight and obese children and young people are increasing in most societies, it is increasingly common in these age groups as well.

Pathophysiology

The onset of T2DM is usually insidious, and the period before the individual becoming symptomatic but during which there is progressive dysfunction of insulin release and glucose metabolism is called **pre-diabetes**. The pre-diabetic period can last for years. T2DM is a complex condition, in which pancreatic β-cells begin to fail, leading eventually to reduced insulin secretion. β-cell failure is thought to be due essentially to overwork – the result of prolonged and excessive insulin production because of prolonged and sustained exposure to excessive blood glucose concentrations. In association with consistently high insulin levels, body cells lose their capacity to respond normally to insulin (**insulin resistance**). Insulin resistance is much more common in obese people than in those of normal weight. The underlying reasons for the abnormal changes are not understood, but the course of the developing disorder generally follows a particular pattern (Fig. 10.15). In the pre-diabetic stage, blood glucose levels initially remain fairly normal because, despite insulin resistance, the pancreatic β-cells produce more insulin to compensate (hyperinsulinaemia). As the pre-diabetic state progresses, and β-cell function deteriorates, insulin levels begin to fall. As this happens, blood glucose levels begin to rise, symptoms

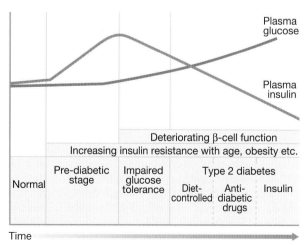

Fig. 10.15 The natural course of T2DM. (Modified from Ralston S, Penman I, Strachan M, et al. (2018) *Davidson's principles and practice of medicine*, 23rd ed, Fig. 20.8. Edinburgh: Elsevier Ltd.)

appear and frank diabetes becomes apparent. Some β-cell function may be retained in many people, who therefore continue to produce some insulin, in contrast to those with T1DM, whose pancreatic islets are completely destroyed and who produce no insulin at all.

The biphasic pattern of normal insulin release in response to rising blood glucose levels may show an initial spike, although this may be lower than normal, and, depending on the degree of pancreatic dysfunction, shows either a depressed or absent second phase. As the disorder progresses, the insulin response diminishes more and more, and in late disease there may be little or no insulin released and no evidence of two distinct phases.

Signs and symptoms

Of all people with T2DM, 60% have no symptoms at the time of diagnosis, but others present with the classic symptoms of polydipsia, polyuria, weight loss, fatigue, and hunger. Others may present with indications of diabetes-induced end-organ damage, such as paraesthesias, deterioration in vision or renal impairment. Diabetic retinopathy generally appears more quickly post-diagnosis in T2DM than type 1 because it is likely the T2DM patient has had a long pre-diabetic period with undetected hyperglycaemia.

Prognosis and management

How well patients do in the long term depends on how well they manage their condition and control their blood glucose levels. Tight glycaemic control delays or even prevents the onset of vascular and neurological complications and slows their progression once they have appeared. Initial management includes attention to lifestyle changes, including weight loss, smoking cessation, limiting alcohol intake, increasing exercise levels, and ensuring a healthy diet. A range of oral anti-diabetic drugs, which reduce blood glucose levels by a range of metabolic actions, is available, although many people eventually require some insulin treatment as well, particularly in times of illness.

HYPERGLYCAEMIA OF PREGNANCY

Pregnancy induces a state of insulin resistance, leading to a tendency to hyperglycaemia and sometimes precipitating frank diabetes. Diabetes that occurs in pregnancy in a previously non-diabetic woman is called **gestational diabetes**. Risk factors include maternal overweight/obesity, having had gestational diabetes in a previous pregnancy and a family history of diabetes, and worldwide affects about 14% of pregnancies.

Pathophysiology

In a healthy pregnancy, elevated levels of oestrogen, progesterone, leptin, and placental hormones induce mild insulin resistance, increasing blood glucose, fatty acid, and amino acid levels to ensure the growing fetus is adequately supplied. The reasons why some women develop gestational diabetes are not clear, but there are likely several contributory factors. For example, β-cells in the pancreas of a healthy pregnant woman increase in size and number to increase insulin secretion to cope with the demands of pregnancy. In gestational diabetes, the β-cells fail to do this, and insulin levels are inadequate to cope with the increased blood glucose levels, leading to hyperglycaemia.

Consequences of hyperglycaemia of pregnancy

This condition affects both mother and baby. It increases the risk of pre-eclampsia and premature birth, and of the development of T2DM and cardiovascular disease in later life in the mother. The baby is likely to be of above-average birth weight and is more likely to need delivery by caesarean section. There is evidence that gestational DM increases the risk of stillbirth and of the child becoming obese and/or developing T2DM in later life.

DIABETES OF OTHER SPECIFIC TYPES

Diabetes can result from a range of specific diseases and conditions. For example, disorders of the pancreas, including pancreatitis, pancreatic cancer, or cystic fibrosis damage pancreatic tissues, including the β-cells. Some hormones (e.g., thyroxine and cortisol) antagonise the actions of insulin and disorders associated with hypersecretion of these hormones lead to diabetes. Hyperthyroidism and Cushing syndrome are therefore associated with DM. Drugs that mimic the actions of adrenaline (β-adrenergic agonists and α-adrenergic agonists) also antagonise the action of insulin because adrenaline itself increases blood glucose levels as part of its action in the stress response. Infections can lead to β-cell-destruction; rubella and mumps, for example, are associated with DM.

THE THYROID GLAND AND ITS DISORDERS

The thyroid gland produces, stores, and secretes two main hormones: **T_3 (tri-iodothyronine)** and **T_4 (thyroxine)**. These hormones are produced by adding three and four atoms of iodine respectively to the amino acid tyrosine, which is then packaged in a protein-rich matrix called **thyroglobulin** into storage units called *thyroid follicles* in the gland. T_4 is the main form produced, stored, and released by the thyroid. However, once released into the circulation, the peripheral tissues convert it into T_3, which is much more biologically active.

Disorders of thyroid secretion are the commonest form of endocrine disease and are more common in women than men.

Actions of thyroid hormones

Thyroid hormones are essential for normal fetal growth and development, and regulate metabolism in nearly all body cells after birth. They increase basal metabolic rate, cell oxygen consumption, and the production of body heat; and they increase blood levels of fuel and nutrient molecules to promote cell division and tissue growth. They stimulate gluconeogenesis (glucose production from non-carbohydrate molecules) in the liver. They break down stored triacylglycerols to release free fatty acids and enhance protein breakdown (mainly from muscle) to release free amino acids. Thyroid hormones are therefore physiological antagonists of insulin.

Control of thyroid hormone levels

The thyroid gland is regulated by the HPA (see Fig. 10.3). The hypothalamus releases thyrotrophin-releasing hormone (TRH) into the capillaries supplying the anterior pituitary, which triggers the release of thyroid stimulating hormone (TSH) into the systemic circulation. TSH in its turn stimulates the release of T_3 and T_4 from the thyroid gland. When thyroid hormone levels exceed normal, this feeds back onto

Table 10.1 Metabolic consequences of abnormally high or low levels of thyroid hormones

High T_3/T_4 level	Low T_3/T_4 level
Increased glucose production (gluconeogenesis and glycogenolysis stimulated)	Reduced glucose production (gluconeogenesis and glycogenolysis inhibited)
Protein synthesis inhibited and protein breakdown stimulated, causing muscle wasting	Protein synthesis stimulated and protein breakdown inhibited
Stored fats broken down, increasing circulating blood lipid concentrations	Fat stores built up, reducing circulating blood lipid concentrations
Increased body temperature	Reduced body temperature

Table 10.2 Signs and symptoms of hyperthyroidism and hypothyroidism*

Hyperthyroidism	Hypothyroidism
Goitre	**Mental slowness**
Heat intolerance	**Dry, puffy, coarse skin and dry, thin, unmanageable hair**
Tachycardia, atrial fibrillation, bounding pulse, flushed and warm skin, hypertension, heart failure, palpitations	**Bradycardia,** hypertension, heart failure, cold peripheries
Thirst, vomiting, and diarrhoea	
Hair loss, onycholysis (separation of the fingernail from the nailbed)	**Slow-relaxing reflexes** Gruff voice
Sweating	Cold intolerance, hypothermia
Pre-tibial myxoedema	Myxoedema
Irritability, restlessness, hyperactivity	Anaemia
Poor concentration, psychosis	Poor memory, depression, psychosis
Muscle weakness and wasting, tremor	Aches and pains, muscle weakness, ataxia, inactivity
Reduced libido, menstrual irregularities including amenorrhoea	Reduced libido, heavy menstrual periods
Weight loss, increased appetite	Weight gain, mild obesity, anorexia, constipation

*Those in bold are most useful in diagnosis. Not all patients show all symptoms.

both the anterior pituitary gland and the hypothalamus, reducing the secretion of TRH and TSH.

HYPERTHYROIDISM

Hyperthyroidism is usually the result of several pathological conditions affecting the thyroid gland but rarely can be caused by disorders of the anterior pituitary or the hypothalamus. The commonest cause is Graves disease. The metabolic consequences of elevated circulating thyroid hormones are summarised in Table 10.1. Because thyroid hormones accelerate the metabolism of virtually all body cells, the signs and symptoms associated with hyperthyroidism are wide-ranging. Excessively high levels of T_3 and T_4 sensitise body tissues to the effects of the sympathetic nervous system, causing cardiovascular effects including hypertension and tachycardia. The increased workload and oxygen consumption of the heart can cause heart failure in untreated hyperthyroid disease. Increased metabolic rate leads to heat intolerance and weight loss. Depending on the aetiology, there may be goitre (swelling of the thyroid gland). The signs and symptoms of hyperthyroidism are summarised in Table 10.2.

Graves disease

This autoimmune condition, sometimes called *thyrotoxicosis*, is the commonest cause of hyperthyroidism, accounting for up to 60% of all cases. The female:male ratio is 10:1, and the disease occurs worldwide. It is commonly associated with other autoimmune disorders, including myasthenia gravis, rheumatoid arthritis, and systemic lupus erythematosus.

Pathophysiology

In Graves disease, the autoantibodies present are directed towards the TSH receptor on the thyroid gland. These autoantibodies act like TSH from the pituitary gland and stimulate the thyroid follicles to synthesise and secrete thyroid hormone (Fig. 10.16). Circulating levels of thyroid hormone therefore rise.

Signs and symptoms

In addition to those listed in Table 10.2, Graves disease is associated with characteristic ophthalmic changes. The incidence of eye involvement increases with age at diagnosis, smoking, and the duration of the disease. The eyes protrude from their sockets (exophthalmos) because the autoantibodies also stimulate the connective tissue that

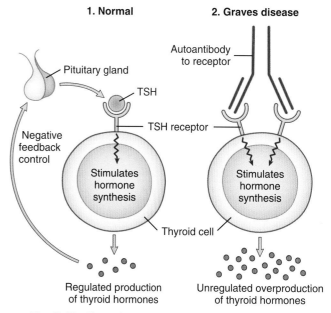

Fig. 10.16 The action of autoantibodies in Graves disease.

cushions and supports the eyeballs in their bony orbits. This becomes inflamed and hypertrophic, and extra fat tissue is laid down. As the volume of this supporting connective tissue expands, it pushes the eyes forward, and they bulge. Not only is this cosmetically difficult for the patient, it may also prevent the eyelids closing properly over the front of the eye and cause corneal dryness and increased risk of corneal damage. In addition, rising pressure in the orbit can compress the optic nerve and cause visual disturbances, and can restrict the movement of the eyeball in its orbit, making it difficult for the patient to direct their gaze towards particular items in their field of vision. These ocular changes usually do not improve even when the patient's thyroid function is regulated because they are caused by the inflammatory/autoimmune changes in the periorbital tissues rather than by the hyperthyroidism itself. In about 5% of people with Graves disease, a similar proliferation of connective tissue occurs in the skin of the shin, and occasionally on the face or arms. The thickening connective tissue attracts water and leads to swelling and thickening in the area. This is called **myxoedema**; when on the front of the shin, it is called *pre-tibial myxoedema.*

The excessive T_3 and T_4 levels in the blood feed back to the anterior pituitary and shut down its release of TSH. Graves disease is therefore characterised by high levels of circulating thyroid hormones but very low levels of TSH.

Management and prognosis

Graves disease tends to follow a relapsing/remitting course, with periods of hyperthyroidism interspersed with periods of more normal thyroid function. Treatment includes radioactive iodine to destroy thyroid tissue and antithyroid drugs. Radioactive iodine usually causes hypothyroidism, which then in turn must be treated with thyroid hormone replacement therapy.

HYPOTHYROIDISM

The metabolic consequences of reduced circulating thyroid hormones are summarised in Table 10.2. Worldwide, the commonest cause of hypothyroidism is iodine deficiency. In populations for which iodine deficiency is not a problem (e.g., because of good diet, iodine-supplemented water, and/or foodstuffs), the commonest cause of hypothyroidism is Hashimoto disease. Other causes of primary hypothyroidism include failure of the thyroid to develop during fetal life (congenital agenesis), thyroid destruction because of cancer, thyroid infections, and certain drugs (e.g., lithium). Treatment for hyperthyroidism (thyroid irradiation, anti-thyroid drugs and radioactive iodine) may all cause hypothyroidism.

Hashimoto thyroiditis

This autoimmune disorder tends to appear in middle age. As with most autoimmune disorders, it is commoner in women than men and is associated with other autoimmune conditions, including coeliac disease and connective tissue diseases. There is a strong familial tendency; the risk to first-degree relatives of a sufferer is several times higher than in the general population.

Pathophysiology

Autoantibodies are produced mainly against the enzyme thyroid peroxidase, which converts T_4 to T_3, leading to a fall in circulating thyroid hormone levels. Autoantibodies to thyroglobulin may also be present. The gland becomes infiltrated with inflammatory cells, including plasma cells, which are probably the source of the autoantibodies, and that cause inflammation and eventual fibrosis, shrinkage, and destruction of the gland.

Signs and symptoms

The disorder usually progresses slowly, and it may be months or even years before signs and symptoms are obvious enough that a diagnosis is made. Its principal features are listed in Table 10.2. Falling levels of thyroid hormone stimulate the anterior pituitary to produce TSH to restore them, and Hashimoto thyroiditis is usually characterised by low levels of T_3 and T_4, despite elevated levels of TSH.

Management and prognosis

The treatment of choice is lifelong hormone replacement therapy.

THE PARATHYROID GLANDS

These four small glands are located on the posterior face of the thyroid gland, two on each lobe. Their combined weight is less than 0.5 g, but without the hormone they produce, parathyroid hormone (also called parathormone, or PTH), the body is unable to regulate calcium or phosphate balance, or synthesise vitamin D.

The role of parathormone

The parathyroid cells that secrete PTH, called chief cells, constantly measure plasma calcium. When blood calcium levels fall, PTH is released, and increases them in two main ways:

- PTH breaks down bone tissue to release calcium (and phosphate)
- PTH stimulates the activation of vitamin D in the kidney.

PTH activity and vitamin D work closely together in the maintenance of plasma calcium levels and in bone health. In the kidney, PTH stimulates the conversion of the inactive form of vitamin D, 25-hydroxyvitamin D, into the active form, 1,25-hydroxyvitamin D. Active vitamin D stimulates calcium uptake in the gastrointestinal tract and reabsorption in the kidney, increasing calcium levels in the bloodstream and therefore increasing the amount of calcium available for deposition in bone. Although the action of vitamin D on bone is complex, normal levels increase bone turnover, essential for normal bone formation and maintenance of good bone health (see also rickets and osteomalacia; p.333). Good bone turnover ensures continuous release of calcium into the bloodstream and maintains blood calcium levels. Fig. 10.17 summarises the interaction between vitamin D and PTH in the regulation of blood calcium and bone turnover. Lack of vitamin D, which in turn causes low blood calcium levels, causes osteomalacia in adults and rickets in children.

HYPERPARATHYROIDISM

High levels of PTH cause breakdown of bone, which may cause bone pain and increase the risk of fracture, and elevated blood calcium levels (hypercalcaemia) as calcium is released from bone into the blood. Hypercalcaemia can cause renal stones because the excess calcium precipitates

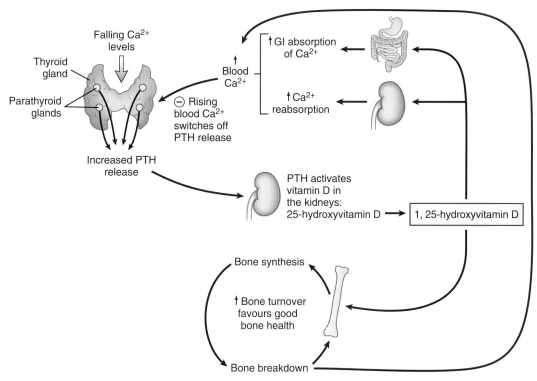

Fig. 10.17   The roles of vitamin D and parathormone in calcium homeostasis.

out in the kidney. Calcium is essential for a wide range of physiological mechanisms, including nerve conduction, blood clotting, muscle contraction and enzyme activity, and excessive levels affect nearly every organ in the body. Hypercalcaemia causes a wide range of non-specific symptoms including nausea and vomiting, muscle aches and pains, fatigue, thirst, polyuria, and neuropsychiatric issues including confusion, depression, and coma. To implement appropriate treatment, it is important to distinguish between primary and secondary hyperparathyroidism.

Primary hyperparathyroidism

This is the uncontrolled, excessive secretion of PTH, usually (90% of cases) caused by a functioning parathyroid adenoma. It is three times as common in women than men, and usually occurs over the age of 50. Sometimes carcinomas elsewhere, including breast, lung, and kidney cancers, secrete PTH.

Secondary hyperparathyroidism

This is increased PTH secondary to uncorrected hypocalcaemia and is usually caused by vitamin D deficiency or chronic kidney disease. The failing kidneys are unable to perform their normal function of converting the inactive form of vitamin D, 25-hydroxyvitamin D, to the active form, 1,25-hydroxyvitamin D, and so the body becomes deficient in vitamin D. This in turn reduces calcium absorption and hypocalcaemia ensues. The parathyroid glands react by increasing PTH secretion, which does not improve renal reabsorption of calcium because the failing kidneys are unable to respond, but parathormone releases calcium and phosphate from bone, leading to demineralisation of the skeleton and weakening of bone tissue (osteomalacia; p.333), a common event in chronic kidney disease.

HYPOPARATHYROIDISM

The commonest cause of reduced parathyroid gland function is injury sustained during thyroid surgery. Without adequate levels of PTH, vitamin D activation is reduced, leading to hypocalcaemia because calcium cannot be extracted from bone and calcium absorption from the GI tract and renal tubules does not take place. Hypocalcaemia impairs muscle contraction and nerve conduction, and can cause heart failure and arrhythmias, bronchospasm, seizures and tetany, prolonged skeletal muscle contraction.

THE ADRENAL GLAND AND ITS DISORDERS

The adrenal glands, located on the upper pole of the kidneys, are enclosed in a protective capsule and the interior is composed of two discrete layers of tissue: the outer cortex and the inner medulla (Fig. 10.18). Both layers function as endocrine glands; the cortex secretes steroid hormones, principally glucocorticoids and mineralocorticoids, and the central medulla is part of the sympathetic nervous system and releases adrenaline.

THE ADRENAL MEDULLA

This forms the core of the gland and represents about 10% of its total mass. The cells here, called *chromaffin cells* or *phaeochromocytes*, synthesise and store adrenaline and noradrenaline (catecholamines), which they release into the bloodstream when stimulated by the sympathetic nervous system.

Phaeochromocytoma

This rare tumour of the adrenal medulla is benign in 90% of patients. Most cases arise randomly, but about 30% are associated with inherited disorders, including neurofibromatosis.

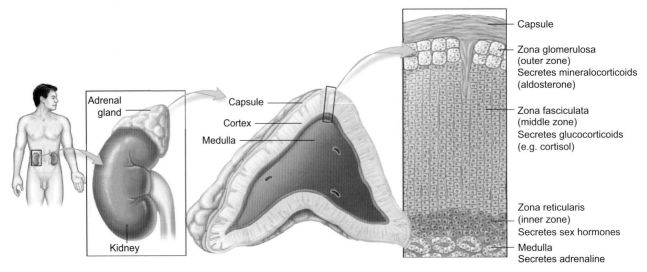

Fig. 10.18   The position and structure of the adrenal glands. (Modified from Moini J, Badolato C, and Ahangari R (2021) *Epidemiology of endocrine tumors*, Fig. 1.20. Philadelphia: Elsevier Inc.)

The main presenting sign is hypertension, which may be severe and immediately life-threatening (hypertensive crisis), but the disorder may be completely asymptomatic if the tumour is non-functioning. It occurs in all races and is most common in the age group 40 to 60 years.

Pathophysiology

Unlike normal adrenal medullary tissue, the tumour is not supplied with sympathetic nerves, and so its secretion of catecholamines is not regulated by the sympathetic nervous system. Its secretory pattern may be sporadic and unpredictable, although there are identifiable trigger factors, including childbirth, exercise, and certain drugs (e.g., beta blockers and opioids).

These tumours are often rich in blood vessels and haemorrhage may be fatal.

Signs and symptoms

These involve multiple body organs because of the wide-ranging actions of the sympathetic nervous system. Sympathetic stimulation of the cardiovascular system causes hypertension, palpitations, and tachycardia and can precipitate heart failure. There may be sweating, anxiety, tremor, hyperglycaemia, headache, pallor, and constipation. Initially, episodes may be infrequent, perhaps once every few weeks, and last only a few seconds, but as the tumour grows, typically the frequency and duration of attacks increases. Elevated catecholamine levels are found in the blood and urine.

Management and prognosis

Drugs that antagonise catecholamines (e.g., alpha and beta blockers) are used to reduce catecholamine stress on the cardiovascular system before surgery, which is the treatment of choice. This is usually curative when the tumour is benign, giving a 5-year survival rate of over 95%. In malignant phaeochromocytoma, the outlook is poorer, with a 5-year survival of less than 50%.

THE ADRENAL CORTEX

The adrenal cortex can be thought of as three separate endocrine glands because it contains three layers of different types of cells secreting three different types of adrenal steroid hormones (Fig. 10.18). The outer layer, the zona glomerulosa, secretes mineralocorticoids and is under the control of the renin-angiotensin system (see Fig. 6.43). The main mineralocorticoid is aldosterone. The middle layer, the zona fasciculata, secretes glucocorticoids (mainly cortisol), and the inner zona reticularis secretes the sex hormones oestrogen, progesterone, and testosterone. These latter two regions are under the control of the HPA.

Mineralocorticoids and disorders of mineralocorticoid secretion

Reduced levels of aldosterone are usually caused by adrenal insufficiency (see below). Elevated levels may be caused by a disorder of the adrenal cortex itself (primary hyperaldosteronism) or secondary to dysfunction of the renin-angiotensin system (see Fig. 6.43), which is the main mechanism by which aldosterone levels are controlled.

Functions of aldosterone

Aldosterone is an important regulator of sodium excretion by the kidney. It acts on the distal convoluted tubule and the collecting duct of the nephron and enhances sodium reabsorption (which passively increases water reabsorption as well) and potassium excretion. Aldosterone therefore increases total body water and sodium.

Hyperaldosteronism

Because of increased sodium and fluid load, hyperaldosteronism causes hypertension and sometimes oedema. Excessive potassium loss can lead to hyperglycaemia and precipitate diabetes because potassium is needed for insulin secretion. Hypokalaemia can also impair muscle function, causing skeletal muscle weakness and cardiac arrhythmias.

Primary hyperaldosteronism. In up to 60% of patients, primary hyperaldosteronism is caused by a functioning adenoma of the zona glomerulosa, which secretes elevated levels of aldosterone. In the majority of the remainder, the overproduction is caused by adrenal gland hyperplasia. Either cause produces a collection of signs and symptoms called

Conn syndrome and affects more women than men. It is the commonest cause of secondary hypertension.

Management and prognosis. Aldosterone receptor antagonists (e.g., spironolactone) are used to block the action of aldosterone. If the cause of the hyperaldosteronism is an adrenal adenoma, the adrenal glands can be removed surgically. Lifelong treatment with steroids is then required. The prognosis is generally good, but in some patients, hypertension persists even after adrenalectomy, probably because of permanent vascular damage sustained during the hypertensive period.

Secondary hyperaldosteronism. This is caused by conditions that reduce blood flow through the kidney, which activates the renin-angiotensin system (see Fig. 6.43). Activation of the renin-angiotensin system increases renin levels, an important distinguishing sign differentiating between primary and secondary hyperaldosteronism. Reduced renal blood flow may be caused by low circulating blood volume, renal arterial disease, or cardiac failure (Fig. 10.19). Treatment should address the underlying cause.

Glucocorticoids and excessive glucocorticoid secretion

Over- or under-secretion of glucocorticoids can be caused by disease of the adrenal glands themselves, but also by disorders of the anterior pituitary or the hypothalamus because secretion from the zona fasciculata is controlled by the HPA.

Functions of cortisol

Complete adrenal cortex failure from any cause is not compatible with life because glucocorticoid hormones are essential to fundamental metabolic pathways and to the body's stress response.

Cortisol (also called *hydrocortisone*) is secreted according to a diurnal rhythm, with blood levels very low overnight, rising towards morning and falling again towards evening. This variation in secretion underpins the primary function of glucocorticoids in preparing the body to manage stress, and stress increases cortisol levels in the blood. Stress in physiology refers to any event that shifts homeostatic balance in the body away from normal, including pathological events such as illness, injury, and infection. Cortisol activates several key metabolic pathways to ensure that, in the face of a threat to homeostasis, body cells have an adequate supply of essential nutrients, and additionally it provides a brake on the inflammatory and immune responses. Nearly all tissues have glucocorticoid receptors, and so the effects of cortisol are widespread. It increases blood sugar levels, blood fatty acid levels, and blood amino acid levels. It restricts the laying down of new body tissues and induces a degree of insulin resistance in body cells, reducing their glucose uptake to maintain adequate supply for the brain. It has profound anti-inflammatory and immunosuppressant properties. Cortisol, additionally, has mineralocorticoid activity, and stimulates sodium and water reabsorption in the kidney. The physiological effects of cortisol are summarised in Table 10.3.

Hypersecretion of glucocorticoids: Cushing disease and Cushing syndrome

Harvey Cushing was an American neurosurgeon credited with several significant advances in medical practice,

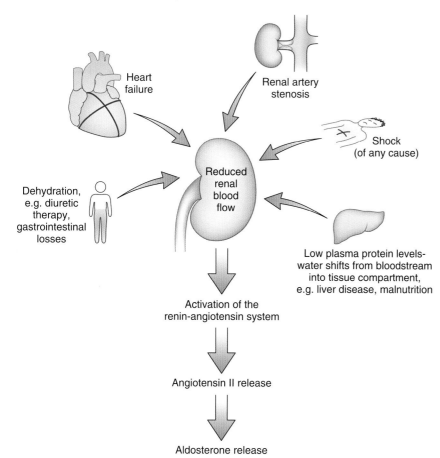

Fig. 10.19 Some causes of secondary hyperaldosteronism.

Heart failure

Renal artery stenosis

Shock (of any cause)

Dehydration, e.g. diuretic therapy, gastrointestinal losses

Reduced renal blood flow

Low plasma protein levels-water shifts from bloodstream into tissue compartment, e.g. liver disease, malnutrition

Activation of the renin-angiotensin system

Angiotensin II release

Aldosterone release

Table 10.3   The physiological effects of cortisol (hydrocortisone)

Cortisol effects	Effect	Mechanisms
-on glucose metabolism	Hyperglycaemia	Insulin resistance, reducing glucose uptake by body cells Inhibition of gluconeogenesis (synthesis of glucose from non-carbohydrate sources, e.g., amino acids and glycerol) in the liver Breakdown of glycogen in the liver and muscle
-on protein metabolism	High blood levels of circulating amino acids	Activates breakdown of muscle (the body's main reservoir of protein) Inhibition of protein synthesis
-on fat metabolism	Hyperlipidaemia	Stimulates breakdown of fat from fat stores; fat is broken down into fatty acids (an additional fuel source) and glycerol (converted into glucose)
-on the inflammatory and immune responses	Suppression	Inhibition of white blood cell migration, secretion, activation, and adhesion Inhibition of synthesis of inflammatory mediators
-on other physiological functions		Inhibits the bone-building function of osteoclasts and the tissue-building activity of fibroblasts

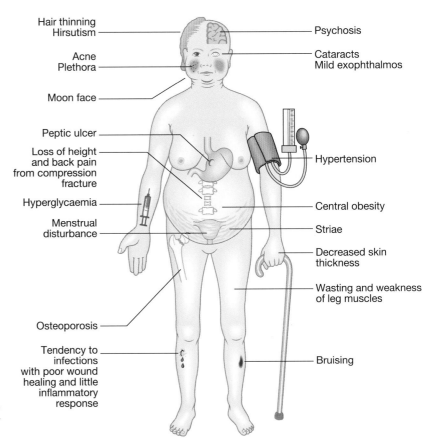

Fig. 10.20   Signs and symptoms of Cushing disease. (Modified from Ralston S, Penman I, Strachan M, et al. (2018) *Davidson's principles and practice of medicine*, 23rd ed, Fig. 18.20. Edinburgh: Elsevier Ltd.)

and who named Cushing disease, a disorder of the pituitary gland, in 1912. The pituitary gland, under the control of the hypothalamus, secretes ACTH, which in turn stimulates cortisol release from the adrenal cortex (see Fig. 10.2). Pituitary oversecretion of ACTH, usually from a benign but functioning pituitary adenoma, causes excessive cortisol release from the adrenal cortex. This causes a constellation of signs and symptoms associated with glucocorticoid excess (Fig. 10.20) and its commonest cause is pituitary disease. An identical clinical picture is seen if the excessive glucocorticoid levels are caused by administration of exogenous steroids, or (rarely) by a functioning adrenal tumour. Some lung tumours may produce ACTH, also giving elevated glucocorticoid levels.

If glucocorticoid hypersecretion is caused by any other cause than pituitary disease, it is referred to as *Cushing syndrome*, not *Cushing disease*.

Adrenocortical insufficiency

Destruction or dysfunction of the adrenal cortex, affecting all regions of the gland, lead to loss of glucocorticoid, mineralocorticoid, and sex steroid secretion. When this is caused by adrenal disease (primary adrenal insufficiency), it is called Addison disease. This is usually of autoimmune origin and commonest in females between 30 and 60 years of age. Other causes include adrenal malignancies, both primary and metastatic, which destroy the gland and infections involving the adrenal gland (e.g., tuberculosis). Patients may present with either glucocorticoid or mineralocorticoid deficiency, although if untreated, they eventually develop signs and symptoms of both. Because there is significant physiological reserve, there may be no indication of disease until over 90% of adrenal tissue is lost. Sometimes a person whose failing adrenal function has not yet been identified can present suddenly and acutely ill (Addisonian crisis) after a precipitating factor (e.g., infection or surgery). In such people, the stress response, which would normally involve a rapid increase in glucocorticoids, is inadequate because of glucocorticoid deficiency, and even a minor stressor can trigger life-threatening cardiovascular collapse.

Secondary adrenal cortex insufficiency may be caused by pituitary or hypothalamic disease, but the most frequent cause is a rapid withdrawal of glucocorticoid therapy. Glucocorticoid treatment suppresses natural glucocorticoid secretion by inhibiting CRH release from the hypothalamus and ACTH release from the anterior pituitary. If steroid treatment is abruptly stopped, plasma levels rapidly fall, and although normal HPA function will eventually re-establish itself over the course of the following weeks, it leaves the individual critically deficient in glucocorticoids in the short term.

Signs and symptoms

In chronically developing adrenal insufficiency, there may be symptoms associated with low aldosterone levels, including hypotension, shock, and hyperkalaemia. Glucocorticoid deficiency leads to hypoglycaemia, hypotension, shock, malaise, weakness, depression, nausea, and vomiting. In Addison disease, the anterior pituitary responds to falling blood glucocorticoid levels by increasing ACTH secretion to increase adrenal gland release of glucocorticoids. Elevated blood ACTH levels cause skin pigmentation because the hormone stimulates melanocytes. In autoimmune Addison disease, circulating autoantibodies destroy melanocytes, causing permanent depigmentation of patches of skin in any part of the body (vitiligo).

In Addisonian crisis, the patient presents in circulatory shock, with hypotension, hypoglycaemia, and serious electrolyte imbalances: hyponatraemia, hyperkalaemia, and hypercalcaemia.

Management and prognosis

Steroid replacement must be initiated, and in the case of addisonian crisis, it must begin immediately. Treatment is lifelong.

BIBLIOGRAPHY AND REFERENCES

Barrett, E. J., Liu, Z., Khamaisi, M., et al. (2017). Diabetic microvascular disease: An endocrine society scientific statement. *The Journal of Cinical Endocrinology and Metabolism, 101*(2), 4343–4410.

Diaz-Valencia, P. A., Bougneres, P., & Valleron, A.-J. (2015). Global epidemiology of type 1 diabetes in young adults and adults: A systematic review. *BMC Public Health, 15*, 255–270.

Dworakowska, D., & Grossman, A. B. (2018). Aggressive and malignant pituitary tumours: State-of-the-art. *Endocrine-Related Cancer, 25*, R559–R575.

Newsholme, P., Cruzat, V., Arfuso, F., & Keane, K. (2014). Nutrient regulation of insulin secretion and action. *Journal of Endocrinology, 221*, R105–R120.

Nicolaides, N. C., Kyratzi, E., Lamprokostopoulou, A., et al. (2015). Stress, the stress system and the role of glucocorticoids. *Neuroimmunomodulation, 22*, 6–19.

Plows, J. F., Stanley, J. L., Baker, P. N., et al. (2018). The pathophysiology of gestational diabetes mellitus. *International Journal of Molecular Sciences, 19*(11), 3342–3363.

United Kingdom Prospective Diabetes Study (UKPDS) Group. (1998). Effect of intensive blood-glucose control with metformin on complications in overweight patients with type 2 diabetes (UKPDS 34). *Lancet, 352*(9131), 854–865.

Zheng, Y., Ley, S. H., & Hu, F. B. (2018). Global aetiology and epidemiology of type 2 diabetes mellitus and its complications. *Nature Reviews Endocrinology, 14*, 88–98.

Useful websites

Diabetes UK global incidence of TIDM: https://www.diabetes.org.uk/about_us/news_landing_page/uk-has-worlds-5th-highest-rate-of-type-1-diabetes-in-children/list-of-countries-by-incidence-of-type-1-diabetes-ages-0-to-14.

International Diabetes Foundation website: https://www.idf.org.

Useful StatsPearls article on gigantism and acromegaly: https://www.ncbi.nlm.nih.gov/books/NBK538261/.

WHO Classification of diabetes mellitus 2019 report at: https://www.who.int/publications-detail/classification-of-diabetes-mellitus.

WHO 2016 Global report on diabetes: https://apps.who.int/iris/bitstream/handle/10665/204871/9789241565257_eng.pdf;jsessionid=AC2DF83D15BF6AEB9C2CF6793EF8DF1D?sequence=1.

11

Disorders of Gastrointestinal Function

CHAPTER OUTLINE

INTRODUCTION
    The organs of the gastrointestinal system
    Control of gastrointestinal motility
    The gastrointestinal microbiome
    gastrointestinal Defences
MOTILITY DISORDERS
    Gastro-oesophageal reflux disorder
    Intestinal pseudo-obstruction
INFECTIONS AND INFLAMMATORY
CONDITIONS OF THE GASTROINTESTINAL TRACT
Oral infections
Gastroenteritis
Cholera
Typhoid fever
Hepatitis
    Viral hepatitis
    Alcoholic liver disease
Gastritis
Peptic ulcer disease

Inflammatory conditions of
    the small and large intestines
    Irritable bowel syndrome
    Inflammatory bowel disease
    Diverticular disease
    Appendicitis
NEOPLASMS OF THE GASTROINTESTINAL
TRACT
    Tumours of the salivary glands
    Oesophageal cancer
    Gastric cancer
    Liver cancer
    Pancreatic cancers
    Colorectal neoplasms
NUTRITIONAL AND MALABSORPTIVE
DISORDERS
    Pancreatitis
    Cholestasis
    Coeliac disease

INTRODUCTION

The gastrointestinal (GI) tract is essentially a long muscular tube linking the mouth and the anus. Foodstuffs passing through the tract are subjected to mechanical and chemical digestion, and essential materials absorbed to meet the body's metabolic needs. Although the different parts of the tract are associated with different functions, and are structurally modified accordingly, the tract wall has the same three layers throughout (Fig. 11.1). It is lined with epithelium, whose specialised modifications for digestion and absorption are described later. The middle layer of the wall of the tract is muscular and provides peristaltic propulsion of gastrointestinal contents on their journey from mouth to anus. The outer layer, the serosa, is a protective coat that isolates the tract from adjacent structures.

THE ORGANS OF THE GASTROINTESTINAL SYSTEM

The main structures along the length of the GI tract, namely the oesophagus, stomach, small and large intestines, and the rectum and anus are shown in Fig. 11.2. Accessory organs (i.e., the salivary glands, pancreas, liver, and gall bladder) add digestive fluids into the tract lumen at various points.

The stomach

The stomach is an expanded pouch between the oesophagus above and the duodenum below. Once in the stomach, material is prevented from passing back up the oesophagus by a ring of circular muscle called the *lower oesophageal sphincter* at the junction between the oesophagus and stomach (Fig. 11.3) and a pinching action of the diaphragm, through which the oesophagus passes. The stomach is mainly concerned with mechanical digestion and regulation of the flow of foodstuffs into the small intestine. Its strong muscular walls contract rhythmically, kneading its contents, liquefying them into a thick fluid called chyme and mixing them with gastric juice.

The stomach produces key hormones, enzymes, and other substances essential to healthy gastrointestinal function. The gastric lining features gastric pits lined with squamous epithelium containing a range of secretory cells, and the different parts of the stomach produce different substances (Fig. 11.3). The epithelium of the body of the stomach contains **parietal cells** that secrete hydrochloric acid. This maintains gastric fluids at a pH value of around 2, highly acidic and an important defence mechanism: most microbes and their toxins are destroyed in this corrosive fluid. The mechanism in the parietal cell membrane that pumps hydrogen

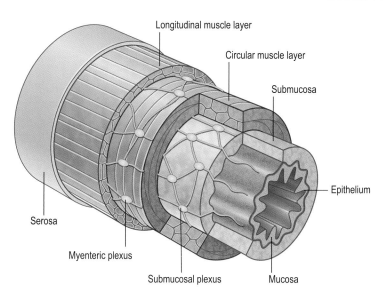

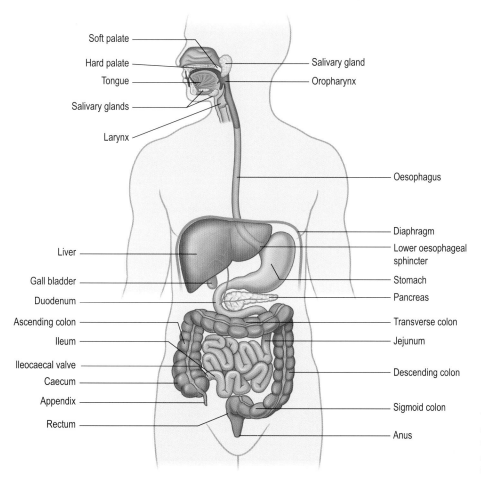

Fig. 11.1 The general structure of the gut wall. (Modified from Waugh A and Grant A (2018) *Ross & Wilson anatomy and physiology in health and illness*, 13th ed, Fig. 12.2. Oxford: Elsevier Ltd.)

Fig. 11.2 The main organs of the gastrointestinal tract and their accessory structures. (Modified from Waugh A and Grant A (2018) *Ross & Wilson anatomy and physiology in health and illness*, 13th ed, Fig. 12.1. Oxford: Elsevier Ltd.)

(H^+) ions into the stomach fluids to decrease its pH is usually referred to simply as the proton pump. Parietal cells also produce intrinsic factor, essential for absorption of vitamin B_{12}. **Chief cells** in the body of the stomach produce pepsin, which initiates protein digestion. This epithelium is also rich in **mucous cells** producing protective mucus.

The epithelium of the antrum contains **G cells**, which produce the hormone gastrin and release it into the bloodstream in response to the arrival of digested proteins in the stomach. Gastrin stimulates the release of hydrochloric acid into the stomach from parietal cells.

Gastric epithelial protection

The acidity of the stomach juices and the digestive action of gastric pepsin would be highly damaging to the living tissues of the stomach, and key protective mechanisms operate to

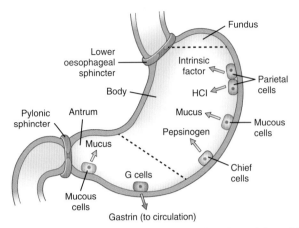

Cell Type	Location	Secretion
Parietal cells	Body	HCl Intrinsic factor
Chief cells	Body	Pepsinogen
G cells	Antrum	Gastrin
Mucous cells	Antrum	Mucus

Fig. 11.3   The regions of the stomach and the secretory functions of the epithelial lining. (Modified from Costanzo L (2018) *Physiology*, 6th ed, Fig. 8.15. Philadelphia: Elsevier Inc.)

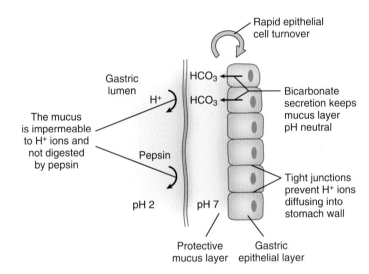

Fig. 11.4   Mechanisms protecting the gastric epithelium.

prevent direct contact and to limit tissue damage caused by excess H⁺ ions diffusing into the epithelial lining (Fig. 11.4). Most epithelial tissues subjected to constant injury protect themselves by producing multiple layers, as in the stratified epithelium of the skin. The gastric mucosal lining is only one cell thick, but the cells are held together with tight junctions (p.10), greatly reducing the movement of substances, including H⁺ ions, into deeper tissues. It is coated with mucus, produced by mucous cells in the epithelium. Mucus is made of polysaccharides and is impermeable to acid, providing a physical barrier separating the stomach tissues from their own secretions. It is also impermeable to pepsin, so this proteolytic enzyme cannot diffuse through the mucus and digest the stomach lining. In addition, the mucus is rich in **bicarbonate**, which neutralises any acid that does diffuse back into the gastric epithelium from the stomach contents. The bicarbonate is a by-product of the same chemical pathway in the gastric parietal cells that produces the acid, ensuring that acid production is matched by protective bicarbonate production. The surface membrane of the gastric epithelial cells is, additionally, adapted to resist the corrosive effect of acid. The rate of gastric epithelial cell turnover is very high (every 2–4 days), rapidly replacing any damaged cells. **Prostaglandins** are key factors contributing to mucosal defences, which explains why non-steroidal anti-inflammatory drugs, which

block prostaglandin production, are significant risk factors in peptic ulcer disease (PUD).

The liver

The liver performs multiple metabolic functions essential in fundamental nutrient and energy pathways. It detoxifies and inactivates potentially harmful compounds, produces plasma proteins, stores essential substances (e.g., iron and glucose), regulates the composition of blood, and produces bile. It produces glucose, ketone bodies, cholesterol, and fatty acids (used to synthesise triacylglycerol, the form in which the body stores fat). The liver is also an important part of the mononuclear phagocyte defence system and possesses populations of macrophages (Kupffer cells), which filter the blood passing through the organ removing, and destroying particulate matter, including cellular and bacterial fragments and worn-out red blood cells. The liver receives blood via two large vessels. The hepatic artery branches off the aorta and brings oxygenated blood to supply the liver's oxygen requirements. The hepatic portal vein drains the stomach and most of the intestines and brings blood laden with the products of digestion directly to the liver, which extracts them for storage or redistribution. Liver cells (hepatocytes) possess complex systems of enzymes that regulate synthetic and detoxifying processes.

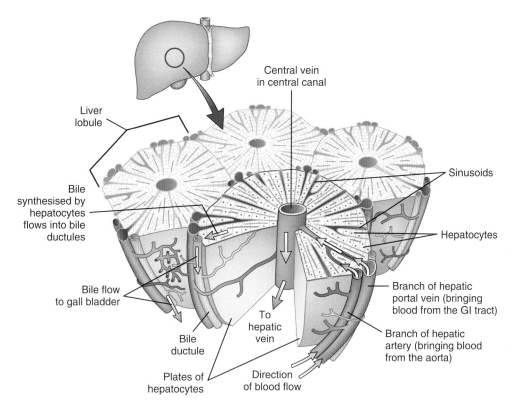

Central vein
in central canal

Liver
lobule

Bile
synthesised by
hepatocytes
flows into bile
ductules

Sinusoids

Hepatocytes

Bile flow
to gall bladder

Branch of hepatic
portal vein (bringing
blood from the GI tract)

Bile
ductule

To
hepatic
vein

Branch of hepatic
artery (bringing blood
from the aorta)

Plates of
hepatocytes

Direction
of blood flow

Fig. 11.5 Liver lobules. (Modified from Mescher LA and Junqueira LCU (2013) *Junqueira's basic histology: text and atlas*. New York: McGraw-Hill Medical.)

Liver lobules

Within liver tissue, hepatocytes are arranged in hexagonal units called lobules (Fig. 11.5). The hexagons are composed of plates of cells radiating out from a central canal containing a central vein, which carries blood away from the lobule. Branches of the hepatic artery and hepatic portal vein, bringing blood into the liver, run together at the corners of the lobules. The blood from these vessels then flows through sinusoids linking them to the central vein. The central veins merge to form the hepatic vein, which returns blood to the inferior vena cava.

The sinusoid walls are made of plates of hepatocytes, which contain all the necessary enzymes to perform the liver's metabolic function, so as the blood flows through the sinusoids, exposed to the hepatocytes, materials are extracted and added, and the composition of the blood adjusted. Hepatic macrophages are found on this epithelial surface as well, performing their defence function. Hepatocytes also secrete bile, which is not passed into the blood, but is drained away in tiny bile ductules that eventually merge to form the bile duct and empty their bile into the gall bladder.

The biliary tract

The anatomical arrangement of the biliary tract and its relationship to associated structures is shown in Fig. 11.6. Bile flows from the liver via the hepatic ducts into the gall bladder, where it is stored and concentrated. When food, especially fatty food, arrives in the duodenum, the gall bladder contracts, and bile flows into the duodenum through the common bile duct.

Bile. Bile is a convenient route for the liver to excrete wastes like **bilirubin**, a yellow-green pigment released as a by-product of haemoglobin breakdown when old erythrocytes are destroyed, and cholesterol. Cholesterol is converted by the liver into **bile acids** (cholic acid and chenodeoxycholic acid) and is excreted in this form in bile. Bile acids act like a detergent, breaking globules of fat up into much smaller droplets (emulsification), which increases the surface area for the action of pancreatic and intestinal lipases. This is important for efficient fat digestion. Bile acids are not very water soluble, so in excess they can precipitate out in the bile and form gallstones.

Jaundice. Jaundice is the yellowish colouration of skin, the sclera, and other body tissues resulting from bilirubin accumulation. This may be caused by excessive rates of haemolysis, for example in newborn babies who have a significantly higher erythrocyte count in the womb because they need to extract oxygen from the mother's bloodstream. After birth, when the baby is breathing independently, the excess erythrocytes are no longer needed and are quickly broken down, releasing a sudden surge of bilirubin into the bloodstream. If bilirubin levels are excessive in the newborn, it causes a form of brain injury called **kernicterus**, which results because bilirubin is neurotoxic. Jaundice is also a common consequence of liver disease or problems with bile flow.

Hepatocytes actively extract bilirubin from the bloodstream for excretion in the bile. If liver function is impaired, bilirubin remains in circulation, causing jaundice. If there is obstruction anywhere in the ducts carrying bile from the liver to the gall bladder, or from the gall bladder to the duodenum, bile backs up into the liver and bilirubin levels in the bloodstream rise, causing jaundice.

The pancreas

This organ performs both endocrine and exocrine roles because it secretes the hormones **insulin** and **glucagon** into the bloodstream (endocrine; see Chapter 10) and digestive enzymes into the duodenum (exocrine). Pancreatic digestive

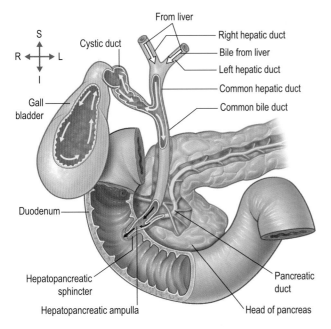

Fig. 11.6 The gall bladder and the direction of bile flow. (Modified from Waugh A and Grant A (2018) *Ross & Wilson anatomy and physiology in health and illness*, 13th ed, Fig. 12.38. Oxford: Elsevier Ltd.)

juice contains proteases, including trypsin, to break down proteins into peptides and amino acids, lipases for the digestion of fats to fatty acids and glycerol and amylase to break down starch into the disaccharide maltose. To protect itself from self-digesting, the pancreas produces its enzymes as inactive precursors that are not activated until they are secreted into the duodenum. The pancreas also secretes bicarbonate, making its digestive juices alkaline and neutralising the acid chyme arriving in the duodenum from the stomach.

The small intestine

The small intestine is about 6 m (15 ft) long and is divided into three segments. The short first segment, the **duodenum**, receives pancreatic enzymes and bile; the second section is called the **jejunum**, and the third and longest section is the **ileum**. The epithelial lining of the small and large intestine is composed of **enterocytes**, with specialised digestive and absorptive functions. The mucosa of the small intestine is folded into ridges called **plicae**. The plicae are covered in a carpet of finger-like villi and the individual enterocytes covering the villi in turn have microvilli on their free surfaces (Fig. 11.7). The result is a 600-fold increase in surface area compared with a tube of the same diameter but without these adaptations. This greatly facilitates absorption.

Between the villi, tubular-shaped glands dip into the deeper tissues; these are the intestinal crypts (sometimes called the *crypts of Lieberkuhn*) and are lined with intestinal epithelium. Specialised adaptations to the crypt epithelial lining include goblet cells secreting lubricating mucus and specialised immune cells that secrete protective and antimicrobial substances. The tips of the enterocytes possess digestive enzymes, including **maltase**, **sucrase**, and **lactase**, which digest small carbohydrates to monosaccharides (single sugar units such as glucose), peptidases that split peptides into amino acids and lipases to digest fats. These enzymes complete the digestion of carbohydrates, proteins and fats

begun in the intestinal lumen by pancreatic enzymes. Water-soluble products of digestion-amino acids from proteins and monosaccharides from carbohydrates-are absorbed directly into the capillary network extending the length of the villus. Fat-soluble substances are absorbed into the lymphatic system via the lacteal running centrally in the villus.

The barrier function of the enterocytes

The small intestine is designed for absorption, but this needs to be selective to ensure that unwanted or potentially toxic materials and microbes do not cross from the intestinal lumen into the blood. The enterocytes provide an essential barrier function; the junctions between cells are tight junctions (p.10), preventing passive diffusion of materials from the intestinal lumen into the bloodstream, and blocking the movement of bacteria and viruses. They also make a range of antimicrobial substances and are coated with antibodies produced by immune cells deeper in the intestinal wall, greatly reducing the possibility that infective cells or toxic substances may penetrate the epithelial lining. This barrier function is impaired in some gastrointestinal disorders (e.g., inflammatory bowel disease).

The large intestine and rectum

The large intestine (colon) is about 1.5 m (5 ft) long. It extends from the ileocaecal junction, where the distal ileum opens into it, to the rectum and anus. Its blind end is a small pouch called the **caecum**, from which the small, closed tube of the appendix also opens. Its main function is water absorption and propelling faecal material towards the rectum for storage until it is convenient to defaecate. The wall is not folded into plicae, nor does it have villi as seen in the small intestine, but the epithelium is still composed of absorptive enterocytes, with goblet cells that produce lubricating mucus. It also possesses crypts, which are deeper than in the small intestine, and there are pockets of lymphoid tissue present, called lymphoid follicles, with a protective function.

CONTROL OF GASTROINTESTINAL MOTILITY

Regulation of GI tract motility is achieved by both neural and hormonal mechanisms. The smooth muscle of the gut wall, from the oesophagus to the anus, is arranged in two layers (except in the stomach, which has three layers of muscle). The innermost layer is composed of circular fibres and the fibres in the outermost layer run longitudinally (Fig. 11.1). Between the two layers is a network of nerve fibres, called the *myenteric plexus* (of Auerbach), part of the so-called *enteric nervous system.* This plexus is influenced by the autonomic nervous system and by circulating hormones, but it generates its own nerve signals and reflexes independently of central nervous system control, giving the gastrointestinal tract autonomy in the regulation of motility, secretion, and digestion. The enteric nervous system contributes to maintenance of basal tone (sustained contraction in an otherwise resting muscle) in the tract wall and responds to the presence (or absence) of foodstuffs and the nature of the foodstuffs in the tract, by increasing (or decreasing) peristaltic activity and adjusting the composition of digestive secretions released.

As in the heart, the smooth muscle of the GI tract displays pacemaker activity. Even in the absence of neural or hormonal stimulation, the GI smooth muscle produces regular,

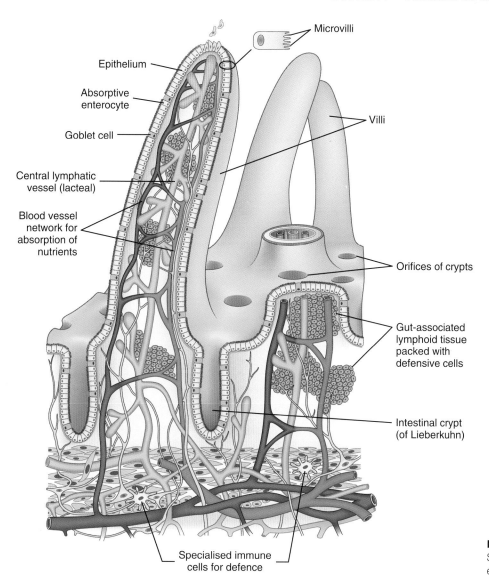

Microvilli

Epithelium

Absorptive
enterocyte

Goblet cell

Villi

Central lymphatic
vessel (lacteal)

Blood vessel
network for
absorption of
nutrients

Orifices of crypts

Gut-associated
lymphoid tissue
packed with
defensive cells

Intestinal crypt
(of Lieberkuhn)

Specialised immune
cells for defence

Fig. 11.7 Intestinal villi. (Modified from Standring S (2021) *Gray's anatomy,* 42nd ed, Fig. 64.20. Oxford: Elsevier Ltd.)

slow, sustained contractions. When material enters the intestines, the rate and strength of the contractions increases.

Transit time is the time taken for swallowed material to reach the anus, and in normal individuals this is very variable. Different foodstuffs travel through the tract at different speeds, and different sections of the tract propel foodstuffs forward at different speeds. A fat-rich meal stays in the stomach far longer than a carbohydrate-rich meal, for example, and materials typically remain in the large intestine for longer than in the small intestine. On average, it takes the stomach 4 to 5 hours to completely empty after a meal, but average colonic transit time is in the order of 30 hours.

THE GASTROINTESTINAL MICROBIOME

The gastrointestinal tract is densely populated with a diverse collection of commensal microbes, including bacteria, fungi, and viruses, forming a significant part of the body's **microbiome** (the total microbial population of the human body). Along with microbial populations found on the skin and colonising other passageways such as the urethra, these microbial communities are intimately involved in a wide range of physiological functions essential to the health of the host. Colonisation of the GI tract begins at birth and goes through clear developmental stages through childhood and into adulthood. The microbial populations that establish themselves at different stages in the growing child reflect the changes in nutritional intake; for example, communities of bacteria capable of digesting plant materials appear when the infant is moved onto a mixed diet.

The evolving microbiome is an important influence on the developing immune system, and disrupting it in childhood, for example by antibiotic use or malnutrition, is associated with a higher risk of asthma and other allergies. In health, the immune system tolerates the gut microbiome, but some disorders (e.g., inflammatory bowel disease) are associated with microbiome-induced immune activation. The microbiome controls the immune and inflammatory responses of the gut wall to non-resident, potentially pathogenic organisms, upregulating and downregulating defence mechanisms as appropriate. It also directs the development of the GI epithelium and the nervous system, and there are links between dysfunctional microbiota and obesity and autism. Obesity is an expanding and global problem, imposing a significant burden on health and health economics. An individual's microbiome profile changes with body mass index, waist-to-hip ratio, blood cholesterol and other blood lipid levels, glycaemic index, and cardiovascular risk. The metabolic activity of the microbiome has significant impact on host metabolism, including influencing the use of glucose and lipids. Dysfunctional microbiomes alter this in some way, leading to a low-grade inflammatory response in the body, insulin resistance and a clearly demonstrated tendency to obesity. The details of how this happens are not understood.

The GI microbiome feeds on the slurry of digested and semi-digested foodstuffs within the gut, producing certain vitamins and digesting otherwise indigestible materials. A healthy microbiome also prevents pathogenic organisms from establishing themselves and potentially causing disease. Microbes and gut epithelial cells constantly interact with each other, to their mutual benefit, regulating proliferation, energy use, endocrine responses, and immune function. Diversity of the microbiome is important to health, and restricted diets change the GI environment and the availability of nutrients, leading to the loss of particular microbial species. Increasingly, the links between the GI microbiome and a whole range of disorders, both gastrointestinal and systemic, are becoming evident; in addition to those mentioned above, they include type 2 diabetes, cardiovascular disease, colorectal cancer and inflammatory bowel disease.

GASTROINTESTINAL DEFENCES

Healthy immune function in the GI tract walks a finely balanced tightrope between immunological tolerance of its resident microbiome and the diversity of antigens consumed as part of a normal varied diet while still responding rapidly and effectively to potentially dangerous antigens when exposed to them. The GI microbiome plays a key part in preventing infection. The GI tract has multiple defence mechanisms in addition to this. The acidic pH of saliva, and the extremely acidic gastric juices, kill microbes and denature protein toxins. The GI tract is rich in defensive immune tissue packed with immune cells, collectively called GALT (gut-associated lymphoid tissue). This includes the tonsils of the mouth and throat, the lymph nodes that filter lymph draining from the tract and scattered patches of immune tissue in the intestine, sometimes called *Peyer's patches*. In addition, resident in the epithelium throughout the intestines is an extensive population of lymphocytes, and as a result the lining of a healthy intestine is a highly effective barrier to microbial penetration.

MOTILITY DISORDERS

The total length of the intestines is about 7.5 m. They rely upon peristalsis to ensure that materials entering from the gastric end arrive at the rectal end for excretion, and physical obstruction or changes in motility can significantly increase or decrease transit time or halt onward movement of gut contents completely. This affects normal digestion and absorption and may be associated with a whole constellation of signs and symptoms, including abdominal pain, bloating, constipation, diarrhoea, obstruction, vomiting and gastro-oesophageal reflux. Often, GI motility issues are secondary to another conditions.

The co-ordinated peristaltic activity of the oesophagus, stomach, and intestines can be altered by a range of physiological and pathophysiological events. Irritants, the presence of high-fibre materials, emotional and psychological states, exercise, many drugs, and increasing age alter GI motility. Two very common features of motility disorders are diarrhoea and constipation.

Diarrhoea

Diarrhoea is defined as the passing of three or more liquid stools a day. It is generally caused by infection, but some inflammatory conditions (e.g., ulcerative colitis (UC)) may also be responsible. Other causes include prolonged periods of stress, overuse of laxatives, some cancers of the gastrointestinal tract, and endocrine disorders such as Addison disease. Acute diarrhoeal disorder lasts fewer than 14 days and is commoner than chronic diarrhoeal disorder, which persists for longer.

Pathophysiology

In gastrointestinal infection, the gut epithelium becomes overwhelmingly secretory. Although absorptive processes are usually preserved, the intestinal lining begins to actively secrete water and electrolytes into the gut lumen. This is likely at least partly because of the generalised inflammatory response caused by the infection. In addition, the epithelium responds specifically to microbial toxins and proteins, which bind to the epithelial cell surface or actively invade the epithelial cells and trigger the secretory response. This is an important defence mechanism by the epithelium as it attempts to wash away or dilute the noxious agent. Fluid loss into the gut lumen can be torrential, and rapidly leads to dehydration. Cytokines released by inflammatory cells recruited into the area in infective or inflammatory conditions stimulate smooth muscle contraction of the gut wall, increasing motility and decreasing transit time, and causing significant abdominal pain.

Management and prognosis

Whatever the underlying cause, fluid replacement is a critical element of treatment. In chronic diarrhoea, the loss of nutrition caused by short transit times and any reduction in appetite must also be addressed. Identifying the cause of the diarrhoea is important, so that appropriate management may be put in place.

Constipation

Constipation is the passing of dry, hard stool, usually fewer than three times a week. It is frequently associated with poor-quality diets lacking in fibre, low fluid intake, low levels of exercise, increasing age, and certain drugs (e.g., opioids and iron supplements), but it may also be an indication of disease, including colorectal cancer, irritable bowel syndrome, multiple sclerosis, or hypothyroidism. It is common in pregnancy because of high circulating levels of progesterone, which relaxes smooth muscle.

Pathophysiology

Intestinal transit times are often extended, allowing nearly all water in the intestinal contents to be absorbed, giving dry, hard faeces. Highly processed diets lacking in fresh fruit, vegetables and other sources of fibre lack bulk, and so the inherent

BOX 11.1 Common causes of constipation

Low-fibre diet	Chronic intestinal pseudo-obstruction	As a side effect of drugs: opiates, iron supplements, drugs with anti-cholinergic side effects	Neurological disorders: multiple sclerosis, Parkinson disease, spinal cord damage, stroke
Low fluid intake	Hypothyroidism	Psychological disorders	Hirschsprung disease
Pregnancy	Hypercalcaemia	Colorectal cancer	Painful defaecation (e.g., haemorrhoids, anal fissures)
Depression	Reduced mobility		

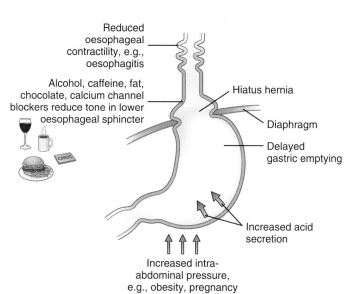

Fig. 11.8 Causes of gastro-oesophageal reflux disease.

stimulus for peristalsis is reduced, increasing transit time. Nervous system disease (e.g., multiple sclerosis) can affect gastrointestinal control and impair motility. Endocrine and metabolic disorders can also reduce GI motility; for example, because thyroxine stimulates peristalsis, hypothyroidism is associated with reduced motility throughout the tract, causing gastro-oesophageal reflux, reduced gastric emptying and constipation. Box 11.1 lists some common causes of constipation.

Management and prognosis
Identifying the cause is important because, although constipation is very common, not usually serious, and often easily managed, significant underlying disease including malignancy needs to be excluded. Improving lifestyle habits such as diet and exercise, and maintaining a good fluid intake, is sometimes all that is required. The use of laxatives can be effective, but chronic use of laxatives in turn impairs GI motility, worsening the problem.

GASTRO-OESOPHAGEAL REFLUX DISORDER

Gastro-oesophageal reflux disorder (GORD) is a common condition caused by reflux of acidic gastric fluid into the oesophagus. GORD may be associated with increased secretion of gastric acid (e.g., in Zollinger-Ellison syndrome), but most people with GORD produce normal levels of acid and the problem arises because the function of the lower oesophageal sphincter is compromised or abdominal pressure is increased (Fig. 11.8). Reduced tone of the lower oesophageal sphincter and low oesophageal motility predispose to reflux. Some drugs, hormones, and foods (e.g., calcium channel

blockers, caffeine, alcohol, and high blood progesterone levels in pregnancy) relax the lower oesophageal sphincter and are known causes of reflux. Abdominal pressure rises in pregnancy, especially late pregnancy, in abdominal obesity, and when gastric emptying is delayed. Delayed gastric emptying is common in people with GORD, but the cause is often not identified. Hiatus hernia, in which the stomach pushes through the diaphragm into the lower chest, also frequently causes reflux symptoms. There is no difference between males and females in the incidence of GORD, but it is much more common in countries with refined, high-fat diets and where obesity rates are high.

Pathophysiology
In health, the junction between the squamous epithelium lining the oesophagus and the columnar epithelium of the stomach is clearly and sharply demarcated (Fig. 11.9A). Because the oesophageal epithelium lacks the protective adaptations against acid present in the stomach, it becomes inflamed and ulcerated when exposed to refluxing gastric contents. Typically, the lower 8 to 10 cm of the oesophagus is affected. When the condition becomes chronic, the damaged oesophageal epithelium becomes thickened and keratinised in an adaptive effort to protect underlying tissues. This can cause stricture, which interferes with effective oesophageal peristalsis and leads to obstruction and difficulty with swallowing. With chronic exposure, the oesophageal epithelium transforms from stratified squamous epithelium to columnar epithelium rich in mucous cells, to protect underlying tissues. This metaplastic change (p.65) is called

Clearly demarcated
gastro-oesophageal junction

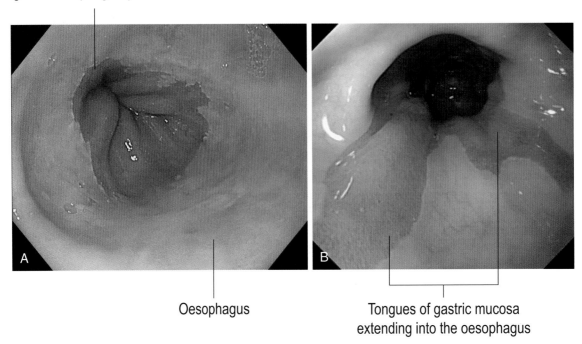

Oesophagus

Tongues of gastric mucosa
extending into the oesophagus

Fig. 11.9 The gastro-oesophageal junction. (A) Normal, showing the clearly demarcated gastro-oesophageal junction. (B) Barrett oesophagus, showing pink tongues of gastric mucosa extending upwards into the oesophagus. (Modified from (A) Brennan PA, Standring S, and Wiseman S (2014) *Gray's surgical anatomy*, Fig. 67.2. London: Elsevier Ltd; and (B) Walker B, Colledge NR, Ralston S, et al. (2014) *Davidson's principles and practice of medicine*, 22nd ed, Fig. 22.28. Oxford: Churchill Livingstone.)

Barrett oesophagus (Fig. 11.9B) and precedes dysplastic change, which in turn may proceed to malignant oesophageal adenocarcinoma. This malignant change is more common in males than females.

Signs and symptoms

Initial symptoms include pain or discomfort behind the sternum, especially when lying down or bending over, and worse after eating. There may be increased salivation (waterbrash), a reflex response to oesophageal irritation. There may be cough and hoarseness, if the inflammatory changes extend upwards to the larynx and upper trachea. In longstanding oesophagitis, anaemia may develop because of low-level but sustained blood loss from ulceration.

Management and prognosis

Weight loss, smoking cessation, and dietary advice are important where relevant. Pharmacological treatment includes antacids, H_2 receptor blockers, and proton pump inhibitors. Domperidone can improve peristalsis and improve gastric emptying. Surgery (e.g., to repair hiatus hernia, or to improve the function of the lower oesophageal sphincter) is also used.

INTESTINAL PSEUDO-OBSTRUCTION

This rare but disabling condition affects all races and both sexes equally. Patients present with symptoms of acute obstruction but with no obvious cause. It is commoner in older (over 80 years) and debilitated people. Affected adults often have additional conditions including diabetes, scleroderma, or malignant disease. It may complicate recovery from abdominal surgery.

Pathophysiology

The cause of the disorder is not known, but most evidence suggests an abnormality in the autonomic nervous system's control of gastrointestinal motility. Increased sympathetic nervous system activity causes spasm of the tract wall, and decreased parasympathetic activity relaxes it, leading to atony. Both situations prevent peristalsis and forward movement of the tract contents. Patients have been successfully treated both with sympathetic blocking drugs and parasympathetic stimulants, so no definitive management protocol has been reached. The small intestine is more often affected than the large intestine.

Signs and symptoms

Acute abdominal pain, nausea, vomiting, abdominal distension, and constipation are common.

Management and prognosis

It is essential to rule out mechanical obstruction before beginning treatment. Sympathetic blockers (e.g., guanethidine) and anti-cholinesterase drugs (to increase parasympathetic activity) are generally considered the most effective approach.

INFECTIONS AND INFLAMMATORY CONDITIONS OF THE GASTROINTESTINAL TRACT

The gastrointestinal system has an important barrier function in protection against ingested toxins and microbes. The gut microbiome is key to this, and the GI tract is equipped with immune and inflammatory defences to deal with potentially harmful materials entering the body via this route. Consumption of foods and fluids that may have significant microbial loads means that gastrointestinal infections are common, despite these multiple defence mechanisms. A wide range of microbes are associated with GI infection, and although many infections are of relatively short duration, causing illness that perhaps lasts only a few days, chronic, repeated, or untreated gastrointestinal infections present a major global problem imposing significant morbidity and mortality. The diarrhoea associated with GI infection and inflammation causes dehydration and malnutrition and is the most common cause of preventable death worldwide in children under 5.

ORAL INFECTIONS

Over 700 species of bacteria colonise the human mouth, growing on the mucous membrane or on the teeth. Microbes can form stable and well-established colonies on the tooth surface because unlike epithelia this does not shed its upper layers. In health, the oral microbiome confers significant benefits; it prevents the growth of pathogenic organisms, prevents the internal environment of the mouth from becoming too acidic, and produces antibacterial and anti-inflammatory substances to reduce the likelihood of infection or inflammatory disorders. Despite the rich and varied bacterial population of the oral surfaces, acute infections of the mouth are relatively rare. Factors including poor oral hygiene, reduced saliva production, treatment with broad-spectrum antibiotics, smoking and diets high in sugar alter the balance of the individual's oral microbiome, and increase the risk of infection and inflammatory conditions. Good oral hygiene removes possibly pathogenic bacteria from the oral surfaces. Loss of saliva caused by disease or as a side effect of certain drugs, dries the oral mucosa and deprives it of saliva's antiseptic, lubricating, and washing benefits. The presence of sugars in the mouth encourages the growth of lactobacilli, which break the sugars down into acids, encouraging dental decay and the proliferation of acid-tolerant bacteria at the expense of normal, acid-neutralising bacteria. This changes the healthy oral microbiome to a less healthy one, predisposing to infection and inflammation especially of the gums, and the development of dental caries. Gingivitis (gum inflammation) and periodontitis (inflammation and destruction of the bone underlying the tooth) are common causes of tooth loss.

Systemic consequences of dental disease

Periodontitis destroys the joint between the tooth and the underlying bone and increases the risk that oral microbes may enter the bloodstream (Fig. 11.10). Organisms may also enter the bloodstream after dental extraction, especially in an unhealthy mouth. Bacterial endocarditis can result from bacteraemia secondary to dental surgery, especially in people with pre-existing cardiac disease. In addition, periodontitis increases the risk of atheroma formation and so is associated with increased risk of stroke and coronary artery disease. As with other chronic infections (e.g., *Helicobacter pylori*; p.288) or chronic respiratory infections, periodontitis increases levels of circulating inflammatory mediators, which trigger the formation of atherosclerotic plaques, and increase the coagulability of the blood. Bacteraemia secondary to dental disease may also cause glomerulonephritis.

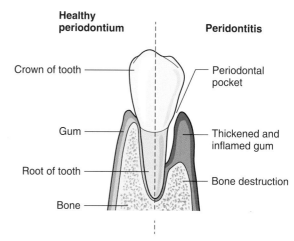

Fig. 11.10 The healthy gum and periodontitis. Periodontitis features gingivitis, bone destruction caused by the ongoing inflammatory response, and the development of pockets between the tooth and the gum, which trap materials and predispose to infection. (Modified from Mascarenhas AK, Okunseri C, Dye B, American Association of Public Health Dentistry (2021) *Burt and Eklund's dentistry, dental practice, and the community*, 7th ed, Fig. 15.1. Philadelphia: Elsevier Inc.)

GASTROENTERITIS

This general term means inflammation of the stomach and small intestine, usually secondary to infection, and globally accounts for 15% of deaths in the under-five age group. Most of these deaths occur in developing countries, but mortality has been steadily falling over recent decades because implementation of oral rehydration programmes has provided a cheap, effective, and easy way to reduce the devastating consequences of the diarrhoea associated with gastroenteritis. Most cases are of relatively short duration and in otherwise healthy people are not usually a threat to life. In debilitated people, or the very young or the very old, it can be much more dangerous. Gastroenteritis commonly causes nausea, vomiting, and diarrhoea, with abdominal pain and cramping of the stomach and intestines. There may be headache and fever, and some forms of food poisoning, involving more aggressive organisms or in vulnerable people, can precipitate liver failure, renal failure, or neurological complications. A range of microbes can cause gastroenteritis, including bacteria, amoebae, protozoa, and viruses, including norovirus and rotavirus.

A pathogen can infect and damage the gastrointestinal tract in one of two main ways: either by directly invading the wall of the tract, or by secreting enterotoxins. Note that of the many groups of micro-organisms associated with GI infection, different members of the same group can have different properties; for example, some species of *Escherichia coli* are invasive while others produce enterotoxins.

Invasive organisms. Some pathogens invade the intestinal wall and elicit a strong inflammatory response there, leading to cytokine release with swelling, bleeding, and tissue destruction. The stool is likely to be bloody and there may be mucus in it (dysentery). Examples include some *Clostridium, Campylobacter, Salmonella,* and *Shigella* species and *Entamoeba histolytica.* From the gut wall, they may spread in the bloodstream or the lymphatics to distant organs.

Enterotoxin secretion. Other organisms do not invade, and their pathogenicity is caused by production and release of

BOX 11.2 Microbes that cause food poisoning

Bacillus cereus	This microbe, common in the environment, grows rapidly at room temperature and contaminates many different foodstuffs: meat, rice, fish, and vegetables. It may also cause respiratory tract, eye, and wound infections. Its toxins are enzymes that directly damage to the intestinal mucosa and although cooking kills the organism, the toxin may survive.
Campylobacter species	Campylobacter infection is more prevalent in summer than winter and is the commonest global cause of infective gastroenteritis. The bacterium lives in the digestive system of poultry, cattle, and other animals. Undercooked chicken and unpasteurised milk are the usual sources of infection, but the organism is robust and can survive on surfaces and in water, and infection can be picked up directly from infected animals, including domestic pets. Cooking and pasteurisation kill the bacteria.
Clostridium perfringens	*C. perfringens* is a common, anaerobic bacterium found in soil, water, faeces, and air and is a frequent cause of food poisoning, usually when large batches of food is being cooked or prepared rather than in the home. Its enterotoxin damages the small intestine, causing diarrhoea, pain, and nausea. The bacterium produces spores that survive inadequate cooking and that proliferate when the food is left to cool at room temperature for extended periods.
Clostridium botulinum	See text
Cryptosporidium species	This is a group of protozoal infections that mainly affects children, in whom it causes sustained diarrhoea that can lead to dehydration and malnourishment. The parasites spread by the faeco-oral route, although waterborne outbreaks (e.g., in fouled swimming pools or lakes) and direct contact with an infected animal are also possible. The organism invades the intestinal epithelial cells, proliferates, and sheds new organisms into the GI tract, which are passed with the stool and infect others. The parasites are hardy, can survive for many months without a host, and are not killed with standard disinfectants. Boiling kills them.
Escherichia coli	Most strains of these bacteria are harmless, and commonly found living in the colon. Some strains (e.g., shiga toxin-producing *E. coli* can cause serious food poisoning with dysentery). It is usually transmitted by the faeco-oral route, and associated with undercooked foodstuffs including meat, raw milk and its products, and unwashed fruit and vegetables tainted with contaminated water.
Norovirus	Worldwide, this virus is the commonest cause of epidemic non-bacterial gastroenteritis and although the illness usually runs a short (24–48 hours) course, it produces profuse and copious watery diarrhoea, projectile vomiting, and very painful abdominal cramps. The virus invades the lining of the stomach and the villi of the small intestine, but not the large intestine. It spreads via the faeco-oral route, or via contaminated airborne droplets, or by direct person-to person contact and is highly contagious. It is stable to extremes of temperature (from freezing to 60°C), disinfection, alcohol, and low pH.
Rotavirus	This virus mainly affects the small intestine, reducing water and nutrient absorption and causing copious diarrhoea, especially in children, who are at particular risk of becoming dehydrated. It is spread by the faeco-oral route or by eating contaminated foods, and the virus is stable without the host for long periods, meaning that infection can be picked up from work surfaces, toys, medical equipment, and a host of other objects.
Salmonella species	*Salmonella* species adhere to and invade intestinal epithelial cells and cause gastrointestinal infections including typhoid fever. Infection is usually spread in contaminated food. The bacterium can remain viable in the body for some time after the host has recovered, and during that time the host is infectious. The incubation period in salmonella food poisoning is between 6 and 48 hours and symptoms begin abruptly, with varying degrees of diarrhoea and abdominal pain. Vomiting is not usual. Severe infection can prostrate the sufferer, with dehydration, hypotension, shock, and renal failure.
Staphylococcus aureus	*S. aureus* is a common commensal on skin and may be transmitted to foodstuffs if food preparation hygiene is inadequate. If food is not stored at low enough temperature or heated adequately during cooking the organism survives and produces a toxin, which causes the signs and symptoms: nausea, vomiting, abdominal cramps and dciarrhoea. Onset is usually rapid, as little as 30 minutes after ingestion but usually resolves within 24 hours.

an enterotoxin, which massively stimulates the secretory function of the intestinal wall. This results in copious, watery diarrhoea that does not contain blood or pus and is not usually accompanied by significant abdominal cramping. Examples of microbes that produce such toxins are *Escherichia coli*, *Staphylococci*, *Cryptosporidium*, *Clostridium perfringens*, and *Bacillus cereus*. Some toxins are stable to cooking and food preservation/processing methods and can cause disease even after the microbe itself has been killed.

Food poisoning

This general term means illness caused by eating contaminated food. Not all food poisoning is infective, for example, eating poisonous mushrooms or foodstuffs contaminated with heavy metals causes food poisoning. Although food poisoning secondary to contamination of food or drink with microbes is very common, it is generally mild and self-limiting, except in vulnerable people. Common organisms include *Escherichia coli*, *Salmonella*, *Clostridium*, and *Campylobacter* species and *Staphylococcus aureus*. Further information about important organisms that cause food poisoning is given in Box 11.2.

Botulism

Clostridium botulinum, an anaerobic bacterium found in inadequately processed foods, produces one of the most toxic poisons known. Botulinum toxin is a potent neurotoxin and in even tiny concentrations can cause lethal respiratory paralysis. Bacterial spores (p.19) are heat resistant and are present in the soil and water sources. Consumption of the spores in adults is not problematic because the immune system destroys them, but eating foods containing the toxin cause botulism. Food preparation, including for preserving for later consumption, must scrupulously follow guidelines to ensure any toxin present is destroyed. Infection is usually secondary to consumption of contaminated foods, in which case it causes severe food poisoning, but can also follow contamination of open wounds. The neurotoxin blocks the release of acetylcholine by nerves in the brain, mainly in the brainstem and in the cranial nerves, and also in the peripheral nervous system. This disrupts normal neural function and can cause respiratory paralysis, visual disturbances (blurred or double vision, drooping eyelids), and progressive skeletal muscle paralysis. Given appropriate medical support, including artificial ventilation, there is usually a full recovery with no residual neurological deficiency, but this can take a long time (up to a year) and mortality rates are about 10%.

Dysentery

Dysentery is generally used to mean gastrointestinal infection, usually of the colon, that produces watery, bloody diarrhoea. It is usually caused by *Shigella* species (bacillary dysentery) or an amoeboid infection, usually *Entamoeba histolytica*. It is associated with organisms that invade the epithelial cells lining the colon, setting up an intense inflammatory reaction and directly damaging the tissue.

Bacillary dysentery

The commonest cause of bacterial dysentery is *Shigella*, but others include *Campylobacter*, *Escherichia coli*, and *Clostridium difficile*. Shigella is a highly virulent bacterium, and fewer than 200 organisms entering the GI tract is enough to cause infection. It is spread by the faeco-oral route and is associated with poverty, poor sanitation, low standards of hygiene, and lack of a clean water supply. As such, it is a significant health problem in developing countries. Symptoms begin a day or two after infection, and although the stool contains blood and mucus the volume is not as great as with an enterotoxin-mediated gastroenteritis, so dehydration is less of a risk. There is fever, abdominal pain, and sometimes vomiting. Except in the vulnerable (e.g., children, undernourished people, people with co-existing chronic conditions, and the immunocompromised), the course of the disease is self-limiting with resolution in a week or so.

Amoebic dysentery

This is usually caused by *Entamoeba histolytica*, an anaerobic parasitic protozoan that causes a gastrointestinal infection called *amoebiasis*. Worldwide, the amoeba is widespread and infects tens of millions of people every year, although only about 10% develop gastrointestinal symptoms. It is common in some South and Central American countries, Asia, and Africa. Humans are its natural host, and it invades the distal small intestine and colon, causing inflammation, diarrhoea, abdominal pain and anorexia and weight loss. The colon may perforate because of the inflammatory damage. From the intestines, the amoeba travels to other organs, significantly the liver, causing abscess formation (Fig. 11.11). The brain, heart, lungs, and genitourinary organs may also be

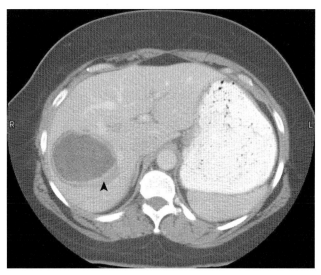

Fig. 11.11   CT scan showing a liver abscess (arrowed) in *Entamoeba histolytica* infection. (Modified from Klatt E (2015) *Robbins and Cotran atlas of pathology*, 3rd ed, Fig. 8.91. Philadelphia: Elsevier Inc.)

Flagellum

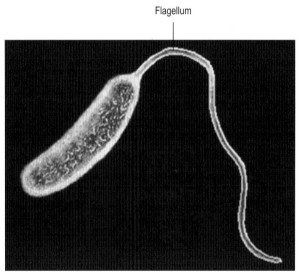

Fig. 11.12   *Vibrio cholerae*. (Modified from Moredun Animal Health, LTD/Science Photo Library/Photo Researchers, Inc.)

infected. Symptoms begin up to 4 weeks after infection, and without treatment infection can be lifelong.

CHOLERA

The causative organism in cholera is *Vibrio cholerae*, a flagellated bacterium (Fig. 11.12) spread by the faeco-oral route. Most cases follow consumption of foodstuffs or water that have been contaminated with infected faecal material. In 1854 a London doctor, John Snow, showed that a contaminated water supply, drawn from the Broad Street public pump, was the source of an ongoing local cholera outbreak that had caused hundreds of deaths. His demonstration was simple: he removed the water pump handle so that the local people had no access to its infected water, and the number of cholera cases immediately reduced to almost nil. Left untreated, the diarrhoea induced by cholera toxin released by the bacterium causes rapid dehydration, and death can

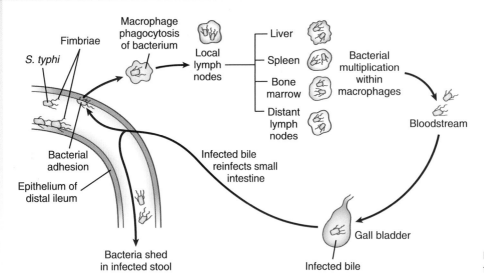

Fig. 11.13 The pathogenesis of typhoid fever.

follow in a matter of hours. The disease causes up to 143,000 deaths worldwide every year and is widespread in impoverished, overcrowded conditions with poor sanitation and no clean water supply. This number is likely to be an underestimate because affected areas are not likely to have accurate recording and monitoring systems in place, and outbreaks are not reported because of the negative impact this can have on business, tourism, and trade.

Pathophysiology
The organism is susceptible to low pH, so gastric acid may prevent infection if the number of bacteria entering the GI tract is small enough. Lower microbe counts are capable of causing infection if they enter in food rather than water, because foodstuffs act as a protective barrier between the bacteria and the acidic gastric juice. Once in the intestines, they produce a virulent enterotoxin that stimulates secretion by the intestinal epithelium, producing watery, electrolyte-rich diarrhoea. Rapidly progressing dehydration caused by diarrhoea reduces circulating blood volume and causes shock, unless there is fluid and electrolyte replacement.

Management and prognosis
Cholera is easily, cheaply, and rapidly treatable with fluid and electrolyte replacement, provided this is available.

TYPHOID FEVER

The causative bacterium, *Salmonella typhi*, is usually spread by consumption of food or water contaminated with infected faecal material. Typhoid (enteric fever) is most prevalent in conditions of overcrowding, poor sanitation, and limited access to clean water. WHO statistics (2018) report the incidence of typhoid fever as 11 to 20 million people worldwide, from which up to 160,000 people die annually. Most cases occur in children and young people. Typhoid is associated with carrier status; that is, recovered individuals who still carry viable bacteria and can infect others. Up to 6% of people remain carriers for considerable lengths of time after recovery. The most notorious typhoid carrier was an Irish woman called Mary Mallon, a cook in New York at the beginning of the 20th century. Her choice of profession was

unfortunate, as she caused typhoid outbreaks wherever she worked and was responsible for at least three deaths. Called Typhoid Mary by a furious public, she had the misfortune to live in the pre-antibiotic era and spent the last 23 years of her life in quarantine to prevent her infecting any more people.

Pathophysiology
The bacteria adhere to the lining of the distal ileum via specialised fimbriae. They are engulfed by macrophages, which carry the bacteria into the lymphatic system, including lymph nodes, the liver, spleen, and bone marrow. *S. typhi* possess an external capsule that does not activate immune or inflammatory cells, so they are not destroyed and multiply within lymphoid tissues and cells. Eventually they spill into the bloodstream and appear in the bile, which in turn reinfects the gastrointestinal tract and produces contaminated faeces, which can pass the infection to others (Fig. 11.13).

Signs and symptoms
Typically, there is fever, headache, anorexia, nausea, abdominal pain, and malaise. Severe cases can suffer intestinal perforation or neurological complications, including convulsions, meningitis, encephalopathy, and schizophrenic psychosis.

Management and prognosis
Typhoid can be treated with antibiotics, although antibiotic resistance is an increasing problem. The first typhoid vaccine was developed in 1896, and two vaccines are currently available, but neither gives long-lasting immunity and neither can be given to children under 2 years old, a high-risk group. Untreated, the death rate is high, and the course of the disease is prolonged over several weeks. A new vaccine that may be given to children under two is currently being trialled.

HEPATITIS

This term means inflammation of the liver and may be caused by infection (usually viral), toxins such as alcohol, or autoimmune disease.

Cirrhosis

Cirrhosis is liver scarring secondary to long-term, repeated liver injury. The liver has a remarkable capacity to regenerate after surgery or necrosis secondary to disease. It does this by a combination of hepatocyte hyperplasia and proliferation and can restore a damaged liver to full size and function. However, if disease or injury to the liver is sustained, eventually the liver lobules are replaced with fibrotic scar tissue, destroying normal liver architecture, and progressively impairing its function. If enough functional liver tissue remains, cirrhosis may cause no clinical problems, but as it proceeds, characteristic symptoms appear, including fatigue, muscle wasting, anorexia, weight loss, and thin and papery skin. Other consequences of cirrhosis are described in Alcoholic liver disease below.

Portal hypertension. Progressive liver fibrosis impedes blood flow through the organ. This increases pressure in the blood vessels supplying it (i.e., the hepatic artery and the hepatic portal vein) and in the vessels supplying them, including the oesophageal veins.

Hepatic encephalopathy. The injured liver's ability to clear toxins and process other blood-borne substances is reduced, and they accumulate in the blood. When this affects the brain, it causes hepatic encephalopathy, which may be fatal.

Increased tendency to bleed. If the liver is unable to produce adequate quantities of clotting proteins, bleeding times increase, and the risk of spontaneous haemorrhage rises.

VIRAL HEPATITIS

One of the WHO's key strategies is global elimination of viral hepatitis by 2030. The death rate for this infection is comparable to tuberculosis and higher than HIV infection; however, unlike these diseases, its incidence is rising. Death in hepatitis is usually caused by the development of hepatic carcinoma or cirrhosis secondary to the infection. Five viruses cause hepatitis in humans: the hepatitis A virus (HAV), hepatitis B virus (HBV), hepatitis C virus (HCV), hepatitis D virus (HDV), and hepatitis E virus (HEV). Hepatitis B and C are responsible for 96% of all hepatitis deaths worldwide. Initial infection causes acute hepatitis, which may become chronic if the virus is not cleared.

Pathophysiology

Some key information relating to each form of hepatitis is given in Table 11.1. The virus invades hepatocytes and triggers apoptosis, leading to hepatocyte death. The liver becomes infiltrated with immune and inflammatory cells, provoking an acute inflammatory response. The liver may be swollen and tender. The greater the extent of tissue death, the more significantly liver function is impaired, and the greater the risk of developing fibrosis, cirrhosis, chronic liver disease, and liver failure. As liver cells are lost, and liver scarring proceeds, the signs and symptoms of cirrhosis may appear.

HBV. This is the commonest chronic viral infection in the world. Much of the liver damage done in HBV infection is secondary to the aggressive immune response mounted to the virus by T cells, which damages healthy liver cells and infected ones. Of all infected adults, 90% develop antibodies to the virus, clear it from the body, and recover fully, although the proportion of children

who manage this is lower. Those who do not clear the virus completely may develop chronic hepatitis, and the virus may reactivate in later life. Chronic hepatitis usually causes fatigue, and flare-ups of the disease cause signs and symptoms of acute hepatitis. Other body systems may become involved; for example, glomerulonephritis in chronic hepatitis is the result of glomerular deposition of the large quantities of immune complex (p.92) formed when antiviral antibodies react with the virus. Chronic HBV hepatitis is a major risk factor for cirrhosis and hepatocellular carcinoma; most hepatocellular carcinoma cases are secondary to HBV infection. The time course of HBV infection is shown in Fig. 11.14.

HCV. Most cases of HCV are asymptomatic, but up to 85% of patients do not clear the infection and may progress to chronic hepatitis. Of these patients, up to 30% develop cirrhosis, and their risk of hepatocellular carcinoma is increased, particularly if there is co-infection with HBV.

Signs and symptoms

These vary greatly between individuals. Mild infection can be asymptomatic. Characteristic symptoms include nausea, vomiting, anorexia, malaise, fatigue, mild fever, and pain in the abdominal right upper quadrant. There may be jaundice, caused by the inability of the infected liver to break down bilirubin released by haemolysis, which causes itch and dark coloured urine. Severe and progressive (fulminant) hepatitis is more likely to be associated with systemic complications, including encephalitis.

ALCOHOLIC LIVER DISEASE

The production and consumption of alcohol (ethanol) in human society date back thousands of years, but the current levels of alcohol consumption worldwide are prime causes of mortality and morbidity and carry a huge economic cost. In addition, alcohol consumption is strongly linked to use of other psychoactive substances, including tobacco, opioids, and benzodiazepines. WHO (2018) data indicate that total global alcohol consumption is equivalent to every person over the age of 15 drinking 6.4 L of pure alcohol in a year. This is not spread evenly between countries; the per capita pure alcohol consumption in Europe is 10 L/year, but in many mainly Muslim countries, this figure is 2.5 L. Alcohol has detrimental effects on many body tissues, including the liver, where it is a common and potent cause of cirrhosis.

A genetic predisposition to alcohol dependence itself is well recognised, but not all heavy drinkers develop serious liver disease. One important risk factor for alcohol-related liver disease is female sex; for any given level of alcohol consumption, the rates of liver disease are higher in women than men.

Pathophysiology

The liver is the main organ responsible for alcohol metabolism, so it is particularly vulnerable to the effects of high alcohol consumption. Hepatocytes contain two main alcohol-metabolising enzymes, alcohol dehydrogenase, responsible for 80% to 90% of ethanol metabolism, and one of the cytochrome P450 enzymes called CYP2E1. Alcohol metabolism produces quantities of acetaldehyde, which is toxic because

Table 11.1 The five types of viral hepatitis

HV type	Incubation period	Disease course	Route of transmission
A	15–45 days	Infection almost always resolves with no long-term complications; not associated with carrier state. Often occurs in epidemics	Usually faeco-oral
B	40–150 days	Associated with carrier state (see text)	Infected blood and blood-contaminated instruments Mother to child around birth Sexual activity
C	8 weeks	Associated with increased risk of hepatocellular carcinoma and chronic cirrhosis (see text)	Infected blood and blood-contaminated instruments IV and intranasal drug use Sexual activity Mother to child around birth
D	45–160 days (coinfection with HBV)	HDV only infects HBV positive people; this coinfection with HBV causes more rapid disease progression and increased risk of chronic liver disease	Intravenous drug use Mother to child around birth Sexual activity
E	2–10 weeks	Particularly dangerous in pregnant women and can cause chronic liver disease but usually full recovery follows infection	Faeco-oral

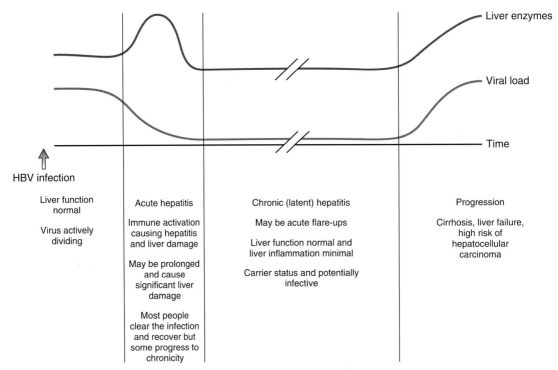

Fig. 11.14 Time course of hepatitis B infection.

it damages proteins, lipids, and nucleic acids. To reduce acetaldehyde levels, the liver oxidises it to acetate (Fig. 11.15). However, when these pathways are in constant use because of high alcohol intake, there are knock-on effects on other pathways; normal aerobic energy production is disrupted and fatty acid production is increased, leading to fat deposition within hepatocytes (fatty liver, also called **steatosis**). In addition, chronic activation of CYP2E1 has the knock-on effect of releasing highly toxic reactive oxygen species (ROS), leading to inflammation and hepatocyte damage.

Fatty liver (Fig. 11.16A) is the earliest sign of alcoholic liver damage. It may be completely reversible if the individual stops drinking. However, progressive fatty change and the ongoing inflammatory changes caused by in part to chronic release of ROS but also to alcohol-induced activation of Kupffer cells, lead to alcoholic hepatitis, in which the hepatocytes become so badly damaged they swell and die. This exacerbates inflammation, as neutrophils and other defence cells arrive to clear up the damaged tissue, and nodular fibrosis and cirrhosis develop (Fig. 11.16B).

There may be bleeding from the upper gastrointestinal tract secondary to the development of **oesophageal varices**. Varices are dilated and weakened areas in veins (haemorrhoids are another example of varices). As the liver becomes

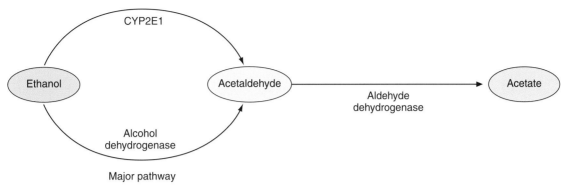

Fig. 11.15 The two main pathways of ethanol metabolism in the liver. (Modified from Waller DG, Renwick A, Hillier K, et al. (2010) *Medical pharmacology and therapeutics*, 3rd ed, Fig. 54.2. Edinburgh: Elsevier Ltd.)

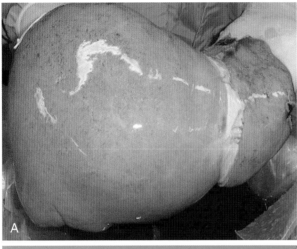

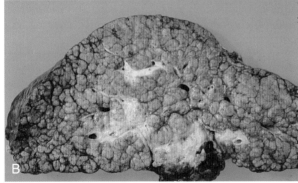

Fig. 11.16 Liver changes seen in alcoholic liver disease. (A) Fatty liver. The liver is swollen and pale yellow in colour. (B) Cirrhosis. Normal liver tissue has been replaced with masses of fat-rich, yellow fibrotic nodules. (From (A) Banasik J (2022) *Pathophysiology*, 7th ed, Fig. 4.3. St Louis: Saunders; and (B) Damjanov I, Perry A, and Perry K (2022) *Pathology for the health professions*, 6th ed, Fig. 11.9. St Louis: Elsevier Inc.)

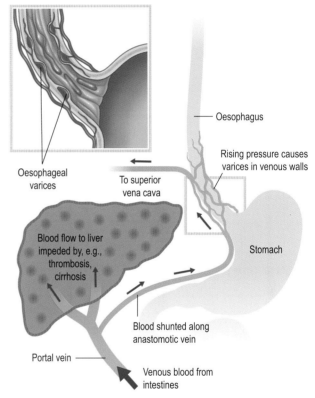

Fig. 11.17 Oesophageal varices. (Modified from Waugh A and Grant A (2018) *Ross & Wilson anatomy and physiology in health and illness*, 13th ed, Fig. 12.47. Oxford: Elsevier Ltd.)

increasingly swollen and fibrotic, blood vessels are physically compressed and resistance to blood flow through the liver rises. Pressure increases in the hepatic artery and the hepatic portal vein as blood backs up (portal hypertension). Rising pressure in the hepatic portal vein in turn backs up into veins draining the oesophagus and stomach, which become swollen and stretched, producing fragile varices that are liable to rupture (Fig. 11.17). Rupture can cause sudden, heavy, and disastrous haemorrhage; it may be spontaneous, or initiated by a traumatic medical procedure such as endoscopy.

Ascites (fluid accumulation in the abdominal cavity) occurs because of portal hypertension and low plasma protein levels. When plasma protein levels fall, the osmotic pressure of the blood is reduced, allowing fluid to escape into other body spaces. Very large volumes of fluid may accumulate in the abdominal cavity, requiring to be drained. Low plasma protein levels may be secondary to low plasma protein production by the liver, and also to poor nutritional status.

Signs and symptoms

The liver may be tender and enlarged, causing abdominal pain in the right upper quadrant. Active hepatitis is associated with fever and systemic indications of inflammation

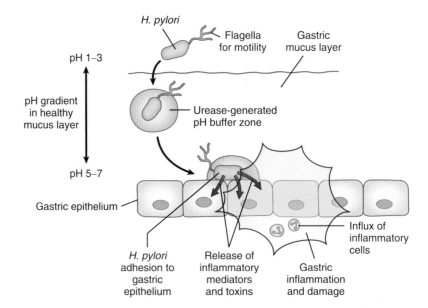

Fig. 11.18 *H. pylori* and gastritis.

(e.g., raised white blood cell numbers and serum inflammatory markers). In addition, there are indications of liver failure, which vary in severity depending on the extent of liver damage. Jaundice occurs because of liver failure to metabolise bilirubin. Liver enzyme levels in the blood rise because they spill from damaged and dying hepatocytes. Bleeding times may be increased because of reduced synthesis of clotting proteins. There may be indications of malnutrition because regular heavy drinkers often fail to eat properly. There may be hepatic encephalopathy, brain injury secondary to high levels of circulating toxins.

Management and prognosis
Pathophysiological changes in the liver (fatty liver, alcoholic hepatitis) are often reversible until there is established cirrhosis, which is permanent. Additionally, there is still significant mortality associated with serious alcoholic hepatitis. Continued alcohol consumption is the main prognostic factor.

GASTRITIS

This is inflammation of the stomach lining. It is very common and results from a wide range of causes, from short-term inflammation after drinking too much alcohol to chronic conditions in which the stomach lining is progressively destroyed by autoimmune mechanisms.

Acute gastritis
Exposure of the gastric mucosa to irritants like alcohol, spicy foods, irritant drugs (e.g., non-steroidal anti-inflammatory drugs), or bacterial toxins in contaminated food causes inflammation. In developing shock, hypotension, and vasoconstriction in tissues and organs not essential for life support, reduce blood flow through the gastrointestinal tract and can lead to gastric ischaemia and acute gastritis, sometimes with significant bleeding.

***Helicobacter pylori (H. pylori)* gastritis**
H. pylori infection of the stomach and intestines is very common, especially in older people, and is probably spread through the faeco-oral route from contaminated water and foods, or from the oral-oral route when kissing. It probably establishes itself in childhood, and about 60% of the world's population are thought to be infected. In most people, *H. pylori* gastritis is asymptomatic, although when examined through an endoscope there is clear evidence of inflammatory changes in the stomach lining. Using its flagellae, the organism travels through the gastric mucus layer and adheres to gastric epithelial cells where it triggers an influx of inflammatory cells, including neutrophils and other white blood cells, which initiate a powerful inflammatory response (Fig. 11.18). It protects itself against the acidic environment of the stomach by producing an enzyme called **urease**, which generates alkaline ammonia, creating a protective buffer zone around itself.

In some people, infection mainly involves the epithelium of the body of the stomach, and the chronic inflammation causes widespread atrophy, including destruction of gastric glands. This steadily reduces gastric acid secretion, and the pH of the gastric fluids increases. The chronic inflammation caused by the infection may trigger metaplastic changes in the gastric lining, a known risk factor for cancer. This, along with the increased pH of the stomach fluids, another risk factor for gastric cancer, may be the reason why *H. pylori* infection increases the risk of gastric carcinoma.

In other cases, *H. pylori* infection predominantly affects the antrum and causes a significant increase in gastrin secretion from the G cells in the antral epithelium. This in turn causes an increase in acid secretion and is strongly associated with peptic ulcer disease.

PEPTIC ULCER DISEASE

This occurs when the protective mechanisms responsible for preventing acidic gastric fluids injuring the stomach or duodenal lining are inadequate. Acidic gastric juice coming into direct contact with the stomach or duodenal lining causes corrosive injury resulting in ulceration. The main risk factors are *Helicobacter pylori* (*H. pylori*) infection and non-steroidal anti-inflammatory drug (NSAID) consumption. Other risk factors include cigarette smoking, a family history and serious illness (e.g., trauma, sepsis, respiratory failure). Occasionally, a condition that causes production of excessive quantities of gastric juice (e.g., gastric carcinoma) is responsible.

Pathophysiology

Ulceration may be caused by a breakdown in the normal mucosal protective mechanisms, or by excessive acid production. Ulcers may be single or appear as a crop. Erosion extends through the mucosa and into deeper layers of the tract wall, which in severe disease may perforate completely, allowing digestive contents to leak into the peritoneal cavity (Fig. 11.19).

H. pylori infection of the antrum of the stomach increases gastrin secretion from G cells. Gastrin stimulates acid secretion by parietal cells (Fig. 11.20). The highly acidic chyme from the stomach arriving in the duodenum cannot be adequately neutralised by duodenal juices, causing duodenal inflammation and injury. The duodenal epithelium undergoes metaplastic change, transforming into gastric epithelium to protect itself. This leads essentially to an extension of gastric lining into the duodenum, bringing *H. pylori* with it, and contributing to the development of duodenal ulcers.

Signs and symptoms

In early or mild disease, there may be upper abdominal burning or pain, and a feeling of fullness after even small meals. Symptoms may vary depending on the location of the ulceration. With gastric ulceration, patients tend to eat less and lose weight because the arrival of food in the stomach immediately triggers gastric juice production and irritates the ulcer, causing pain. With duodenal ulcers, however, patients may

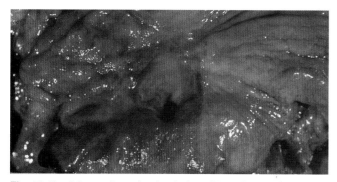

Fig. 11.19 A large, deep duodenal ulcer. (From Goldblum J, Lamps L, McKenney J, et al. (2018) *Rosai and Ackerman's surgical pathology*, 11th ed, Fig. 15.18. Philadelphia: Elsevier Inc.)

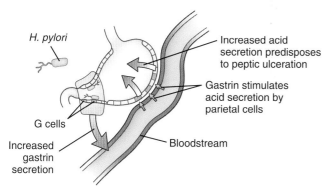

Fig. 11.20 *H. pylori* infection and peptic ulcer disease.

eat more and actually put on weight because the presence of food dilutes the acidic content of the chyme arriving in the duodenum and makes it less irritant. They are likely to complain of pain 2 or 3 hours after eating, when the acidic chyme is being delivered into the duodenum. The patient may be anaemic because of chronic bleeding from the ulcer.

Management and prognosis

Eradication of *H. pylori*, usually with a combination of antibiotics and a proton pump inhibitor to reduce acid production, is a priority and eradication of the infection usually allows the ulcer to heal. The rate of re-infection and re-ulceration is high, however. Discontinuation of an NSAID, or introduction of a proton pump inhibitor to reduce acid production, also helps healing.

INFLAMMATORY CONDITIONS OF THE SMALL AND LARGE INTESTINES

As a group, these conditions are very common.

IRRITABLE BOWEL SYNDROME

Irritable bowel syndrome (IBS) is common, affecting twice to three times as many women as men and usually manifesting before the age of 40. There is often a family history and there is a link with certain personality traits, such as neuroticism, and other disorders, including depression and fibromyalgia.

Pathophysiology

The underlying aetiology of IBS is not clear, although various factors including changes in the gastrointestinal microbiome and food intolerances have been described. IBS may sometimes follow a bout of gastroenteritis. The tract may be hypersensitive to distension, although the reason is not understood, and abnormal response of the gastrointestinal muscle to stress may also be involved, although again the link is currently vague.

Signs and symptoms

These are variable. Some people experience mainly diarrhoea, although others experience mainly constipation, and others experience both. There may be bloating and abdominal pain or discomfort. The disorder features periods of normal bowel function interspersed with symptomatic bouts of illness, which may be triggered by stress or antibiotic use.

Prognosis and management

Reassurance, support, and the provision of educational material regarding IBS are very important. Some patients find reducing certain dietary carbohydrates reduces bloating and improves symptoms. Caffeine stimulates intestinal motility and is best avoided, or intake limited when diarrhoea is a significant feature. Pain, constipation, and diarrhoea can all be controlled by appropriate drugs. Psychotherapy is useful in both regulating gastrointestinal function and improving the overall quality of life.

INFLAMMATORY BOWEL DISEASE

This general term, usually abbreviated as IBD, usually includes two main conditions: UC and Crohn disease and the key features of these conditions are summarised in Box 11.3.

BOX 11.3 Key features of Crohn disease and ulcerative colitis

	Crohn disease	Ulcerative colitis
Sex	M = F	F>M
Genetic tendency	Yes	Yes
Link with GI cancer	Yes	Yes
Tissues in gut wall affected	Mucosa only, with ulceration and loss of crypts and goblet cells.	All layers affected, with fissuring, fistula formation, and granulomatous inflammation
Areas of GI tract affected	Anywhere; colon and ileum most frequently affected. Skip lesions seen.	Colon only, spreading continously from rectum.
Extraintestinal manifestations	Common	Common
Recurrence after surgery	Common	No

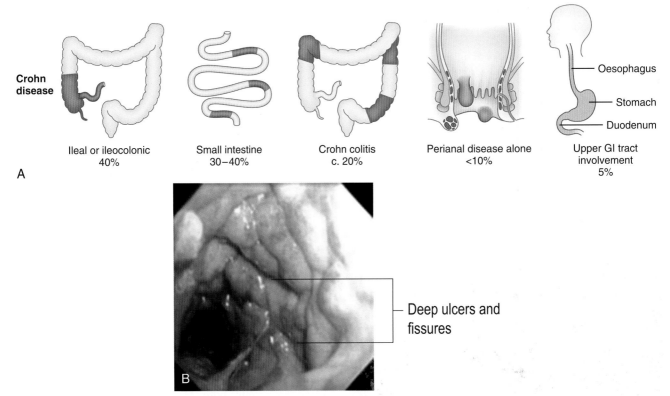

Fig. 11.21   Crohn disease. (A) Typical distribution of lesions, showing skip lesion pattern. (B) 'Cobblestone' appearance of the mucosal surface caused by deep and extensive fissures and ulcers. (B, Modified from Goldman L and Schafer A (2012) *Goldman's Cecil medicine*, 24th ed, Fig. 143.1. Philadelphia: Elsevier Inc.)

Both have a genetic predisposition, and both increase the risk of gastrointestinal cancer. The Global Burden of Disease study (2017) reported that the worldwide prevalence of IBD has increased from 79.5 to 84.3 per 100,000 population between 1990 and 2017. Rates are rising fastest in wealthy countries, particularly the UK and North America and are highest in people with high socioeconomic status. The increasing incidence is due mainly to a rise in the incidence of Crohn disease; the incidence of UC is stable.

Crohn disease

The colon, ileum, and perianal region are the regions most frequently affected in Crohn disease, but any part of the tract may be involved, from the mouth to the anus (Fig. 11.21A). The cause is unknown, but there is a familial tendency, and several genes that increase susceptibility have been identified. It is thought that environmental and lifestyle factors, including smoking, a diet low in plant-based foods and high in meat, long-term use of anti-inflammatory drugs, and exposure to pollution can trigger disease in genetically susceptible people. Having been breastfed is protective. The gut microbiome is altered, and the range of gut flora is reduced, with increased populations of some bacteria associated with pathogenicity. Diet can affect this; certain food additives and artificial sweeteners, and diets low in high-fibre foods reduce the diversity of the microbiome and are associated with increased risk. The disease is most common in urban areas in developed countries, but the incidence is increasing in developing nations. It usually appears in young

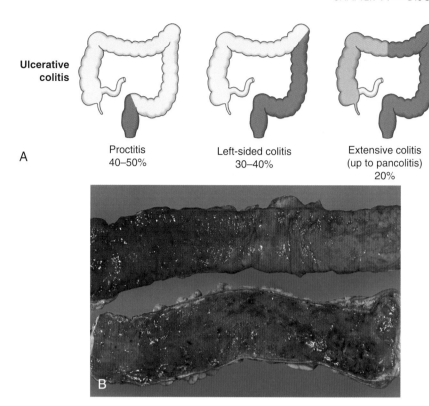

Ulcerative colitis

Proctitis
40–50%

Left-sided colitis
30–40%

Extensive colitis
(up to pancolitis)
20%

A

B

Fig. 11.22 Ulcerative colitis. (A) Typical distribution of lesions, showing continuous spread from the rectum. (B) Mucosal ulceration, bleeding, oedema, and inflammation in UC. (Reproduced from Cooke R, Stewart B (2004) Colour atlas of anatomical pathology, 3rd ed. Oxford: Elsevier Ltd.)

adulthood, although an increasing number of cases are being diagnosed in children.

Pathophysiology

The whole thickness of the intestinal wall is inflamed and oedematous. The cause of the inflammation is not known, but it appears to be an abnormal immune response to the gastrointestinal microbiome. T cells are thought to be particularly important in this dysregulated immune response, releasing a raft of inflammatory mediators which directly injure intestinal tissues. Initially, the crypts within the mucosal lining become inflamed and develop abscesses, which then ulcerate. Ulcers often develop longitudinally, producing deep fissures and giving the surface a cobblestone appearance (Fig. 11.21B). Developing and enlarging ulcers erode into the deeper layers of the bowel wall and can cause perforation, leading to fistula formation between the lumen of the tract and nearby structures, including adjacent loops of bowel, the vagina, the bladder and even through the skin to the body surface. The bowel wall is invaded with lymphocytes and plasma cells, characteristic of a chronic inflammatory response, and granulomas form. The inflamed regions are usually not continuous, giving a patchy distribution with segments of uninvolved tissue in between; these are called **skip lesions**. There may be strictures, leading to obstruction, and adhesions, limiting bowel motility.

Signs and symptoms

Diarrhoea and cramping pain are characteristic of the commonest lesion pattern affecting the colon and ileum. In the 5% in whom higher parts of the tract are affected, nausea, vomiting, and anorexia are frequent. There may be urgency, constipation, and bloody or mucus-rich stool.

In addition to gastrointestinal involvement, about 30% of patients have extraintestinal manifestations, with inflammatory changes affecting the joints, eyes and skin. There is also an increased risk of gallstones because bile acids are poorly reabsorbed across the inflamed tract wall, reducing levels of bile acids in the gallbladder. Because they are important in keeping cholesterol in solution in the bile, lack of bile acids causes cholesterol to precipitate out of solution in the bile and form stones. The incidence of kidney stones is also increased because reduced bile salt levels reduces fat absorption in the intestine. This indirectly increases oxalate reabsorption into the bloodstream, increasing oxalate levels in the renal tubules and favouring stone formation.

Management and prognosis

Crohn disease is associated with increased mortality, partly through the increased risk of malignancy, but also because of complications of the disorder itself, including haemorrhage, perforation, and infection. Steroids, non-steroidal anti-inflammatory drugs, and immunomodulators are used to relieve pain and inflammation, and antibiotics are used to manage infections. Surgery is generally reserved for the management of complications (e.g., fistulas or strictures).

Ulcerative colitis

UC involves only the large intestine. It begins in the rectum and spreads continuously towards the proximal colon, with no gaps, and can eventually affect the entire large intestine (Fig. 11.22A). Worldwide, UC is the commonest form of IBD, and affects 1 in 200 people in the developed world. It usually manifests before the age of 30, although there is a second peak of occurrence between 50 and 70 years. As with Crohn disease, incidence correlates with higher socioeconomic status and living in an industrialised area. However, smoking and removal of the appendix while young reduce the risk of UC.

Pathophysiology

UC is characterised by periods of relapse and remission. The pathophysiology is not well understood but probably involves some environmental factor in genetically susceptible individuals. The basis is probably immunological, with failure of the normal barrier function of the intestinal wall, allowing dendritic cells (defensive immune cells) within the intestinal wall to come into contact with normal intestinal bacteria living on the mucosal surface. This causes an abnormal and inappropriate immune response and ongoing colonic inflammation. Normally, only the mucosa is involved (Fig. 11.22B). On endoscopy, colorectal mucosa is swollen and inflamed, and histological examination of biopsy tissue shows a chronic lymphocytic infiltrate, damaged and distorted crypts, fibrosis, and abscesses. Significant inflammation can reduce motility and peristalsis. These less motile regions become distended (toxic megacolon) and can perforate.

Signs and symptoms

Diarrhoea, with or without blood and/or mucus, and abdominal pain are usual symptoms. The disorder begins with rectal bleeding and faecal urgency. There is usually weight loss and nutritional status may be poor because of malabsorption. In some patients, UC is associated with other inflammatory disorders with an immune component, including joint, liver, skin, and eye conditions.

Management and prognosis

The disease may be managed in some people with diet and anti-inflammatory drugs, but a significant minority (up to 30%) need surgery. Complete removal of the colon cures the disease but leaves the patient with a stoma. UC increases the risk of malignant change and the development of adenocarcinoma of the colon.

DIVERTICULAR DISEASE

This condition, and the related disorder diverticulitis, affects the large intestine. A diverticulum is a pouch lined with mucosa that pushes out through the muscle layer of the colon wall (Fig. 11.23). Diverticular disease increases in frequency with increasing age and is more common in people whose diet contains a great deal of refined foods and is poor in fibre. This is associated with smaller, dry faecal mass, which needs higher pressures in the gut lumen to move along the tract. This higher pressure is considered the main reason the outpouchings develop.

Pathophysiology

When there are no symptoms, the condition is called **diverticulosis**. However, faecal material can become lodged in the diverticulum, causing inflammation, bleeding, and sometimes perforation. When inflammation is a feature, the condition is referred to as **diverticulitis**. Chronic inflammation can lead to fibrotic changes and thickening in the colon wall, with possible obstruction. There may be significant bleeding if the inflammation erodes local blood vessels. The diverticuli can erode into local structures, e.g., the bladder,

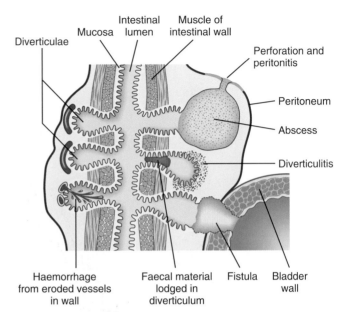

Fig. 11.23 Diverticular disease and its complications. (Modified from Cross S (2019) *Underwood's pathology: a clinical approach*, 7th ed, Fig. 15.20. Oxford: Elsevier Ltd.)

forming a fistula, or through the peritoneal membrane and cause peritonitis. Infection can lead to abscess formation.

Signs and symptoms

There is often constipation and abdominal cramps, and the colon may be swollen and tender to palpate. Periods of active inflammation are associated with diarrhoea and sometimes rectal bleeding.

APPENDICITIS

The blind-ended hollow appendix opens from the caecum. Its narrow neck is a common site for impaction by faecal material, local lymphatic swelling or, sometimes, worms. This leads to inflammation, necrosis, and infection (mainly by *E. coli*). Acute appendicitis is a medical emergency because of the risk of perforation. As the organ swells, its blood supply is compromised, its tissues become necrotic, and pus accumulates at the site. Classically, there is lower right quadrant pain, nausea, vomiting, anorexia, and fever. Surgical removal is essential in acute appendicitis.

NEOPLASMS OF THE GASTROINTESTINAL TRACT

Cancers of the gastrointestinal tract are very common and can arise at any location. Colorectal, liver, stomach, oesophageal, and pancreatic cancers were the third, fourth, fifth, eighth, and ninth most common causes of cancer-related deaths, respectively, globally in 2020. There is considerable geographical variation, however, and the incidence of some GI cancers is actually falling in some countries.

TUMOURS OF THE SALIVARY GLANDS

Most salivary gland tumours are benign but are usually removed because there is a small chance of malignant transformation. Malignant tumours arise either in the acinar cells, which produce saliva, or the mucoepidermal cells lining the

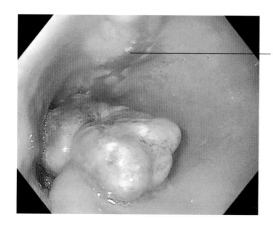

— Barrett oesophagus

Fig. 11.24   Oesophageal carcinoma; extending up the oesophageal wall above the tumour is a tongue of Barrett oesophagus (see also Fig. 11.9). (Modified from Kuipers E (2020) *Encyclopedia of gastroenterology*, 2nd ed, Fig 5. Philadelphia:, Elsevier Inc.)

gland. Risk factors include increasing age; benign tumours usually appear before 40 years, whereas tumours arising in later life are more likely to be malignant. Smoking, a strong risk factor for most head and neck cancers, is not associated with salivary tumours, but there is evidence that radiation exposure and exposure to certain carcinogens such as nitrosamines, found in cigarette smoke and some preserved foods, may increase risk.

About 80% of salivary tumours arise in the parotid glands, and about 80% of parotid tumours are benign pleomorphic adenomas, of which fewer than 1% undergo malignant change. Surgery is usually curative, but some tumours may recur.

OESOPHAGEAL CANCER

Globally, four-fifths of cases of oesophageal cancer occur in less wealthy nations, including Latin America, Asia, and Africa. This is usually an aggressive cancer with a poor prognosis. Males are twice as likely as females to develop the disease. Clearly identified risk factors include smoking, human papilloma virus infection, obesity, and alcohol consumption. Smoking and alcohol together are particularly strong risk factors. Alcohol is thought to damage the oesophageal lining, allowing the carcinogens in tobacco smoke to enter cells and damage their DNA. Chronic irritation of the oesophageal lining in gastro-oesophageal reflux disease is thought to underlie the increased risk of oesophageal cancer in this condition. There is limited evidence that eating plenty of fruit and vegetables and higher levels of physical activity are protective.

Pathophysiology

The two main types of oesophageal cancer, squamous cell carcinoma and adenocarcinoma, arise from the epithelial cells and the glandular tissue, respectively, of the oesophageal lining. Squamous cell carcinoma is the commonest type of oesophageal cancer (88%). It usually arises in the upper portion of the oesophagus, whereas adenocarcinomas usually develop close to the gastro-oesophageal junction, which is rich in glandular tissue. The main risk factor for adenocarcinoma, the incidence of which is rising in richer countries, is reflux disease, associated with chronic irritation of the lower oesophagus by the backwash of acidic gastric contents and Barrett oesophagus (see Fig. 11.9).

Signs and symptoms

Difficulty swallowing (dysphagia) is usually an early symptom, and initially affects solids but as the oesophageal lumen gets narrower and narrower, will eventually also make swallowing liquids a problem. Fig. 11.24 shows an oesophageal carcinoma partially blocking the oesophagus and clear evidence of Barrett oesophagus. There may be pain behind the sternum or in the epigastric region, cough if the tumour grows into the airways, and hoarseness if the tumour grows into the recurrent laryngeal nerve.

Management and prognosis

The diagnosis is usually late, meaning that the prognosis is frequently poor. The 5-year survival rate in Europe is only 10%. Surgery, chemotherapy, and radiotherapy may all be treatment options.

GASTRIC CANCER

Although gastric cancer is a major global health issue, its incidence is declining in many countries, including some with the highest rates, such as Japan. Globally, Japan and South Korea have the highest incidence, which is eight times higher than North America and Europe, where incidence is the lowest. The strongest risk factors include *Helicobacter pylori* infection, smoking, and obesity. There is an association with diets rich in salty, pickled, and processed foods. The falling incidence seen in many developed countries is thought to be caused by changing dietary and smoking habits and decreasing rates of *H. pylori* infection. Some stomach cancers have a hereditable component; for example, people with mutations in *BRCA1* and *BRCA2* (p.84) may have an increased risk. Epstein-Barr viral infections, male sex, and type A blood are also risk factors.

Pathophysiology

The commonest gastric cancer is adenocarcinoma, and most of these arise in the antrum, mainly on the lesser curvature. Based on the appearance of the tumour and the cells within it and molecular and genetic abnormalities, gastric adenocarcinomas are divided into two main groups: intestinal tumours, which tend to develop as bulky solid masses that may ulcerate and perforate the stomach wall (Fig. 11.25); and diffuse cancers, which grow as invasive individual cells that infiltrate the stomach wall.

Intestinal tumours. These are very strongly associated with *H. pylori* infection and the chronic inflammation caused by this organism, and unlike diffuse stomach cancer, this type of stomach cancer is falling sharply, accounting for the reduction in the overall incidence of the disease. *p53* mutations (p.75) are frequently found in intestinal tumours,

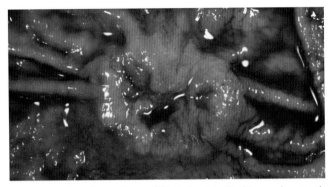

Fig. 11.25 Gastric carcinoma. This bulky intestinal type adenocarcinoma shows central ulceration. (From Kumar V, Singh M, Abbas A, et al. (2022) *Robbins & Cotran Pathologic Basis of Disease*, 10th ed: South Asia Edition, Volume 1, Fig. 17.18. New Delhi: RELX India Pvt. Ltd.)

along with mutations in several other tumour suppressor genes. These tumours usually develop from precursor lesions, including benign adenomas, gastritis and dysplastic changes, and screening programmes in high-risk countries have successfully reduced mortality rates by identifying and treating these lesions at an early stage.

Diffuse tumours. These are not associated with clear precursor changes, and the most common genetic mutation found is in a tumour suppressor gene called *CDH1*. This gene codes for an adhesion protein called **cadherin**. When the gene mutates, cadherin production is reduced, cells lose their ability to adhere to each other and infiltrate locally.

Signs and symptoms

Early signs and symptoms are often non-specific; they include dyspepsia, weight loss, anorexia, fullness even after small meals and abdominal discomfort. More advanced symptoms include vomiting, sometimes with blood, abdominal pain, abdominal distension, faecal blood, and anaemia caused by chronic bleeding.

Management and prognosis

This cancer is often diagnosed at a late stage, so the prognosis is poor and mortality rates are correspondingly high. Five-year survival rates vary depending on the stage at diagnosis and on the medical care available. Most patients (up to 80%) present with metastatic disease. If there are distant metastases, 5-year survival is almost zero, and even if the spread is local, 5-year survival is still only in the region of 10% to 15%. If the patient presents with apparently localised disease, and undergoes surgery with the intention of cure, recurrence rates can approach 50%. Chemotherapy in conjunction with surgery may extend life but significant remission is rare.

LIVER CANCER

Because of the liver's enormous physiological reserve, and its remarkable ability to regenerate after injury, it is often the case that liver tumours are diagnosed late and at a point where most of the liver has been destroyed by the disease. Secondary tumours of the liver are far more common than any primary liver cancer. The commonest cancers that metastasise to the liver originate in the colon, lung, pancreas, and breast. Primary liver cancer may arise from the liver cells themselves (hepatocellular carcinoma, HCC) or from the biliary system (cholangiocarcinoma). In 2020 liver cancer accounted for 4.7% of all primary cancers globally, but incidence and mortality rates vary significantly from country to country (Fig. 11.26).

Hepatocellular carcinoma

Fig. 11.27 shows a large hepatocellular carcinoma (HCC). HCC accounts for over 80% of all liver malignancies and is very strongly associated with hepatitis B (HBV) and hepatitis C (HCV) infection. The rates of HCC vary from country to country, but closely mirror infection patterns. Of all HCC cases, 85% are found in low- and middle-income countries, where the disease is usually diagnosed in the 30 to 60 years age group, compared with over 60 years in wealthy countries. Rates are rising in the developed world, thought to be caused by the increasing rates of hepatitis C and alcohol use and obesity. Reducing or clearing the viral load in viral hepatitis with antiviral drugs reduces the risk of HCC.

HBV is the main cause of HCC in East Asia and most of Africa, whereas HBC predominates in the USA, Europe, North Africa, Japan, and the Middle East. Other risk factors include high alcohol intake and cirrhosis, obesity-related fatty liver disease, diabetes, and certain food-borne toxins, such as aflatoxins, fungal toxins that contaminate some cereals and are powerfully carcinogenic to the liver. Aflatoxins are important contributors to HCC rates in, for example, West Africa, whereas they are of minimal importance in Western countries because food processing eliminates them.

Pathophysiology

HCC can be categorised into several subgroups depending on the genetic abnormalities present in the tumour cells. As with other cancers, identifying the molecular and genetic characteristics of specific tumours is becoming increasingly important for treatment choices. However, mutations that deactivate the tumour suppressor gene *p53* (p.75) are common. Another frequent mutation is found in the *β-catenin* gene, increasing the level of β-catenin protein, which deregulates liver cell growth controls. Cirrhosis increases the likelihood of malignancy because of the ongoing cycle of inflammation, fibrosis, and cellular proliferation in the affected liver. Sometimes, HCC is preceded by clearly identified changes in the liver tissue, including non-malignant hepatocellular adenoma and varying degrees of dysplasia, including dysplastic nodules.

Signs and symptoms

Non-specific indications include abdominal pain, fatigue, weight loss, and anorexia. There may be oedema and ascites because the failing liver is unable to maintain normal plasma protein levels, leading to reduced blood osmotic pressure and fluid shift into the tissues and peritoneal cavity. There may be oesophageal varices caused by rising pressure in the anastomotic vessels linking the oesophageal veins and the hepatic portal system (see Fig. 11.17). Jaundice occurs because the failing liver does not metabolise bilirubin as normal, which then accumulates in the bloodstream. Bleeding times may be extended if liver production of clotting factors is reduced. Sometimes confusion and mental changes occur as toxins accumulate in the bloodstream. Blood alpha-fetoprotein (AFP) levels rise in 60% of HCC, but this is not an HCC-specific marker because it occurs in other conditions including ovarian and testicular cancer and

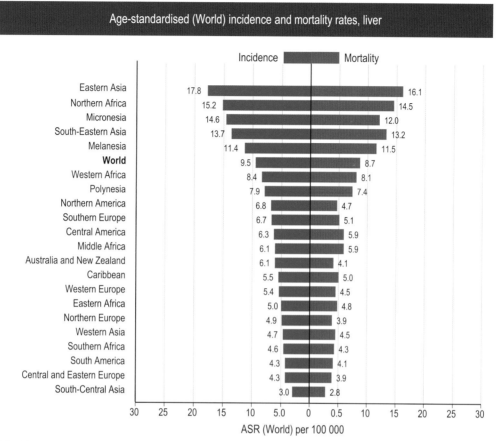

Fig. 11.26 Global incidence and mortality rates for liver cancer, 2020. (From https://gco.iarc.fr/today/data/factsheets/cancers/11-Liver-fact-sheet.pdf.)

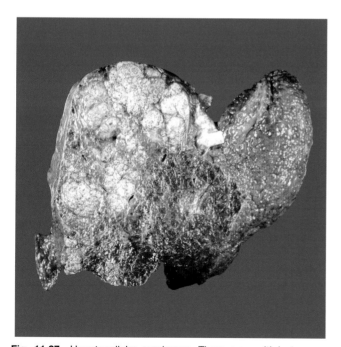

Fig. 11.27 Hepatocellular carcinoma. There are multiple tumours visible; the liver itself is cirrhotic. (From Lamps LW, Westerhoff M, and Kakar S (2022) *Diagnostic pathology: hepatobiliary and pancreas*, 3rd ed, Fig. 76.855. Philadelphia: Elsevier Inc.)

hepatitis. However, changing AFP levels in a confirmed case of HCC correlate with disease progression so can be used to monitor the success or otherwise of treatment and identify recurrences early.

Management and prognosis

Survival times are significantly longer in certain countries (e.g., Taiwan and Japan) whose healthcare systems incorporate early screening and regular monitoring in higher-risk individuals. Surgical removal of the tumour is usually the best option for improved survival; most tumours are relatively resistant to radiotherapy and chemotherapy. Prognosis is generally poor, even in countries with well-funded medical systems, and the overall 5-year survival rate is around 15%.

Cholangiocarcinoma

These are the second most common liver malignancies and arise from the epithelial lining of the biliary tract. There are multiple risk factors for these cancers, all of which relate to inflammatory changes within the biliary tree and include infestation with liver flukes, hepatitis, cirrhosis, gall stones, and chronic pancreatitis. Only 10% of cholangiocarcinomas arise in ducts within the liver itself (intrahepatic disease) and for unknown reasons the incidence of these tumours is rising globally. The remaining are extrahepatic. However, the prognosis is very poor across the board in these cancers;

average survival time is only about 6 months because most patients present with inoperable disease.

PANCREATIC CANCERS

Pancreatic adenocarcinoma is the commonest pancreatic cancer and one of the most lethal malignancies; survival rates have changed little since the 1960s. Globally, it is the 11th commonest cancer but the seventh commonest cause of cancer-related death. Risk factors include smoking, obesity, chronic pancreatitis, diabetes, and family history. The diagnosis is usually made between 60 and 80 years of age, and it is commoner in black people than white people.

Pathophysiology

Most pancreatic adenocarcinomas are aggressive and poorly differentiated, and rapidly infiltrate the pancreas and adjacent structures. Of all tumours, 70% arise in the head of the pancreas, 20% in the body and the remainder in the tail. Tumour location affects the functional consequences of the disorder. Tumours in the head can quickly obstruct the common bile duct, blocking the flow of bile from the gall bladder to the duodenum and causing jaundice. This usually means they are detected more quickly than tumours in the body or tail of the organ, which can grow to a significant size without detection. Pancreatic cancers spread quickly into adjacent organs, including the spleen, stomach, and transverse colon. They often grow along blood vessels and nerves, and distant metastases are most commonly found in lung and liver. Venous thromboembolism occurs in a proportion of patients; pancreatic cancer, in common with some other malignancies, induces a hypercoagulable state, although the reason why is not clear. Mutations in a range of tumour suppressor and tumour promoter genes have been identified in this disease. The commonest mutation is in *KRas,* one of the *Ras* family of tumour promoter genes, seen in 90% of cases. Familial pancreatic cancer is associated with *BRCA1* and *BRCA2* mutations (p.84). As with other cancers, identifying the molecular characteristics of individual cancers is used to inform treatment decisions. Recent research suggests that the invasive carcinoma stage is a late event in a long sequence of precursor events that can take decades to develop. This suggests that there may be an extended window for early detection if a suitable screening method could be found.

Signs and symptoms

These are often vague and non-specific, especially in the early stages of the disease; they include epigastric pain that may radiate to the back, anorexia, nausea, and weight loss.

Management and prognosis

The prognosis is usually dismal, with a median survival time of 4 to 6 months. The overall 5-year survival rate is only 9%; even those whose disease is localised at diagnosis and have the best prognosis only have an expected 5-year survival rate of 28%. Over half of patients already have secondary disease when they present. Surgery provides the only possibility of cure, but even small, well-differentiated tumours have a very high recurrence rate after removal.

Tumours of the endocrine pancreas

Rarely, tumours arise not from the glands that secrete digestive enzymes but from the islets, responsible for hormone secretion. The commonest are **insulinomas**, which are often asymptomatic but which can produce enough insulin to cause troublesome hypoglycaemic episodes. **Gastrinomas** are gastrin-secreting tumours, which may develop in the duodenum and the pancreas. The gastrin they produce stimulates excessive gastric acid production, so these tumours are associated with peptic ulceration. This triad of characteristics—pancreatic islet lesions, excessive gastric acid production and peptic ulceration—is called Zollinger-Ellison syndrome.

COLORECTAL NEOPLASMS

Colorectal carcinoma is discussed in detail on p.85.

NUTRITIONAL AND MALABSORPTIVE DISORDERS

Food and drink passing through the tract from mouth to anus are subjected to a series of digestive processes that break complex molecules into smaller, simpler ones for absorption across the tract wall. Deficiency of key digestive enzymes and other agents (e.g., in pancreatitis or pancreatic cancer, cystic fibrosis or cholestasis) or damage to the intestinal epithelium causing reduced absorption (e.g., coeliac disease or chronic diarrhoea) can all significantly reduce absorption and lead to poor nutritional status.

PANCREATITIS

Pancreatitis may be acute or chronic.

Acute pancreatitis

This is caused by inappropriate activation of pancreatic enzymes, which are normally secreted into the duodenum as inactive precursors to avoid auto-digestion of the pancreas. The main enzyme involved is the protein-digesting enzyme trypsin. Acute pancreatitis is usually related to high alcohol intake, or to gallstones. There is a genetic tendency, and there is an association between cystic fibrosis and both acute and chronic pancreatitis. Alcohol-related disease is commoner in males than females, and pancreatitis related to biliary tract disease is commoner in females than males.

Pathophysiology

Inappropriate activation of trypsin and other enzymes within the pancreas initiates autodigestion of the organ, activating a powerful inflammatory response with inflammatory cell infiltration, bleeding, swelling, and necrosis. Leakage of digestive enzymes into the peritoneal cavity degrades and injures local tissues. The increased permeability of local blood vessels caused by the ongoing inflammatory response can allow the enzymes to leak into the bloodstream and circulate to distant tissues, where they can cause serious damage, for example in the lung and kidney (Fig. 11.28). The ongoing inflammatory response triggers the clotting cascade, with increased risk of inappropriate clotting. Severe disease causes shock and multiorgan failure and carries a mortality rate of up to 30%.

Signs and symptoms

Abdominal pain is the main symptom-constant, severe, aching, of sudden onset and often radiating to the back. There

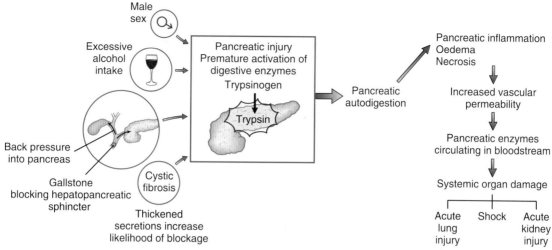

Fig. 11.28   The pathogenesis of acute pancreatitis.

is likely to be nausea and vomiting, and there may be hyperglycaemia if the islet cells are damaged and insulin production is reduced.

Management and prognosis

There is a 10% to 15% mortality rate associated with pancreatitis, with the risk of death higher in more severe cases. Developing shock needs to be managed, pain relief offered, and anti-thrombotic support given as needed. Identifying and treating any underlying cause (e.g., gallstones) is important.

Chronic pancreatitis

This is strongly associated (60% of cases) with alcohol use but may also be associated with chronic gallstones or a tumour blocking the pancreatic duct. It is sometimes associated with autoimmune disease and circulating autoantibodies. Familial pancreatitis accounts for only 1% of cases. The perpetual inflammatory changes in the organ cause atrophy and replacement of functional pancreatic tissue with fibrotic tissue, with pancreatic failure. The scarred and stiffened organ may also block the duodenum or bile duct.

Signs and symptoms

There is usually severe abdominal pain, often intermittent, which may radiate to the back. As the disorder progresses, and the endocrine and exocrine functions of the pancreas are lost, diabetes develops, and poor digestion of fats leads to weight loss, diarrhoea, and fatty stool (steatorrhoea). In advanced disease, there may also be evidence of protein malabsorption.

Management and prognosis

The 10-year survival rate after diagnosis is 70%. Alcohol avoidance, pain relief, and dietary support to improve nutritional status are important. A low-fat diet is used because of poor fat digestion, and pancreatic enzyme supplements are prescribed to improve digestion of foodstuffs.

CHOLESTASIS

This term means the obstruction of bile flow anywhere between the liver and the duodenum, or an abnormality of

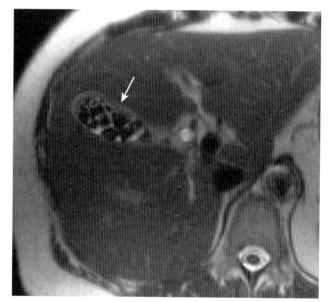

Fig. 11.29   Gallstones. Magnetic resonance image showing several stones in the gallbladder (arrowed). (From Gore RM and Levine M (2015) *Textbook of gastrointestinal radiology*, 4th ed, Fig. 77.10. Philadelphia: Elsevier Inc.)

bile production, either of which leads to the accumulation of bile in the liver. Possible causes include a tumour obstructing the biliary ducts (see Fig. 11.6), cystic fibrosis, or liver cirrhosis or fibrosis in which bile passageways within the liver are compressed by shrunken, stiffened, and scarred liver tissue. The commonest cause of bile duct obstruction is gallstones. The consequences of reduced bile delivery to the duodenum are impaired fat digestion and absorption, which also reduces absorption of the fat-soluble vitamins A, D, E, and K. In addition, jaundice develops, and this is associated with pruritis, because bilirubin irritates free nerve endings in the skin.

Gallstones (cholelithiasis)

Gallstones originate in the gallbladder (Fig. 11.29) and may cause no problems. However, when the gallbladder contracts in response to food, especially fatty food, in the

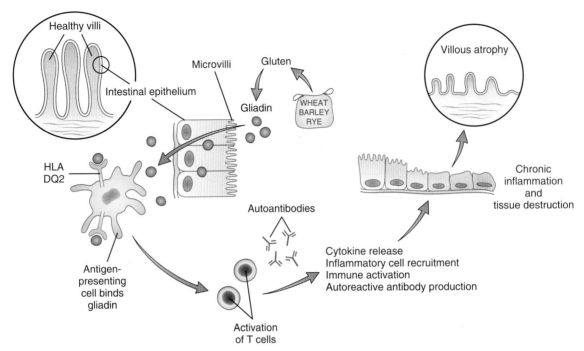

Fig. 11.30 The pathogenesis of coeliac disease.

duodenum, stones can pass into the biliary tree. Here they can lodge and obstruct bile flow into the duodenum (choledocholithiasis). The main presenting symptom is pain: acute, unrelenting and prolonged, and usually felt in the upper centre of the abdomen but also sometimes the lower chest, and often radiating to between the shoulderblades or the tip of the right scapula.

Stones form in the gallbladder when the concentration of dissolved substances, mainly cholesterol and bilirubin, exceeds the capacity of the bile to keep them in solution. They then precipitate out of solution, initially as tiny crystals that over time grow and fuse to produce stones. In general, the risk of developing gallstones increases with age and is commoner in Europe and the United States than in Africa, Asia, and the Far East. Stones may contain predominantly cholesterol or be mainly bilirubin (in the form of calcium bilirubinate) but many stones contain both (mixed composition). Cholesterol stones are the commonest form in most countries, and are more frequent in women than men, especially women of reproductive age, because oestrogen increases cholesterol excretion in the bile. Bilirubin (pigment) stones are usually associated with infection of the gallbladder by liver flukes.

Cholecystitis

This is inflammation of the gall bladder. It may be acute or chronic, and both are almost always caused by gallstones, which provoke an ongoing inflammatory reaction in the gallbladder epithelium. If this is complicated with infection, the gallbladder may fill with pus and perforate, causing acute peritonitis.

COELIAC DISEASE

The protein content of barley, wheat, and rye is called **gluten**. Coeliac disease is an immune-mediated inflammatory disease of the small intestine in which the individual becomes intolerant of gluten-derived proteins, including a protein called **gliadin**. The disorder may present in infancy or childhood, or in the individual's 20s or 30s. It is estimated that about 1% of Western peoples are affected, but about half of them are asymptomatic and undiagnosed. However, the incidence varies significantly: for example, about 2 in 100 Finnish people are affected. There is a strong genetic component: risk is elevated in first-degree relatives of affected people.

Pathophysiology

The immunological basis of coeliac disease seems to lie with two MHC class II molecules, HLA-DQ2 or HLA-DQ8. The importance of the MHC complex in determining immune tolerance is discussed on p.91. DQ2 and DQ8 are produced on antigen presenting cells (APCs) in the gastrointestinal epithelium. Gliadin crosses the epithelial barrier of the epithelium, binds to DQ2 and DQ8 and activates the APC. This stimulates an immune response, triggering inflammation and the production of cytotoxic T cells and autoreactive antibodies that destroy the gastrointestinal epithelium (Fig. 11.30). Over time, intestinal villi are destroyed, leading to malabsorption.

Most DQ2 and DQ8 positive people do not develop coeliac disease, so additional risk factors must be required; it is not known what these risk factors are, nor whether they are genetic or environmental. Coeliac disease is also associated with other autoimmune disorders, including type 1 diabetes, thyroid disease, and myasthenia gravis, underlining its immunological aetiology.

Signs and symptoms

Babies and children fail to thrive, develop diarrhoea, and become malnourished because absorption from the damaged small intestine is impaired. Older children and adults may suffer from delayed puberty, tiredness, mouth ulcers, and diarrhoea, and show indications of malabsorption such as iron and folic acid deficiency.

Management and prognosis

Dietary elimination of gluten-containing grains is the cornerstone of management. This usually resolves the symptoms but is not always easy to achieve because wheat, barley, and rye are used so widely. Supplementation of the diet to replace nutritional deficiency is important.

BIBLIOGRAPHY AND REFERENCES

Ford, A. C., Moayyedi, P., & Hanauer, S. B. (2013). Ulcerative colitis. *BMJ, 346*, f432.

GBD 2107 Inflammatory Disease Collaborators. (2019). The global, regional and national burden of inflammatory bowel disease in 195 countries and territories, 1990–2017: A systematic analysis for the Global Burden of Disease Study 2017. *Lancet Gastroenterology and Hepatology, 5*(1), 17–30.

Heiman, M. L., & Greenway, F. L. (2016). A healthy gastrointestinal microbiome is dependent on dietary diversity. *Molecular Metabolism, 5*, 317–320.

Hills, R. D., Pontefract, B. A., Mishcon, H. R., et al. (2019). Gut microbiome: profound implications for diet and disease. *Nutrients, 11*, 1613–1653.

Khan, S. A., Tavolari, S., & Brandi, G. (2019). Cholangiocarcinoma: Epidemiology and risk factors. *Liver International, 39*(51), 19–31.

Kilian, M., Chapple, I. L. C., Hannig, M., et al. (2016). The oral microbiome: An update for oral healthcare professionals. *British Dental Journal, 221*(10), 657–666.

Mak, W. Y., Hart, Al, & Ng, S. C. (2019). Crohns disease. *Inflammatory Bowel Disease, 47*(6), 377–387.

McColl, K. E. L. (2011). The elegance of the gastric mucosal barrier: Designed by nature for nature. *Gut.* https://doi.org/10.1136/gutjnl-2011-301612

Narayanan, M., Reddy, K. M., & Marsicano, E. (2018). Peptic ulcer disease and *Helicobacter pylori* infection. *Mo Med, 115*(3), 219–224.

Osna, N. A., Donohue, T. M., & Kharbanda, K. K. (2017). Alcoholic liver disease: Pathogenesis and current management. *Alcohol Res, 38*(2), 147–181.

Tack, J., & Pandolino, J. E. (2018). Pathophysiology of gastroesophageal reflux disease. *Gastroenterology, 154*, 277–288.

Yang, J. D., Hainaut, P., Gores, G. J., et al. (2019). A global view of hepatocellular carcinoma: Trends, risk, prevention and management. *Nature Reviews Gastroenterology and Hepatology, 16*, 589–604.

Useful websites

Cancer Research Fund/American Institute for Cancer Research report: Diet, nutrition, physical activity and oesophageal cancer. (2018). https://www.wcrf.org/sites/default/files/Oesophageal-cancer-report.pdf.

IARC statistics on liver disease. (2018). https://gco.iarc.fr/today/data/factsheets/cancers/11-Liver-fact-sheet.pdf

NICE information on gastroenteritis: https://cks.nice.org.uk/gastroenteritis#!topicSummary.

WHO global hepatitis report. (2017). https://apps.who.int/iris/bitstream/handle/10665/255016/9789241565455-eng.pdf;jsessionid=234A29307C1E8FD368ABF52199C16D2E?sequence=1

WHO fact sheet on cholera: https://www.who.int/news-room/factsheets/detail/cholera.

WHO Global status report on alcohol and health. (2018). https://www.who.int/substance_abuse/publications/global_alcohol_report/en/

12 Disorders of Renal Function

CHAPTER OUTLINE

INTRODUCTION
Gross structure of the kidney
The renal nephron
    The main parts of the nephron
    Regulation of renal blood flow and glomerular filtration rate
    The composition of urine
The lower urinary tract
    The ureters
    The urinary bladder
HYPERTENSION AND THE KIDNEY
GLOMERULAR DISORDERS
Glomerulonephritis
    Acute glomerulonephritis
    Chronic glomerulonephritis

INFECTIONS AND INFLAMMATORY CONDITIONS
    Urethritis and cystitis
    Pyelonephritis
URINARY TRACT TUMOURS
Renal tumours
    Renal cancer
Bladder cancer
CONGENITAL, INHERITED, AND DEVELOPMENTAL DISORDERS
    Congenital disorders
    Polycystic kidney disease
URINARY CALCULI
ACUTE KIDNEY INJURY
CHRONIC KIDNEY DISEASE

INTRODUCTION

The kidneys excrete wastes and regulate the composition of body fluids. Each kidney, about the size of the adult human fist, sits behind the peritoneum against the posterior body wall. They receive between 20% and 25% of the cardiac output and produce between 800 and 2000 mL of urine daily, depending on fluid loss from other sources and fluid intake. Urine drains from the kidney along paired, muscular-walled ureters into the urinary bladder, where it is stored until it is convenient to urinate. Urine passes from the bladder to the exterior along the urethra (Fig. 12.1).

GROSS STRUCTURE OF THE KIDNEY

Each kidney is enclosed in a tough, inelastic, reddish-brown capsule. The indentation of the kidney that gives it its bean shape is called the hilum (Fig. 12.2A). Here the renal artery enters, and the renal vein and lymphatic vessels leave. The ureter exits the kidney here as well, draining the urine produced by the renal processes described below into the ureters.

On visual inspection, the cut face of the kidney shows a darker outer layer (the **cortex**) and roughly triangular shaped lighter areas of tissue (the **medullary pyramids**), which are separated from each other by fingers of cortex extending down between them. The region of the kidney adjacent to the hilum is a hollow area called the *renal pelvis*.

Urine drains from the tips of the pyramids (each tip is called a *papilla*) into open spaces called calyces, which open directly into the pelvis. Each kidney contains about 1.2 million nephrons, its functional units.

THE RENAL NEPHRON

A nephron is basically a tiny but highly folded tubule, with a blood filtration unit (the renal corpuscle, containing the **glomerulus**) at one end, and the other end opening into a drainage channel called a **collecting duct**. Networks of blood capillaries wrap around the nephron to reabsorb important materials from the filtrate and to secrete unwanted substances from the blood directly into the tubule for excretion. As the fluid filtered from the bloodstream in the glomerulus passes through the tubule, its composition is adjusted, so that by the time it has passed through the collecting duct all essential substances have been reclaimed and waste materials have been added. At this stage, the fluid is no longer called filtrate, but urine.

THE MAIN PARTS OF THE NEPHRON

The renal corpuscle is a tiny (about 200 µm in diameter) pea-shaped structure. Corpuscles are in the renal cortex (see Fig. 12.2B). The corpuscle is composed of the hollow, cup-shaped Bowman capsule (glomerular capsule), and the **glomerulus**, a tuft of blood capillaries that brings blood under pressure from the renal artery into the Bowman capsule

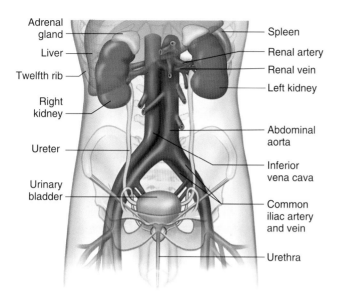

Fig. 12.1 The main organs of the urinary system. (Modified from Thibodeau GA and Patton KT (2008) *Anatomy & physiology*, 8th ed. St. Louis: Mosby.)

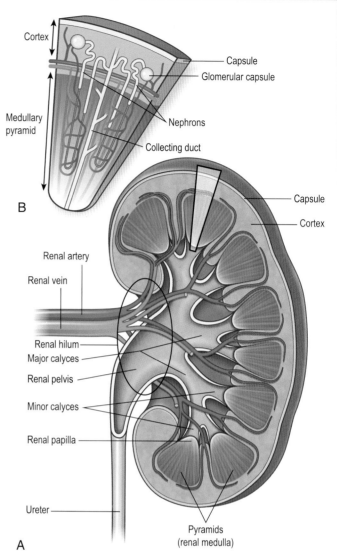

Fig. 12.2 Frontal section of the kidney. (A) Gross. (B) Detail showing the orientation of nephrons within the kidney. (Modified from Waugh A and Grant A (2018) *Ross & Wilson anatomy and physiology in health and illness*, 13th ed, Fig. 13.3. Oxford: Elsevier Ltd.)

(Fig. 12.3). The glomerular capsule opens into the **proximal convoluted tubule** (PCT), which in turn opens into a hairpin section called the loop of Henle (the loop of the nephron). The loops dip into the medulla of the kidney (see Fig. 12.2B). Some run deeper than others: those that penetrate furthest into the medulla are particularly important for concentrating urine. The ascending limb of the loop emerges from the medulla back into the cortex and continues into the **distal convoluted tubule** (DCT), which empties into a larger passageway called a **collecting duct**. Collecting ducts collect filtrate from multiple nephrons and drain it into the renal pelvis, from where it passes via the ureter to the urinary bladder for storage.

The structure and permeability of the nephron wall, and the pumps and carriers embedded in it, vary in different parts of the nephron so that essential substances can be reabsorbed into the blood from the filtrate, and unwanted substances can be excreted from the blood into the filtrate. In this way the kidney can precisely regulate urine composition.

The renal corpuscles

A detailed cross-section of a glomerulus and its associated Bowman capsule is shown in Fig. 12.4. The capillary walls are composed of a single layer of endothelial cells sitting on a basement membrane. The glomerular capillaries form loops, into which blood flows from the afferent arteriole and then exits via the efferent arteriole. The capillaries are embedded in a specialised connective tissue matrix produced by mesangial cells, which sit between the capillary loops. In close association with the glomerular capillaries are podocytes, epithelial cells with lots of tiny extensions called foot processes, which wrap around the capillaries. The tiny gaps between adjacent foot processes are called filtration slits, and filtered fluid passes between them from the bloodstream and into the glomerular capsule. From the capsular space, the filtrate flows into the PCT.

Filtration is the first stage in the production of urine. Blood pressure in the glomerular capillaries, about 55 mm Hg,

is higher than in other capillary beds, because the efferent arteriole, carrying blood away from the glomerulus, is narrower than the afferent arteriole bringing blood in (see Fig. 12.4). This keeps the pressure high to drive filtration through the glomerular walls and into the capsule space. Materials small enough to pass through the filtration slits, for example glucose, water, electrolytes, amino acids and urea, end up in the filtrate. Blood cells and large molecular weight substances, such as plasma proteins, are too big to be filtered, remain in the bloodstream and exit the glomerulus in the efferent arteriole. The efferent arteriole then splits into a network of capillaries that track alongside the remaining sections of its nephron, wrapping closely around it for exchange of substances between the blood and the filtrate.

Proximal convoluted tubule

Filtrate from the glomerular capsule passes into the PCT. Like the renal corpuscle, the PCT is located in the renal cortex. The epithelium lining this section of tubule possesses a carpet of microvilli (see Fig. 12.4), which increases the surface area of the cell membrane in direct contact with the filtrate fluid to increase reabsorption. About two-thirds of filtrate volume is actively reabsorbed here, including electrolytes, glucose, amino acids, and water. In addition, unwanted substances that are either too big to pass through the glomerular filter (e.g., creatinine and penicillin) or that are still present in excess quantities in the blood after it leaves the glomerulus (e.g., excess H^+ ions) are actively pumped

out of the blood and into the nephron. This is called *secretion*, the third essential process in urine formation.

Loop of the nephron

This section forms a deep hairpin loop dipping into the medulla of the kidney, still closely followed by capillaries from its efferent arteriole. Reabsorption of salts and water continues here, but the main function of the loop is to concentrate the filtrate, which enters the loop at the same osmotic concentration as the interstitial fluid bathing the kidney cells but which needs to be significantly concentrated to reduce water losses from the body.

Distal convoluted tubule and collecting duct

By the time the filtrate arrives in the DCT, the main essential substance remaining to be reabsorbed is water, although some electrolytes (e.g., sodium, potassium, and chloride) are also reabsorbed here. Antidiuretic hormone (ADH) and aldosterone, two key hormones in the regulation of salt and water balance, act on these regions of the nephron to control sodium and water reabsorption according to the body's needs. Secretion of excess electrolytes (e.g., potassium) occurs here. The DCT lies very close to the PCT at its origin at the renal corpuscle, forming the juxtaglomerular apparatus.

REGULATION OF RENAL BLOOD FLOW AND GLOMERULAR FILTRATION RATE

The glomerular filtration membrane possesses no specific pumps or carrier mechanisms for transferring materials from the blood into the filtrate. The quantity and composition of the filtrate depend entirely upon the pressure difference across the glomerular membrane, the health of the glomerular membrane, and the size of the molecules or particles in the bloodstream. Fig. 12.5 shows normal pressures operating at the glomerular membrane. Blood (hydrostatic) pressure in the glomerular capillary is usually around 55 mm Hg, forcing fluid through the filtration membrane into the

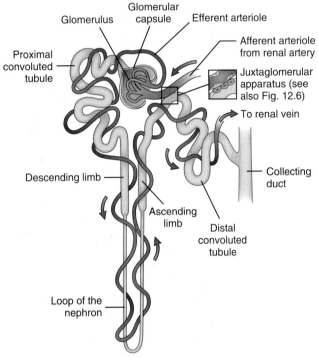

Fig. 12.3 A representative nephron and its associated blood vessels. Arrows indicate direction of blood flow. (Modified from Applegate E (2011) *The anatomy and physiology learning system,* 4th ed, Fig. 18.4. Philadelphia: Elsevier Inc.)

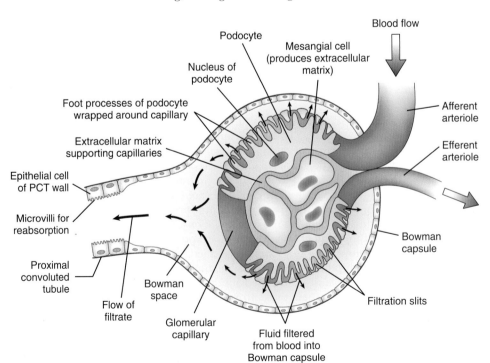

Fig. 12.4 A glomerulus within its Bowman capsule. Only one capillary is shown for clarity. Foot processes of podocytes wrap round the capillary, forming filtration slits. The capillary network is embedded in a matrix produced by mesangial cells.

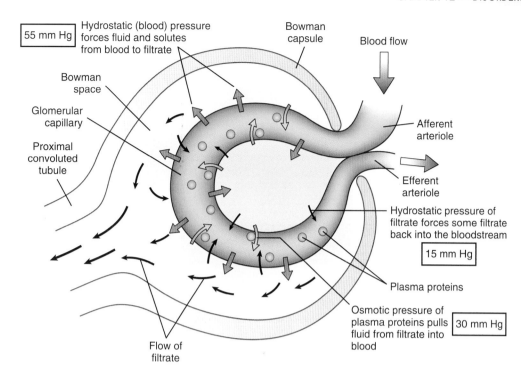

Fig. 12.5 Filtration pressures across the glomerular membrane.

capsular space. The fluid within the capsular space exerts back pressure on the filtration membrane, but because it is continuously draining away into the proximal convoluted tubule, its pressure stays low, only about 15 mm Hg. The other main factor determining the net filtration rate is the plasma osmotic pressure, which is mainly caused by the plasma protein content of the blood. Because plasma proteins are too big to escape through the filtration slits, they are retained in the blood, and the osmotic pressure they exert pulls water molecules back through the filtration membrane. Osmotic pressure of the bloodstream contributes about 30 mm Hg of pressure returning fluid from the capsule into the bloodstream. The net filtration rate and direction of filtration are therefore determined by the capillary hydrostatic pressure, forcing fluid and small molecules into the capsule, less the hydrostatic pressure of the capsular fluid and the osmotic pull of plasma proteins retained in the bloodstream:

$$55 \text{ mm Hg} - (15 \text{ mm Hg} + 30 \text{ mm Hg}) = 10 \text{ mm Hg}$$

This relatively small pressure difference of only 10 mm Hg is enough to drive net filtration from the glomerular capillary into the capsular space. If the filtrate cannot drain quickly away, perhaps because of a blockage somewhere beyond the glomerulus, and filtrate builds up in the tubule, the capsular hydrostatic pressure increases, reducing the filtration pressure difference and reducing filtration. This will lead eventually to kidney failure.

Glomerular filtration rate (GFR). The GFR is the volume of filtrate formed by both kidneys in a given period of time. On average, it is about 125 mL/min, equivalent to about 180 L/day, or in other words, the kidneys process the entire blood volume between 30 and 35 times every single day. This high filtration rate allows the kidneys to control body fluid level and composition very accurately. GFR rises if glomerular blood pressure rises, or if blood plasma protein levels fall,

because this changes the balance of pressures across the glomerular membrane (see Fig. 12.5). GFR falls if glomerular blood pressure falls, if the glomerular filter becomes clogged with cell debris—for example, in autoimmune-mediated glomerular damage—or if fluid pressure in the tubule itself rises.

Autoregulation and GFR

As discussed above, the key factor driving GFR is blood pressure in the glomerulus, and the pressure difference driving filtration across the normal healthy filtration membrane is very small: only 10 mm Hg. Systemic blood pressure fluctuates continually in health, with significant spikes, for example, during periods of exercise or emotional stress and falls of up to 20% at night when asleep. It is essential that these changes are not transmitted to the glomerular capillaries because this would cause inappropriate changes in GFR, adjusting fluid and electrolyte loss without regard for the body's fluid and electrolyte needs. In addition, even transiently high blood pressure could damage the fragile glomeruli. For example, consider fluid and electrolyte requirements during exercise. The body loses large amounts of fluid and salts in sweat and respiration during exercise, so it is important that the kidneys compensate for this by reducing GFR to reduce urinary fluid and electrolyte loss. But blood pressure rises in exercise, which would lead to the opposite by increasing glomerular capillary blood pressure, GFR and urine production, worsening the body's fluid and electrolyte loss. The kidneys must therefore be able to prevent this systemic rise in BP from being transmitted to the glomerular capillaries. Their ability to do just that—to isolate themselves from changes in systemic blood pressure and internally manage pressure and flow within the renal vasculature—is an example of **autoregulation**, in which the juxtaglomerular apparatus and macula densa are key players.

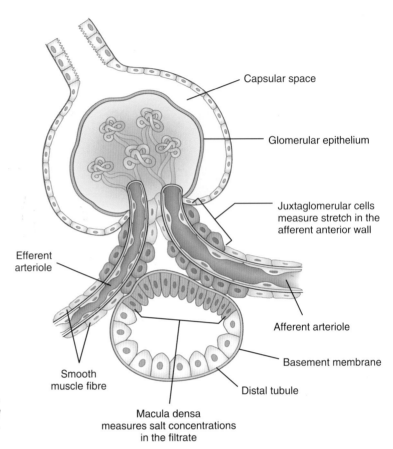

Fig. 12.6 The juxtaglomerular apparatus and macula densa. (Modified from Hall JE and Hall ME (2021) *Guyton and Hall textbook of medical physiology*, 14th ed, Fig. 27.10. Philadelphia: Elsevier Inc.)

The juxtaglomerular apparatus and macula densa

The juxtaglomerular apparatus (JGA) is a specialised collection of cells found at the entrance to the glomerulus, where the afferent and efferent arterioles enter and leave, and in direct contact with the distal convoluted tubule belonging to the same nephron as the glomerulus (see Figs. 12.3 and 12.6). The JGA contains specialised cells that measure the stretch in the wall of the afferent arteriole (and therefore the blood pressure here) and the macula densa contains chemosensitive cells that measure sodium and chloride levels in the filtrate within the tubule. These key measurements are essential for autoregulation.

Renal autoregulation

The kidneys control the diameter of both the afferent and efferent arteriole, allowing very precise regulation of glomerular capillary pressure and therefore GFR. In the healthy nephron, the afferent arteriole supplying the glomerular capillaries is wider than the efferent arteriole, so that more blood arrives in the glomerulus than can drain away, increasing pressure in the glomerular capillaries to drive filtration. The healthy kidney controls blood flow into the glomerulus mainly by adjusting the diameter of the afferent arteriole. Vasodilation here increases flow and pressure, and vasoconstriction reduces flow and pressure. There are two key mechanisms here: one mediated by the stretch receptors in the JGA, and the other by the macula densa chemoreceptors, which respond to the concentration of sodium and chloride ions in the filtrate. A rise in blood pressure, for example in exercise, is detected by stretch receptors in the JGA, which in turn constricts the afferent arterioles, reducing flow and preventing pressure rising in the glomerulus, and maintaining a constant GFR. If perfusion pressure in the renal artery falls—for example, in heart failure, causing a sustained fall in blood flow to body organs including the kidneys—this is also detected by stretch receptors in the JGA, which dilates the afferent arterioles and increases blood flow into the glomerulus to protect GFR. This mechanism involves the release of vasodilatory prostaglandins. This is likely to be one reason why non-steroidal anti-inflammatory agents, such as ibuprofen and aspirin, can be significantly nephrotoxic in some people, especially in those with a pre-existing degree of kidney impairment.

In addition to the reflex vasoconstriction of the afferent arteriole to stretch when pressure rises, sodium and chloride concentrations in the filtrate of the distal convoluted tubule are constantly measured by the macula densa. Rising levels of these electrolytes stimulate vasoconstriction of the afferent arteriole, reducing GFR and reducing the loss of these electrolytes in the urine.

THE COMPOSITION OF URINE

In the healthy adult, the average daily urine output, with a fluid intake of about 2 L/day, is usually between 800 and 2000 mL. Urinary pH is generally slightly acid, usually around 6, giving it bacteriocidal properties, although the normal range, depending on what is being excreted in the urine, is 4.5 to 8. Urine is normally at least 95% water, containing a range of waste products such as urea, urobilinogen, uric acid, creatinine, and excess minerals such as sodium, calcium, potassium, chloride, oxalates, and sulphates.

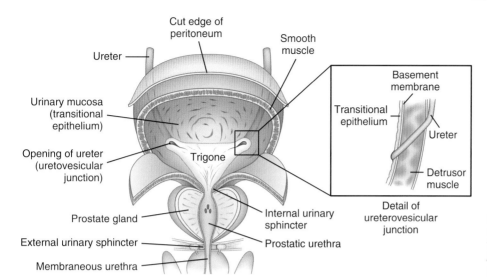

Fig. 12.7 The structure of the bladder and the uretovesicular junction. (Modified from Patton K and Thibodeau G (2014) *The human body in health & disease*, 6th ed, Fig. 20.7. St. Louis: Mosby.)

THE LOWER URINARY TRACT

This is composed of the ureters, urinary bladder, and urethra. They are lined with a specialised epithelium, called the urothelium, which varies in thickness depending on where it is located. Urothelium permits dilation and stretching during peristaltic movement of urine from the renal pelvis through the tract and presents a stable, effective barrier protecting underlying tissue from any potential toxic substances present in the urine.

THE URETERS

The ureters, usually 25 to 30 cm long, contain three layers of muscle in their walls: two layers of longitudinal muscle with a layer of circular muscle in between. This arrangement allows for regular peristaltic contractions to sweep down the ureters, actively driving urine draining from the kidneys into the urinary bladder.

The ureterovesicular junction

In health, urine flows in one direction, from the kidney to the bladder, and the area where the ureter empties into the bladder is called the **ureterovesicular junction** (Fig. 12.7). Reflux of urine along the ureters from the bladder to the kidney is prevented by two main features of the ureterovesicular junction:

- The angle of the ureter where it inserts into the bladder is acute, forming a valve-like structure. Rising pressure in a filling bladder compresses it, sealing the opening.
- The ureter passes through the bladder wall at an oblique angle so that, when the detrusor muscle of the bladder contracts, it compresses and closes off a significant length of the ureter, making an effective seal.

Anatomical abnormalities of the ureterovesicular junction increase the incidence of reflux, which is associated with repeated urinary tract infections from an early age. Sometimes this can be picked up on antenatal scans. As children grow, it may improve, but is a significant cause of reflux nephropathy, renal scarring, hypertension, and end-stage kidney disease in children.

THE URINARY BLADDER

The urothelium of the urinary bladder is a transitional epithelium that stretches without damage as the bladder fills. Below the urothelium lies the detrusor muscle, a layer of smooth muscle that remains relaxed to allow the bladder to fill with comfort, but which contracts to expel urine during urination (see Fig. 12.7).

HYPERTENSION AND THE KIDNEY

The kidney is intimately involved with the control of blood pressure and, by regulating water excretion, total body water, which on average, represents 60% of body weight. Because water moves freely in and out of cells and in and out of extracellular spaces including blood vessels, total body water is an important determinant of blood volume. Total body sodium, which is closely associated with total body water, is also controlled by the kidney; increased sodium retention by the kidney also increases water retention. If the kidney reabsorbs more water, this expands blood volume and tends to increase blood pressure, and if it increases water excretion, this reduces blood volume and blood pressure. In addition, the kidney stimulates the release of hormones, including angiotensin II, that control blood vessel diameter, a key regulator of blood pressure. The juxtaglomerular apparatus and macula densa, as described above, constantly monitor pressure in the afferent arteriole and the osmotic concentration of the filtrate in the distal convoluted tubule. If blood pressure falls in the afferent arteriole, or sodium and chloride concentrations fall in the filtrate, the kidney activates the renin-angiotensin system to increase sodium and water reabsorption, which in turn increases total body water, including blood volume, and therefore increases blood pressure. This is discussed in more detail in Chapter 6 (see p.165 and Fig. 6.43).

GLOMERULAR DISORDERS

Glomerular function is reduced in a wide range of conditions. The clinical presentation of the disorders varies

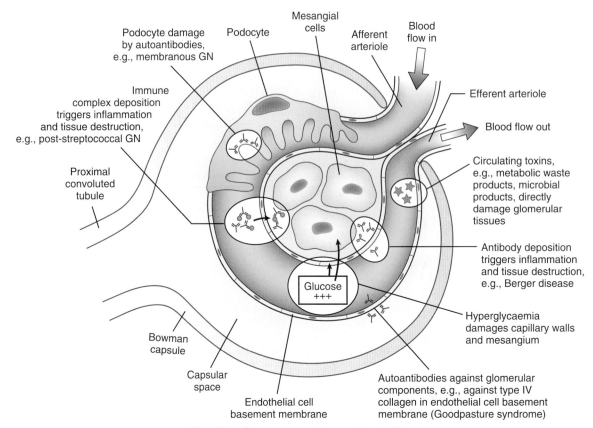

Fig. 12.8 Some causes of glomerulonephritis.

depending on the underlying pathophysiological changes, so it is important to understand these processes. Acute conditions may resolve, either completely or with some residual impairment of glomerular function, but frequently lead to chronic conditions that may in turn develop into chronic kidney disease.

GLOMERULONEPHRITIS

Glomerulonephritis (GN) is inflammation of the glomeruli, impairing their ability to selectively filter the blood. It is associated with a wide range of disorders. In primary GN, the defect is inherent to the kidney, and in secondary GN it is caused by a systemic disorder. Additionally, GN may be acute or chronic. A wide range of pathological events may injure the glomeruli or reduce glomerular function (Fig. 12.8). Immunological injury is the commonest mechanism of glomerular damage. Tissue-specific autoantibodies may target glomerular structures, or the glomeruli may be damaged when immune complexes, formed elsewhere in the bloodstream, are deposited in the glomerular tissues and trigger inflammation. Hyperglycaemia, in poorly controlled diabetes, damages the glomerular mesangium and causes inflammatory changes. The glomerular capillaries may also be damaged by circulating toxins or waste products, for example, in metabolic disorders or infections.

The terms **glomerulonephritis** and **glomerulonephropathy** are sometimes used interchangeably, although technically speaking, glomerulonephritis implies an inflammatory component to the disorder. Whatever the underlying pathophysiological processes, glomerular damage impairs the

filtering action of the glomerular membrane, allowing substances normally retained in the blood, such as plasma proteins and blood cells, to escape into the filtrate and appear in the urine. Progressive destruction of glomeruli reduces glomerular filtration rate and steadily reduces the ability of the kidney to clear wastes and to retain substances essential to the body's needs.

ACUTE GLOMERULONEPHRITIS

Acute GN is usually associated with glomerular damage secondary either to direct attack by autoantibodies produced against glomerular components or by deposition of immune complexes formed elsewhere and transported in the bloodstream to the kidney. Vasculitis affecting the renal glomeruli can also be the source of injury. Globally, the commonest cause of acute GN is Berger disease, caused by IgA deposition. Before this, the commonest cause was post-streptococcal GN, but this is now in decline in most countries.

Pathophysiology

The target of the immune attack may be the endothelium of the glomerular capillaries, the mesangial cells that produce their supporting matrix, or the podocytes of the glomerular membrane. This determines the signs and symptoms of the condition. The glomeruli are inflamed, swollen, and infiltrated with leukocytes. Cellular proliferation (of the capillary endothelial cells, the mesangial cells and podocyte epithelial cells) enlarges the glomeruli, resulting in swelling and enlargement of the kidney, which may be half again its normal size. The basement membrane on which the endothelial cells rest is thickened. Whatever the nature of the injury, if it is prolonged or repeated, the healing process causes permanent sclerotic changes in the glomerular capillaries which become stiff and scarred, with deposition of connective tissues such as collagen. Once the glomerular capillaries are effectively destroyed by these sclerotic changes, with loss of their filtering capacity, the remainder of its nephron atrophies. Chronic kidney disease is a common development in many cases of acute GN. Some of the mechanisms by which acute GN arises are described here.

Berger disease

This condition is caused by the deposition of blood-borne antibody, usually IgA, in the glomerular mesangium. This sets up an inflammatory response, with mesangial cell proliferation, activation of complement and recruitment of inflammatory cells, leading to glomerular injury and necrosis. The incidence of the disorder is higher in conditions associated with raised IgA levels, such as some liver disease, systemic lupus erythematosus, ankylosing spondylitis, and some cancers. Its geographical distribution is not even; it is four times as common in Asia than in the United States. It is up to six times commoner in males than females, and usually manifests between the ages of 10 and 30. The patient usually presents with haematuria and proteinuria. Protein levels in the urine can be very high. In the systemic condition Henoch-Schönlein purpura, circulating IgA deposits in other tissues as well, including joints, intestines, and skin, in which case the glomerulonephritis is considered part of that disorder.

Post-streptococcal GN

Renal symptoms arise between 1 and 3 weeks after a type A streptococcal infection, usually of the skin or throat, and usually in children. The inflammatory response to the infection includes production of antibodies to streptococcal proteins, forming immune complexes that are then actively transported through the glomerular capillary filtration membranes and trapped in the interstitial spaces, where they set up a powerful inflammatory response (Fig. 12.9). Recruitment of inflammatory cells and the release of a range of inflammatory cytokines injure the glomerulus, leading to ongoing glomerular damage. It is thought that children are more frequently affected than adults because the filtration slits in the immature kidney are larger than in the mature kidney, with enough room for the immune complex to get through the glomerular membrane. Males are more commonly affected than females, and all races are equally affected. There is usually haematuria and often heavy proteinuria as well.

Membranous GN

In this common form of glomerular injury, also sometimes called *membranous nephropathy*, the podocytes are damaged by IgG autoantibody attack (see Fig. 12.8). In up to four-fifths of patients, the autoantibodies are formed against a specific protein, the phospholipase A_2 receptor, on the podocyte plasma membrane. This generates immune complexes that activate complement and trigger an ongoing inflammatory response which thickens the glomerular capillary wall (leading to the term membranous glomerulonephritis) and eventually causes glomerular sclerosis and permanent glomerular damage. In the remaining 20% of patients, the disorder is usually secondary to a systemic immune disorder, such as systemic lupus erythematosus, infection, or malignancy. In all these conditions, antibodies are produced to an antigen: antinuclear antibodies in SLE, microbial proteins in infection, and tumour antigens in cancer. Binding of these antibodies to their antigen generates immune complexes, which deposit in the glomerular capillaries, activate complement and an inflammatory reaction, and destroy the glomeruli.

Membranous GN may resolve spontaneously, progress to end-stage kidney disease, or follow a course somewhere in between, with a degree of kidney impairment that can remain stable for the rest of the individual's life. It is more common in white people than in black people or Asians and is twice as common in men than women. Incidence increases with age.

Autoimmune anti-basement membrane disease

In this form of glomerulonephritis, autoantibodies are made against type IV collagen in the basement membrane of the glomerular capillaries. Patients, often young adults, present with acute GN. In **Goodpasture syndrome,** the circulating anti-type IV collagen autoantibodies attack basement membrane in both the lungs and the kidneys (see Fig. 12.8). Without treatment, there is massive pulmonary inflammation and haemorrhage, and progressive renal failure.

Glomerular capillary vasculitis

Systemic vasculitis disorders (e.g., Henoch-Schonlein purpura) cause inflammation and necrosis of blood vessels, compromising blood flow to the tissues they supply. When

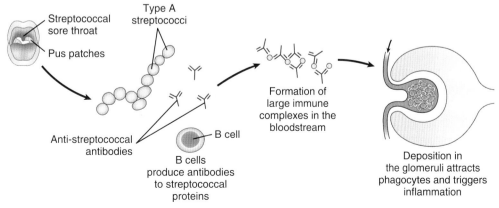

Fig. 12.9 The pathogenesis of post-streptococcal glomerulonephritis.

the glomerular capillaries are affected, renal function is progressively impaired. Most cases of renal vasculitis are associated with an autoantibody called ANCA (anti-neutrophil cytoplasmic antibody), which targets neutrophils. ANCA binds to and activates neutrophils in the bloodstream, triggering the release of cytoplasmic enzymes from neutrophil granules, recruitment and activation of more inflammatory cells, and migration of activated neutrophils out of the blood and into the tissues. This causes vascular inflammation, which shuts down blood flow through the glomeruli and leads to glomerular necrosis. Serum markers of inflammation, including C-reactive protein, are elevated. The risk of developing ANCA-mediated GN increases with age, and it usually appears as acute kidney injury.

Signs and symptoms

Acute GN usually presents with haematuria, often with proteinuria, as a result of the damaged filtration membrane. There may be hypoalbuminaemia, if protein loss in the urine is significant. Blood levels of urea and creatinine, important waste products, rise as glomerular function fails. Hypertension occurs, because falling blood flow through the kidney activates the renin-angiotensin system. Rapidly advancing disease may be accompanied by oliguria or even anuria because of rapid failure of glomerular filtration.

Management and prognosis

Acute GN significantly predisposes to chronic kidney disease. A poorer prognosis is associated with male sex and co-existing hypertension. Management of GN depends on the underlying cause. GN with a significant immune component may respond well to steroids.

CHRONIC GLOMERULONEPHRITIS

This umbrella term includes any form of glomerular disorder or disease with a long-term, sustained course. It is often not diagnosed until it is well advanced because the kidneys have significant reserve, and in the initial stages, nephrons that are still healthy enlarge and compensate for those that are diseased. The cause may never be firmly established, but

known causes include diabetic nephropathy and systemic lupus erythematosus.

Diabetic nephropathy

Diabetes mellitus (DM) causes vascular disease, which commonly affects the renal arterial system and the glomerular capillaries. About 40% of diabetic people develop some degree of renal impairment, and globally, diabetic kidney damage is one of the most frequent causes of end-stage kidney disease. Good glycaemic control, not smoking, managing blood lipid levels, and controlling hypertension are all key factors in reducing the risk of developing diabetic nephropathy, and in slowing its progression if it does develop.

Pathophysiology

The aetiology is complex, and the renal blood vessels, including the glomerular capillaries, are damaged by a combination of pathological processes secondary to DM (Fig. 12.10). Hypertension, associated with atherosclerosis, is common in DM. The glomeruli of the kidney are particularly vulnerable to the effects of sustained hypertension.

Hypertension-induced atherosclerosis in the renal arterioles reduces blood flow into the glomeruli. Initially, the kidneys respond to this by dilating the afferent arteriole (autoregulation; see above). This increases pressure in the glomerular capillaries and initially actually increases GFR. However, this increased pressure accelerates the developing atherosclerosis and the rate at which the glomerular capillaries are damaged. As they become progressively atherosclerotic and narrowed, blood flow through the arterioles supplying the glomeruli falls, interfering with autoregulation, causing ischaemia of the glomerular tissues, and reducing GFR (see Fig. 12.10A). Additionally, hyperglycaemia directly damages the walls of glomerular capillaries, reducing blood flow and reducing GFR (see Fig. 12.10B). Excess glucose in the bloodstream stimulates expansion of the mesangial tissues, and it deposits in the basement membrane and extracellular matrix as substances called **advanced glycosylation end-products (AGEs)**. This thickens the basement membrane, damages the filtration membrane, and allows much larger particles than normal to pass from the bloodstream

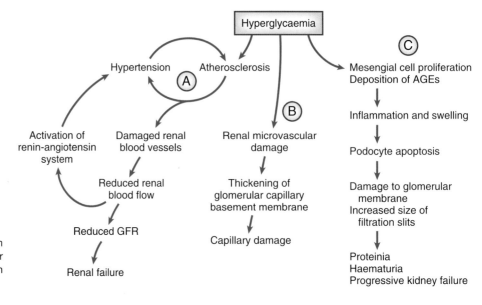

Fig. 12.10 Renovascular disease in diabetic nephropathy. *GFR,* Glomerular filtration rate; *AGEs,* advanced glycation end products.

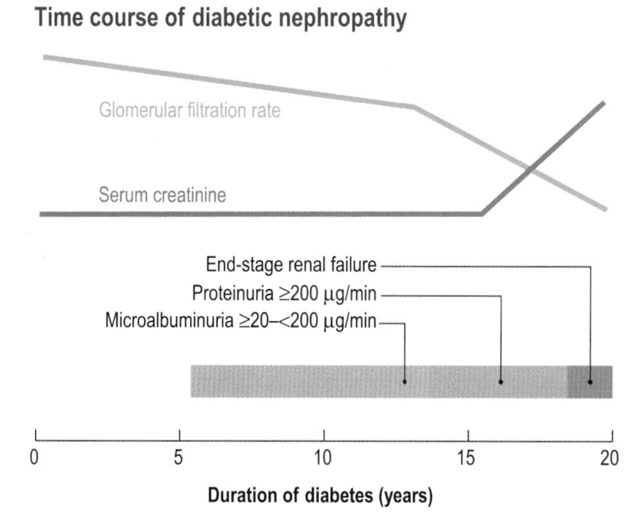

Time course of diabetic nephropathy

Fig. 12.11 The time course of diabetic nephropathy. (Modified from Thomas S and Karalliedde J (2015) Diabetic nephropathy, *Medicine* 43(1): 20–25. https://doi.org/10.1016/j.mpmed.2014.10.007.)

into the filtrate. The kidney becomes infiltrated with inflammatory cells, including lymphocytes and macrophages, which sustain an ongoing inflammatory environment that leads to podocyte death, which disrupts the glomerular filter, and eventually to ischaemia and death of the renal tubules as well (see Fig. 10.12C).

Signs and symptoms

In the early stages, there is microalbuminuria, low but measurable with sensitive tests, and persistent levels of protein in the urine. As the condition progresses and the glomerular filter becomes steadily more permeable, protein levels in the urine rise. This typically develops over several years in type 1 DM but may be present at diagnosis in type 2 DM (because the disease has probably been present for a long time before diagnosis). Once at the stage of persistent macroalbuminuria (i.e., over 300 mg in 24 hours), the GFR progressively declines, and serum creatinine rises as the glomerular filter continues to deteriorate. Once at this stage, most people will progress to end-stage renal failure. A typical time-course of diabetic nephropathy is shown in Fig. 12.11. However, it is important to note that the degree of proteinuria varies between individuals and significant renal compromise can actually be present even without clinically evident proteinuria. Worsening hypertension is an additional indication of deteriorating kidney function.

Management and prognosis

Prevention is clearly the ideal, wherever possible, by careful diabetes management. Tight glycaemic control, weight management, maintaining a normal blood lipid profile and blood pressure are all important and can slow progression in developing renal nephropathy. Angiotensin converting enzyme inhibitors are usually the first choice in managing hypertension. Once macroalbuminuria is established however, end-stage renal failure is usually eventually inevitable.

INFECTIONS AND INFLAMMATORY CONDITIONS

The urethra opens to the exterior at the external urethral orifice, at the penile tip in males and between the labia minora in the female perineum. Microbial colonisation of the distal urethra is normal in healthy individuals, but proximal structures, including the ureters and kidneys, should contain no pathogenic bacteria. The urinary bladder, until recently, has also been believed to be sterile except in infection, but evidence now suggests that it is populated in many healthy, asymptomatic women with microbes also found in the vagina.

There are multiple risk factors for urinary tract infection (UTI; Fig. 12.12). Infection may occur anywhere along the tract, but the incidence is higher in women than in men because the urethral opening to the exterior in females is close to the anal opening, and contamination is easy. In addition, the female urethra is shorter than in the male, making ascending infections more likely to reach the bladder and cause cystitis. From the bladder, infection can spread up the ureter to reach the kidney, and lead to pyelonephritis. In general, conditions that obstruct urine flow or contribute to urinary stasis predispose to UTI.

The risk of UTI is increased in pregnancy because raised circulating progesterone relaxes the smooth muscle of the bladder and the ureter, reducing peristalsis in the ureters and increasing bladder capacity. This predisposes to urinary stasis. In addition, the expanding uterus can compress and block the ureters, obstructing urine flow and increasing pressure in the renal pelvis. Diabetes increases risk because glycosuria provides conditions favourable for bacterial growth in the urine; in addition, there may be neuropathy of the bladder, impairing effective emptying. Conditions that obstruct urine flow increase the risk of infection: renal calculi, urethral compression by prostatic enlargement or a local tumour, and constipation, especially in children, can all restrict urine flow and cause urine pooling behind the obstruction, with increased risk of infection. Other high-risk groups include premature babies and older people and those with structural or functional abnormalities of the urinary tract (e.g., single kidney and polycystic kidney disease). Risk is also increased with indwelling catheters, surgical procedures involving the urinary tract and in sexually active individuals, especially those with multiple partners. The female menopause can increase risk because oestrogen helps maintain a healthy urothelium, presenting an effective barrier to microbial invasion.

UTI is usually caused by ascending infection, from the urethra, up to the bladder, and potentially up the ureters to the kidneys themselves. The commonest organism in ascending UTI is *Escherichia coli* because this organism, present in faeces, contaminates the perineal area. Other microbes include other enterococci (bacteria from the gastrointestinal tract present on the perineum), and *Klebsiella* and *Pseudomonas* species.

URETHRITIS AND CYSTITIS

Microbes ascending from the distal urethra can colonise the upper urethra and find their way into the bladder, causing

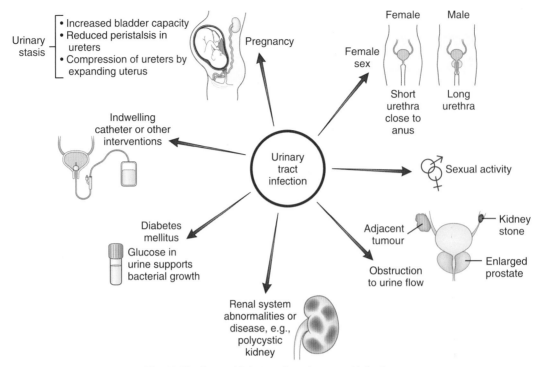

Fig. 12.12 Some risk factors for urinary tract infection.

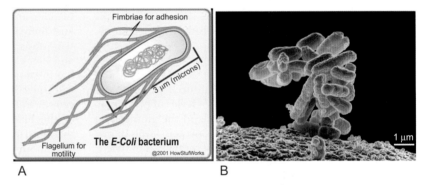

Fig. 12.13 *E. coli.* (A) Drawing showing the flagellum and fimbriae of *E. coli.* (B) Low power electron micrograph of a cluster of *E. coli.* (Photo by Eric Erbe, digital colourisation by Christopher Pooley, both of USDA, ARS, EMU. Credit: http://commons.wikimedia.org/wiki/File:E_coli_at_10000x_original.jpg.)

cystitis, the commonest form of UTI. Up to 50% of women will experience a UTI during their lifetime.

Pathophysiology

Escherichia coli is an effective coloniser of the urinary tract because it has flagellae for motility and fimbriae that allow it to fasten to the epithelium of the urinary tract, resisting flushing away by urine flow (Fig. 12.13). The microbe penetrates the epithelial cells, triggering an inflammatory reaction that causes swelling, erythema, and bladder irritability.

Signs and symptoms

There may be significant bacterial load in the urine without symptoms, but common presenting complaints include urgency and frequency of urination and pain while urinating. The urine is cloudy, and possibly bloodstained, with a deeply offensive smell.

Management and prognosis

A good fluid intake and managing identified causative factors are all important. Most infections resolve with treatment, which may include acidification of the urine (which inhibits bacterial growth) and antibiotics. Repeated infections with no apparent predisposing factors suggest that there is an underlying cause that has not yet been identified.

Non–infection-related cystitis

Infection is not the only cause of an acute inflammatory change in the urothelium of the bladder. Radiation injury and trauma—for example, during a medical procedure—can both cause a sterile cystitis. Interstitial cystitis is a chronic inflammatory condition not associated with identified infection and which is sometimes called *painful bladder syndrome* because of the significant element of lower abdominal pain associated with the condition. It is more common in females than males. The underlying pathophysiology is not understood, although it is likely to be multifactorial. One theory is that the barrier function of the urothelium in the bladder is impaired in some way, allowing urinary solutes to migrate into deeper tissues, irritating muscle and nerves and accounting for the pain, urgency, frequency, and sometimes painful sexual intercourse characteristic of the condition.

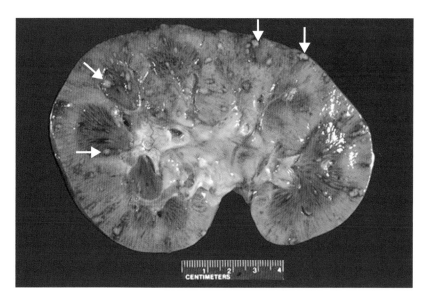

Fig. 12.14 Acute pyelonephritis with multiple abscess formation (arrows). (Modified from Klatt E (2015) *Robbins and Cotran atlas of pathology*, 3rd ed, Fig. 10.63. Philadelphia, Elsevier Inc.)

PYELONEPHRITIS

Pyelonephritis is infection of the kidney. Infection usually ascends from the lower urinary tract, which in turn is usually associated with vesicoureteric reflux (reflux of urine from the bladder back up the ureters into the kidneys, normally prevented by an anatomically and functionally normal ureterovesicular junction; see Fig. 12.7). This may be caused by a structural abnormality that allows reflux, or an obstruction in the tract that increases pressure upstream of the bladder and urinary stasis.

Acute pyelonephritis

This is caused by bacterial infection in the kidney, usually caused by ascending infection from the bladder (and therefore usually *E. coli*) but sometimes caused by blood-borne infection (e.g., in intravenous drug users or from bacterial vegetations in endocarditis). In blood-borne spread, the organism is most often a staphylococcus, but the range of possible microbes is wide.

Pathophysiology

In ascending infection, the microbes spread from the ureter into the renal tissues, where they establish foci of infection, usually in the renal pelvis, the calyces and medullary tissues. Severe ascending infection may reach the glomeruli in the cortex, but this does not usually happen: the glomeruli are not usually involved. However, if the source of infection is the bloodstream, circulating microbes attach to renal tissues as they pass through the kidney, and infection is distributed as multiple abscesses within the renal cortex, where the blood flow is higher than in the medulla (Fig. 12.14). Infection triggers an immune and inflammatory response, and there is dense infiltration of renal tissues with neutrophils and other white blood cells, causing oedema and swelling of the kidney. Abscess formation, renal tubule necrosis and deposition of fibrous scar tissue may all occur. The ongoing inflammatory response is in itself potentially damaging to the kidney.

Some microbes inhibit phagocyte activity, therefore impairing immune defences. Some strains of *E. coli* and *Proteus* species break down urea in the urine to produce energy. This reaction releases ammonia, which is directly toxic to the kidneys, but it also increases the pH of the urine and makes it alkaline, reducing its antiseptic properties and inhibiting the phagocytic action of neutrophils and other defence cells. The change in pH from the normally acid urine to alkaline also increases the precipitation of salts, forming staghorn stones that can lead to loss of the entire kidney (see Renal calculi below).

Signs and symptoms

There is usually fever, malaise, loin pain, haematuria, nausea, and vomiting. Pus appears in the urine.

Management and prognosis

Antibiotic treatment is the first line of management and supportive treatment to manage other symptoms. In healthy people with uncomplicated pyelonephritis, the prospects of full recovery are usually excellent. If there are complicating factors, such as the development of renal abscesses or sepsis, the outlook is much more variable. Prognosis is also poorer in individuals with co-existing chronic disease such as diabetes. Occasionally, acute kidney injury may develop from an episode of acute pyelonephritis, which delays recovery. Sometimes the kidney does not fully heal and is left scarred.

Chronic pyelonephritis (reflux nephropathy)

This is usually caused by persistent vesicoureteric reflux or obstruction; it is most common in young children with anatomical abnormalities that cause vesicoureteric reflux and who have repeated UTIs caused by this. Repeated episodes of pyelonephritis damage and scar the kidneys. Although there is usually a history of obstruction or reflux, the condition otherwise develops silently, and presents as chronic kidney disease (p.318).

Pathophysiology

When the valve at the ureterovesicular junction is incompetent, bladder contraction and increased pressure in the bladder during urination sends a jet of urine back up the ureters towards the kidney. If the urine is sterile, this may not cause significant kidney damage and this reflux usually disappears as the child grows. However, the risk of UTI is increased because the urine refluxed into the ureter drains

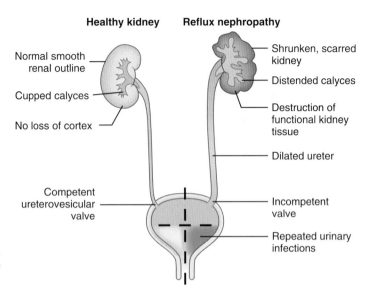

Fig. 12.15 Features of reflux nephropathy. (Modified from Feather A, Randall D, and Waterhouse M (2021) *Kumar and Clark's clinical medicine*, 10th ed, Fig. 36.39. Edinburgh: Elsevier Ltd.)

back into the bladder after urination so that the bladder never fully empties, predisposing to repeated infection. When the condition is caused by obstruction in the urinary tract, the renal calyces and, depending on the location of the obstruction, the ureters become distended. The kidney becomes scarred and shrunken because of tubular necrosis and atrophy, and the renal tissues are infiltrated with lymphocytes and other inflammatory cells characteristic of chronic inflammation (as opposed to the neutrophil-rich infiltrate of acute pyelonephritis). Losing healthy tubules leads to progressive impairment of kidney function and predisposes to the development of end-stage kidney disease. Fig. 12.15 shows the abnormalities associated with reflux nephropathy.

Signs and symptoms
The renal damage sustained in this chronic condition predisposes to hypertension because the damage and scarring that results from it obstructs arterial blood flow into the kidney, activating the renin-angiotensin system (p.165), which in turn increases fluid retention and blood volume, and predisposes to systemic vasoconstriction. However, the condition may be silent even although significant renal damage is developing, except during episodes of active infection, which give signs and symptoms of UTI.

Management and prognosis
Aggressive management of infection, with continuous antibiotic therapy, can greatly reduce the long-term kidney damage associated with this condition, but significantly increases the risk of infection caused by antibiotic-resistant strains of bacteria. Because the condition often resolves spontaneously as the child grows, surgical intervention is not usually needed. Control of hypertension, if present, is important, and if nephrectomy is needed to remove a badly damaged or abnormal kidney, this may resolve it.

URINARY TRACT TUMOURS

The organs and tissues of the urinary system can produce both benign and malignant neoplasms.

RENAL TUMOURS

Benign tumours of the kidney are relatively rare. The commonest are renal adenomas, which are small and slow growing but may be premalignant, and care must be taken not to miss a diagnosis of renal carcinoma.

RENAL CANCER

World Cancer Research Fund statistics (2020) showed that cancer of the kidney was the 14th most common cancer worldwide and the incidence is rising, although global distribution is not equal. The highest rates (for both sexes) are found in central eastern European countries such as Belarus and Estonia, and the lowest rates in Australia, Belgium, and Singapore. Nearly all renal malignancies originate in the epithelial lining of the nephron; a very small proportion arise in the collecting ducts or other renal tissues.

Renal cell carcinoma

This is the commonest kidney malignancy, accounting for up to 90% cases of renal cancer. Risk factors include cigarette smoking, long-term use of non-steroidal anti-inflammatory drugs, chronic kidney disease, male sex, hypertension, obesity, arsenic exposure, and heredity. Heritable kidney cancer tends to manifest at a younger age (below 46 years) than the average age (mid-60s). There are many different cancers in this group, the commonest being clear cell carcinoma.

Pathophysiology
The cell of origin in renal cell carcinoma is the epithelial lining of the proximal convoluted tubule. A wide range of gene mutations, on a range of chromosomes, are associated with the disease. Mutation of one particular gene, the tumour suppressor gene *VHL* on chromosome 3, is found in almost all cases of clear cell carcinoma. Other genes shown to be abnormal in some cases of renal cell carcinoma include *BRCA* (p.84).

Signs and symptoms
A silent clinical course is characteristic of this disease, with few or no warning signs, especially in the early stages. There

may be a palpable mass and/or loin pain. Other signs and symptoms include haematuria, weight loss, malaise, and night sweats. Hypertension arises because the growing tumour secretes renin, activating the renin-angiotensin system. Anaemia also occurs because the diseased kidney's production of erythropoietin steadily falls. Renal cell carcinoma is associated with a high incidence of paraneoplastic syndromes (p.80), causing a wide range of non-kidney-related signs and symptoms. One example is hypercalcaemia, seen in 5% of patients and thought to be caused by the tumour cells producing a protein very similar to parathyroid hormone.

This cancer metastasises most frequently to the lungs and bone.

Management and prognosis

Prognosis is much better for patients who present at an early stage, when the tumour is confined to the kidney. In these patients, removal of the kidney is the treatment of choice and 5-year survival rates are in the region of 95%. However, only a third of patients are diagnosed before metastatic disease has occurred. If the cancer has spread to other organs, survival rates are much poorer and although surgical removal of the primary tumour, plus isolated metastatic growths, can extend life, it is not considered curative. Additional treatment, including targeted chemotherapy, can also prolong life in metastatic disease. Identification of the specific genetic mutation responsible for an individual's renal cell carcinoma identifies the abnormal proteins and the molecular pathways used by the tumour cells, and treatment can be geared specifically towards targeting and interrupting these pathways. Identification of the *VHL* gene and its role in these cancers, for example, has led to advances in targeted treatments in metastatic disease.

Nephroblastoma (Wilms tumour)

Nephroblastoma is the commonest abdominal tumour of childhood. It affects approximately 1 in 10,000 children of white American and European descent. Globally, it is least common in children of Asian background and most common in those from Africa. It is usually diagnosed before the age of 3 years, although if both kidneys are involved, it is usually diagnosed earlier.

Pathophysiology

The origin of the tumour is a nest of embryonic renal cells that persists even after the fetal kidney has fully formed before birth. These embryonic cells (called a **rest**) may disappear spontaneously, but in some children they proliferate and give rise to nephroblastoma. Mutation in any one of a wide range of genes can underlie the malignant transformation. One example is the *WT1* gene; abnormalities in this gene are associated not only with Wilms tumour, but also with a p.314 range of genitourinary abnormalities e.g. renal agenesis.

Signs and symptoms

It usually presents as an abdominal mass. The child may have abdominal pain, fever, and haematuria. There may be secondary spread at the time of diagnosis, and the commonest locations for metastatic growth are the local lymph nodes and peritoneum, and lung and brain.

Management and prognosis

Cure rates for tumours that have not metastasised are over 90%, and even disease that has spread is curable in over 75% of children. Treatment is multimodal, using a combination of surgery, radiotherapy, and chemotherapy.

BLADDER CANCER

This is a common disease, significantly more common in males than females (a ratio of 5:2), with 550,000 new cases worldwide in 2018. It predominantly affects the elderly, with peak incidence in the seventh and eighth decades of life. Risk factors include smoking, exposure to chemicals such as arsenic and chemicals used in the plastic and other industries, and some infections. The parasitic infection schistosomiasis is a major risk factor and contributes to the significantly higher risks for bladder cancer in countries where the causative organism, *Schistosoma haematoblum*, is endemic. This includes Africa and the Middle East.

Pathophysiology

Most bladder cancers (90%) originate in the transitional cells of the urothelium, the lining of the bladder, which is exposed to high concentrations of carcinogens excreted in the urine. Transitional cell tumours usually grow in finger-like projections into the bladder space-these are called papillary tumours (Fig. 12.16). As they enlarge, they may penetrate the basement membrane and grow into the muscle of the bladder wall. There are often multiple tumours present, but most are low grade, slow growing, and observe the boundary of their basement membrane. Only about 20% grow through their basement membrane into the detrusor muscle below. These tumours tend to be aggressive and are associated with a poorer outcome.

A small minority of bladder tumours originate from squamous epithelial cells found in the urothelium. These squamous cell carcinomas are associated with chronic inflammation, such as in chronic infections (including schistosomiasis as described previously) or after long-term catheterisation. Squamous cell bladder cancers are usually more aggressive

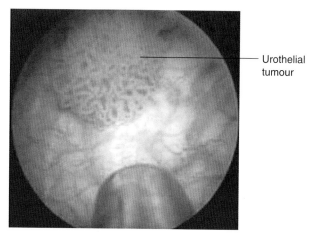

— Urothelial tumour

Fig. 12.16 Endoscopic view of a urothelial bladder tumour. (Modified from Schäfauer C and Ettori D (2013) Detection of bladder urothelial carcinoma using in vivo non-contact, ultraviolet excited autofluorescence measurements converted into simple color-coded images: a feasibility study, *Journal of Urology* 190(1), 271–277, Fig. 7.)

than transitional cell tumours, appear in younger people and are likely to be more advanced at diagnosis.

A wide range of genetic abnormalities has been found in bladder cancer. Mutations in the tumour suppressor gene *p53* (p.75) are common, both in invasive and non-invasive tumours: *p53* abnormalities are found in 60% of invasive bladder cancers. Abnormalities in the genes *GSTM1* and *NAT2* have also been found. These genes code for the production of the enzymes glutathione-S-transferase and n-acetyltransferase respectively, which detoxify a range of carcinogens, including those found in cigarette smoke. Reduced production of these enzymes therefore increases carcinogen levels, which are excreted in the urine, accounting for their association with bladder cancer.

Signs and symptoms

Nearly all patients experience haematuria, and a high proportion have symptoms of an irritable bladder: frequency, urgency, and pain on urination. There may be pelvic pain.

Management and prognosis

As with other cancers, how advanced the tumour is at diagnosis is directly related to the outcome. *p53* mutation is a poor prognostic factor. Although most urothelial cancers are slow growing and not particularly invasive, they are more likely to recur after treatment, and they may in time transform into more malignant disease. Tumours can be surgically removed or treated with chemotherapy and/or radiotherapy.

CONGENITAL, INHERITED, AND DEVELOPMENTAL DISORDERS

Structural abnormalities of the urinary tract include developmental abnormalities and the development of cystic lesions. Congenital abnormalities of the urinary system are very common, affecting 1 in 10 births, and are a common reason for kidney disease in children.

CONGENITAL DISORDERS

Some congenital disorders have an inherited component, but most are caused by an acquired abnormality during intrauterine life: for example, maternal use of ACE inhibitors in pregnancy is associated with a range of developmental abnormalities in the fetal kidney. There is a range of abnormalities, which vary considerably in severity. Many are completely asymptomatic and are only discovered as an incidental finding during investigations for unrelated issues. Some, however, are life threatening or incompatible with life. The kidneys may be small and underdeveloped, with fewer nephrons than normal, or the kidney may be displaced and out of position, for example sitting in the pelvis rather than the abdomen. There may be two ureters on each side, or a single ureter that does not insert in the normal site through the bladder wall, which may obstruct urine drainage into the bladder and increase the risk of infection. Very rarely, there may be more than one bladder, or a normal bladder may be located on the surface of the body at birth.

Renal agenesis

Agenesis means failure of organ development. If one kidney develops normally but the other is absent at birth, the outcome is often excellent, with the remaining kidney coping well and performing the function of two. This condition is relatively common, affecting up to 1 in 500 live births. The individual may be asymptomatic and lead a normal life, although there is predisposition to hypertension and renal disorders. If both kidneys fail to develop during pregnancy (bilateral renal agenesis), the baby cannot survive and stillbirth is a likely outcome. The incidence of this condition is 1 in 5000 pregnancies. It is usually associated with other developmental defects, including failure of lung or limb development, and has been associated with several chromosomal abnormalities, including trisomy 21 (p.58) and Turner syndrome. The underlying cause is not known, although it is certain to be complex, as the cooperation and coordinated function of multiple genes is required for normal embryonic development. Many mutations in a range of genes have been reported, including the *WT1* gene associated with Wilms tumour. Male children are more likely to be affected than females.

Horseshoe kidney

This is an anatomical abnormality rather than a disease; the kidneys are fused into one, usually at the lower poles, giving the characteristic horseshoe shape (Fig. 12.17). Only about a third of people with this condition experience problems, which may include increased incidence of urinary tract obstruction and certain tumours (e.g., Wilms tumour), urinary tract infections, and kidney stones. It is found in up to 1 in 400 live births and is more common in identical twins and in siblings.

POLYCYSTIC KIDNEY DISEASE

Cysts, small fluid filled spaces within the renal tissue, develop in a large proportion of normal healthy kidneys as part of the ageing process. However, cystic disorders have detrimental effects on renal function and some cysts may have malignant potential. Long-term haemodialysis can cause cysts to form in both the cortex and medulla of the kidney. Such cysts often cause no trouble, but they can bleed, causing pain, and they increase the risk of renal cell carcinoma in long-term dialysis patients.

Autosomal dominant polycystic kidney disease

This inherited disorder (p.47) accounts for a significant proportion of individuals developing end-stage renal failure and those requiring dialysis. Estimates of incidence vary but may be as high as 1 in 400 in some populations.

URINARY CALCULI

The deposition of minerals as calculi (urinary stones) in the kidneys, bladder, or urinary passageways, also called **urolithiasis**, can cause serious obstruction, trauma, and inflammation in the urinary tract. More men than women are affected and there is a familial predisposition. Risk factors include high levels of stone-forming minerals in the blood or urine, including calcium and uric acid, usually because of overproduction, increased intake, or impaired excretion; however, urolithiasis occurs in many individuals with none of these risk factors. There is often a family history.

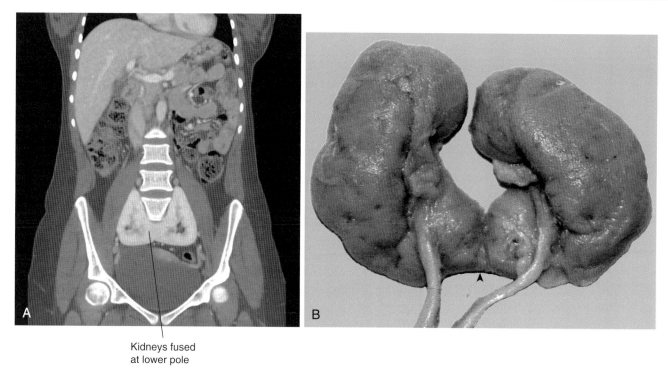

Kidneys fused
at lower pole

Fig. 12.17 Horseshoe kidney, showing fusion at the lower poles. (A) CT scan. (B) Gross anatomy. (Modified from (A) Dighe M, Grajo JR, and Lee L (2022) *Abdominal imaging*, Fig. 24.2. Philadelphia: Elsevier Inc; and (B) Klatt E (2020) *Robbins and Cotran atlas of pathology*, 4th ed, Fig. 10.13. Philadelphia: Elsevier Inc.)

Pathophysiology

Stones form when the concentration of a mineral dissolved in the urine exceeds its solubility, and the mineral precipitates out as crystalline particles. This may be because the levels of dissolved minerals are higher than normal, but another contributing factor is low urine volume, which concentrates urinary solutes and may trigger crystallisation. Another important factor is urinary pH, because rising pH (an alkaline urine) or falling pH (acidification of the urine) changes the solubility of stone-forming chemicals. Factors that affect urinary pH include diet: foods that lower urinary pH include fish, coffee, sugary food and high-protein food, and foods that increase it include vegetables, nuts, and many fruits. Urinary tract infections increase pH because of the action of urea-splitting bacteria, which produce ammonia that alkalinises the urine. Prolonged vomiting alkalinises the urine because of the loss of gastric acid. Acidification of the urine can happen in diabetic ketoacidosis, starvation, and prolonged diarrhoea, which eliminates alkaline intestinal secretions from the body.

Certain chemicals found in urine inhibit crystallisation of minerals and stone formation. These substances include citrate, glycosaminoglycans, pyrophosphate, and a glycoprotein called *nephrocalcin*. Deficiency of these inhibitors may be at least partly responsible for stone formation in those people who do not have recognised risk factors such as hyperuricaemia or impaired purine metabolism.

Urinary stones can be categorised according to their composition. There are four main types: calcium/phosphate stones, uric acid stones, sycstine stones, and struvite stones.

Calcium/phosphate stones. Up to 70% of urinary calculi are made of calcium oxalate, with a variable phosphate content (Fig. 12.18A). Renal excretion of calcium rises if the nephrons are intrinsically unable to reabsorb calcium normally, increasing calcium content in the urine and predisposing to calcium stone formation. However, the problem may lie elsewhere: in some cases, calcium absorption from the gastrointestinal tract is excessive, leading to increased calcium content in the urine as the kidneys clear it from the blood to keep blood calcium levels normal. Acidification of the urine also reduces calcium solubility and predisposes to calcium stones.

Uric acid stones. Uric acid is released when the body breaks down purines, key constituents of nucleic acids such as DNA and RNA. Body tissues therefore contain significant amounts of waste uric acid, which must be excreted by the kidneys. If purine levels rise, uric acid levels also rise. This increases the concentration of uric acid in urine, which may precipitate out as uric acid stones. Conditions in which cell turnover, and therefore purine metabolism, is very high, such as leukaemia, are associated with uric acid calculi. Purines are found in high concentrations in non-dairy animal products (whose cells are also rich in nucleic acids): certain meats (e.g., bacon, turkey, venison and liver) and some fish (e.g., trout, haddock, anchovies, sardines, herring and mussels) are particularly rich in purines. All alcoholic drinks, especially beer, also contain high purine levels. It follows then that diets rich in these foodstuffs predispose to uric acid stones. The incidence of these calculi is increased in gout, a condition associated with high blood uric acid levels (hyperuricaemia). Not everyone with gout develops urinary stones, but they are a common consequence in this condition. Uric acid is not soluble in acidic fluids, so acidification of the urine is a significant predisposing factor; note that the presence of uric acid itself in the urine decreases urinary pH and promotes stone formation.

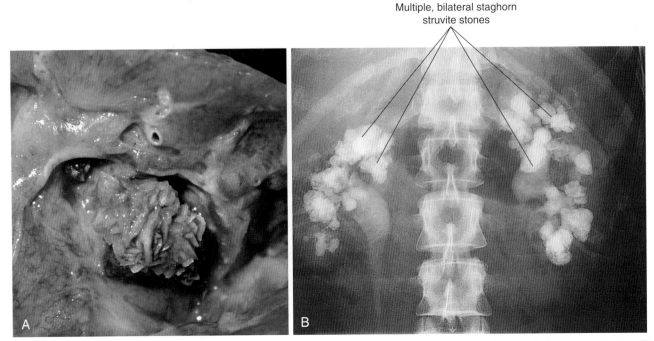

Fig. 12.18   Urinary stones. (A) Calcium stone. (B) Multiple staghorn calculi in both kidneys in a patient with a bacterial urinary infection. The alkaline conditions produced by the microbes favoured precipitation of struvite and the formation of struvite stones. (From (A) Sens MA and Hughes R (2021) *Diagnostic pathology: forensic autopsy*, Fig. 17.222. Philadelphia: Elsevier Inc; and (B) Walker B, Colledge NR, Ralston S, et al. (2010) *Davidson's principles and practice of medicine*, 21st ed, Fig. 17.36. Oxford: Churchill Livingstone.)

Cystine stones. Cystinuria, an inborn error of metabolism that leads to increased excretion of the amino acid cysteine, is associated with the production of cystine stones. Acidification of the urine accelerates stone formation.

Struvite stones. Struvite is magnesium ammonium phosphate, which is insoluble in alkaline urine. These stones are therefore strongly associated with repeated urinary tract infections because urine is alkalinised in urinary tract infections by bacteria that produce alkaline ammonia from urea. Struvite stones are more common in women than men, reflecting the higher incidence of UTIs in females than males. The calculi can form in the kidney itself, filling the renal pelvis and extending into the calyces, giving a large, branched stone called a *staghorn calculus* (see Fig. 12.18B). Most staghorn calculi are struvite stones and associated with infection.

Signs and symptoms
The pain caused by stones caught in the urinary tract is excruciating. Although some stones are smooth, others are sharp, irregular, and rough. Peristaltic contractions of the walls of the tract move the stone towards the exterior and can cause significant trauma. Haematuria is a frequent symptom, and urinary stasis caused by obstruction and the tissue injury predispose to infection. Complete obstruction causes backing up of urine behind the stone, which, depending on where the stone is lodged, can dilate the urinary passageways and cause **hydronephrosis** (dilation of the renal pelvis and calyces caused by accumulation of urine).

Prognosis and management
Maintaining good fluid intake is important in all types of stone because production of high volumes of dilute urine helps to keep substances in solution. It also helps buffer

swings in urinary pH that can predispose to stone deposition. Limiting dietary intake of purine-rich foods helps to prevent uric acid stones, and administration of bicarbonate, which is excreted in the urine and increases its pH, is an effective strategy in preventing stone formation in people at risk. Sometimes small stones can be left to work their way out of the tract, provided adequate analgesia is given, but larger or more troublesome calculi can be broken up with ultrasound, dissolved by adjusting the pH of the urine, or surgically removed. Recurrence in susceptible people is common.

ACUTE KIDNEY INJURY

Acute kidney injury (AKI, previously called *acute renal failure* (ARF)) is an umbrella term describing sudden deterioration in renal function after any one or more of a wide range of events or diseases. **Pre-renal causes** refer to causes of AKI caused by reduced blood flow to the kidney, for example after haemorrhage. **Intrinsic renal causes** relate directly to some impairment of renal function, for example caused by nephrotoxic drugs. **Post-renal causes** are caused by obstruction of urine flow somewhere between the kidney and the exterior, for example, prostatic enlargement (Fig. 12.19). Risk factors include chronic conditions like diabetes, liver disease, hypertension, heart failure, hospitalisation, and autoimmune disorders, all of which can significantly affect kidney function.

Pathophysiology
The pathophysiological changes in the affected kidney depend on the cause. In all types of AKI, the GFR falls, although the reasons for this are different depending on the nature of the original insult.

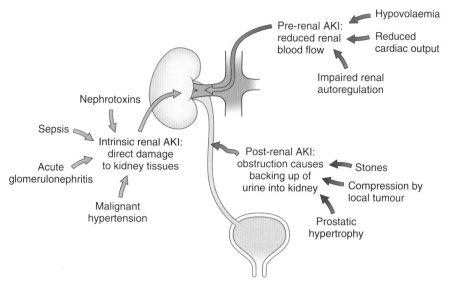

Fig. 12.19   Categories of acute kidney injury.

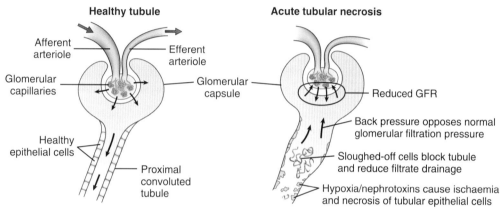

Fig. 12.20   Acute tubular necrosis in pre-renal AKI. The figure shows injury to the proximal convoluted tubule, but ATN can affect any part of the nephron.

Pre-renal AKI. Events that reduce blood flow to the kidney cause ischaemia and necrosis of renal tissue, including the tubules themselves, and are an important cause of acute tubular necrosis (ATN), in which the tubular epithelial cells die, lose their normal cell-cell attachments, and detach from their basement membrane. They slough off into the tubular lumen, blocking filtrate flow, increasing pressure in the tubule and reducing filtration in the glomeruli (Fig. 12.20).

Normal blood flow through the glomerulus is shown in Fig. 12.21A. Increased blood pressure is maintained in the glomerular capillaries because outflow is restricted by the narrow efferent arteriole, and this maintains filtration pressures. Reduced blood flow to the kidney reduces perfusion pressure in the glomeruli. Initially, autoregulation maintains GFR despite falling pressure in the afferent arteriole, and the efferent arteriole constricts to keep pressure high in the glomerulus (see Fig. 12.21B). However, once efferent arteriole constriction reaches its limit, autoregulation can help no further and blood pressure in the glomerulus starts to fall. This reduces glomerular filtration rate (see Fig. 12.21C), and impairs the clearance of waste products, including creatinine. Reduced circulating blood volume (as in serious dehydration, burns, excessive diuresis or haemorrhage), poor heart function (as in heart failure or cardiac tamponade)

and conditions with significant systemic vasodilation causing a drop in blood pressure (as in sepsis, anaphylaxis or the use of vasodilator drugs) all restrict renal perfusion. Pre-renal AKI is therefore usually associated with hypotension, thirst, tachycardia (as the heart attempts to maintain blood pressure and tissue perfusion), and poor blood flow to the extremities.

Renal (intrinsic) AKI. Insults to the kidney itself are the commonest reason for AKI, and GFR falls because the ongoing kidney damage, whatever the aetiology, releases vasoconstrictor mediators, constricting afferent arterioles, reducing renal perfusion, glomerular blood flow and therefore GFR. Causes include nephrotoxic drugs (e.g., furosemide, radiocontrast media, gentamicin, non-steroidal anti-inflammatory drugs, lithium), glomerulonephritis, sepsis, renal infections, and renal ischaemia. Renal ischaemia leads to ATN and is the commonest cause of intrinsic AKI. Signs and symptoms reflect the underlying cause: for example, in AKI secondary to glomerulonephritis, there may be oedema, haematuria and hypertension.

Post-renal AKI. Obstruction to urine flow characterises post-renal AKI. Urine backs up behind the obstruction, eventually backing up all the way through the renal pelvis to the tubules themselves, increasing pressure in the nephrons

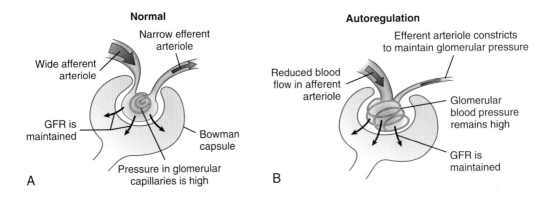

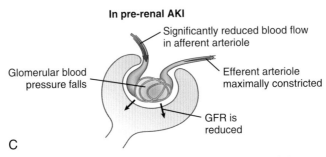

Fig. 12.21 Loss of glomerular filtration pressure in pre-renal acute kidney injury. (A) Normal. (B) Autoregulation may initially maintain GFR. (C) When the ability of autoregulation to maintain perfusion pressure in the glomerulus is exhausted, glomerular blood pressure falls and GFR falls.

and reducing GFR. Obstruction may be caused by expanding tumours, either associated with the urinary tract itself (e.g., bladder cancer, benign prostatic hypertrophy or prostate enlargement) or nearby (cervical cancer). Renal stones may obstruct the tract. Signs and symptoms reflect the underlying cause: for example, renal stones may cause pain, or in developing prostatic enlargement, the patient may report hesitancy, frequency, and urgency of urination.

Management and prognosis

With appropriate treatment, most cases of AKI resolve, although a proportion of patients do not recover and develop end-stage renal disease. Fluid balance must be corrected; hypovolaemia is reversed with fluid replacement and fluid overload is managed with diuretics. Identifying and treating underlying conditions is essential, for example, discontinuing nephrotoxic drugs, treating infection, and clearing any post-renal obstruction.

CHRONIC KIDNEY DISEASE

Chronic kidney disease (CKD; previously called *chronic renal failure*) is a frequent consequence of systemic disorders and insults that adversely affect kidney health and is a significant cause of morbidity and mortality worldwide. The kidneys possess significant reserve, and the initial stages of renal impairment are generally masked by compensatory mechanisms, but the diagnosis is made on the basis of haematuria or proteinuria, and/or a reduction in GFR to less than 60 mL/min/1.73 m² that has persisted for 3 months or more. Once the kidney's ability to compensate is exhausted, the loss of functional nephrons causes a progressive decline in

BOX 12.1 Causes of chronic kidney disease

Renal disorders	Non-renal disorders
Glomerular disease	Diabetes mellitus
Polycystic kidney disease	Hypertension
Recurrent kidney stones	Autoimmune disorders (e.g., SLE, RA, amyloidosis)
Drugs (e.g., NSAIDs, gold, heroin)	Infections (e.g., syphilis, parasitic infections, HIV)
Urinary tract obstruction	Vascular disease
Renal artery thrombosis	Metabolic disorders (e.g., hypokalaemia or hypercalcaemia)
Radiation damage	Malignant disease
Renal trauma	Hyperlipidaemia

renal function and can be tracked by a progressively falling GFR and deterioration in other markers of kidney function. Risk factors include increasing age and a very wide range of systemic disorders, presented in Box 12.1. In up to one-fifth of patients, the underlying cause is never determined. Whatever the underlying aetiology, once over half of the nephrons are lost, the degenerative changes occurring in the remaining nephrons follow a common course. Typically, the disorder develops over decades and although a small proportion of patients (2%–3%) progress to end-stage renal disease, renal function stabilises in many people. Several causes of CKD have been discussed above, including diabetic nephropathy and autoimmune disorders.

In 2002, the United States National Kidney Foundation produced a framework for classifying CKD. This has been adopted internationally, because it provides a consistent set of terms and guidelines that replaced the confusing and variable terminology and practices used beforehand. Table 12.1 summarises the five stages of CKD according to declining GFR as given in the report and indicates the key pathophysiological changes associated with each.

Pathophysiology

The pathophysiology is complex, not only because of the wide range of causative factors, but because renal impairment has many knock-on effects in so many other aspects of body function, mainly caused by **azotemia**, the accumulation of urea and creatinine in the blood (Fig. 12.22). In the early stages of developing renal injury, the kidney compensates and so GFR remains normal and may even be elevated. This happens because as nephron loss occurs as a result of the injury, renal blood flow is directed through steadily reducing numbers of healthy nephrons, which hypertrophy in response, maintaining normal kidney function. However, as the proportion of damaged and non-functional nephrons increases, the ability of the remaining healthy nephrons to maintain this high filtration rate is exhausted, and indications of declining renal function appear. It is likely that the high blood flow through healthy nephrons damages the delicate glomerular capillaries, so that in addition to dysfunction caused by the original disorder, destruction of healthy nephrons is accelerated by the high hyperperfusion pressures to which they are exposed. The plasma levels of

Table 12.1   National Kidney Foundation stages of CKD (2002)

Stage	Severity	GFR (mL/min/1.73 m²)	Comment
1	Renal function normal	≥90 (may actually be above normal because of compensatory mechanisms)	Usually no symptoms
2	Mild renal impairment	60–89	There may be hypertension. PTH levels rise and there may be evidence of bone damage. Raised plasma urea and creatinine.
3	Moderate renal impairment	30–59	Anaemia present, caused by erythropoietin deficiency Raised plasma urea and creatinine.
4	Severe renal impairment	15–29	Hyperkalaemia, acidosis, sodium and water retention. Raised plasma urea and creatinine.
5	End-stage renal failure	<15	Severe hypertension, anaemia, hyperphosphataemia. Death is likely without dialysis or transplant.

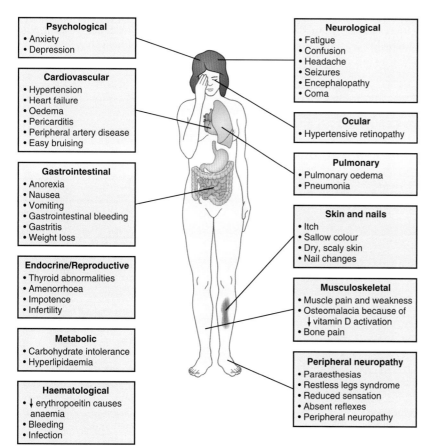

Psychological
- Anxiety
- Depression

Cardiovascular
- Hypertension
- Heart failure
- Oedema
- Pericarditis
- Peripheral artery disease
- Easy bruising

Gastrointestinal
- Anorexia
- Nausea
- Vomiting
- Gastrointestinal bleeding
- Gastritis
- Weight loss

Endocrine/Reproductive
- Thyroid abnormalities
- Amenorrhoea
- Impotence
- Infertility

Metabolic
- Carbohydrate intolerance
- Hyperlipidaemia

Haematological
- ↓ erythropoeitin causes anaemia
- Bleeding
- Infection

Neurological
- Fatigue
- Confusion
- Headache
- Seizures
- Encephalopathy
- Coma

Ocular
- Hypertensive retinopathy

Pulmonary
- Pulmonary oedema
- Pneumonia

Skin and nails
- Itch
- Sallow colour
- Dry, scaly skin
- Nail changes

Musculoskeletal
- Muscle pain and weakness
- Osteomalacia because of ↓ vitamin D activation
- Bone pain

Peripheral neuropathy
- Paraesthesias
- Restless legs syndrome
- Reduced sensation
- Absent reflexes
- Peripheral neuropathy

Fig. 12.22 Systemic manifestations of chronic kidney disease. (Modified from Brown D, Edwards H, Buckley T, et al. (2020) *Lewis's medical-surgical nursing*, 5th ed, Fig. 45.2. Sydney: Elsevier Australia.)

nitrogenous wastes creatinine and urea begin to rise, and protein loss across the filtration membrane appears, causing proteinuria. Some of this protein deposits in the interstitial tissues of the nephron, setting up an inflammatory response that provokes fibrosis and accelerates nephron loss.

CKD and bone health. Advancing CKD is associated with hyperparathyroidism and bone disease because the failing kidneys lose the ability to regulate calcium balance. The range of bone abnormalities that develops secondary to CKD is called renal osteodystrophy. The failing kidneys cannot retain calcium, which is lost in the urine. In response to the consequent hypocalcaemia, the parathyroid glands secrete parathyroid hormone (PTH), and raised blood PTH levels are commonly found in progressing CKD. PTH stimulates bone breakdown, releasing calcium and phosphate into the blood to restore circulating calcium levels. This depletes the bone calcium content and leads to osteomalacia. In addition, the kidneys are responsible for activation of vitamin D, which declines in the failing kidneys. Vitamin D is needed for calcium absorption in the intestine, and its deficiency further worsens the hypocalcaemia, increasing PTH levels and promoting bone loss and degenerative bone changes.

In addition, blood phosphate levels rise because the kidneys cannot excrete it. Hyperphosphataemia also has a detrimental effect on bone health because it suppresses vitamin D activation in the kidney, further reducing calcium absorption and plasma calcium levels. This in turn increases PTH levels and the leaching of calcium from bone. The effect of CKD on bone health is summarised in Fig. 12.23.

CKD and fluid and electrolyte balance. In mild to moderate disease, fluid and electrolyte levels often remain within normal levels, but as the disorder advances, sodium and water retention usually develop, with oedema and increased blood pressure. A small proportion of patients actually lose sodium and water and may require salt supplements and attention to maintaining hydration. The later stages of CKD are also usually associated with renal inability to excrete potassium, causing hyperkalaemia. This can be worse in diabetes, because potassium movement between the blood and the intracellular fluid is affected by insulin-mediated glucose uptake by cells. Insulin increases cellular permeability to potassium, decreasing blood potassium levels. If there is inadequate insulin administration, or an inadequate response to insulin, potassium shifts from inside cells into the extracellular fluids (which of course includes plasma). This makes the hyperkalaemia worse. Hyperkalaemia depresses muscle contractility, including the heart and respiratory muscles, and can cause cardiac arrhythmias, cardiac arrest, and respiratory arrest.

Nitrogenous waste products, including urea and creatinine, begin to rise in the plasma even in the early stages of CKD, but they do not usually cause symptoms until disease is relatively advanced. Accumulation of acids causes a metabolic acidosis. This affects body physiology and biochemistry in a variety of ways, including deteriorating bone health, impairing protein use and production (which can contribute to poor nutritional health, muscle wasting and muscle weakness), and further damages the kidneys themselves.

CKD and anaemia. Anaemia is a very common symptom in CKD. Its prevalence has been calculated at twice that of the general population (15.4% compared with 7.6%), and the incidence increases with the stage of disease. The kidneys produce erythropoietin, the principal hormone involved in the production of red blood cells. Erythropoietin levels fall in CKD, leading to a reduction in erythrocyte production and anaemia. Other factors that may contribute to anaemia of CKD include increased red cell loss in haemodialysis, poor dietary intake if the patient is nauseated or anorexic, and the toxic effects of uraemia on erythrocytes.

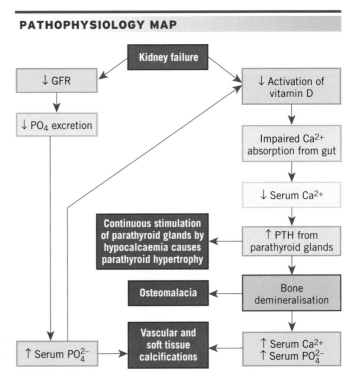

PATHOPHYSIOLOGY MAP

Fig. 12.23 The effect of chronic kidney disease on bone health. (Modified from Barry M, Goodridge D, Lewis S, et al. (2014) *Medical-surgical nursing in Canada*, 3rd ed, Fig. 49.4. Toronto: Elsevier Inc.)

Signs and symptoms

Patients can be asymptomatic even in the face of severely reduced GFR (less than 30 mL/min/1.73 m^2). However, early symptoms include increased urine production, as the kidneys lose the ability to concentrate the filtrate, which usually manifests itself as nocturia because the patient needs to empty his bladder more frequently than usual. As GFR continues to fall, and the patient becomes progressively azotemic, there is pruritis, nausea, oliguria, vomiting and anorexia. Anaemia causes tiredness, breathlessness, and reduced exercise tolerance. With accumulation of toxic wastes in the blood, there is acidosis, drowsiness, seizures, and coma.

Management and prognosis

Identifying and managing underlying aetiology and risk factors is important (e.g., early diagnosis and good management of diabetes delays the development of CKD in these patients). Iron supplements and erythropoietin treatment is useful in reversing anaemia. Correction and management of electrolyte and fluid imbalance is essential. Good nutrition, including dietary restriction or supplementation as required, can help protect bone health and improve physical and mental well-being. Identification and minimisation of cardiovascular risk factors is important (e.g., managing hypertension and hyperlipidaemia) because this slows the rate of kidney deterioration. Dialysis and/or renal transplantation are indicated in very advanced disease.

BIBLIOGRAPHY AND REFERENCES

Basile, D. P., Anderson, M. D., & Sutton, T. A. (2012) Pathophysiology of acute kidney injury. *Comprehensive Physiology, 2*(2):1303–1353.

Carlstrom, M., Wilcox, C. S., & Arendshorst, W. J. (2015). Renal autoregulation in health and disease. *Physiological Reviews, 95,* 405–511.

Couser, W. G. (2017). Glomerular disease. *Clinical Journal of the American Society of Nephrology, 12,* 983–997.

Lange, D., & Scotland, K. (Eds.). (2019). *The role of bacteria in urology* (2nd ed.). Springer.

Lim, A. K. H. (2014). Diabetic nephropathy: Complications and treatment. *International Journal of Nephrology and Renovascular Disease, 7,* 361–381.

Nabi, S., Kessler, E. R., Bernard, B., et al. (2018). Renal cell carcinoma: A review of biology and pathophysiology. *F1000Research, 7,* 307. 10.12688/f1000research.13179.1.

Schnaper, H. W. (2014). Remnant nephron physiology and the progression of chronic kidney disease. *Pediatric Nephrology, 29*(2). https://doi.org/10.1007/s00467-013-2494-8.

Stauffer, M. E., & Fan, T. (2014). Prevalence of anemia in chronic kidney disease in the United States. *PLoS One, 9*(1):E84943.

Szychot, E., Apps, J., & Pritchard-Jones, K. (2014). Wilms' tumour: Biology, diagnosis and treatment. *Translational Pediatrics, 3*(1), 12–24.

Thomas-White, K., Forster, S. C., Kumar, N., et al. (2018). Culturing of female bladder bacteria reveals an interconnected urogenital microbiota. *Nature Communications, 9.* 1557. https://doi.org/10.1038/s41467-018-03968-5.

Useful websites

Hill, M. A. Embryology Renal system: Abnormalities: https://embryology.med.unsw.edu.au/embryology/index.php/Renal_System_-_Abnormalities

Kidney Disease: Improving Global Outcomes 2012 clinical practice guideline for the evaluation and management of chronic kidney disease (CKD): https://kdigo.org/guidelines/ckd-evaluation-and-management/

UNC School of Medicine: Information on membranous nephropathy: https://unckidneycenter.org/kidneyhealthlibrary/glomerular-disease/membranous-nephropathy/

WCRF bladder cancer report (2015, revised 2018): https://www.wcrf.org/sites/default/files/Bladder-cancer-report.pdf

13 Disorders of Musculoskeletal Function

CHAPTER OUTLINE

INTRODUCTION
Skeletal muscle
  Skeletal muscle
Bone
  Classification of bones
  Bone cells
  Compact and spongy bone
  Embryonic development of bone
Joints
  The structure of synovial joints
DISORDERS OF SKELETAL MUSCLE
Autoimmune disorders
  Myasthenia gravis
Muscle tumours
  Rhabdomyosarcoma
The myopathies
  The muscular dystrophies
  Acquired myopathies
DISORDERS OF BONE
Structural and degenerative
  disorders
  Osteogenesis imperfecta
  Osteoporosis
  Paget disease
  Osteomalacia and rickets
  Endocrine-related bone conditions
Osteomyelitis
Tumours of bone and cartilage

Benign tumours
Secondary tumours of bone
Osteosarcoma
Chondrosarcoma
Spinal Deformity
DISORDERS OF JOINTS
  Osteoarthritis (osteoarthrosis)
  Rheumatoid arthritis
  Juvenile idiopathic arthritis
  Infective (septic) arthritis
  Spondyloarthritis
  Crystal-Induced arthritis
DISORDERS OF CONNECTIVE TISSUE
  Ehlers-Danlos syndrome
  The mucopolysaccharidoses
SPRAINS, FRACTURES, AND OTHER
MECHANICAL INJURY
  Low back pain
  Plantar fasciitis
  Tennis elbow (lateral epicondylitis)
Muscle injury
  Rotator cuff injury
Bone injury
  Types of fracture
  Bone fracture and its healing
Joint injury
  Sprained ankle

INTRODUCTION

The musculoskeletal system includes the tissues and structures of the skeleton and its associated musculature. Its basic functions include body movement, maintenance of posture, and protection of internal organs. In addition, bone tissue is the main reservoir of calcium and phosphate, and the red bone marrow contained within spongy bone produces blood cells (**haemopoiesis**). In addition to bone and skeletal muscle, key connective tissues such as collagen and cartilage are essential to the structure and function of the system and some disorders affecting these tissues will also be considered here. Chapter 1 discusses the biology of connective tissue, including cartilage, collagen and glycosaminoglycans.

Some systemic disorders—such as systemic lupus erythematosus, systemic sclerosis (scleroderma), and psoriasis—can feature significant musculoskeletal involvement but are considered in other chapters.

SKELETAL MUSCLE

Most skeletal muscle, as the name suggests, is attached to the bones of the skeleton by collagenous inelastic tendons. The skeletal muscles of the body come in a wide variety of shapes and sizes. The smallest is the tiny stapedius muscle of the middle ear, whose job is to anchor the stapes bone to

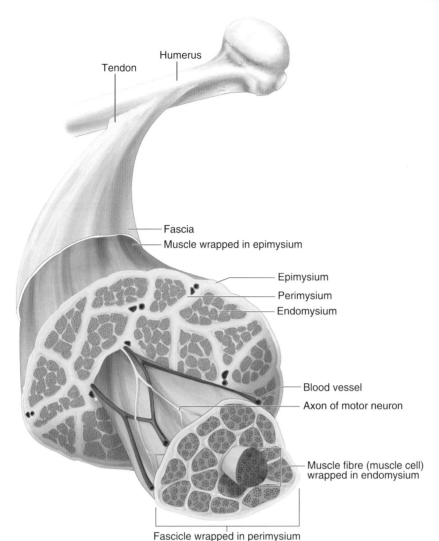

Tendon

Humerus

Fascia
Muscle wrapped in epimysium

Epimysium
Perimysium
Endomysium

Blood vessel
Axon of motor neuron

Muscle fibre (muscle cell)
wrapped in endomysium

Fascicle wrapped in perimysium

Fig. 13.1 The structure of a skeletal muscle. (Modified from Patton K, Thibodeau G, and Douglas M (2012) *Essentials of anatomy and physiology*, Fig. 10.1. St Louis: Mosby.)

the inner wall of the middle ear cavity and prevent it from extreme vibration in very noisy environments. The largest by volume is the gluteus maximus of the buttock.

SKELETAL MUSCLE

Each individual muscle is an organ in its own right and is enclosed in a protective outer wrapping of connective tissue called the **epimysium**, formed mainly from type I collagen fibres (Fig. 13.1). Muscle cells (also called *fibres*) are individually wrapped in a delicate layer of connective tissue called **endomysium** and packaged together in bundles called **fascicles**; each fascicle can contain up to 150 muscle cells and is wrapped in a connective tissue sheath called **perimysium**. The capacity of skeletal muscle cells to repair after damage is limited because mature cells cannot divide, but muscle tissue contains populations of stem cells called **satellite cells**, which proliferate after injury. New cells produced by satellite cell division can fuse with each other to form brand new muscle cells, or with existing damaged muscle cells, to repair them.

Skeletal muscle cell structure

Skeletal muscle cells are cylindrical in shape, non-branching, and multinucleate. Within the cell membrane (the

sarcolemma), the cytoplasm is packed with the contractile proteins actin and myosin, which are responsible for cell shortening and the generation of tension when the muscle is stimulated by its associated motor nerve. The cells are rich in mitochondria for energy production and contain myoglobin, which, like haemoglobin in erythrocytes, binds oxygen and provides an immediate oxygen reservoir to resist hypoxia in an exercising muscle.

The neuromuscular junction

Individual skeletal muscle fibres are supplied by a branch of a motor nerve, part of the voluntary (somatic) nervous system. The synapse between the motor nerve and a skeletal muscle fibre is called the *neuromuscular junction* (Fig. 13.2), and the neurotransmitter released is always acetylcholine. Acetylcholine is synthesised in the nerve terminal and stored in vesicles (1). Upon the arrival of an action potential, calcium channels open in the nerve terminal membrane and calcium enters from the extracellular fluid, causing the vesicles to fuse with the presynaptic membrane of the nerve ending. This releases ACh into the synaptic cleft (2), which diffuses rapidly across this narrow gap, only 50 nm wide, and binds to ACh receptors embedded on the post-synaptic muscle membrane (3). The ACh receptors found at the

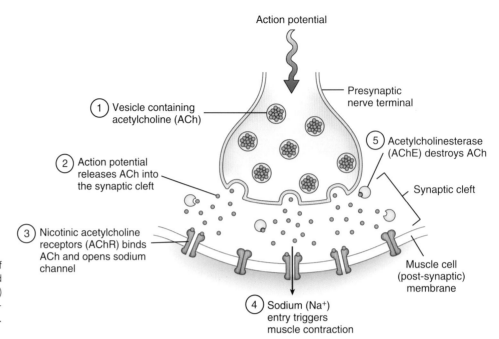

Fig. 13.2 Structure and operation of the neuromuscular junction. (Modified from Fitzmaurice S and Nind F (2010) *Saunders solutions in veterinary practice: small animal neurology*, Fig. 44.1. Edinburgh: Elsevier Ltd.)

neuromuscular junction are called *nicotinic muscarinic receptors* and are tightly linked to sodium channels. When ACh binds, the sodium channels open, allowing a rapid influx of sodium into the skeletal muscle cell and generating an action potential, which spreads through the skeletal muscle cell and triggers contraction (4). ACh is rapidly cleared from the synapse through enzymatic breakdown. Acetylcholinesterase (AChE), the enzyme responsible, is present in the muscle membrane close to the ACh receptors to ensure rapid destruction of ACh after it has activated its receptors and triggered contraction of the muscle cell (5).

BONE

Bone is a strong, rigid, non-deformable connective tissue. Although a third of bone mass is composed of calcium and phosphate salts, and nearly all of the remainder is composed of type 1 collagen fibres, it is a living and dynamic tissue, with a rich blood supply and specialised populations of cells that maintain and repair it. The slow but continuous turnover of bone ensures the skeleton is continually renewing itself. Bones that experience higher mechanical stresses self-renew faster; for example, in a healthy young adult, complete replacement of the bone of the femur occurs over about 12 months.

CLASSIFICATION OF BONES

The bones of the body are classified according to their general shape (Fig. 13.3). Irrespective of their shape, bones are constructed with an outer shell of dense compact bone tissue and spongy bone within.

Structure of a long bone

This is shown in Fig. 13.4. Note the outer compact bone shell and the spongy bone filling the bone ends. The medullary cavity runs up the centre of the shaft of the bone. The inner bone surfaces are lined with a membrane called **endosteum**, and the outer surface of the bone, except for surfaces that form joints, is covered with a fibrous protective

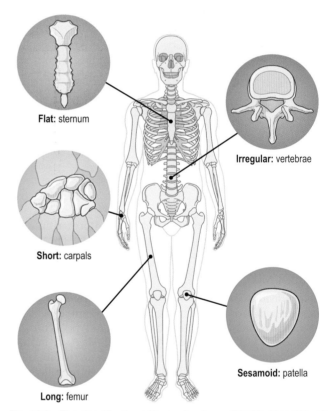

Fig. 13.3 The classification of bones by shape. (Modified from Waugh A and Grant A (2018) *Ross & Wilson anatomy and physiology in health and illness*, 13th ed, Fig. 16.1. Oxford: Elsevier Ltd.)

membrane called the **periosteum**. These membranes are important in bone repair and remodelling because they are rich in the cells responsible for producing new bone and for removing old or diseased bone. The periosteum also provides channels for the distribution of blood vessels that supply the bone. Surfaces involved in joint formation are covered in hyaline (joint) cartilage.

BONE CELLS

The cells that build, maintain, and break down bone are shown in Fig. 13.5. **Osteoprogenitor cells** are stem cells that live in the membranes that line and cover bone (i.e., in the endosteum and below the periosteum). After bone damage, they are activated, differentiate into osteoblasts, and begin laying down new bone tissue. **Osteoblasts** are bone-building cells. They lay down the collagen matrix first (this is called *osteoid*), and then mineralise it by depositing calcium and phosphate salts, converting it into mature bone tissue. They

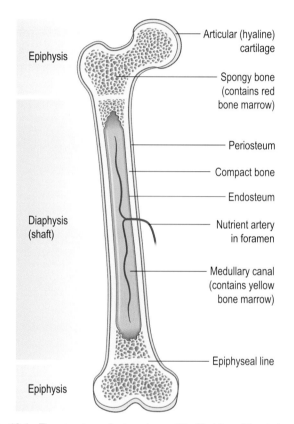

Fig. 13.4   The structure of a long bone. (Modified from Waugh A and Grant A (2018) *Ross & Wilson anatomy and physiology in health and illness*, 13th ed, Fig. 16.2. Oxford: Elsevier Ltd.)

construct this new bone all around themselves, encasing themselves and sealing themselves into pockets called *lacunae*. At this stage, they become **osteocytes**, mature bone cells, and act as caretakers of the bone in their local vicinity, monitoring and performing minor repairs as required. In the event of bone injury, these osteocytes de-differentiate into osteoblasts again and become active builders of bone once more.

Osteoclasts arise from a different cell line from osteoprogenitor cells, osteoblasts, and osteocytes. They are related to cells of the monocyte-macrophage lineage and, like these cells, are responsible for the removal of unwanted material, in this case bone tissue. Osteoclasts are large cells with multiple nuclei, because at an early stage in their development they are formed by the fusion of up to 200 individual monocyte-like cells. They dissolve bone using acids and collagenases stored in their lysosomes. This is essential for routine maintenance of bone and in bone healing and remodelling.

COMPACT AND SPONGY BONE

These are the two main types of bone tissue. The ultrastructure of both these bone tissues is shown in Fig. 13.6. In both compact and spongy bone, the bone tissue is laid down in layers (**lamellae**) by osteoblasts, which, once trapped inside the bone they have formed, become osteocytes living in their lacunae. Although osteocytes live in these individual pockets, they communicate directly with one another via thread-like extensions of their cytoplasm extended into tiny channels in the bone called **canaliculi**, which directly link individual lacunae (Fig. 13.7). However, the lamellae are arranged differently in compact and spongy bone. In compact bone, concentric lamellae are formed encircling a central canal, like the rings of a tree, forming cylindrical structures called **osteons**. These osteons are packed together, along the long axis of the bone; there are about 21 million osteons in the average human skeleton. The central canal carries blood vessels and nerves that supply the bone tissue. Connecting channels called *Volkmann's canals*, carrying branches of blood vessels, link central canals throughout the bone with the marrow cavity and allow the vascular system to form a communicating network of vessels throughout compact bone.

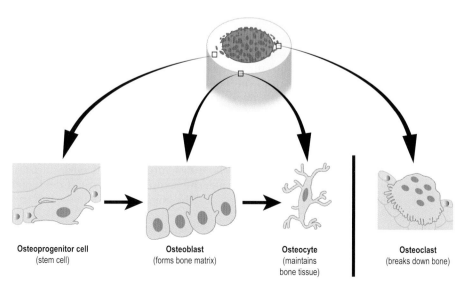

Osteoprogenitor cell	Osteoblast	Osteocyte	Osteoclast
(stem cell)	(forms bone matrix)	(maintains bone tissue)	(breaks down bone)

Fig. 13.5   Bone cells. (Modified from Shankar N and Vaz M (2015) *Textbook of applied anatomy and applied physiology for nurses*, 2nd ed, Fig. 20.5. New Delhi: Elsevier India.)

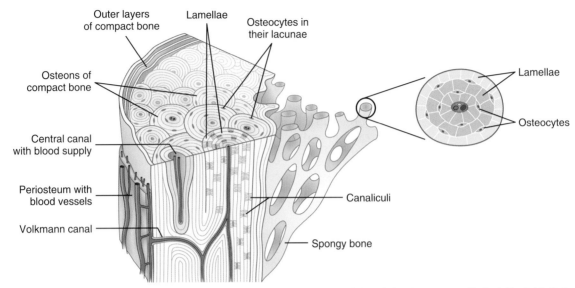

Fig. 13.6   The ultrastructure of compact and spongy bone. (Modified from Standring S (2021) *Gray's anatomy,* 42nd ed, Fig. 5.16. Oxford: Elsevier Ltd.)

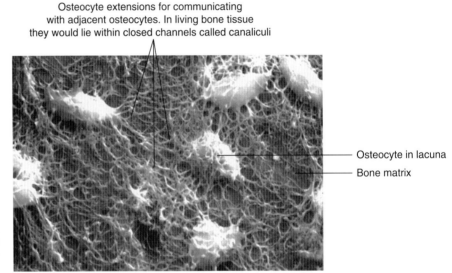

Osteocyte extensions for communicating with adjacent osteocytes. In living bone tissue they would lie within closed channels called canaliculi

Osteocyte in lacuna

Bone matrix

Fig. 13.7   Scanning electron micrograph of osteocytes in bone tissue. (Modified from Bullough PG (2010) *Orthopedic pathology,* 5th ed, Fig. 1.29. St Louis: Mosby.)

Spongy bone lacks osteons. Instead, the bone, laid down in lamellae like compact bone, is built in branching plates, pillars and bars of bone that form a honeycomb-like open framework. The osteocytes, living in their lacunae between the lamellae, are interconnected by tiny canaliculi as in compact bone, but these canaliculi open onto the surface of the bone and cells obtain their oxygen and nutrients by diffusion from tissue fluids circulating in these tiny passages. The spaces in the spongy bone are filled with red bone marrow, whose function of haemopoiesis is described on p.110.

EMBRYONIC DEVELOPMENT OF BONE

A template of the skeleton is laid down in the first few weeks after conception in the form of rods and plates of hyaline cartilage, produced by chondrocytes. The plates convert to bone and become the flat bones of the skeleton. The conversion of soft tissue to bone is called **ossification**. The rods are converted into the long bones of the limbs. Initially, they are surrounded with a dense membrane, an early form of the periosteum, containing osteoprogenitor cells (Fig. 13.8A). These cells differentiate into osteoblasts and begin to synthesise compact bone within the primary centre of ossification, producing a thin outer collar that encloses and supports the cartilage model (Fig. 13.7B). As the bone grows, it requires its own blood supply. Vascular bud cells migrate into the bone tissue and a blood vessel network begins to develop (Fig. 13.7C). Secondary centres of ossification appear within each end of the cartilage rod, and bone tissue is laid down here too (Fig. 13.7D). Bear in mind that the chondrocytes in the developing bone are constantly producing new cartilage that is continuously converted to bone so that the whole structure is steadily enlarging. Osteoclast activity creates the medullary cavity, and the blood vessel network expands. The bone continues to thicken and lengthen as fetal development progresses, with thickening and strengthening of the outer layer of compact bone, and remodelling as required to give shape, form and internal structure. At birth, the baby's skeleton contains 300 bones, compared with the adult complement of only 206, and the

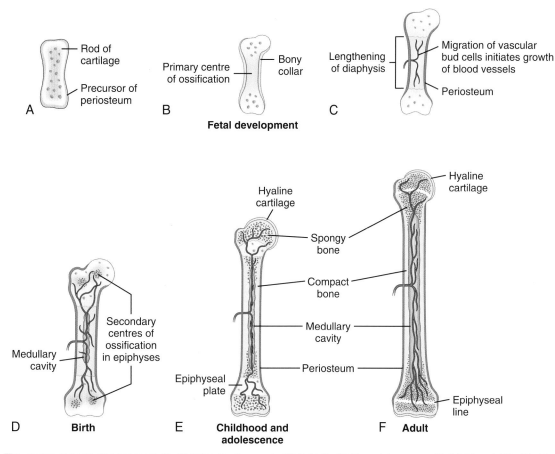

Fig. 13.8 The stages of bone development. (A–C) Fetal development. (D) At birth. (E) Pre-adolescence. (F) Adulthood. (Modified from Waugh A, and Grant A (2018) *Ross & Wilson anatomy and physiology in health and illness*, 13th ed, Fig. 16.7. Oxford: Elsevier Ltd.)

cartilage content is much higher than in the adult. Fusion of some of these individual smaller bones occurs post-natally, along with progressive ossification: for example, the bones of the neonatal skull are separated by fibrous joint material, which converts to bone in the months after birth, forming the continuous bony structure of the cranium.

At either end of the long bone in the newborn is a plate of cartilage, separating the bone ends from the bone shaft (Fig. 13.7E). These are called the growth plates or **epiphyseal plates**, and they allow the long bones of the skeleton to continue to lengthen during childhood. The chondrocytes continue to manufacture cartilage, but the growth plate does not thicken because as fast as the new cartilage is laid down, it is converted to bone at the interface between the growth plate and the shaft of the bone. As long as this continues, the bone continues to lengthen and the child grows in height. At puberty, under the influence of the sex hormones testosterone (in boys) and oestrogen (in girls), the activity of osteoblasts in the growth plate is increased. This accelerates the process of bone deposition, so that the cartilage is converted to bone faster than new cartilage is produced to replace it. Over a period of a few months, the growth plate is completely replaced by bone, marked on X-rays by a thin pale line, but no longer functional as a growth zone (Fig. 13.7F).

Maintenance of mature bone tissue

Mature bone is maintained and repaired by the co-ordinated activities of osteoblasts and osteoclasts. Adequate dietary calcium and phosphate intake is required for bone mineralisation. At any one time, only about 1% of total body calcium is found in the blood, the remainder being mainly incorporated into bone, which functions as a reservoir and storage site for calcium. Blood calcium levels are maintained between 2.20 and 2.65 mmol/L. Values outside of this range affect cardiac and nerve function, because calcium is an essential electrolyte in the generation of action potentials, the electrical stability of cell membranes and for neurotransmitter release. As a result, when blood calcium levels fall, osteoclast activity increases, breaking down bone tissue to release calcium into the bloodstream, and when calcium levels rise, the excess is extracted and laid down into bone.

The hormones **calcitonin** and **parathormone** regulate calcium homeostasis. Vitamin D is essential for calcium absorption from the small intestine and reabsorption in the kidney (see Fig. 10.17) and stimulates differentiation of both osteoblasts and osteoclasts. Vitamin C is required for collagen synthesis. Deficiency of either vitamin impairs bone growth.

JOINTS

A joint is a structure formed where two or more bones are held together by connective tissues. Some joints permit movement, whereas the structure of others holds the bones together so firmly that no movement is possible.

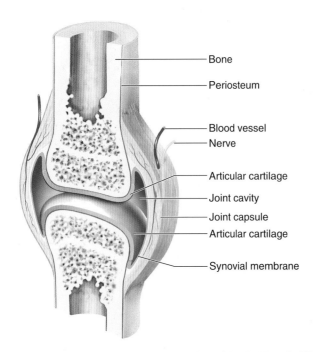

Fig. 13.9   The main features of a synovial joint. (Modified from Bell F, Patton KT, Williamson P et al (2024) *The human body in health & disease*, 8th ed, Fig. 8.28. St. Louis: Elsevier Inc.)

THE STRUCTURE OF SYNOVIAL JOINTS

The main features of a synovial joint are shown in Fig. 13.9. The bone ends are held together by a sleeve of connective tissue, continuous with the periosteum of the participating bones. Supporting ligaments, tough, fibrous cartilaginous bands, directly link the bones of the joint and further protect and stabilise it. These external structures of the joint sleeve enclose a cavity, called the **synovial cavity**, which is filled with a small amount of viscous, slippery **synovial fluid** that lubricates the joint and nourishes those internal joint structures lacking their own blood supply. The internal joint surfaces that do not directly bear weight are lined with a delicate membrane called the **synovial membrane**, which produces the synovial fluid by filtering blood plasma into the synovial space. The viscous, slippery quality of the fluid is caused by the addition of hyaluronan, made and secreted by the synovial cells.

Joint cartilage

Hyaline cartilage coats the surfaces of bones in direct apposition to one another, enlarging the joint space, preventing damaging bone-bone contact, and minimising friction when the joint moves. Joint cartilage is porous, and synovial fluid soaks into it, providing additional cushioning when the joint is loaded and the bone ends are forced together. Joint cartilage is made primarily of type I collagen, produced by chondrocytes, the only cells in cartilage. Chondrocytes also synthesise other essential molecules, including proteoglycans, the second-most abundant substance in cartilage. Collagen makes joint cartilage tough and durable, and proteoglycans regulate the water content of cartilage and give it shock-absorbing properties.

DISORDERS OF SKELETAL MUSCLE

The number of skeletal muscle cells present in an individual is genetically determined and remains fairly constant throughout life, unless there is loss associated with damage or disease.

AUTOIMMUNE DISORDERS

Many systemic autoimmune disorders affect skeletal muscle, and skeletal muscle inflammation, destruction, and weakness are features of the clinical picture. They include systemic lupus erythematosus and systemic sclerosis.

MYASTHENIA GRAVIS

Myasthenia gravis (MG) was first described and named in 1672 by the English physician Thomas Willis, who also described and named the anatomical arrangement of the circle of Willis (circulus arteriosus) in the brain. MG is a rare, acquired (i.e., it does not have a hereditable component and does not run in families) autoimmune disease caused by autoantibody-mediated destruction of acetylcholine receptors on skeletal muscle. It affects 1 to 2 in every 10,000 people, with no significant racial predisposition. Most cases are diagnosed in the 20 to 30 years age bracket. There is a sex difference, with a female:male ratio of around 3:2, although this shifts to a slight male predominance in older onset adults.

Pathophysiology
Acetylcholine (ACh) released from motor nerve endings at the neuromuscular junction binds to post-synaptic ACh receptors on the muscle membrane to initiate muscle contraction. Most patients with MG produce autoantibodies to the nicotinic ACh receptor, which bind to the receptor and activate complement and other immune-mediated defence mechanisms, destroying the receptor and damaging the adjacent cell membrane (Fig. 13.10A). In a minority (15%) of cases, the autoantibodies are directed against other muscle proteins, but the end result is the same: blockade of neuromuscular transmission because of reduced numbers of ACh receptors, and progressive damage to skeletal muscle.

Most people with MG have associated thymic abnormalities, including thymic hypertrophy and thymomas. In embryonic development, the thymus gland eliminates autoreactive T cells; that is, it destroys any T cells that possess receptors that would allow them to attach to self-antigens on body cells and trigger an autoimmune response. The thymus is also important in the production of regulatory T cells, which control and limit the immune response. The production of autoantibodies in MG is strongly associated with a deficiency in thymus gland function.

Signs and symptoms
The initial stages are associated with fluctuating muscle weakness and rapid muscle fatigability, which often gets worse with exercise and as the day goes on (Fig. 13.10B). Commonly, the extraocular muscles are affected early in the disorder, so diplopia (double vision) and ptosis (drooping eyelids) may be the presenting symptoms. Between 15% and 25% of patients only ever have ocular symptoms, but the disease usually progresses to more widespread skeletal muscle

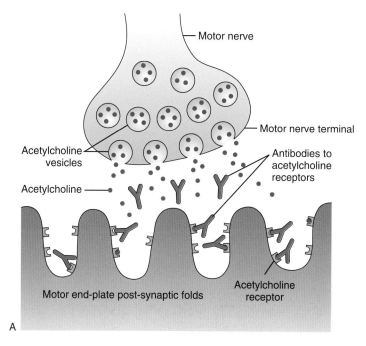

CLINICAL SIGNS

- Ocular ptosis and/or diplopia
- Facial muscle weakness
- Dysarthria
- Dysphagia
- Neck flexor weakness
- Shoulder girdle weakness
- Respiratory muscle weakness
- Forearm weakness
- Hand weakness
- Lower limb weakness

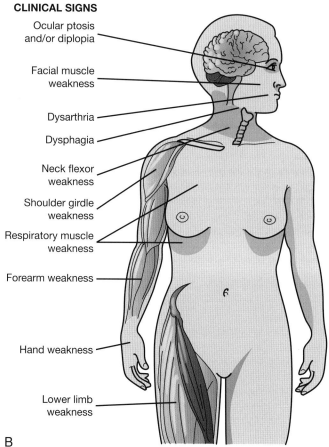

SYMPTOMS

- Drooping of upper eyelids
- Double vision
- Diminished expression
- Slurred speech
- Difficulty swallowing
- Shoulder tiredness
- Exhaustion, decrease in respiration
- Arm fatigue and/or weakness

Fig. 13.10 Myasthenia gravis. (A) Acetylcholine receptors on skeletal muscle are destroyed by autoantibodies so that ACh can no longer stimulate the muscle. (B) Possible manifestations of myasthenia gravis. (Modified from (A) Banasik J (2018) *Pathophysiology*, 6th ed, Fig. 10.3. St Louis: Saunders; and (B) Knights K, Rowland A, and Darroch S (2019) *Pharmacology for health professionals*, 5th ed, Fig. 17.3. Sydney: Elsevier Australia.)

involvement, with generalised weakness, which generally worsens with time. Involvement of the respiratory muscles (the diaphragm and intercostal muscles are skeletal muscles, even though they are not under complete voluntary control) may be life threatening. Symptoms often get worse with stress (infection, surgery, emotional stress), a wide range of drugs, menstruation, pregnancy, and warm weather.

Management and prognosis

Current management options can give a normal or near-normal lifespan. Anticholinesterase drugs, which block the breakdown of acetylcholine and prolong its action at the neuromuscular junction, are useful. Thymectomy can help some patients, sometimes inducing complete remission, especially those with thymic tumours. Immunosuppressants reduce the levels of circulating autoantibodies. Supportive treatment includes artificial ventilation during episodes of respiratory muscle paralysis and prompt treatment of respiratory infections. MG-related death is generally caused by respiratory failure.

MUSCLE TUMOURS

Muscle tumours are rare because the rate of cell turnover is low in healthy muscle tissue. Malignant tumours of muscle are sarcomas, reflecting their embryonic tissue of origin, and benign neoplasms are called *myomas*. Rhabdomyoma (which should not be confused with rhabdomyosarcoma, described below) is a rare benign skeletal muscle tumour.

RHABDOMYOSARCOMA

This malignant skeletal muscle tumour is usually diagnosed before the age of 6. It is the commonest sarcoma of childhood, accounting for 3% of all childhood tumours, although it also occurs in adolescents and adults. There is a 1.5:1 male:female ratio. There are three main subtypes, which vary in the underlying genetic abnormality, age of presentation and degree of cell differentiation, but all are aggressive and progressive.

Pathophysiology
The cell of origin is a primitive precursor of skeletal muscle. In children, the tumour usually appears in the head or neck region, or in the genitourinary tract. In adolescents and adults, a wider range of tissues may be affected, including the limbs. Because the cells are precursors, they are not cylindrical in shape like mature muscle cells but vary greatly in shape and size and usually lack any sign of the normal skeletal muscle striations. They lack the molecular markers of mature skeletal muscle and possess a range of genetic abnormalities (depending on the subtype of disease present). Common sites of metastatic spread include lymph nodes, bone marrow, and lung.

Signs and symptoms
The cancer usually presents as a growing mass at the site of origin. Genitourinary tumours can cause haematuria and/or urinary obstruction.

Management and prognosis
Treatment is usually with surgery and chemotherapy, sometimes with radiotherapy. The average 5-year survival rate in children is 61% and in adults 27%, but in cases where metastatic disease was present at diagnosis, the average 5-year survival is usually less than 25%.

THE MYOPATHIES

Myopathy is an umbrella term simply meaning disease of muscle, so a wide range of muscle disorders with different underlying causes fall into this category, including congenital or inherited disorders, and diseases caused by inflammatory conditions, toxins, infections, or metabolic changes. They do not include any muscular issues of neurological origin, in which the muscle itself is normal, but cannot function because of impaired nerve supply. Myopathies usually reduce muscle strength, and often cause pain or muscle

tenderness. Several systemic autoimmune and inflammatory conditions frequently feature myopathy in their clinical pictures, including sarcoidosis, systemic lupus erythematosus, and rheumatoid arthritis.

THE MUSCULAR DYSTROPHIES

This group of more than 30 inherited diseases is characterised by progressive skeletal muscle atrophy. They are caused by mutations in key genes essential for the production of proteins essential to skeletal muscle development and function. There is no cure for any of the muscular dystrophies, but supportive treatments, including physiotherapy, mobility aids, and specific interventions for particular problems (e.g., surgery for scoliosis) can reduce the impact of the resultant disabilities. The commonest muscular dystrophy, Duchenne muscular dystrophy, is discussed on p.41.

FACIOSCAPULOHUMERAL DYSTROPHY

The faulty gene in this disorder lies on the long arm of chromosome 4. Called *DUX4*, it is usually silent in most adult tissues. The mutation in facioscapulohumeral dystrophy activates this gene, but how this leads to the pathological changes of the disease is not understood. As the name of the disease suggests, muscles of the face, shoulder, and upper arm are most significantly affected, with progressive loss of muscle fibres and muscle mass over time. Symptoms usually start in adolescence, and because the disease is inherited in an autosomal dominant fashion, it affects both sexes equally. Facial muscle weakness can prevent full closing of the eyelids, leading to dry eye and increased risk of corneal injury. The affected person may struggle to drink through a straw or smile because of facial muscle weakness. Upper body weakness makes simple actions such as throwing a ball or pulling clothing on or off over the head difficult or impossible. Some individuals suffer more serious disease than others, and widespread muscle weakness can cause skeletal deformities such as lordosis because muscles become too weak to support the skeleton. About 20% of affected individuals eventually require the use of a wheelchair. In other people, the disease progresses much more slowly and may cause only minor difficulties throughout life.

Myotonic dystrophy

This is the commonest adult-onset muscular dystrophy, usually presenting between the ages of 20 and 30. Globally, the prevalence is estimated at about 1 in 8000 people, but there are population differences. There are two main forms—type 1 and type 2—each with a specific gene mutation, and both are inherited in an autosomal dominant fashion, so both sexes are equally affected. As with facioscapulohumeral muscular dystrophy, the functions of the abnormal proteins produced by the mutated genes are not known, but skeletal muscle is not the only tissue affected in this disorder-affected people often have other systemic disorders, such as cataract, heart defects, and diabetes. Skeletal muscle cells, when viewed under the microscope, are histologically abnormal and there is a progressive loss of cell numbers and skeletal muscle mass. Muscle weakness is also accompanied by episodes of myotonia-prolonged muscle contraction, which may, for example, mean that having picked something up, a person may not then immediately be able to release it. The disorder progresses with age. Disease-related mortality is usually from cardiac or respiratory impairment, but some people, usually those with type 2 disease, may have a normal lifespan.

ACQUIRED MYOPATHIES

Inflammatory myopathy, as described previously, is a well-recognised feature in many autoimmune and systemic inflammatory disorders. In dermatomyositis, a rare auto-immune disorder affecting mainly the skin and muscle, muscle is progressively destroyed by an ongoing abnormal inflammatory process, driven by activated T cells and macrophages, although the antigenic stimulus that initiated their activation is not known. Occasionally myositis (muscle inflammation) may appear as an idiopathic condition, with no associated disorder, with swollen, painful and weakened skeletal muscles. Other causes of myopathy include a wide range of therapeutic drugs (statins, opioid analgesics, statins, quinine, amiodarone, and glucocorticoids among others). The inherited mitochondrial disorders can have profound effects on muscle function because muscle tissue has such high energy requirements. Alcohol is toxic to muscle tissue, as are other drugs of abuse, including cocaine. Also, the circulating inflammatory mediators released by some malignancies can cause inflammation and atrophy of muscle.

DISORDERS OF BONE

Bone health is generally optimal in young adults (25–30 years of age) and tends to deteriorate as people get older. A range of factors, including metabolic disturbances, infection, and malignancy, can lead to bone disease.

STRUCTURAL AND DEGENERATIVE DISORDERS

Bone is laid down in the embryonic skeleton as cartilage models that are gradually ossified during the embryonic and early post-natal periods. Bone health is maintained in adult life by a range of homeostatic mechanisms, and failure in any of these causes or accelerates degenerative changes that may cause frank disease.

OSTEOGENESIS IMPERFECTA

This condition (also called *brittle bone disease*, p.46) occurs because of inherited faults in type I collagen production. With the loss of the collagen infrastructure of bone, the relatively overmineralised tissue becomes brittle and liable to fracture and shatter.

OSTEOPOROSIS

Osteopenia means a loss of bone mass in the skeleton, despite normal mineralisation. This is a natural age-related phenomenon, affecting both sexes equally, and it can be slowed considerably by lifestyle factors, including not smoking, low to moderate alcohol intake, maintaining a healthy diet, and taking plenty of weight-bearing exercise, which stimulates bone deposition. When osteopenia reaches the point at which the bone is weakened enough to fracture, the condition is termed **osteoporosis**. This is a common disorder, representing the most frequently diagnosed metabolic bone disorder worldwide and thought to affect over 200

million people globally. Female sex and increasing age are important risk factors, and the disorder occurs in all racial populations, although northern European white women and Asian women report the highest incidence.

Pathophysiology

Healthy bone is in a constant state of remodelling, as osteoclasts dissolve bone tissue and osteoblasts replace it. These two processes co-operate to ensure that bone loss is at least matched by bone replacement to maintain bone volume in the skeleton. In osteoporosis, the usual homeostatic balance between osteoblast bone-building activity and osteoclast bone-destroying activity is disrupted, and osteoclast activity predominates. Consequently, the rate at which bone is lost outstrips the rate at which it is replaced, and the bone mass of the skeleton falls. The bone becomes porous and brittle because of its loss of tissue, but the collagen:mineral ratio remains within the normal range (compare with **osteomalacia**). Osteoporosis is confirmed when bone mineral density is two standard deviations less that would be expected in a young healthy adult of the same sex.

Either a reduction in osteoblast activity or an increase in osteoclast activity may account for the developing imbalance. Osteoporosis is a complex disorder, with multiple risk factors and therefore multiple contributory mechanisms. However, increasing age and the activity of steroid sex hormones are the most significant risk factors. Oestrogen is an important stimulator of osteoblast activity, and in premenopausal women, it maintains bone mass. Loss of oestrogen at the menopause has dramatic detrimental effects on bone. Although both osteoclast and osteoblast activity are upregulated, osteoclast activity exceeds osteoblast activity, and bone mass declines. Ageing, the other main risk factor, seems to lead to loss of bone mass because the supply of osteoprogenitor cells, which produce osteoblasts, declines.

Other important factors that diminish bone mass include dietary deficiencies: low calcium and/or phosphate intake stimulates bone breakdown to maintain circulating blood levels of these electrolytes. In response to low blood calcium levels, the parathyroid gland releases parathormone to release calcium from bone. Likewise, vitamin D deficiency limits calcium absorption from the small intestine, even if dietary calcium is sufficient. There is a genetic predisposition in some people. Pre-natal health, birthweight, and maternal health all relate to the incidence of osteoporosis in later life. Extended use of glucocorticoids predisposes to osteoporosis because they suppress the activity of connective tissue building cells, including osteoblasts. Low body weight, frailty, and poor general health are also all associated with earlier onset of osteoporosis.

Signs and symptoms

The condition may be asymptomatic at diagnosis and picked up as an incidental finding (e.g., minor fracture on an X-ray). Presentation in symptomatic people depends on which bones are affected. The spine is a common site, particularly the lumbar and thoracic spine, which bear the greatest loads. Osteoporotic vertebrae are compressible (Fig. 13.11), leading to loss of height, and vertebral fractures may occur. Spinal deformity, such as kyphoscoliosis and lordosis, can result from weakening of the vertebral column. There is increased incidence of fractured neck of femur and of pelvic

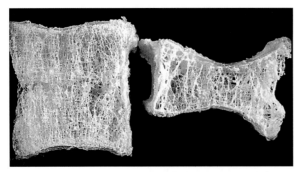

Fig. 13.11 Reduction in mass and thickness of osteoporotic vertebra (right) compared with normal (left). (Modified from Kumar V, Singh M, Abbas A, and Aster J (2020) *Robbins & Cotran pathologic basis of disease: South Asia edition*, 10th ed, Fig. 26.10. India: Elsevier India.)

fractures. Postmenopausal women have increased risk of osteoporosis-related fracture, especially neck of femur, and for both sexes, 80% of fractures in the over-50s are in individuals with some degree of osteoporosis.

Management and prognosis

Prevention is very important, especially in youth. Optimising bone health when young to allow bone density to reach its maximum gives the bone significant reserves against age and disease-related deterioration. Regular weight bearing exercise, a varied and healthy diet, not smoking and moderating alcohol intake are all protective. Osteoporosis is a progressive disorder, but even after diagnosis, bone health can be improved by following these bone-friendly lifestyle principles. A range of drugs that slow or reverse the progress of osteoporosis is available, including bisphosphonates, which improve the mineralisation of bone rather than increasing bone mass, dietary supplements, hormone replacement therapy in postmenopausal women, and parathormone treatment.

PAGET DISEASE

Paget disease is named for Sir James Paget, who described it (calling it *osteitis deformans*) in 1877. This is the second most common bone disease in older people after osteoporosis. There is a male:female ratio of 1.8:1, and significant geographical variation worldwide. It is common in Northern Europe and the United States, with a prevalence of between 2% and 4%, although in Norway and Sweden the prevalence is only 0.3%. It is rare in Asia, the Middle East, and Africa; for example, in sub-Saharan Africa, the prevalence is 0.01% to 0.02%. In all populations, incidence rises significantly with age. Worldwide, the incidence of the disease is falling. The cause of Paget disease is not known, but there is often a hereditable component, and there is clear evidence of geographical clustering, even within the same country, so an environmental factor is also likely. Viral infection has been suggested as a possible trigger.

Pathophysiology

The disease may appear in localised areas in one bone, in multiple bones or may affect an entire bone. It can arise anywhere, but the bones of the axial skeleton (skull, vertebra, and ribs) are most frequently involved and the hands and feet almost never. Bone remodelling is excessive and abnormal. Osteoclast activity accelerates, and as a result the rate of bone degradation increases. In response, osteoblastic

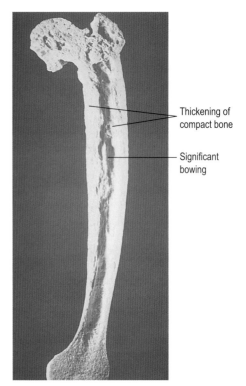

Thickening of compact bone

Significant bowing

Fig. 13.12 Photograph of femur affected by Paget disease. The compact bone is thickened, the bone is enlarged, and bowing of the shaft is evident. (Modified from Wold L, Krishnan Unni K, Sim F, et al. (2008) *Atlas of orthopedic pathology*, 3rd ed, Fig. 7.8. Philadelphia: Elsevier Inc.)

activity also increases, but the new bone laid down is not constructed properly, and is disorganised, undermineralised, and weak. Affected bones may enlarge because of the abnormal remodelling (patients may report that they need bigger hats than before!) and deform (Fig. 13.12). Bone turnover rate can increase by as much as 20-fold. The bone marrow is infiltrated with fibrotic tissue and newly formed blood vessels and may even itself become mineralised. The disease generally evolves into an inactive stage, during which the excessive bone remodelling ceases and the disorder becomes quiescent.

Signs and symptoms

Often, patients are asymptomatic; the condition might be discovered by accident during investigations for other reasons. Symptomatic patients present with bone pain, fractures, and deformity. Swelling and pain over an involved site can occur. Vertebral involvement can compress spinal nerves, and deafness may develop if the temporal bone of the skull is involved, because it is important in conducting sound waves into the middle ear. Recent work suggests that Beethoven's deafness, which developed in his 40s and was complete by the time he reached the age of 45, was caused by Paget disease.

Management and prognosis

Many patients do not need treatment. Pain relief is important, and bisphosphonates, which inhibit osteoclast activity and bone breakdown, may be used. About 1% of people with Paget disease develop osteosarcoma.

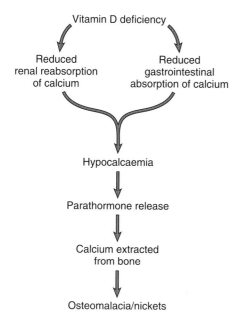

Fig. 13.13 The relationship between vitamin D deficiency and osteomalacia/rickets.

OSTEOMALACIA AND RICKETS

Osteoporosis and osteomalacia may be confused because the terminology is similar. Osteoporosis, as described previously, is caused by reduced deposition or increased breakdown of otherwise normal bone tissue, reducing the mass of the skeleton and giving porous, brittle, weakened bones. Osteomalacia is caused by undermineralisation of the collagenous framework of adult bone, giving soft and pliable bones not strong or rigid enough to resist the normal mechanical demands placed on the skeleton. Rickets is caused by undermineralisation of growing bones in which the growth plates are still active, leading to a weakened and deformed skeleton.

Vitamin D is essential for calcium absorption in the GI tract and in the kidney, and vitamin D deficiency is the usual cause of osteomalacia and rickets, usually secondary to dietary deficiency or poor absorption (Fig. 13.13; see also Fig. 10.17). Because vitamin D is synthesised in the skin on exposure to ultraviolet B (UVB) rays in sunlight, deficiency is commoner in people living in northern latitudes, and shows a seasonal pattern: it is worse in the winter months and improves in the summer. Kidney disease can also lead to calcium deficiency because the kidney normally metabolises inactive 25-hydroxyvitamin D into its active derivative 1,25-hydroxyvitamin D required for calcium absorption in the small intestine and the renal tubules. Bone hypomineralisation is a well-recognised consequence of chronic kidney disease (see Fig. 12.23) and is caused by inadequate renal synthesis of vitamin D.

Rickets was once a very common disorder in children of families living in poverty in northern countries, where diet was poor and there was not enough sunlight to synthesise adequate vitamin D in the skin. Vitamin D and its ability to prevent rickets were discovered in the 1930s, and since the link has been understood, improvements in diet (cod liver oil administration to children was a common if unpopular ritual in many families) and fortification of foodstuffs with vitamins have greatly reduced the incidence of rickets.

Osteomalacia remains a common finding in older people who spend most of their time indoors and have a poor diet.

Pathophysiology

Healthy mineralisation of the osteoid framework of bone depends on an adequate supply of calcium and phosphate. Rickets and osteomalacia are both caused by calcium deficiency, usually because of a lack of vitamin D, but manifest differently because they are associated with different stages of skeletal formation: in children, the lack of calcium means that ossification of the cartilage-rich skeleton cannot proceed, but in adults, whose bone is already fully ossified, demineralisation weakens and softens the skeleton.

Secondary hyperparathyroidism accompanies this disorder because low calcium levels stimulate the parathyroid gland to release parathormone, which stimulates osteoclast activity and bone breakdown in an effort to maintain normal blood calcium concentrations (see Fig. 10.17).

Signs and symptoms

These depend on whether a child or adult is affected. In rickets, the bones are soft and easily deformed. For example, pressure from lying in a cot can flatten the skull, and once the child begins to walk, the leg bones become curved because they are not strong enough to support the weight of the upper body.

In osteomalacia, bone pain and spontaneous incomplete fractures, particularly in the long bones and pelvis, are common.

Management and prognosis

Vitamin D supplements are usually curative, provided the underlying problem is a straightforward vitamin deficiency. If the issue lies with vitamin D activation, for example, in renal failure, then vitamin D supplementation will not resolve the disorder, and the activated form of the vitamin, 1,25-hydroxyvitamin D must be administered.

ENDOCRINE-RELATED BONE CONDITIONS

Many hormones affect bone health and homeostasis (see also Ch. 10).

Parathormone

Plasma calcium levels are controlled mainly by parathormone (PTH) from the parathyroid glands. Disorders of PTH secretion therefore have implications for bone physiology. PTH is secreted into the blood in response to hypocalcaemia and increases blood calcium levels to within the normal range by four main mechanisms: it increases calcium absorption in the small intestine, increases calcium reabsorption in the renal tubules, activates vitamin D in the kidney, and increases osteoclast activity and bone breakdown (Fig. 13.14 and see also p. 266). Hyperparathyroidism, which is almost always caused by vitamin D deficiency, depletes bone of its mineral content in an attempt to maintain blood calcium levels. In hypoparathyroidism, there is inadequate parathormone to maintain blood calcium levels, causing hypocalcaemia, a low bone mineral content, and increased risk of fractures.

Steroid hormones

The sex hormones testosterone and oestrogen promote bone deposition. This accounts for the increased risk of

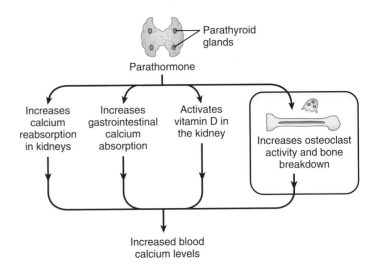

Fig. 13.14 The role of parathormone in demineralising bone.

osteoporosis in postmenopausal women, not matched in men of similar age because testosterone levels remain high in males even into relatively old age.

Glucocorticoids are the body's stress hormones and have multiple systemic effects primarily targeted at shutting down much of the body's normal tissue maintenance activity (e.g., bone turnover) and increasing the availability of glucose and fats (for energy) and other nutrients (e.g., amino acids) in response to a stressor such as infection or trauma. In long-term glucocorticoid therapy (e.g., after an organ transplant) or in adrenal gland disease (e.g., Cushing disease), sustained elevation of plasma glucocorticoid levels results in long-term suppression of osteoblast activity and osteoclast stimulation, with an overall loss of bone mass. This causes osteoporosis and increased risk of fracture.

Sympathetic hormones

There is evidence that excessive exposure to adrenaline (e.g., in phaeochromocytoma) decreases bone density by increasing osteoclast activity. β-blocker treatment has been reported to be osteoprotective because it inhibits bone resorption.

Aldosterone

Primary aldosteronism significantly affects the renal and cardiovascular systems, increasing blood volume and commonly causing secondary hypertension. High levels of aldosterone also increase the risk of fracture, particularly in the vertebrae. The reasons for this are not clear, but bone cells possess receptors for mineralocorticoids such as aldosterone, and so are presumably capable of responding directly to these hormones, which must affect their behaviour in ways yet to be explained.

Growth hormone

Growth hormone (GH) is essential for normal development and growth of body tissues, including bone. It is released from the anterior pituitary and stimulates proliferation of cartilage and bone. Deficiency in childhood causes skeletal growth to fail, leading to the clinical syndrome called *dwarfism*. General Tom Thumb, who achieved fame as a circus performer in the 19th century, suffered from pituitary dwarfism and attained an adult height of only 99 cm. At the other extreme, excess in childhood (e.g., in a pituitary tumour) causes gigantism. Excess GH in adulthood causes acromegaly.

OSTEOMYELITIS

Osteomyelitis is bone inflammation and destruction secondary to infection. Bone is not normally exposed to the external environment, but infection can arise either from septicaemia, where live organisms circulating in the bloodstream colonise the bone, or from contamination of an open fracture or wound, including after surgery or dental work. Diabetic foot infections are another important source of bacteraemia that may lead to osteomyelitis. The pathogenic organism may be bacterial, viral, fungal, or parasitic in nature.

The risk of osteomyelitis increases in poor health or immunosuppression, and with increasing virulence of the microbe. Most cases occur in children, usually because of a skin infection such as a boil, or entry of organisms via a minor skin breach. The organism in this case is usually *Staphylococcus aureus*, but a number of other pathogens are clinically important (e.g., *Klebsiella* species are often found in intravenous drug users and in individuals whose osteomyelitis is secondary to a genitourinary infection). Syphilis and tuberculosis can also involve bone. The incidence in adults is rising because of increasing age of the population, intravenous drug use, and the increased use of devices implanted or inserted into body tissues for medical reasons (e.g., intravascular stents and bone fixation materials).

Pathophysiology

Not all parts of a bone are equally vulnerable to infection. Parts with a generous blood supply receive a higher-than-average pathogen load and are more likely to be colonised. Hence, in children, in whom the bone ends and epiphyseal plates are highly active and therefore receive a rich blood supply, infections of the ends of long bones are common. In adults, common sites of infection are the vertebrae, long bones, pelvis, and clavicle. Affected bone is progressively destroyed by the ongoing inflammatory and immune response within the bone. The pathogens may travel throughout the bone, using the central canals of the osteons and the open

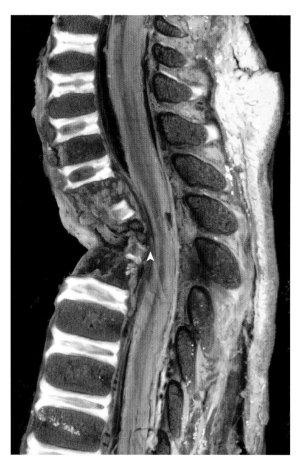

Fig. 13.15 Osteomyelitis of T8 and T9 caused by systemic tuberculosis. There is extensive vertebral destruction. (From Klatt EC (2021) *Robbins and Cotran atlas of pathology*, 4th ed, Fig. 17.28. Philadelphia: Elsevier Inc.)

spaces in spongy bone, and so the infection spreads within the bone. In response, neutrophils and other inflammatory cells including lymphocytes infiltrate the bone and release a raft of cytokines and mediators that initiate a powerful inflammatory reaction. This, and pathogenic activity of the infecting organism, leads to bone necrosis (Fig. 13.15). If the infection tracks to the periosteum, pus and other infective material accumulate between it and the bone underneath, separating the bone from its blood supply because blood vessels supplying the bone run through the periosteum. This accelerates the necrotic changes in the area of infection. Sinuses can form between the infected bone and the surface of the skin, allowing pus and other inflammatory materials to drain away.

Signs and symptoms
Bone pain and sometimes local redness, swelling, and tenderness are seen. There is also fever, malaise, fatigue, and anorexia.

Management and prognosis
Antibiotics and surgical drainage are the cornerstone of management. In about 25% of individuals, the condition relapses and becomes chronic, with recurring infections that may appear years after the initial event.

TUMOURS OF BONE AND CARTILAGE

Primary tumours of bone and cartilage are relatively rare because of the fairly low rate of proliferation of these tissues.

Those that do occur usually arise in the first few decades of life. Both benign and malignant tumours occur, and both cause pain, fractures, and swelling; benign tumours are much more common than malignancies. Malignant tumours, however, tend to be aggressive and fast growing.

BENIGN TUMOURS

These include osteoma and osteoblastoma, bone-forming tumours associated with adolescence that are mainly treated with radiotherapy and surgical excision, respectively. Chondromas and osteochondromas are benign tumours of cartilage. Chondromas usually arise in the age range 30 to 50 years and affect the bones of the hands and feet. They can be surgically removed if they are troublesome. Osteochondromas are bony extensions with a cartilage cap, projecting from the parent bone (usually the ends of long bones) by a bony stalk. They are the commonest benign tumour of bone, and usually cause no problems. Those that are large enough to cause pain or deformity are removed surgically.

SECONDARY TUMOURS OF BONE

Bone tissue is a common site for growth of metastatic tumours that have seeded from a primary elsewhere. They are generally widespread and indicate a poor prognosis. The commonest primary sites are breast, prostate, lung, and kidney, and the preferred sites for bone metastases involve the vertebrae, pelvis, ribs, sternum, and skull.

Bone is a common site for spread of a primary cancer because many malignant cells express appropriate receptors for bone tissue, allowing them to attach and establish new growths. In addition, the bone marrow receives a rich blood supply, and blood flows slowly here, increasing the likelihood that blood-borne cancer cells can adhere, survive, and grow. Most metastatic growths destroy bone tissue (**lytic metastases**), whereas others stimulate bone growth (**blastic metastases**), and some feature both. In either case, the architecture of the bone becomes abnormal, and the bone becomes weaker. As bone is broken down, calcium levels in the blood rise, causing the symptoms of hypercalcaemia, including fatigue, muscle pain and weakness, headache, nausea, and vomiting. Growing tumours in the vertebrae can compress the spinal cord or spinal nerves.

OSTEOSARCOMA

The oldest known case of malignant disease in the human fossil record is an osteosarcoma, identified in a toe bone from a *Homo sapiens* relative found near Johannesburg, South Africa, and dated from 1.7 million years ago. Nowadays, it is the commonest solid malignant tumour of bone, although it is a rare disease. It is slightly commoner in black people than white, and in males than females. Globally, its incidence is 3.4 cases per million people, with the highest rates in children between the ages of 5 and 15 years, although there is a second peak in older adults, often associated with Paget disease. Any bone can be affected, but most cases arise in the ends of long bones, particularly (42%) in the femur.

Pathophysiology
The tumour presents as a rapidly expanding mass progressively destroying the parent bone, with both lytic and blastic features. It frequently grows from the interior of the bone and through the bone surface, separating the periosteum from the bone below; this activates the osteoprogenitor cells and osteoblasts in the periosteum resident there, triggering

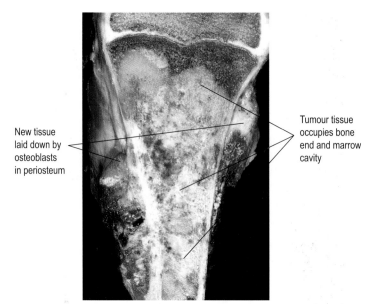

New tissue laid down by osteoblasts in periosteum

Tumour tissue occupies bone end and marrow cavity

Fig. 13.16 Osteosarcoma of the proximal tibia. The normal architecture of the bone end is destroyed, and the tumour extends into the medullary cavity. (Modified from Kumar V, Abbas A, Aster JC, et al. (2021) *Robbins essential pathology*, Fig. 18.6. Philadelphia: Elsevier Inc.)

the production of new bone (Fig. 13.16). This causes swelling and deformity. Early metastasis to the lungs is common.

Signs and symptoms

Pain and swelling are common, and sometimes pathological fractures occur.

Management and prognosis

The outlook in this disorder has improved enormously in recent years, with an average 50% cure rate after surgery and chemotherapy. The prognosis is better in younger patients; the average 5-year survival rate for those over 60 years is only 24%.

CHONDROSARCOMA

This is a family of malignant tumours of cartilage, most of which are relatively slow growing and reasonably well differentiated, so they are histologically quite similar to normal cartilage. The commonest form, conventional chondrosarcoma, represents 90% of cases, with a slight male predominance and appears mainly in people over 50 years old. They arise mainly in the pelvis and ribs and are usually removed surgically.

SPINAL DEFORMITY

The vertebral column is a stack of 33 vertebrae: 7 cervical, 12 thoracic, 5 lumbar, 5 (fused) sacral, and 4 (fused) coccygeal, stabilised with intervertebral discs, ligaments, and muscles. The spine is not a truly vertical structure. It possesses four curves: two primary curves, the thoracic and sacral curvatures, which are established before birth; and two secondary curves, the cervical and lumbar curvatures, which are present in later fetal development and fully established once the child learns to support his head and gets up on his feet to walk (Fig. 13.17A). The thoracic and sacral curves are called the kyphotic curves, and the cervical and lumbar curves are called the *lordotic curves*.

Lordosis

This means excessive concavity of the lumbar curvature; it is also called *swayback* (Fig. 13.17B). It may be secondary to obesity or pregnancy, in which the body's centre of gravity is shifted forward by the increased mass of the abdomen. It may also be secondary to vertebral disease, such as osteoporosis, where the weakened vertebrae are compressed in response to forces applied through the spine, causing fractures and vertebral collapse.

Kyphosis

This is excessive curvature of the thoracic spine (Fig. 13.17C). It may be caused by poor posture, or by vertebral disease such as osteoporosis. Congenital kyphosis can occur if spinal development does not follow normal patterns in the developing fetus. Kyphosis can cause pain and, if severe, can affect the integrity of the spinal cord and cause neurological problems of the spinal nerves exiting the vertebral column from between affected vertebrae.

Scoliosis

This is a lateral deformity of the spine, giving an S or C shape when viewed from the back, but also often involving a degree of twisting of the vertebral column as well (Fig. 13.17D). It may be idiopathic or secondary to connective tissue disorders such as Marfan syndrome or neuromuscular disorders such as cerebral palsy. It can cause back pain and inhibit normal expansion of the ribcage during breathing.

DISORDERS OF JOINTS

A wide range of conditions cause inflammatory and degenerative changes in joints. Inflammatory conditions of joints (arthritis) are common and there is a range of aetiologies. The patterns of joint involvement are often characteristic of the different forms of arthritis (Fig. 13.18).

OSTEOARTHRITIS (OSTEOARTHROSIS)

This degenerative disorder is found in all populations and is the commonest form of joint disease worldwide. It is more common with advancing age and is a significant cause of pain, disability, cost to healthcare systems, and lost working days. It is estimated that more than four-fifths of individuals over 65 years have some degree of osteoarthritis (OA), although if mild, people may remain asymptomatic

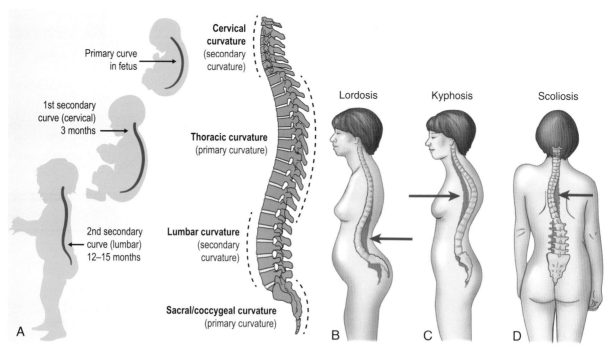

Fig. 13.17 Spinal curves. (A) The primary and secondary spinal curves. (B) Lordosis. (C) Kyphosis. (D) Scoliosis. (Modified from (A) Waugh A, and Grant A (2018) *Ross & Wilson anatomy and physiology in health and illness*, 13th ed, Oxford, Elsevier Ltd; Fig. 16.28; (B–D) Thibodeau GA, and Patton K (2024) *The human body in health and disease*, 8th ed, St Louis, Mosby; Fig. 8.18.)

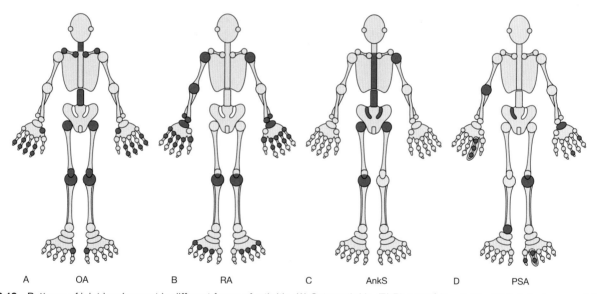

Fig. 13.18 Patterns of joint involvement in different forms of arthritis. (A) Osteoarthritis. (B) Rheumatoid arthritis. (C) Ankylosing spondylitis. (D) Psoriatic arthritis. (Modified from Ralston S, Penman I, Strachan M, et al. (2018) *Davidson's principles and practice of medicine*, 23rd ed, Edinburgh, Elsevier Ltd; Fig. 24.10.)

throughout their lives. It is commoner in women than men. There is a hereditable component, and individual risk is increased if there is a family history. Other risk factors include low levels of the sex hormones (which are osteoprotective), infection or trauma to the joint, repetitive and heavy use of the joint, diabetes and pre-existing bone disease, or weakness. Obesity is linked to OA of the knees.

Pathophysiology
The actual cause of OA is not known, but mechanical stress and trauma seem to be important in initiation of the disease

process. The most frequently affected joints are the hip, spine, and knee, which bear most weight (Fig. 13.18A). The underlying pathological change in OA is a biochemical breakdown of joint cartilage, which thins, flakes, and loses its smooth surface. As the cartilage wears away, the joint space between the bone ends gets smaller and smaller, increasing the pressure in the joint capsule and increasing the mechanical stress to which the joint structures, including the cartilage itself, is subjected. Eventually, the bone underneath is exposed, leading to direct bone-bone contact, subjecting the bone to mechanical stress from which the

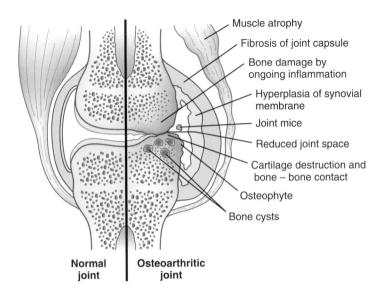

Muscle atrophy

Fibrosis of joint capsule

Bone damage by ongoing inflammation

Hyperplasia of synovial membrane

Joint mice

Reduced joint space

Cartilage destruction and bone – bone contact

Osteophyte

Bone cysts

Normal joint **Osteoarthritic joint**

Fig. 13.19   The osteoarthritic joint.

cartilage normally protects it. The bone responds by thickening and forming bony projections (osteophytes), which may break off into the joint space as bony fragments called *joint mice*. These loose bodies, trapped between the bone ends, cause further damage to the joint surfaces when the joint is loaded and the bone ends forced together. The damaged bone may also develop cavities, called *cysts* or *geodes*, weakening the bone (Fig. 13.19).

Traditionally, OA is considered a disorder of the synovial cartilage, but as described previously, changes are also seen in the bone underlying the cartilage, and also in the synovial fluid and in the tissues of the joint capsule, which can contribute to deformity of the joint. OA is generally considered a non-inflammatory arthritis, but measurable levels of inflammatory cytokines, including interleukins and prostaglandins, are found in the synovial fluid. In addition, the synovial fluid contains significant levels of **metalloproteinases**, degradative enzymes responsible for breaking down the matrix of joint tissues. In the early stages, the joint cartilage swells and its cellular activity increases, as chondrocytes respond to, and attempt to repair, the damage. This stage may be prolonged (over years) in mild disease, during which time the individual is asymptomatic. Later, however, the ability of the chondrocytes to compensate for the ongoing pathological changes is exhausted. The production of new cartilage slows, and the cartilage becomes fissured, flaky, and soft. Its proteoglycan content is reduced, progressively compromising the ability of the residual cartilage to cope with mechanical stress.

Signs and symptoms
The wide range of joints that may be affected, and the range of severity of the disease gives a wide spectrum of clinical presentations. Pain is very common, as is morning stiffness and limited range of movement. There may be indications of systemic inflammation, with increases in some acute phase reactants and in erythrocyte sedimentation rate. There may be joint effusions, deformity, and instability because of erosion of the joint surfaces. Involvement of the interphalangeal joints and the carpometacarpal joints can manifest as painless swellings at the joint site (**Heberden nodules** at the distal interphalangeal joints and **Bouchard nodules** at the

proximal joints). **Crepitus**, a crunching or cracking noise when the joint is moved, is caused by the debris present in the joint fluid and the roughened surfaces of the joint structures grating together.

Management and prognosis
Management is symptomatic: controlling pain with non-steroidal anti-inflammatories and steroids, ice and heat treatments, and massage can all help. Weight loss if the knees are affected is important. There are no interventions proven to halt, reverse or prevent this disease.

RHEUMATOID ARTHRITIS

This is a chronic, progressive, systemic inflammatory condition of autoimmune origin. Rheumatoid disease can affect multiple organs (e.g., the heart [rheumatic heart disease]), but the joints are the main target. The female:male ratio is about 3:1, and the peak age of onset between 30 and 50 years. A positive family history with first-degree relatives increases risk, but the concordance in identical twins is less than 20%, showing that environmental factors are strong modifiers of this. There are racial differences in prevalence, although rheumatoid arthritis (RA) affects all populations across the world and its incidence is falling. Globally, the incidence is 3 in 10,000 people, but this is much higher in some races (5–6 in 100 people in some native American peoples, but very low in people of Chinese origin). Smoking is a recognised risk factor.

Pathophysiology
Specifically, the joint tissue targeted by the autoimmune processes in RA is the synovial membrane, which becomes inflamed and hyperproliferative because of the ongoing autoimmune response. The antigen in the synovial membrane responsible for generating the autoimmune response has not yet been identified. The synovial membrane is infiltrated with inflammatory and immune cells, including macrophages and T and B cells, which release a range of cytokines and mediators, including interleukins and TNFα. Osteoclasts are activated, promoting bone breakdown. Within the synovial membrane, B cells produce autoantibodies, including rheumatoid factor (RF). The autoantibodies and their

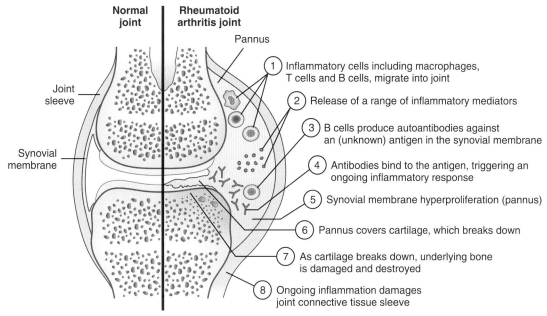

Fig. 13.20   Events in the rheumatoid joint.

target antigen form immune complexes (p.92) that deposit in the synovium, activating inflammatory cells and complement, and progressive synovial membrane hyperproliferation. B cells play a pivotal role in this disease, and therapies that suppress them also cause remission of RA.

The inflamed synovial membrane thickens and swells, filling the spaces in the joint cavity and initiating blood vessel growth into the expanding mass of new tissue (called **pannus**). It covers the joint cartilage, separating it from the synovial fluid that nourishes it and supplies it with oxygen, so the cartilage degrades, exposing the underlying bone, which then breaks down. It involves the connective tissues forming the joint sleeve, causing swelling and deformity. The uncontrolled inflammatory response therefore involves all joint structures, and the joint becomes swollen and painful, often with effusions of fluid collecting within (Fig. 13.20).

Signs and symptoms

Rheumatoid factors (RFs) are autoantibodies directed against IgG and are found in 75% of RA patients, although they are not diagnostic for this disorder because they are also found in other connective tissue autoimmune disorders including Sjögren syndrome and systemic lupus erythematosus. They are also found in up to 5% of healthy individuals. It is thought they are important in a healthy immune response for helping to clear immune complexes from the blood, but their function is not really understood. Their value in RA is as a prognostic indicator: the higher the RF levels, the more severe the disease.

There are indications of a systemic inflammatory response: C-reactive protein levels and erythrocyte sedimentation rates are elevated. Affected joints are swollen, red, painful, and limited in movement, and there may be rheumatoid nodules, firm swollen areas of soft tissue, usually at pressure points. Both sides of the body are usually affected. Most commonly, the small joints of the hands, wrists, and feet are involved initially, particularly the distal interphalangeal joints (Fig. 13.18B), but any synovial joint may be involved, with wasting

of associated muscles. Morning stiffness tends to improve with mobilisation as the day goes on. Deformity develops because of the swelling of the ongoing inflammatory process but also because the structures supporting the joint weaken and are unable to resist forces applied when the joint is loaded. Bursitis and tendinitis are often seen.

There may be extra-articular indications: interstitial lung disease, vasculitis, pericarditis, Sjögren syndrome, and carpal tunnel syndrome. Skeletal muscle wasting, related both to underuse and to muscle destruction caused by the systemic inflammatory response, is seen in two-thirds of cases.

Management and prognosis

There is no cure. Early diagnosis and prompt interventions can slow the progression of the disease and delay and/or limit disability. Although the disease is usually chronic and progressive, in some patients remission can be achieved, often for extended periods. Anti-inflammatory treatment with non-steroidal anti-inflammatory drugs and steroids are used. Disease-modifying anti-rheumatic drugs (DMARDs), especially methotrexate, slow down joint destruction by inhibiting one or more of the autoimmune mechanisms operating. Newer biologics, such as etanercept, block TNF-α.

JUVENILE IDIOPATHIC ARTHRITIS

Juvenile idiopathic arthritis (JIA) is an umbrella term including several acquired, heterogenous conditions featuring inflammatory joint changes that occur before 16 years of age and persist for more than 6 weeks. Included in this group are oligoarthritis, juvenile rheumatoid arthritis, psoriatic arthritis, and a range of less well-categorised conditions. Different subtypes of JIA have different underlying immune mechanisms, but irrespective of the underlying aetiology, the arthritis can cause permanent deformity and disability and may be associated with significant impact on normal psychological, social, physical, and educational development. Controlling the inflammatory response to prevent permanent joint deformity and damage is essential. Identifying the subtype of arthritis is important for therapeutic decision-making. Some forms of the disease can persist into adulthood, but the commonest form, oligoarthritis, which accounts for up to 60% of cases, usually resolves completely or goes into long-term remission, with no permanent disability.

INFECTIVE (SEPTIC) ARTHRITIS

A wide range of organisms may infect joints, introduced either from the bloodstream or from the external environment after trauma or surgical procedures. Bacterial infections are usually the most destructive. Identifying the causative organism so that appropriate antimicrobial treatment can be initiated is essential. The rates of infective arthritis rise with age, and risk factors include immunosuppression (e.g., with glucocorticoid therapy) and co-existing bone or joint disease/injury. Overall, *Staphylococcus aureus* is the most common culprit in acute cases at all ages.

Pathophysiology

Colonisation of joints by blood-borne organisms is not a random event, and some organisms are much more likely to establish themselves in joints than others. Microbes that possess surface receptors that match the adhesion factors present on the surface of joint tissues are most likely to be able to colonise here. *S. aureus*, for example, binds to a variety of connective tissues (including bone) because it expresses specific tissue adhesion molecules on its surface. Once infection is established, the inflammatory response that follows and the microbe's own pathogenic activity damages joint cartilage and the synovial membrane. This leads to pannus formation, further erosion of joint structures, effusions, and necrosis of the bone as blood supply is compromised.

Haematogenous (blood-borne) spread

This may arise when pathogens causing a range of infections elsewhere in the body—including tuberculosis, sexually transmitted diseases, and infective endocarditis—travel in the bloodstream, lodge in joint tissues, and establish new foci of infection. The commonest sexually transmitted organism causing infective arthritis is *Neisseria gonorrhoeae*. Intravenous drug users are most likely to develop *Pseudomonas aeruginosa* infective arthritis. **Lyme disease** is caused by the spirochaete *Borrelia burgdorferi*, which is carried by ticks that feed on mammals such as deer and sheep, but which also bite humans, transmitting the infection via their contaminated saliva. Up to 80% of people with untreated Lyme disease develop arthritis, which usually responds well to antibiotics.

Traumatic infection

This includes infection introduced after joint surgery and the implantation of prosthetics. The latter is the commonest cause of infective arthritis, and the incidence of infection post-joint replacement with an artificial joint is between 2% and 10% of patients. Traumatic injury to the joint is most likely to produce infection with a mixed culture or with anaerobic organisms.

SPONDYLOARTHRITIS

The spondyloarthritides are a group of chronic inflammatory joint conditions that do not feature significant synovial membrane involvement but in which the ligaments that hold the joint together, and the tendons that anchor associated muscles into the bones forming the joint, are inflamed. The term given to inflammation of the attachment sites of ligaments or tendons into bone is **enthesitis**, and this is a key feature of the spondyloarthropathies. They are immune-mediated, largely driven by an abnormal T-cell response to an antigen that has not yet been identified, but that may be an infecting organism. Risk is increased in people who express a particular type of HLA (p.91), HLA-B27.

Ankylosing spondylitis

This is the commonest spondyloarthropathy, affecting 0.1% to 1.4% of people worldwide, with a strong association with the HLA-B27 gene. There is a 3:1 male:female ratio and family clustering, and it usually arises before the age of 40. It is a systemic disorder, affecting organs and tissues throughout the body, and the joints usually involved are the sacroiliac joints and intervertebral joints (see Fig. 13.8C). There is significant enthesitis of the affected joints, with chronic joint inflammation, progressive destruction and fibrosis of joint tissues and ossification of joint structures. As ossification proceeds, the joint becomes progressively less mobile.

Signs and symptoms

Back pain is commonly the presenting symptom, along with spinal rigidity (Fig. 13.21). Involvement of the sacroiliac joint is characteristic of the disorder. Back pain and stiffness, usually worse in the morning, improve with exercise and as the day goes on. Non-joint-related problems include uveitis, cardiac conduction abnormalities, and respiratory problems caused by chest wall rigidity because of ossification of the cartilages attaching the ribs to the sternum.

Management and prognosis

Early diagnosis is very important for a good outcome because with a prescribed exercise programme, joint mobility and associated muscle strength can be maintained and the formation of bony tissue in the joint, responsible for much of the pain and limitation of joint range of movement, can be prevented. If this is achieved, prognosis is very good. Anti-inflammatory drugs and disease-modifying biologics including etanercept substantially reduce joint inflammation and improve function.

Psoriatic arthritis

Psoriasis, a common autoimmune inflammatory skin condition, involves the joints in about 10% of cases. There is a genetic component, particularly in HLA-B27 positive people. The pattern of joint involvement usually shows a polyarthritis (see Fig. 13.8D), with joints of the hands and feet frequently involved, particularly the proximal interphalangeal joints, where tissue destruction shows as a typical 'pencil in cup' appearance on X-ray. Use of standard anti-inflammatories must be carefully monitored because some (e.g., corticosteroids) may make the psoriasis worse. Methotrexate and TNF inhibitors such as etanercept are used and can generally induce extended remission.

Reactive arthritis

This is a sterile arthritis, an inflammatory reaction in joints secondary to a systemic infection. Such infections include *Salmonella*, *Shigella*, *Yersinia*, and *Chlamydia* species. Males are more often affected than females, and there is a strong

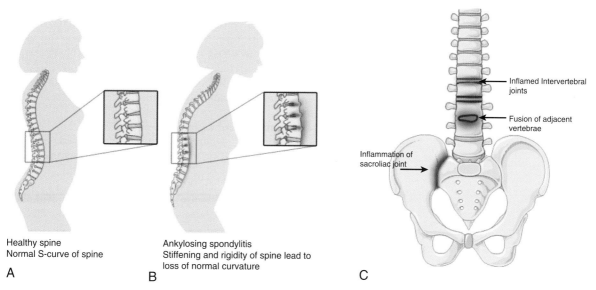

Fig. 13.21 Ankylosing spondylitis of the spine. (A) Normal. (B) Inflammation and fibrosis of the intervertebral joints distort the spine with loss of normal curvature. (C) Intervertebral joints and the sacroiliac joint are commonly affected. (Modified from Groen SS, Sinkeviciute D, Bay-Jensen A-C, et al. (2021) Exploring IL-17 in spondyloarthritis for development of novel treatments and biomarkers, *Autoimmunity Reviews* 20(3): 102760. https:// doi.org/10.1016/j.autrev.2021.102760.)

association with individuals carrying the HLA-B27 gene. It is thought that T cells in the affected individual, activated by the infection, mistakenly attack certain other body tissues, including the joints. Joints of the lower limb are usually affected, with pronounced enthesitis. Of all people with reactive arthritis, 70% recover fully but the condition may grumble on with the development of chronic arthritis. Recurrence is common, with up to 50% of cases relapsing, perhaps in response to reinfection or another stressor.

CRYSTAL-INDUCED ARTHRITIS

Crystals in the synovial fluid may arise for several reasons. Whatever the origin, the tiny crystals are ingested by phagocytes, triggering release of a range of inflammatory mediators and initiation of an ongoing inflammatory response.

Gout

Hyperuricaemia causes precipitation of uric acid crystals in various tissues, including the joint spaces. Arthritis caused by uric acid deposition in the joints is called *gout*. It is five times more common in men than women, usually presents after the age of 50, runs in families, and is associated with obesity, diabetes, and high-protein, fat, and sugar diets. The reason diet is important in the pathogenesis of gout is that uric acid is the end breakdown product of purines, found in high concentrations in rich foods.

Hyperuricaemia may be caused by reduced excretion of uric acid, often as a result of diuretic therapy (because, in order to increase water excretion, diuretics disturb the function of pumps and carriers in the nephron, including inhibiting uric acid excretion). It may also occur because of increased production of uric acid. This may be secondary to a diet high in purines and alcohol, which increases uric acid levels because of their metabolism, or some cancers. Some individuals have inherited conditions that impair uric acid excretion or increase its production.

Pathophysiology

The joint usually affected is the first metatarsophalangeal joint (i.e., the joint at the base of the big toe). The crystals stimulate phagocytic activity in the joint; the activated phagocytes release a raft of inflammatory mediators, which initiate and perpetuate a powerful inflammatory response. **Tophi**, white deposits of uric acid crystals, develop around the joint and may also appear at other body sites: the skin of the ear or the fingers, or over the Achilles tendon, for example. They are painful and unsightly and may ulcerate.

Signs and symptoms

The presentation is usually of acutely painful localised arthritis. The joint is swollen, red, and excruciatingly tender. Other consequences include uric acid kidney stones, as uric acid precipitates out in the kidney, ureters, or bladder, and about 20% of people with gouty arthritis eventually develop renal failure.

Management and prognosis

If not treated, gout completely obliterates the joint. Anti-inflammatory drugs are useful, as is colchicine, which works by inhibiting phagocyte activity and therefore dampening down the inflammatory response. Dietary controls are essential, limiting intake of red meat, shellfish and other seafood, alcohol, and sugary foods and drinks. Weight control is important.

Pseudogout

In this condition, the crystals precipitating into the joint are of calcium pyrophosphate. The cause is not known, although there is an association with hyperparathyroidism, but incidence increases with age.

Pathophysiology

Possible aetiological mechanisms include age-related decline in proteoglycan content of joint cartilage. Proteoglycans inhibit mineral deposition, and so a reduction in proteoglycan content could allow minerals to be deposited in the joint and to crystallise out into synovial fluid and joint tissues. As with gout, the activation of phagocytic cells to remove the crystals leads to a self-sustaining inflammatory reaction. This disorder usually involves multiple joints, although it can be monoarticular, and a wide range of joints can be affected, most commonly the knee.

Management and prognosis

There is no cure, and no treatments proven to inhibit crystal formation. Treatment is supportive, and ultimately the disorder can lead to significant joint destruction, deformity, and loss of function.

Other crystal-related arthritides

Degeneration of intraarticular prosthetic structures can seed synovial fluid with tiny particles that elicit a similar inflammatory response to uric acid and calcium pyrophosphate crystals.

In health, soft tissues—muscle, tendons, cartilage, ligaments—are not mineralised. If normal inhibitors of mineralisation fail (e.g., if proteoglycan content of these tissues falls), then calcium phosphate salts, the normal minerals deposited in bone, can be laid down inappropriately in other tissues. If joint-related structures such as joint cartilage, tendons, or ligaments are involved, it produces a form of arthritis called *basic calcium phosphate deposition disease*. The inflammatory changes follow a similar process to those already described previously.

DISORDERS OF CONNECTIVE TISSUE

Connective tissue plays an essential part in supporting and protecting the muscle and bone of the musculoskeletal system, and its biology is discussed in Chapter 1. Osteogenesis imperfecta, an inherited disorder of type I collagen, is described on p.46. Marfan syndrome is described on p.44.

EHLERS-DANLOS SYNDROME

This group of at least 19 different disorders is caused by the production of faulty collagen, classified into 13 different types. The disorders are inherited, and each is characterised by a different genetic mutation and a different collagen defect. As a result, each disorder has a different clinical presentation. It is rare; the incidence is estimated at 1 in 400,000 people. It is equally distributed between the sexes, and there is no significant racial predisposition.

Pathophysiology

The commonest form of Ehlers-Danlos syndrome, joint hypermobility syndrome, is classified as type III and is associated with faulty types II and IV collagens. In many people, the hypermobility causes no problems but in others it causes joint dislocations and musculoskeletal pain. Type IV Ehlers-Danlos is also called the *vascular type* because it affects type III collagen and leads to fragile blood vessel, uterine, and gastrointestinal walls.

Signs and symptoms

Joint hypermobility is common. The skin may be fragile and hyperextensible. If blood vessels are involved, there may be postural hypotension because blood vessel walls are more distensible than normal and so the normal baroreceptor reflex does not adequately compensate for the fall in blood pressure when standing up suddenly. There may be problems with balance, locomotor control, and bladder control. Tooth development is poor (collagen is a key ingredient of dental enamel and the gum tissue).

Management and prognosis

There is no cure. Treatment, if required, manages symptoms, including analgesics and physiotherapy.

THE MUCOPOLYSACCHARIDOSES

Glycosaminoglycans (GAGs; p.4) were originally called *mucopolysaccharides*, and the group of inherited disorders caused by faulty GAG breakdown are called the *mucopolysaccharidoses*. There are seven variants, numbered I to VII, each of which is caused by a fault in a particular gene that codes for a specific enzyme in the pathways that degrade GAGs. The best characterised, and one of the most severe, is Hurler syndrome, a subtype of type I. The conditions are associated with accumulation of GAGs in the tissues, causing coarsening and thickening, joint stiffness, skeletal deformities, mental retardation, and corneal clouding. The disorders are progressive, and affected babies may appear normal at birth but begin to show developmental delays and abnormalities in the first few months of life. All but one (Hunter syndrome, which is sex-linked and classified as type II mucopolysaccharidosis) are inherited as autosomal recessive conditions. Affected children usually die before the age of 10, usually because of cardiovascular complications caused by the abnormal connective tissue architecture.

SPRAINS, FRACTURES, AND OTHER MECHANICAL INJURY

Mechanical injury to musculoskeletal tissues is common because they are constantly subject to physical stressors. It should be noted, however, that under normal physiological conditions, these stressors are essential for maintaining healthy bone and muscle. Exercise strengthens muscle tissue; the forces applied through bone from the pull of muscles and high-impact exercise increases bone deposition, thickening and strengthening it. Muscle that does not work atrophies and weakens; bone that is not subjected to physical stress loses mass and is prone to fracture. Bone and muscle tissue both have a generous blood supply and should heal well after injury, whereas tendons and ligaments have no intrinsic blood supply and rely on diffusion of nutrients from extracellular fluids. Although this section considers mechanical injury and repair of the musculoskeletal tissues separately, bear in mind that often injury to one involves injury to others.

LOW BACK PAIN

Back pain is one of the commonest events that takes an individual to a medical professional and, in the Western world, is the most frequent reason given for taking time off work. This reflects the global picture; worldwide, more disability is caused by low back pain than any other condition. It is estimated that four out of five human beings experience low back pain at some time in their lives. The costs to society in lost workdays and healthcare interventions are enormous and, as the global population ages, will continue to rise.

Most low back pain is caused by strain or sprain of the musculoskeletal structures in the lower back (muscle, ligaments, tendons, intervertebral discs) by age-related degeneration or vertebral fracture. Other, rarer, causes include metastatic deposits, Paget disease, the temporary spinal loading associated with pregnancy, or arthritis of the intervertebral joints. The condition may present as a short-lived acute event, usually secondary to an identified injury, or, more commonly, as a chronic and relapsing condition. Risk factors include overweight or obesity, and activities associated with an unhealthy lifestyle (smoking, poor diet, high alcohol consumption, poor sleep, and a sedentary lifestyle) are all associated with an increased risk of low back pain.

Pathophysiology

The lumbar spine is subject to constant loading because it bears the weight of the upper body plus any objects being carried. In addition, it experiences constant mechanical stress associated with spinal flexion, extension, and rotation. Forward bending, particularly if associated with twisting and/or lifting a heavy object with outstretched arms, places the greatest stress on the lower spine. The intervertebral discs are compressed, and the muscles and ligaments supporting the spinal column are stretched and strained. Even minor tears or damage in these structures elicit a local inflammatory response, which is likely to become chronic because the loading continues. In addition, it has been shown that injury to vertebral discs sensitise local nerves to mechanical stimuli, enhancing their response and increasing inflammation and pain. If discs are swollen or prolapsed, their associated spinal nerves may be compressed, with shooting pains into the buttock or down the leg.

Management and prognosis

Management of the condition varies enormously depending on the severity of the condition and the resources available. Most individuals recover fully in 2 to 4 weeks from acute events, with rest, non-steroidal anti-inflammatories, application of ice or heat, and gradual remobilisation.

PLANTAR FASCIITIS

This condition, which can cause disabling heel pain, is caused by inflammation of the insertion of the plantar ligament, the thick, web-shaped ligament into the calcaneus of the heel. It links the calcaneal tuberosity to the heads of the metatarsals at the metatarsophalangeal joints (Fig. 13.22). This ligament maintains the arched shape of the foot, acts as a shock absorber in walking and running, and contributes to transmission of forces through the bones of the foot in normal locomotion. If it stretches and loosens, the arch of the foot sinks, giving flat foot. In plantar fasciitis, the ligament is damaged, usually because of repetitive microinjuries, associated for example with high-impact sports such as running. Other risk factors include obesity, poorly supportive footwear, and ageing. In sport-related injury, the surface underfoot plays a part: softer surfaces, for instance grass in football, are less likely than hard surfaces (e.g., as in clay court tennis) to be associated with the condition.

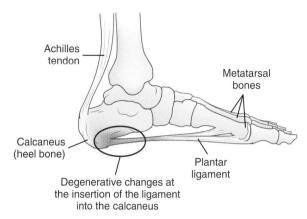

Fig. 13.22 The plantar ligament in plantar fasciitis.

Pathophysiology

The condition presents, often very suddenly, with acute heel pain on the under surface of the heel because this is the area of the ligament, at the ligament/bone interface, that is affected. Plantar fasciitis, like tennis elbow (see below) and the spondyloarthropathies (see previous), is therefore an enthesopathy. There is little inflammatory contribution to this disorder, however, and the pathological changes are primarily degenerative. Over time, with repeated mechanical stress, the ligament degenerates and becomes fibrotic, losing its ability to absorb shock and to contribute to the biomechanics of normal walking and running.

Signs and symptoms

Pain is usually experienced with the first few steps after rest and improves with ambulation. In more severe cases, however, pain may worsen again over the course of the day, especially if the individual is walking or standing for long periods. Pain is relieved by unloading the affected foot but worsened by walking barefoot or on hard surfaces.

Management and prognosis

With appropriate treatment (orthotics and taping for support, stretching exercises, steroid injections, and occasionally surgery) the prognosis is usually excellent and the condition resolves completely.

TENNIS ELBOW (LATERAL EPICONDYLITIS)

This condition is caused by repetitive and excessive mechanical loading of tendons that attach muscles that extend the wrist and supinate the forearm, including the extensor carpi radialis brevis and the extensor carpi ulnaris (Fig. 13.23). The muscles that pull on these tendons produce wrist extension and forearm supination, and excessive, repetitive use of these muscles causes microtrauma in the tendons that attach them to the lateral epicondyle of the humerus. Although commonly called *tennis elbow* because it is relatively frequent in tennis players, any activities that involve repetitive arm movements, including golf, computer use, heavy lifting, or gardening also predispose. There is pain, stiffness, and tenderness of the affected joint, but, as with plantar fasciitis, the principal pathological changes are degenerative, not inflammatory. The condition usually resolves completely with rest, ice, and anti-inflammatory treatment.

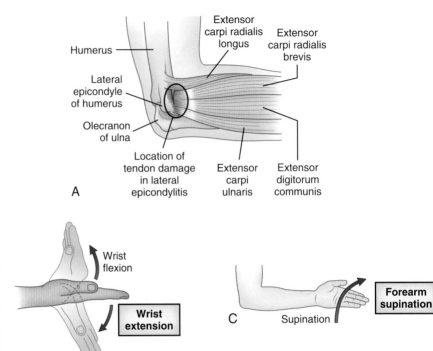

Fig. 13.23 The structures affected in lateral epicondylitis. (Modified from (A) Mansfield P and Neumann D (2019) *Essentials of kinesiology for the physical therapist assistant*, 3rd ed, Fig. 6.16. St Louis: Mosby; (B) Mosby (2022) *Mosby's medical dictionary*, 11th ed, Fig. 18.21. St Louis: Mosby; (C) Mansfield P and Neumann D (2019) *Essentials of kinesiology for the physical therapist assistant*, 3rd ed, Fig. 1.14. St Louis: Mosby.)

MUSCLE INJURY

Skeletal muscle tissue is cemented into bone by tendons. Tendon and bone are both more robust tissues than muscle, and muscle injury is common. Muscle tissue can suffer an acute injury, from a single traumatic event that directly damages the muscle (e.g., overstretching, crushing, or cutting). Much muscle injury, however, is caused by chronic wear and tear, especially in repetitive exercise, and this results in microtrauma, with multiple microtears in the muscle.

Muscle strain. Muscle strain is muscle tearing caused by excessive mechanical loading. The muscle cells themselves are ruptured. Minor strains involve only a small number of fibres within the muscle, so although it is painful, function is preserved. Severe strains involve complete separation of the muscle fibres from their tendon, or complete tearing of the muscle into two separate parts, usually across the belly of the muscle. In this situation, it completely loses function.

ROTATOR CUFF INJURY

The rotator cuff muscles and their tendons form a supportive sleeve around the glenohumeral (shoulder) joint, formed by the head of the humerus and the glenoid cavity of the scapula. This ball-and-socket joint is the body's least stable joint, the downside of having the greatest range of motion. As a result, it is the most frequently dislocated. The four muscles forming the rotator cuff are the **supraspinatus**, the **infraspinatus**, the **teres minor**, and the **subscapularis** muscles. All four have their origins on the scapula, and their insertion on the humerus, helping hold the head of the humerus firmly in the shallow cup of the glenoid cavity (Fig. 13.24). They are used in a range of arm movements, and injury is common. Increasing age is a risk factor, but repetitive overhead movement (e.g., in tennis or volleyball players, house painters, or carpenters) can cause chronic injury even in younger people.

BONE INJURY

Healthy bone is highly resistant to damage because its high inorganic crystal content makes it very strong, and its internal scaffolding of collagen fibres allows it to absorb shocks and reduces the risk of shattering. However, it breaks if enough force is applied, particularly at vulnerable points (e.g., the neck of femur) or with a lateral blow to the shaft of a long bone. A break in bone, even if it does not completely separate the bone into two or more pieces, is called a *fracture*.

TYPES OF FRACTURE

Fractures are classified according to the cleanness of the break, the angle of the fracture, and whether the broken bone ends emerge through the skin. These are summarised in Fig. 13.25.

Stress fractures. Bone is continually subjected to mechanical stress. In healthy bone, the continued turnover of bone replaces older, less strong bone with new bone. However, repetitive activity, especially with heavy loading (e.g., in intensive sports training), allows minor trauma to accumulate with inadequate time to repair. Eventually, the bone becomes so weak it fractures. This is called a *stress fracture*, and the commonest sites for these fractures are the lower limbs because they receive the greatest degree of mechanical loading. Risk factors include female sex (testosterone enhances bone deposition), poor nutritional status, and low body weight (bone and muscle mass are reduced in light people because they are subjected to less force than in those with higher body weight). Treatment is rest, physiotherapy, and gradual remobilisation.

Pathological fractures. These are fractures resulting from pre-existing bone disease in which the bone is already weakened and predisposed to fracture. Examples include metastatic bone disease, Paget disease, and osteoporosis.

Fractures involving an active growth plate. In a growing child's bone, a fracture involving the growth plate can

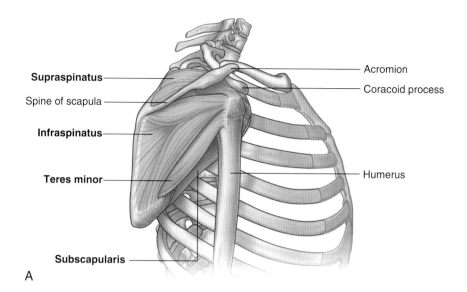

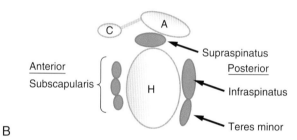

Fig. 13.24 The muscles of the rotator cuff. (A) Viewed from the side. (B) Sagittal section showing the relationship of the muscles to the head of humerus (H), coracoid process of the clavicle (C), and acromion of the scapula (A). (Modified from (A) Drake R, Vogl AW, and Mitchell A (2020) *Gray's anatomy for students*, 4th ed, Fig. 7.9. Philadelphia: Elsevier Inc; and (B) Helms C (2020) *Fundamentals of skeletal radiology*, 5th ed, Fig. 10.1. Philadelphia: Elsevier Inc.)

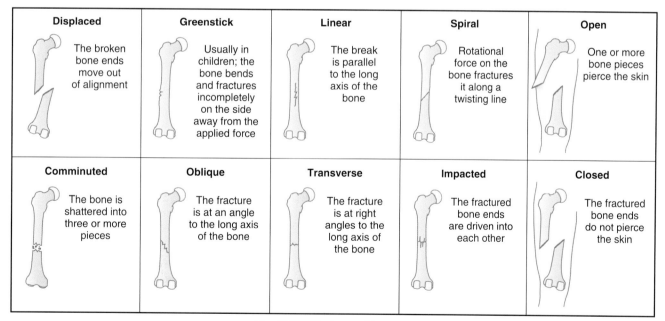

Fig. 13.25 The types of fractures.

disrupt normal bone development, leading to deformity or shortening of the bone. This is more likely if the child is young, with many growing years in front of him, and in major fractures with serious damage to a growth plate.

BONE FRACTURE AND ITS HEALING

The stages of fracture healing are illustrated in Fig. 13.26. In Fig. 13.26A, immediately after fracture, there is bleeding at the fracture site, forming a large mass of clotted blood called a *haematoma*. Depending on the extent of the injury and the degree of blood vessel damage, parts of the local bone, deprived of its blood supply, becomes ischaemic and then necrotic. An intense inflammatory response leads to vasodilation, local swelling, and recruitment of large numbers of inflammatory cells—including lymphocytes, neutrophils, mast cells, and macrophages—into the site. In Fig. 13.26B,

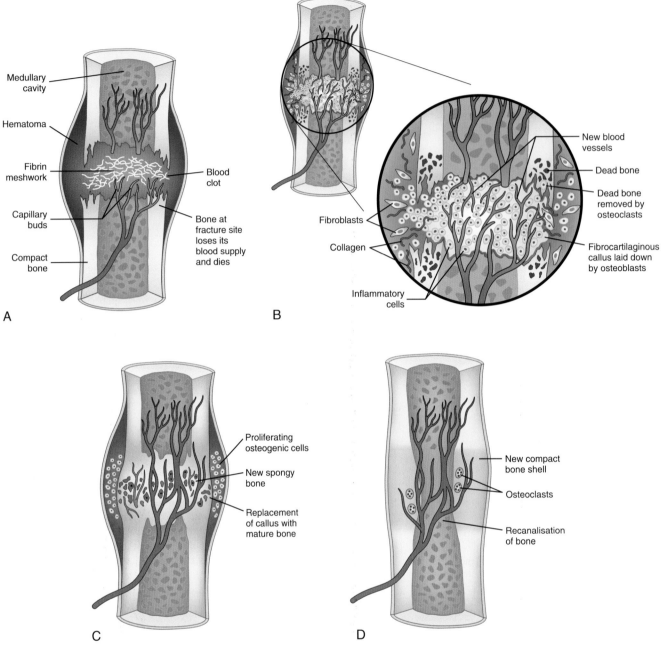

Fig. 13.26 The stages of fracture healing. (A) Immediately post-fracture haematoma formation. (B) Callus deposition at the fracture site. (C) Conversion of callus to mature bone. (D) Restoration of original bone structure.

the haematoma provides a framework for ingrowth of new blood vessels. In addition, the platelets within the clot and infiltrating fibroblasts, lymphocytes, and macrophages release growth factors such as platelet-derived growth factor and fibroblast growth factor that stimulate osteoprogenitor cells in the bone linings to differentiate into osteoblasts. In addition, osteoclast activity is increased, to rapidly break down and clear away damaged bone. Osteoblasts lay down large quantities of new cartilaginous matrix called *callus*, which will be converted into bone later in the repair, and the osteoclasts remove dead and dying bone to make way for the new tissue being produced. In Fig. 13.26C, callus linking the ends of the fractured bone is converted to mature spongy bone. The blood vessel network continues to develop and

mature. In Fig. 13.26D, usually about 2 weeks post-fracture, the architecture of the original bone is restored, with compact bone laid down around the bone perimeter, gradually strengthening the repair. Over the following weeks, the callus is remodelled to the bone's original form with recanalisation of the central cavity and repair of the bone lining (endosteum) and the bone covering (periosteum). Repair usually takes 4 to 6 weeks, but this can be extended in serious fracture and when there are factors present that interfere with healing.

Factors that interfere with fracture healing

Uncomplicated healing of bone fracture usually restores full function, although final remodelling can take years and there may always be some swelling or deformity at the fracture site. Factors interfering with healing include the following:

Poor blood supply. This may be because a major artery was damaged by the fracture so that a large area of bone tissue is deprived of its blood supply, or because the fractured bone had a poor blood supply to start with (e.g., the lower tibia).

Infection. Infection delays healing because an ongoing immune response directed at eliminating infection opposes repair processes. Open fractures are much more likely than closed fractures to become infected: up to half of open fractures become infected, compared with 2% of closed fractures. *Staphylococcus aureus*, a common skin commensal, is a frequent cause of open fracture infection, and other organisms either present in the local environment (e.g., soil organisms if soil has contaminated the wound) and hospital-acquired pathogens are also potential culprits.

Displaced, separated, or mobile bone ends. If the ends of the fractured bone are not close together, or if they are separated by damaged soft tissues, foreign bodies from the injury or fragments of bone, the healing process cannot adequately bridge the gap. If the displaced bone ends are not well aligned, healing may not take place, and even if it does, the healed bone may be deformed. Movement of the bone ends relative to one another during healing damages the new blood vessel network, reducing the blood supply and slowing the healing process. In addition, it breaks up the callus forming in the gap, interrupting the union of the bone ends.

Poor bone health. Bone in poor health before fracture heals more slowly than healthier bone, and fractures in older people heal more slowly than in youth.

Nutritional and lifestyle factors. Fractures in smokers heal more slowly than in non-smokers. Non-steroidal anti-inflammatory drugs and corticosteroids both inhibit healing and slow fracture repair. Individuals with poor nutritional status heal more slowly than normal.

Delayed union or non-union

Slower-than-normal healing (also called *delayed union*) can be a result of any of the factors described previously. Non-union is defined as a failure of the bone ends to form a bony union after a period of 6 months, usually because they are too far apart. If the bone ends are otherwise healthy, surgical intervention to bring them into proper alignment can lead to healing.

JOINT INJURY

Repetitive joint movements cause wear and tear of joint surfaces and can weaken and stretch joint ligaments.

Sprains. A sprain is a stretching or twisting injury to a ligament, usually because the joint in question has been taken beyond its normal range of motion.

SPRAINED ANKLE

The commonest joint that suffers sprains is the ankle. The connective tissues of the joint hold the distal ends of the tibia and fibula against the talus, the most proximal tarsal bone. These bones fit tightly together and limit the movement of the joint to flexion and extension of the foot. This joint transmits the entire weight of the body through the foot to the ground and is highly stable, provided that body weight loads the joint centrally (e.g., in normal walking). However, if the body weight is shifted laterally or medially, causing the foot to turn inwards or outwards, this stretches the medial and lateral ligaments. This can be an acute injury, such as an awkward landing in sport, or can result from an accumulation of wear and tear, again, an injury most commonly sustained in sports. Recovery usually restores full function, although there is an increased likelihood of future sprains as the damaged ligaments are generally slightly stretched and looser than before.

BIBLIOGRAPHY AND REFERENCES

Berrih-Aknin, S. (2017). Role of the thymus in autoimmune myasthenia gravis. *Clinical and Experimental Neuroimmunology, 7,* 226–237.

Bertrand, J., & Held, A. (2017). Role of proteoglycans in osteoarthritis. In S. Grässel, & A. Aszódi (Eds.), *Cartilage volume 2: Pathophysiology.* Springer.

Buchanan, B. K., & Varacallo, M. (2020). *Tennis elbow (lateral epicondylitis), StatPearls 2020.* https://www.ncbi.nlm.nih.gov/books/NBK431092/.

Gdowski, A. S., Ranjan, A., & Vishwanatha, J. K. (2017). Current concepts in bone metastasis, contemporary therapeutic strategies and ongoing clinical trials. *Journal of Experimental & Clinical Cancer Research, 36,* 108.

Kim, B. J., Lee, S. H., & Koh, J.-M. (2018). Bone health in adrenal disorders. *Endocrinology and Metabolism, 33,* 1–8.

Lips, P., & van Schoor, N. M. (2011). The effect of vitamin D on bone and osteoporosis. *Best Practice & Research Clinical Endocrinology & Metabolism, 25,* 585–591.

Macedo, F., Ladeira, K., Pinho, F., et al. (2017). Bone metastases: An overview. *Oncology Reviews, 11,* 321.

Misaghi, A., Goldin, A., Awad, M., & Kulidjian, A. A. (2018). Osteosarcoma: A comprehensive review. *SICOT-J, 4*(12). https://doi.org/10.1051/sicotj/2017028.

Nyary, T., & Scammell, B. (2018). Principles of bone and joint injuries and their healing. *Surgery, 36*(1), 7–14.

Orchard, J. (2012). Plantar fasciitis. *BMJ, 345,* 34–40.

Prakken, B., Albani, S., & Martini, A. (2011). Juvenile idiopathic arthritis. *Lancet, 377,* 2138–2149.

14 Disorders of Reproductive Function

CHAPTER OUTLINE

INTRODUCTION
The female reproductive system
 Female reproductive anatomy
 The female reproductive cycle
 The breast
The male reproductive system
 Male reproductive anatomy
 Regulation of sperm production
 The penis
SEXUALLY TRANSMITTED INFECTION
Bacterial sexually transmitted infections
 Chlamydia
 Gonorrhoea
 Syphilis
Viral sexually transmitted infections
 Genital herpes simplex
 Human papilloma virus
Parasitic sexually transmitted infections
 Trichomoniasis
DISORDERS OF FEMALE REPRODUCTION
Disorders of hormonal function
 Menstrual disorders
 Polycystic ovarian syndrome

Developmental and structural abnormalities
 Endometriosis
 Uterine prolapse
Inflammatory conditions
 Pelvic inflammatory disease
 Bartholinitis
 Cervicitis, vaginitis and vulvitis
Growths and tumours
 Uterine tumours
 Breast tumours
 Ovarian cysts and tumours
DISORDERS OF MALE REPRODUCTION
Developmental and structural abnormalities
 Cryptorchidism (undescended testes)
 Phimosis and paraphimosis
 Testicular torsion
Inflammatory conditions
 Prostatitis
 Orchitis and epididymitis
Growths and tumours
 The penis
 The scrotum and testes
 The prostate gland

INTRODUCTION

Human beings reproduce sexually: that is, new individuals are created by fusing two gametes, one from the father and one from the mother, each of whom contributes a selection of his or her own genetic material to their new baby. Sexual reproduction ensures genetic diversity because each gamete from each parent contains an essentially random selection of that parent's genes, so that every newborn baby (with the exception of identical siblings) has a different assortment of genetic material than any other human being who has ever lived. Because sexual reproduction allows a species to evolve and adapt in response to changing environmental conditions, it favours the survival of that species.

The male and female reproductive organs, collectively, are designed for three main functions:

- Production and storage of gametes: the female ova and the male sperm
- Transmission of male sperm into the female reproductive tract, where fertilisation of the female ovum takes place
- Provision of a safe environment for the development and delivery of a healthy full-term fetus

THE FEMALE REPRODUCTIVE SYSTEM

The external genitalia are collectively called the *vulva* (Fig. 14.1A). The internal reproductive tract includes the ovaries, the uterine tubes, the uterus (including the uterine cervix), and the vagina (Fig. 14.1B).

FEMALE REPRODUCTIVE ANATOMY

The organs of the internal reproductive tract are nestled in the pelvic cavity, supported by the muscles and ligaments of

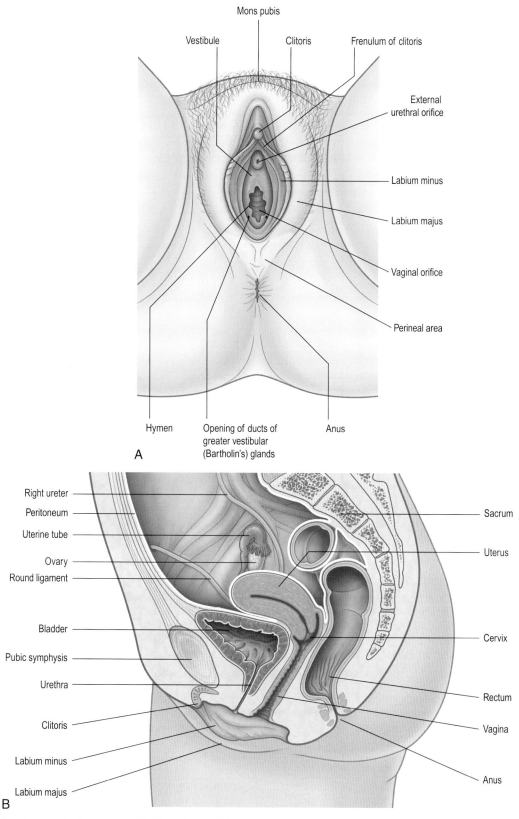

Fig. 14.1   The female reproductive system. (A) The vulva. (B) The internal organs. (Modified from Waugh A and Grant A (2018) *Ross & Wilson anatomy and physiology in health and illness*, 13th ed, Figs. 18.2 and 18.3, Oxford: Elsevier Ltd.)

the pelvic floor, and anchored to each other and the inside of the body wall by a range of ligaments and membranes. The urethra and vagina pass through the pelvic floor on their way to the exterior.

The vulva

The vulva (Fig. 14.1A) consists of the **labia minora** and the **labia majora**, folds of skin that enclose the vaginal opening, the urethral opening, and the glans clitoris. The glans clitoris, analogous to the male penis, is a small body of erectile tissue richly supplied with sensory nerves and important for sexual pleasure. The greater vestibular glands (of Bartholin) are paired glands lying one each side of the vagina, whose ducts open into the vaginal orifice and which secretes mucus to lubricate it during sexual intercourse.

The vagina

This fibromuscular tube, about 10 cm long, extends from the exterior to the cervix, which protrudes into the distal end of the vagina at an angle (Fig. 14.1B). This means the anterior vaginal wall is shorter (7.5 cm) than the posterior wall (9 cm). It is lined with stratified epithelium for protection.

The uterus and uterine cervix

The uterus is a pear-shaped organ anchored in the pelvic cavity by ligamentous attachments (Fig. 14.2). It is sandwiched between the urinary bladder in front and the rectum behind, and is tilted forward, curving over the upper surface of the bladder (Fig. 14.1B) Its walls are mainly composed of smooth muscle, the **myometrium**, and are lined with **endometrium**, composed of glandular tissue and a complex, cell-rich supporting stroma (Fig. 14.2B). The endometrium is made up of two layers: the functional layer, which proliferates and sheds regularly with the menstrual cycle; and the basal layer, which is not shed and is responsible for generating the functional layer in response to circulating sex hormones. The outer layer of the uterus, the serosa or **perimetrium**, encloses the organ in a protective pouch.

For convenient description, the uterus is divided into two sections: the upper two thirds, or body of the uterus; and the lower third, the cervix (neck) of the uterus, which is narrower than the body and provides the channel through which sperm travel and a baby is delivered. The myometrium of the body of the uterus is thick, to produce the powerful contractions required at delivery, but the cervix has little smooth muscle and is composed mainly of elastic and fibrous connective tissue. The opening into the cervix is called the **cervical os** and leads into the internal cervical canal (the **endocervix**). The portion of the cervix facing into the vagina is called the **ectocervix**.

The squamocolumnar junction and cervical erosion

The endocervix is lined with columnar epithelium rich in mucus-secreting glands. However, this is unsuitable for covering the ectocervix and lining the vagina because these structures are exposed to the friction and physical abrasion of sexual intercourse. They are therefore lined with a more robust stratified squamous epithelium, which is better suited for protection. The junction between the two is called the **squamocolumnar junction**, and the change

from one epithelial cell type to another is very clear under the microscope (Fig. 14.3A). In prepubescent girls, it lies within the cervical canal (Fig. 14.3B). However, at puberty, under the influence of oestrogen, the glandular columnar epithelium becomes more extensive, and can appear on the ectocervix as a reddened area around the os (Fig. 14.3C). This is sometimes referred to as a cervical erosion, although the tissue is not damaged in any way: it is simply an extension of the normal columnar epithelium of the endocervix.

The low pH of the vagina irritates the columnar epithelium exposed on the ectocervix and induces hyperplasia and metaplastic changes (p. 65). This region of transformed cells, called the *cervical transformation zone* (Fig. 14.3C), is less stable, and vulnerable to further neoplastic change: this is the most common site for the development of cervical carcinoma (see below p. 366).

Positions of the uterus

In most women, the uterus is **anteverted**, meaning that it leans forward relative to the vagina, resting on the superior surface of the urinary bladder. There is also an angle between the body of the uterus and the cervix, contributing to its forward—leaning position—this is called **anteflexion**. In 10% to 15% of women, the uterus leans backwards relative to the vagina: this is called **retroversion**. If there is also a backwards bend on the cervix-body junction, this is called **retroflexion** (Fig. 14.4).

The ovary

The female gonads, called the *ovaries*, are paired organs suspended within the pelvic cavity by folds of peritoneum and anchored to the uterus by the ovarian ligament. They lie one on each side of the uterus and are formed of a central area of tissue called the *medulla* surrounded by the outer layer, called the *cortex*. At birth, the cortex contains large numbers of **primordial follicles**, each of which contains a primary oocyte, from which the secondary oocyte is released at ovulation during a normal reproductive cycle (Fig. 14.5). After puberty and establishment of a regular menstrual cycle, maturation of the primordial follicles is controlled by hypothalamic and anterior pituitary hormones, and the follicles themselves become mini endocrine glands, secreting sex steroids. Generally, at any one time, several primordial follicles are undergoing maturation but usually only one develops into the tertiary follicle that releases its oocyte mid-cycle at ovulation.

THE FEMALE REPRODUCTIVE CYCLE

Puberty initiates multiple, significant changes in a young woman's reproductive physiology. Under the influence of hormones from the hypothalamus and pituitary gland, the breasts develop and enlarge, and pubic and axillary hair appear. The reproductive cycle, including the ovarian and uterine (menstrual) cycles, are established (Fig. 14.6). The average reproductive cycle lasts 28 days and is usually measured from the first day of the menstrual period, but in health the duration of the cycle can vary from 21 to 35 days. During the first half of the cycle, one or more primordial follicles in the ovary reach maturity; at about day 14 of a 28-day cycle the secondary oocyte is released in the process of ovulation. The empty follicle, now called the

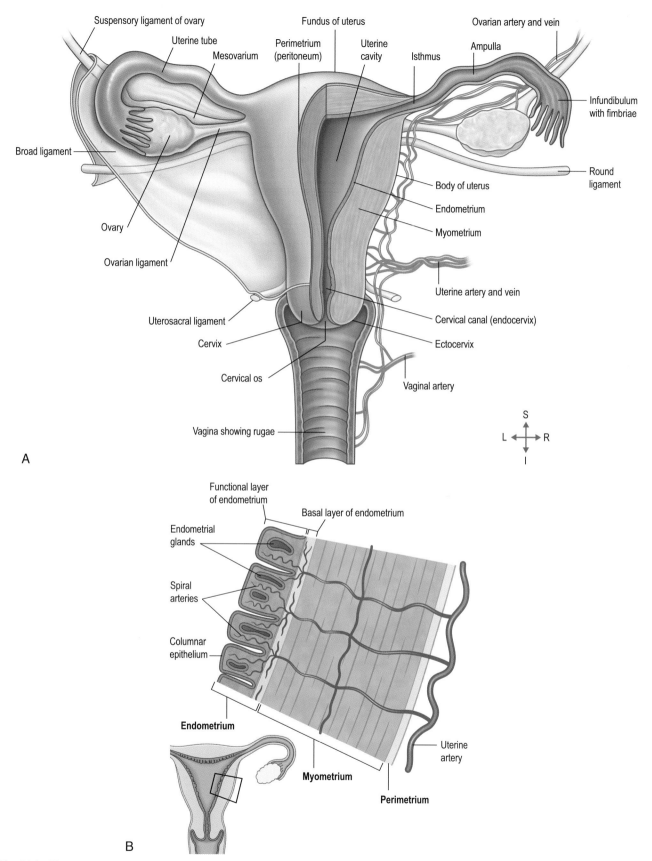

Fig. 14.2 The structure of the uterus. (A) The uterus and its associated structures. (B) Section through the uterine wall. (Modified from Waugh A and Grant A (2018) *Ross & Wilson anatomy and physiology in health and illness*, 13th ed, Figs. 18.4 and 18.5, Oxford: Elsevier Ltd.)

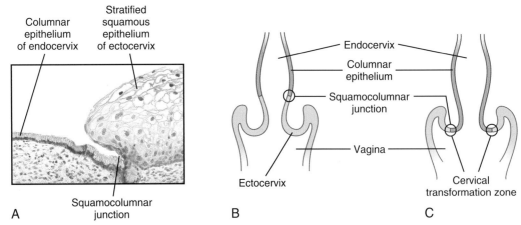

Fig. 14.3 The squamocolumnar junction. (A) The clear transition between the columnar epithelium of the endocervix and the stratified epithelium of the ectocervix. (B) Before puberty, the squamocolumnar junction is located within the cervical canal. (C) After puberty, the squamocolumnar junction is located on the ectocervix. ((A) Modified from Bibbo M and Wilbur D (2009) *Comprehensive cytopathology*, 3rd ed, Fig. 8.1, Edinburgh: Saunders.)

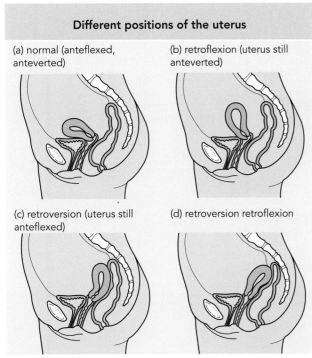

Different positions of the uterus

(a) normal (anteflexed, anteverted)

(b) retroflexion (uterus still anteverted)

(c) retroversion (uterus still anteflexed)

(d) retroversion retroflexion

Fig. 14.4 Positions of the uterus. (A) Normal: forward tilt (anteversion) and slightly bent forwards (anteflexion). (B and C) Retroversion and anteflexion: tilted backwards but with a slight forward bend. (D) Retroversion and retroflexion: tilted and bent backwards. (Modified from Epstein O, Perkin GD, Cookson J, et al. (2008) *Clinical examination*, 4th ed, Fig. 8.32. Edinburgh: Mosby Ltd.)

corpus luteum, is visible on the ovarian surface, and, assuming no pregnancy results from ovulation, degenerates into a small white scar (corpus albicans) over the remaining fourteen or so days of the cycle (Figs. 14.5 and 14.6A). The uterine endometrium thickens and becomes rich in nutrient-secreting glandular tissue to receive and nourish any fertilised oocyte, but if there is no resulting pregnancy, it degenerates and is shed as the monthly period (Fig. 14.6C). Towards the end of the cycle, the breasts may become swollen and engorged, which is usually relieved with the onset of menstruation.

Hormones and regulation of the female reproductive cycle

The ovarian, uterine and breast changes of the reproductive cycle summarised previously are regulated by a range of hormones secreted by the hypothalamus, the anterior pituitary, and the follicles in the ovarian cortex. Hypothalamic hormones, travelling through the portal circulation of capillaries linking the hypothalamus to the anterior pituitary, stimulate the release of key hormones from this gland, which in turn regulate follicular development and ovulation. As the follicle develops throughout one reproductive cycle, it releases the oestrogen and progesterone that initiate changes in the breast and uterine lining associated with the different stages of the cycle.

The ovarian cycle

During a 28-day cycle, one or more follicles proceed towards maturity in the first 14 days. This is driven by follicle stimulating hormone (FSH), released from the anterior pituitary, in response to hypothalamic release of gonadotrophin releasing hormone (GnRH; see Fig. 10.3). As the follicle develops and enlarges, it releases increasing quantities of oestrogen (Fig. 14.6B), which feeds back on the pituitary and stimulates continued release of FSH. About day 12, oestrogen levels become so high that they trigger a change in pituitary secretion, and the pituitary releases a surge of luteinising hormone (LH), which triggers ovulation (Fig. 14.6C).

The empty follicle, now called the *corpus luteum*, continues to function as a mini endocrine gland, but although it releases some oestrogen, its main hormonal product is progesterone. Rising progesterone and oestrogen levels suppress the anterior pituitary, and FSH levels drop. This is important, as the egg may have been fertilised and there may be a pregnancy on the way, in which case follicular development needs to be temporarily suspended. If pregnancy does not occur, the corpus luteum begins to degenerate and progesterone and oestrogen levels start to fall. The pituitary, released from their inhibitory influence, begins to produce FSH again and a new cycle begins.

The menstrual cycle

The uterus also undergoes clear cyclical changes in parallel with the ovarian cycle (Fig. 14.6D). In the first half

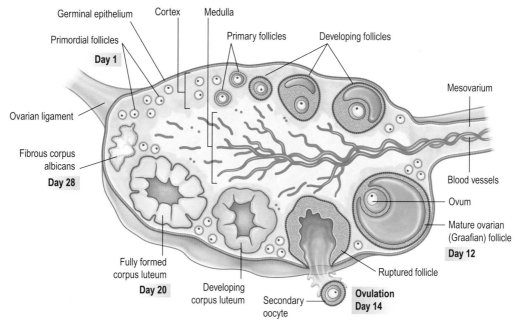

Fig. 14.5   Internal structure of the ovary. The development of a follicle during one ovarian cycle is shown. (Modified from Waugh A and Grant A (2018) *Ross & Wilson anatomy and physiology in health and illness*, 13th ed, Fig. 18.7. Oxford; Elsevier Ltd.)

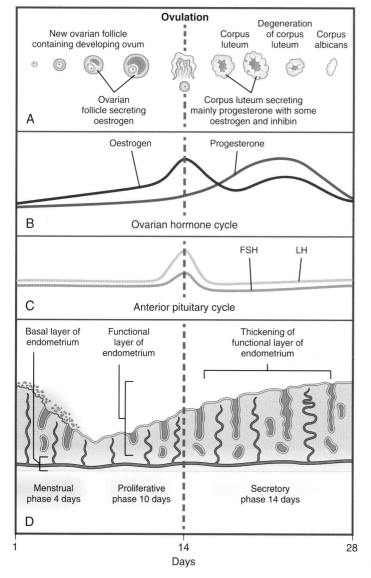

Fig. 14.6   Events of the female reproductive cycle. (A) Ovarian cycle: maturation of follicle and development of the corpus luteum. (B) Ovarian hormone cycle: oestrogen and progesterone levels. (C) Anterior pituitary cycle: luteinising hormone (LH) and follicle stimulating hormone (FSH) levels. (D) Uterine cycle: menstrual, proliferative, and secretory phases. (Modified from Waugh A and Grant A (2018) *Ross & Wilson anatomy and physiology in health and illness*, 13th ed, Fig. 18.10. Oxford; Elsevier Ltd.)

of the cycle, under the influence of rising oestrogen, the functional layer of the uterine lining rapidly thickens and becomes more vascular. This is called the *proliferative phase.* After ovulation, in response to rising progesterone levels, the nature of the functional layer changes: proliferation stops, glycogen is deposited, and the endometrium becomes highly glandular, producing nutritious secretions in anticipation of implantation of a fertilised egg. This is called the *secretory phase.* If pregnancy does not occur, falling hormone levels from the dying corpus luteum leads to shedding of the functional layer as the menstrual period.

THE BREAST

Both males and females have breasts, but the male breast has no reproductive function. The female breast contains a large number of secretory lobules that produce milk, numerous lactiferous ducts to carry the milk to the nipple, and supporting adipose tissue and ligaments (Fig. 14.7). The ducts and glands are lined with epithelium, which is frequently the site of malignant change in breast cancer.

The shape, size, and feel of the breast vary significantly with each stage of the reproductive cycle because oestrogen triggers changes in breast tissue. In the days just before the onset of menstruation, the breast may be swollen and engorged and even painful because of oestrogen-induced breast oedema. Oestrogen also induces cell division in the breast, peaking at around day 22 to 24 of an average 28-day cycle, although increased apoptosis at the end of the cycle returns cell numbers to normal.

THE MALE REPRODUCTIVE SYSTEM

The main structures of the male reproductive system are shown in Fig. 14.8.

MALE REPRODUCTIVE ANATOMY

Males produce sperm in paired organs called **testes**, suspended in the scrotal pouch from the front of the body by the **spermatic cords**. Spermatozoa are stored in the **epididymis** until ejaculation, at which time they are forcibly ejected

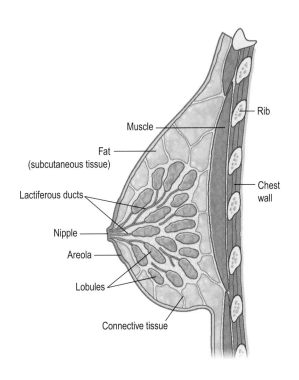

Fig. 14.7 The female breast. (Modified from Waugh A and Grant A (2018) *Ross & Wilson anatomy and physiology in health and illness*, 13th ed, Fig. 18.12. Oxford; Elsevier Ltd.)

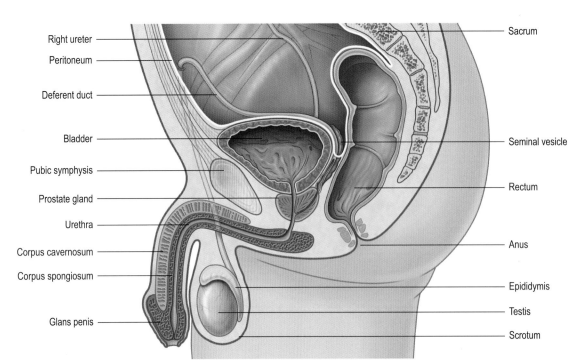

Fig. 14.8 The male reproductive system. (Modified from Waugh A and Grant A (2018) *Ross & Wilson anatomy and physiology in health and illness*, 13th ed, Fig. 18.13. Oxford; Elsevier Ltd.)

from the reproductive tract by co-ordinated contractions of the muscular walls of the passageways of the tract: from the epididymis, through the vas deferens (deferent duct), the ejaculatory duct and the urethra. The prostate gland, the seminal vesicles, and the bulbourethral glands add specialised fluid to the ejaculate.

The testes

The testis is suspended in its scrotal sac by the spermatic cord, which is anchored in the groin. It runs through the inguinal canal and carries the arteries, veins, nerves and lymphatic vessels supplying structures in the scrotum, plus the deferent duct, bundled in a sheath of connective tissue. Each testis contains about 250 lobules, separated from each other by sheets of connective tissue called septa. Each lobule contains between one and four **seminiferous tubules**, coiled tubes in which spermatozoa are produced from germ cells called **spermatogonia**. The seminiferous tubules are embedded in interstitial tissue that contains blood vessels and smooth muscle, which propels the spermatozoa from the testes towards the epididymis. Here also are specialised Leydig cells that produce testosterone (Fig. 14.9).

Each testis is wrapped in three membranous layers. The outermost layer, the **tunica vaginalis**, is a double layer that is the remnants of the pouch of peritoneal membrane in which the testis descends during fetal development. The outer (parietal) layer of the tunica vaginalis, which lines the inside of the scrotal sac, is simply a continuation of its inner (visceral) layer. The tunica vaginalis therefore forms a closed bag into which the testis is pushed like a fist into a water balloon. Collections of fluid in this closed bag cause hydrocele. The **tunica albuginea**, lying within the tunica vaginalis, is a tough, collagen-rich membrane for protection, and is lined by the **tunica vasculosa**, a delicate layer of loose connective tissue rich in blood vessels.

Testosterone

This is the principal androgen (male sex hormone). It is produced in boys in increasing amounts, mainly by the developing testis, triggering puberty, and drives the development and maturation of the male internal and external genitalia, the development of male secondary sexual characteristics and the production of spermatozoa in the seminiferous tubules. It stimulates anabolic tissue growth, driving the growth spurt seen at puberty, and maintains bone mass and muscle mass in the adult male. It is the key hormone in maintaining male libido. In certain body organs, including the prostate gland and the liver, testosterone is metabolised to dihydrotestosterone (DHT) by the enzyme 5α-reductase. DHT is significantly (about nine times) more potent than testosterone itself and is important in the pathogenesis of benign prostatic hypertrophy. Testosterone levels decline slowly with age, but there

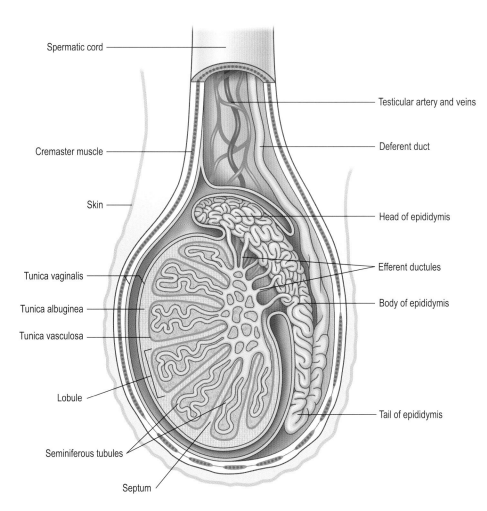

Spermatic cord

Cremaster muscle

Skin

Tunica vaginalis

Tunica albuginea

Tunica vasculosa

Lobule

Seminiferous tubules

Septum

Testicular artery and veins

Deferent duct

Head of epididymis

Efferent ductules

Body of epididymis

Tail of epididymis

Fig. 14.9 The testis. (Modified from Waugh A and Grant A (2018) *Ross & Wilson anatomy and physiology in health and illness*, 13th ed, Fig. 18.14. Oxford; Elsevier Ltd.)

is no equivalent of the female menopause, and healthy males may remain fertile well into old age.

THE PROSTATE GLAND

This gland, about the size of a walnut, sits immediately below the urinary bladder (Fig. 14.8). It consists of glandular tissue bedded in a stroma containing fibrous connective tissue and smooth muscle, which propels its secretions into the urethra during ejaculation. The urethra passes through it on its way to the penis, and so does the ejaculatory duct, formed when the deferent duct and the duct from the seminal vesicle unite. Prostatic secretions contribute about a third of the total volume of semen, are slightly acidic, and contain prostate specific antigen (PSA), an enzyme that liquefies the coagulated semen when it is deposited in the vagina, to facilitate the swimming action of the sperm and allow them to travel into the uterus.

REGULATION OF SPERM PRODUCTION

In the healthy male, from puberty onwards, sperm are produced from the **spermatogonia** lining the seminiferous tubules. Continual spermatogonia cell division both maintains their population and provides a constant supply of spermatogonia that enter the spermatozoa differentiation cycle. In the testes, under the influence of testosterone, spermatogonia differentiate into **spermatocytes**. Spermatocytes undergo meiotic division (p. 54) to produce **spermatids**. Under the influence of Sertoli cells, sometimes called *nurse cells*, spermatids further mature into **spermatozoa**, which undergo final maturation, including acquiring full motility, in the epididymis. Overall, producing a mature spermatozoon from its originator spermatogonium cell takes about 64 days.

THE PENIS

The penis consists of two main sections: the glans penis (the head of the penis) and the shaft. The glans penis is covered with a retractable sleeve of tissue, called the prepuce or foreskin. Below the foreskin is a large number of small sebaceous glands that secrete smegma, a creamy white oily substance that mixes with dead skin cells and lubricates the movement of the foreskin over the glans. The root of the penis, the attachment of the penis to the body, anchors it to the pubic symphysis by two suspensory ligaments. The penis contains two elongated **corpora cavernosa**, which contain spongy erectile tissue and run together from the perineum down the shaft of the penis. They fill with blood during sexual activity, to bring the penis to its erect state. Lying immediately below these paired chambers is the **corpus spongiosum**, which is also composed of spongy erectile tissue, and encloses the urethra, which runs from the urinary bladder in the pelvis, down the shaft of the penis, and opens to the exterior at the tip of the glans penis at the external urethral meatus (Fig. 14.10). The urethra provides the pathway for excretion of urine and also for the ejaculation of semen at sexual climax.

SEXUALLY TRANSMITTED INFECTION

Sexually transmitted infection (STI) is an increasing global problem, with the incidence rising in all countries, in all socioeconomic groups and in all age groups. World Health Organisation data (2021) estimates that 1 million new cases of STIs arise daily, of which the main ones are chlamydia, gonorrhoea, syphilis and trichomoniasis. STI transmitted from mother to child infects the next generation, sometimes with devastating results, including stillbirth, neonatal death, congenital deformities and life-threatening infections in the baby. Although STIs primarily affect the reproductive organs, causing local inflammation and sometimes infertility, many also have systemic effects, destroying other organs and tissues of the body. The risk of bacterial STI increases the risk of contracting HIV threefold or more, and the sexually transmitted human papilloma virus (HPV) is a direct cause of cervical and head and neck cancer. Effective treatment of STI is increasingly hampered by emerging microbial resistance to the main antimicrobials used, especially by strains of *Neisseria gonorrhoeae*. Identification and appropriate treatment can be delayed or missed altogether if the infection

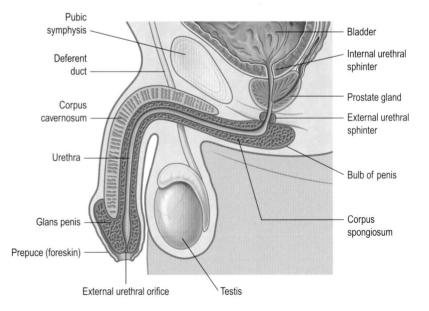

Fig. 14.10 Internal structure of the penis. (Modified from Waugh A and Grant A (2018) *Ross & Wilson anatomy and physiology in health and illness*, 13th ed, Fig. 18.17B. Oxford; Elsevier Ltd.)

is asymptomatic, which is often the case in many STI, especially in the early stages. Embarrassment and fear of social stigma may also deter people from seeking early help.

The risk of contracting an STI is directly related to increasing numbers of sexual partners, engaging in high-risk activity such as not using barrier contraception, and in the selection of high-risk partners. STI may be transmitted by intimate contact, not necessarily involving full sexual intercourse, and all these factors contribute to the high rates of STI occurring in adolescents and young people. Adolescent females in particular are at particular risk because of cervical cell immaturity. Rates of most STIs fall in people in their 30s and 40s, reflecting a reduction in the number of sexual partners as many people enter long term monogamous relationships, but increase again in older people, who may be on the dating scene again after divorce or the death of a long-term partner. Older people are also less likely to consider themselves at risk and are immunologically more susceptible because of age-related decline in immune function.

BACTERIAL SEXUALLY TRANSMITTED INFECTIONS

Globally, the majority of clinically significant STI is of bacterial origin.

CHLAMYDIA

Worldwide, this is the commonest STI, and is the commonest cause of blindness. It is caused by members of the *Chlamydia* genus of bacteria, of which *C. trachomatis* is the main one involved in STI. There are 18 strains of *C. trachomatis*, of which subtypes A, B, and C are associated with conjunctivitis and D–K with reproductive tract infections.

Pathophysiology

Chlamydiae are obligate intracellular parasites, meaning they need to be inside another living cell to grow and divide. These bacteria have a unique (for bacteria) life cycle (Fig. 14.11): their metabolically active, reproductive stage takes place within a host cell, on which they rely for a nutrient supply and for their ATP (energy) production. Chlamydial cells exist in two main forms, the elementary body and the reticulate body. The elementary body is highly infectious, survives outwith host cells, but cannot divide. Elementary bodies attach to receptors on the target host cell and are endocytosed (transported into the host cell). Within their host cell they convert to reticulate bodies, which multiply. This produces up to 1,000 new elementary bodies. When the host cell is lysed by its expanding bacterial load, it releases elementary bodies into the local environment. These attach to neighbouring body cells and are endocytosed through the new host cell plasma membrane, where their development cycle begins again.

After an incubation period of 5 to 10 days, there is an acute, purulent, exudative inflammatory response in infected tissues. The organism preferentially infects columnar epithelium, so the lining of the respiratory and genitourinary tracts, and the conjunctiva, are favoured sites. The inflammatory response leads to fibrosis and scarring, causing problems in ocular infections and permanently blocking tubes and passageways in both male and female reproductive tracts. Many cases are asymptomatic.

In both sexes, the inflammation is widespread within the genitourinary tracts: urethritis, cervicitis, endometritis, salpingitis and pelvic inflammatory disease in women and urethritis, proctitis, and epididymitis in men. In pregnancy, infection can cause abortion, miscarriage, or premature birth.

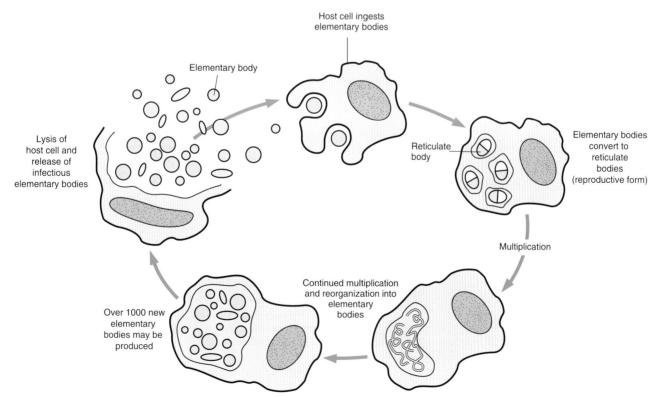

Fig. 14.11 The life cycle of chlamydia. (Modified from Mahon C and Lehman D (2019) *Textbook of diagnostic microbiology*, 6th ed, Fig. 24.1. St. Louis; Saunders.)

Signs and symptoms

The infection is asymptomatic in up to 75% of women and 50% of men. In women, it causes a purulent cervical discharge, which bleeds more readily on gentle probing than normal, so there may be post-coital bleeding. The infection may spread upwards and involve the endometrium and uterine tubes, causing pelvic inflammatory disease. The first indication of the infection may be failure to conceive because of tubal fibrosis and stricture. The risk of ectopic pregnancy rises because the ovum travels more slowly through a restricted and narrowed uterine tube, and implantation of a fertilised ovum occurs before it reaches the uterus. In men, urethritis may cause pain or discomfort on urination, and upward spread of the organisms, with fibrosis of the reproductive tubing, can reduce fertility.

Management and prognosis

Prompt antibiotic treatment, usually with azithromycin or doxycycline, is generally curative. Some cases resolve spontaneously but leave the genitourinary tract permanently damaged. Post-infection complications include reduced fertility, infertility, and arthritis. A baby born to an affected mother can be infected as it passes through the birth canal at delivery, with neonatal eye infection and pneumonia the most common complications. Current research in the hunt for a vaccine, some of which is at the stage of clinical trials in human volunteers, appears increasingly promising.

GONORRHOEA

This STI generally follows a more severe clinical course than chlamydia. The causative organism, *Neisseria gonorrhoeae*, is quite selective in the tissue it infects: it colonises superficial mucosal membranes lined with columnar epithelium, which includes the upper respiratory tract, the conjunctiva and much of the genitourinary tracts (excluding the vagina, except in younger girls whose vaginal epithelium is immature). The term gonorrhoea derives from the Greek terms for gonos (seed) and rhoia (flow, seen in other terms such as *amenorrhoea* and *diarrhoea*), referring to the constant

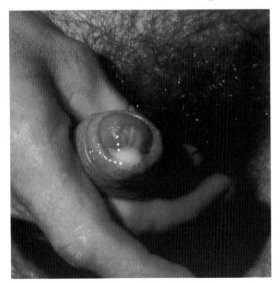

Fig. 14.12 Gonorrhoea. Mucopurulent discharge from the penis. (From Harris P, Nagy S, and Vardaxis N (2010) *Mosby's dictionary of medicine, nursing and health professions: Australian & New Zealand edition*, 2nd ed, Fig. 7.61. Sydney; Mosby Australia.)

discharge of purulent material from the penile tip (Fig. 14.12).

Pathophysiology

There are different subtypes of *N. gonorrhoeae*, which differ in their virulence and in their sensitivity to different antibiotics. The incubation period is short, less than a week.

Signs and symptoms

Shortly after infection, males and females experience discharge from the penis or the vagina respectively, or from other body orifices involved in sexual activity (the throat or the anus). Sometimes, in females, the anus may be infected because of its proximity to the vaginal opening, even without anal penetration. In females, upward spread from the infected cervix leads to uteritis, salpingitis, and pelvic inflammatory disease, with abdominal pain and sometimes fever. Because the distal ends of the uterine tubes open directly into the peritoneal cavity, organisms have direct access into the peritoneal space, and can cause abscess formation, peritonitis, and hepatitis. Newborns may be infected during childbirth, including neonatal conjunctivitis and respiratory infections. In men, the urethritis causes pain on urination, and sometimes haematuria. Ascending infection in the male tract causes epididymitis. In either sex, anal involvement leads to proctitis, pruritis and rectal discharge. Contamination of the eye causes conjunctivitis. The organism may spread in the bloodstream and cause dermatitis, septic arthritis, meningitis, or pericarditis.

Management and prognosis

Antibiotic treatment can be curative, but microbial resistance is an increasing problem. Penicillin, the original drug of choice, is used less and less because penicillin-resistant strains of the organism are now ubiquitous. Post-infective complications include reduced or lost fertility. There may be residual complications secondary to arthritis, meningitis, pericarditis, or other systemic manifestations of the infection. Affected babies may be blinded by the conjunctival infection unless it is rapidly treated.

SYPHILIS

This disorder is caused by the bacterium *Treponema pallidum*. Bacteria from the genus *Treponema* also include *T. pertenue*, which causes the tropical infection yaws. *Treponema* species are spirochaetes, meaning they are long, slender, corkscrew-shaped, single-celled organisms. The first documented outbreak occurred in Naples in the 1490s, suggesting that Christopher Columbus brought the disease back to Europe from the Americas earlier in that decade, after which it spread very rapidly in a population with no natural resistance. Although it is contracted mainly by sexual activity, transmission can also follow direct contact with contaminated body fluids, contaminated blood transfusions, and vertical mother to child in utero infection (congenital syphilis). Syphilis is a multisystem disorder associated with widespread and progressive tissue destruction of any of the body's organs. The incidence of syphilis had been declining since the beginning of the twentieth century, accelerated by the discovery of penicillin, although it is rising again in many parts of the world, including the United States.

Pathophysiology

T. pallidum was first isolated in 1905 but does not survive without its human hosts, including in laboratory conditions. This makes it difficult to study and explains why such intimate contact or direct transmission of contaminated fluids or tissues is required for infection. *Treponema* are actively motile bacteria, possessing whip-like flagellae at one end, helping its dissemination through body tissues, usually through lymphatic channels. The organism can be detected in tissues distant from the site of infection very quickly after infection, showing how fast it can travel in a short time. The incubation period from infection to the appearance of the first sign, usually a painless sore (chancre) on the genital area at the site of inoculation, is usually 2 to 3 weeks but can be up to 3 months. Damage to arteries, including the aorta, is a common feature of all stages of syphilis, and impairs blood supply to affected organs. The progress of the disease usually follows three stages: primary, secondary, and tertiary syphilis (Fig. 14.13).

Primary syphilis. This is the initial **chancre**, a painless lesion with raised edges, and is highly infectious. Associated lymph nodes may also swell. The chancre heals in the following weeks.

Secondary syphilis. The next stage follows 4 to 10 weeks after the appearance of the primary chancre. In the intervening time, the spirochaete has been proliferating and invading body organs, and the clinical picture in secondary syphilis can be quite variable. There may be systemic manifestations, including fever, fatigue, and malaise, but localised problems depend on which organs are most significantly colonised. Of all patients with secondary syphilis, 75% present with a rash featuring small, reddish brown macular lesions that may extend to the palms of the hands and the soles of the feet. Half of patients have generalised lymphadenopathy, reflecting the widespread distribution of the bacteria. There may be meningitis, alopecia, hepatitis, and gastrointestinal inflammation. The signs and symptoms of secondary syphilis subside within a few months and the disease becomes quiescent (the latent phase). In the later stages of latency, the patient becomes non-sexually infectious, although *T. pallidum* is still detectable in the blood and the infection may still be transmitted transplacentally to a fetus. About two-thirds of patients experience no further symptoms.

Tertiary syphilis. A minority of patients progress from secondary to tertiary syphilis, sometimes after a latency of many years. This is characterised by chronic inflammatory tissue destruction and the appearance of **gummas**, granulomatous lesions with rubbery edges and a central necrotic area, which are very slow to heal. Gummas can affect tissues throughout the body, including bone, mucous membranes, testes, and liver. About 80% of cases involve the cardiovascular system, particularly the aorta and the aortic valve. Up to 10% experience chronic neurological destruction (neurosyphilis), either because the spirochaete has directly invaded the central nervous system, or because it has damaged the arteries supplying it.

Immunological changes in syphilis

Although affected people usually develop some immunity to the disease, including the production of anti-*Treponema* antibodies, it is incomplete and is inadequate to clear the infection. This immune response can become disordered; some of the tissue damage (e.g., gummas) seen in late syphilis is caused by a delayed type (type IV) hypersensitivity response to a range of tissue antigens. Syphilis sufferers produce a selection of autoantibodies, including rheumatoid factor and antibodies to blood cells.

Management and prognosis

Untreated syphilis causes significant morbidity and mortality-syphilis is one of the very few STIs capable of killing its host. If treated at either the primary or secondary stage, the prognosis is usually good. Tertiary syphilis responds less reliably to antibiotic treatment, and tissue damage is irreversible. The antibiotic of choice is penicillin.

Congenital syphilis. *T. pallidum* crosses the placenta after the first trimester of pregnancy and can cause miscarriage or stillbirth. Untreated maternal syphilis results in 90% transmission. If the baby is born alive, indications of infection can be evident at birth or become evident as the baby gets older. Because the spirochaete does not cross the placenta during the first trimester, the key period for organogenesis, the body systems and organs are all laid down

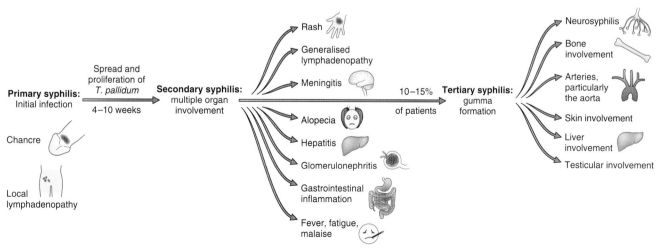

Fig. 14.13 The stages of syphilis.

before infection and so affected babies show the same sort of clinical pattern as in secondary syphilis. Congenital manifestations include a range of skeletal abnormalities from intrauterine bone infection, skin rashes, deafness from damage to the 8th cranial nerve, and visual defects from damage to the retina and cornea. The baby may have ongoing infections, such as meningitis and bone/cartilage infections.

VIRAL SEXUALLY TRANSMITTED INFECTIONS

Viruses are generally fragile and survive poorly without their host cells, so the direct exchange of body fluids in the intimate activity of sexual intercourse facilitates their transmission.

GENITAL HERPES SIMPLEX

Herpes simplex virus (HSV) is a member of the herpesvirus family (p. 21). Two closely related subtypes of HSV cause head and neck and genital infections. Both have worldwide distribution. HSV-2 is associated with genital herpes. HSV-1 is more usually associated with cold sores but may also cause genital herpes, especially in some subpopulations, including young people. HSV-2 tends to be more virulent and reactivates more frequently and more severely. Genital herpes infection is more likely in immunocompromised people and in those with large numbers of sexual partners, and reactivation is associated with periods of stress, such as cold weather, infection or other illness, sunlight, psychological stress or menstruation. In turn, HSV infection increases the risk of contracting other STIs, including HIV. Women are more likely to be infected than men because male-female transmission is more likely than female-male during sexual intercourse.

Pathophysiology

The latent period is usually less than a week, but it can be as long as 3 weeks. Many cases are subclinical and produce no significant symptoms. On initial infection, there may be fever, malaise, and headache. HSV replicates within epithelial cells, creating painful or itchy characteristic blister-like vesicles of the genital epithelium that rupture to form intensely painful ulcers (Fig. 14.14) Herpetic vesicles may occur wherever contaminated sexual fluids come into contact with the skin surfaces: on the external genitalia, including the vulva in women and the penis in men, and the anus and perineum if anal intercourse is practiced. Both sexes may experience urethritis and dysuria, and the genital area becomes swollen and inflamed. The virus migrates from the initial site of infection to local sensory nerves, and travels by axonal transport to the sacral root ganglia, where it is protected from attack by the immune system. Periodic reactivation leads to further outbreaks of blistering. Active disease may be associated with local lymph node enlargement. Occasionally, HSV-2 causes encephalitis, which is potentially life-threatening. Neonatal HSV infection is very serious and needs prompt treatment. It is almost always acquired when the baby passes through an infected birth canal at delivery. Untreated, over half of affected babies die. Even with anti-viral treatment at birth, the child can be left with significant neurological deficit, develop sepsis and/or infections, primarily of the liver and respiratory tract.

Management and prognosis

There is no cure, although anti-viral treatment can alleviate attacks. Prevention is not straightforward because the virus is so widespread, full sexual intercourse is not required for infection and barrier contraceptives are not fully protective.

HUMAN PAPILLOMA VIRUS

As with HSV, human papilloma virus (HPV) infection is widespread and often asymptomatic. There are several subtypes, all of which invade epithelial cells and induce proliferation, producing warts in different areas of the body (e.g., the common verruca and genital warts). The most serious consequence of HPV infection is cancer. Worldwide, 4.5% of all cancers are attributable to HPV, with a significant female preponderance of 8.6% compared with 0.8% in men. HPV causes nearly all cases of cervical cancer, and a significant number of other anogenital cancers (vulval, vaginal and anal malignancies) and oropharyngeal cancers.

Pathophysiology

HPV triggers the production of multiple flat warts on the genitalia, most frequently in the anal areas (Fig. 14.15), but also on the penis, labia, clitoris, and perineum. Orogenital sexual contact can lead to orolaryngeal warts (increasing the risk of orolaryngeal squamous cell cancer associated with this infection). They are usually painless, but they can be itchy, bleed easily, and interfere with sexual penetration, and they can become very large and unsightly, with a cauliflower-type growth pattern.

Management and prognosis

Anti-HPV vaccination has already proven to be cost-effective in countries where it has been implemented, including the UK, Canada, and Australia. Rates of HPV infection, plus the incidence of anogenital warts and pre-cancerous cervical changes, have plummeted. Prevention is clearly the ideal. Current WHO recommendations are to vaccinate girls in the 9 to 14 age bracket, with the aim of inducing immunity

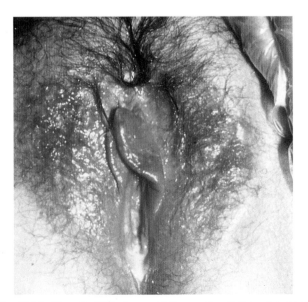

Fig. 14.14 Herpetic blistering and inflammation of the vulva. (From Mutter G and Prat J (2014) *Pathology of the female reproductive tract*, 3rd ed, Fig. 3.34. Oxford; Churchill Livingstone.)

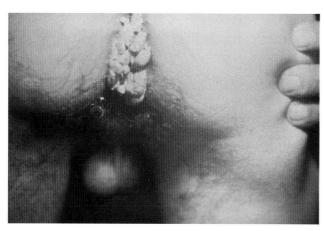

Fig. 14.15 Human papilloma virus induced anal warts. (Courtesy Dr. Wiesner, Centers for Disease Control and Prevention, Public Health Image Library, Atlanta, GA.)

to the virus before their becoming sexually active. Existing warts may be treated with cryotherapy or surgically removed, or treated with salicylic acid, acetic acid, or other preparations, which may eliminate them but may also simply reduce them in size.

PARASITIC SEXUALLY TRANSMITTED INFECTIONS

TRICHOMONIASIS

The causative organism, *Trichomonas vaginalis*, is a flagellated anaerobic protozoan which mainly infects squamous epithelial tissue. It thrives in the vaginal environment but is also occasionally found in the urethra (in both men and women). The parasite attaches itself to the epithelium and causes inflammation, associated with a foul-smelling yellow/green discharge, pruritis and pain. The standard treatment is a single dose of the antimicrobial drug metronidazole.

DISORDERS OF FEMALE REPRODUCTION

Physiologically, the female reproductive tract, and control of female reproductive function, is more complex than the male. This, along with the consequences of reproductive disease on the fetus, gives a wide range of female reproductive disorders.

DISORDERS OF HORMONAL FUNCTION

The regulation of the female reproductive cycle, described previously, relies on a sophisticated network of communication between the key structures involved. The hypothalamus, anterior pituitary and ovary are responsible for synthesis and release of the key female sex hormones, which control structural and functional changes of the ovary, uterus, and breast. Disturbance of this carefully regulated crosstalk by a faulty endocrine response can disrupt the system so badly that fertility is lost.

MENSTRUAL DISORDERS

On average, during the normal monthly period, about 40 mL of blood is lost, although this is highly variable. Excessive flow (over 80 mL) can be caused by high circulating oestrogen or may be associated with uterine fibroids or infection. Persistent heavy flow can quickly lead to anaemia, unless steps are taken to replace the iron being lost. Dysmenorrhoea (painful cramping associated usually with the onset of a period) in the absence of an identified cause, is thought to be associated with high levels of prostaglandin $F2_\alpha$ released in the uterine wall during menstruation. Because of this, non-steroidal anti-inflammatory drugs are generally effective in treating the pain because they work by inhibiting prostaglandin production. Underlying conditions that can cause dysmenorrhoea include endometriosis, pelvic inflammatory disease, infection (including infection caused by an intrauterine device) and uterine fibroids.

Amenorrhoea

Amenorrhoea, the absence of monthly bleeding, may be classified as primary or secondary. **Primary amenorrhoea** is the failure of menstruation to begin in girls under the age of 16. **Secondary amenorrhoea** is when menstruation stops for 6 months or more in a woman who had previously been menstruating normally since puberty. It occurs naturally in pregnancy, after the menopause, and during breast feeding, and may also be a consequence of rapid weight loss and a low BMI, emotional stress or intensive sports training because these events all suppress the hypothalamus and the release of gonadotrophin releasing hormone.

Pathophysiology

In primary amenorrhoea, failure to begin menstruating is occasionally caused by physical obstruction or other abnormality of the tract. The hymen is a thin membrane covering the vaginal opening, which usually canalises in the late stages of fetal development to open the vagina to the exterior. When this does not happen (imperforate hymen) menstrual blood backs up behind the membrane (**haematometrocolpos**; Fig. 14.16) and can cause infection and adhesions. Imperforate hymen occurs in 1 in 1000 births and usually requires surgical intervention to create a normal opening. Rarely, failure of uterine or vaginal development means that even if ovarian function is normal (and the girl is therefore developing other secondary sexual characteristics), menstruation cannot take place because there is no functional or patent reproductive tract.

In either primary or secondary amenorrhoea, the underlying cause usually lies with one or more of the hierarchy of hormones on which the menstrual cycle depends.

Hypothalamic failure to secrete gonadotrophin releasing hormone. If the hypothalamus fails for any reason, the whole system below it also fails, because without GnRH from the hypothalamus, the anterior pituitary does not secrete LH or FSH, and the ovary in turn does not produce oestrogen because there is no follicular development (see Fig. 10.3). Hypothalamic suppression may be caused by excessive sports training, undernutrition, very low body fat content, significant psychological stress and/or psychiatric illness. Anorexia nervosa can cause either primary or secondary amenorrhoea.

Failure of the pituitary gland to secrete FSH and LH. Failure of the pituitary gland may be caused by an inability of the anterior pituitary to respond to hypothalamic hormones because the pituitary cells have a genetic defect in the gene that makes the appropriate hormone receptors. More com-

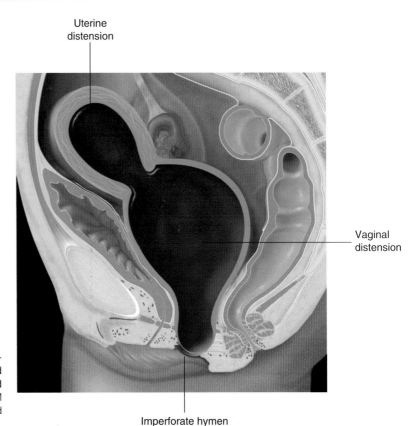

Fig. 14.16 Haematometrocolpos with imperforate hymen. Unable to pass to the exterior, menstrual blood collects in the vagina and uterus, causing distension and displacement of the uterus. (Modified from Shaaban AM and Rogers D (2022) *Diagnostic imaging: gynecology*, 3rd ed, Fig. 56.1084. Philadelphia; Elsevier Inc.)

monly, pituitary failure is caused by a pituitary tumour, or by compression of the pituitary by hydrocephalus or a tumour growing in the adjacent area of the brain.

Failure of the ovary to secrete oestrogen. If the ovaries fail to develop, or the germ cells that will develop into oocytes fail to develop, the ovarian follicles responsible for oestrogen production never develop. The commonest cause of this is Turner syndrome (p. 59), in which the ovaries may be no more than a small mass of fibrous tissue. In this syndrome, although oestrogen is not produced, the levels of FSH and LH are very high, as the pituitary tries to kick-start the inactive ovaries into action.

POLYCYSTIC OVARIAN SYNDROME

This common condition is associated with significant disturbance of sex hormone secretion and is therefore a major cause of infertility. Despite the name, ovarian cysts are not seen in all women and the presence of ovarian cysts is not diagnostic for the disorder because 20% to 30% of non-affected women also have them. In addition, ovarian cysts are also associated with some other endocrine disorders, including thyroid disease, adrenal disease and Cushing disease. The reason for this is not clear.

Polycystic ovarian syndrome (PCOS) is actually a group of disorders that may follow a very mild clinical course, or a much more aggressive one. Depending on the diagnostic criteria used, its prevalence may be as high as 15% in women of reproductive age.

Pathophysiology

PCOS is a complex endocrine disorder, characterised by high circulating levels of LH, oestrogen and testosterone,

insulin resistance, and high blood insulin levels. The condition usually manifests at puberty, when the woman's reproductive cycle begins to establish itself. The ovarian follicles themselves are the source of the excess testosterone. In healthy females, it is normal to have a low level of circulating testosterone, which increases bone and muscle mass and contributes to libido. Normally, oestrogen is by far the predominant sex hormone in women. However, the biosynthesis of oestrogen and testosterone are intimately linked: they share key steps in their biosynthesis from cholesterol, and both are produced from the precursor molecule androstenedione. In addition, testosterone is converted directly to oestrogen by the enzyme aromatase (Fig. 14.17). In PCOS, for reasons that are not understood, the biosynthetic balance is altered in favour of the testosterone pathway and large quantities of this androgen are produced. However, PCOS ovaries are hyper-responsive to LH, so their secretion of both oestrogen and testosterone is excessive. In addition, some of the testosterone is then converted to oestrogen in the tissues, contributing to high oestrogen levels.

Despite high circulating oestrogen levels, the excess testosterone characteristic of the disorder inhibits ovulation. Recall from the description of the normal cycle that high levels of oestrogen directly stimulate the anterior pituitary, keeping FSH and LH levels high and triggering ovulation. In health, the developing follicle in the first half of the cycle secretes increasing quantities of oestrogen, which triggers the LH surge that stimulates ovulation. However, in PCOS, despite oestrogen and LH levels being high, testosterone prevents ovulation and the follicle in the ovary simply continues to expand, filling with fluid and producing

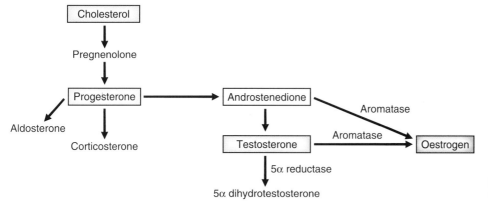

Fig. 14.17 The biosynthesis of oestrogen and testosterone.

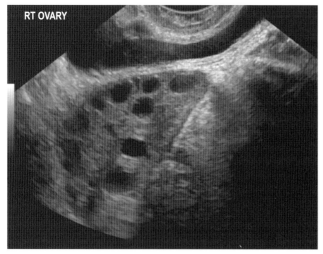

Fig. 14.18 Polycystic ovary. Ultrasound image showing multiple cysts. (From Feather A, Randall D, and Waterhouse M (2021) *Kumar and Clark's clinical medicine*, 10th ed, Fig. 21.29. Edinburgh; Elsevier Ltd.)

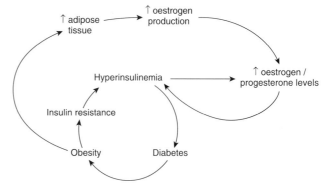

Fig. 14.19 The relationship between hyperinsulinaemia and high circulating sex hormone levels in PCOS.

the characteristic cysts. Most affected women have multiple ovarian cysts (Fig. 14.18), and the ovaries themselves are enlarged.

Hyperinsulinaemia, a frequent finding in PCOS patients, contributes to the hyperandrogenism of the condition because insulin increases ovarian sensitivity to LH, increasing testosterone production. Hyperinsulinaemia and insulin resistance account for the very high rates of obesity and type 2 diabetes associated with the condition, and obesity in turn exacerbates the insulin resistance, so there are positive feedback pathways in PCOS in which hyperinsulinaemia and high levels of circulating androgens reinforce one another (Fig. 14.19). Obesity is also associated with increased circulating oestrogen levels because adipose tissue produces oestrogen.

The cause of the disease is not known, although it is multifactorial, with both genetic and environmental contributory factors. There is a familial tendency, and mutations in genes that code for enzymes essential to steroid synthesis and related to insulin resistance have been identified. Environmental factors, such as hormone exposure in utero are probably also important.

Signs and symptoms
The reduced or suppressed ovulation of PCOS causes infertility or subfertility, and amenorrhoea or very erratic menstruation. Testosterone also causes hirsutism and acne. Diabetes and obesity affect up to two thirds of patients. Insulin resistance may also cause the skin pigment disorder acanthosis nigricans, in which epidermal proliferation is triggered by excess circulating insulin. Affected skin is thickened and dark, and patches commonly appear in the armpits, groin, neck, and elbows, among other sites.

Management and prognosis
A combination of hormone therapy, to counteract the excessive testosterone and to re-establish ovulation, is used. Metformin is used to improve insulin sensitivity and manage diabetes. There is increased risk of cardiovascular disease and endometrial carcinoma in later life.

DEVELOPMENTAL AND STRUCTURAL ABNORMALITIES

Developmental abnormalities arising during embryogenesis may be minor or may lead to complete absence of a functional reproductive tract. Occasionally, only one side of a reproductive organ may have developed normally, with the other half missing; in these circumstances because it arises from the same tissue in embryonic development, the kidney on the affected side is also missing. In some instances, structures may be duplicated (e.g., a double uterus or vagina), or the uterus may be divided in two by a central septum. Sometimes such abnormalities are picked up only when a girl fails to menstruate at puberty, or when she is trying to conceive or has become pregnant.

ENDOMETRIOSIS

This distressing and painful disorder affects women of childbearing age of all races. In endometriosis, patches of endometrium are implanted in organs other than the uterus, mainly in the pelvic and abdominal cavities, and this tissue responds to oestrogen, thickening and degenerating with the menstrual cycle. It is estimated that 1% to 2% of women suffer from some degree of endometriosis, although about a third of cases are asymptomatic. It is a major cause of infertility, subfertility, pelvic pain, and painful sexual intercourse. The cause is not known, although there is a genetic predisposition in some women. There are a number of theories regarding the aetiology of the condition, none of which is entirely satisfactory on its own. For example, one theory suggests that the endometrial tissue seeds the pelvic and abdominal cavities when menstrual flow manages to flow backwards (retrograde flow), through the uterine tubes and into the peritoneal cavity. Although this may sound intuitively attractive, it does not explain why some women develop endometriosis after hysterectomy. Another theory suggests that the endometrial tissue travels through the lymphatic circulation to distant tissues, and another idea is that the endometrial patches represent metaplastic change (p. 65) in the host tissue itself, rather than the arrival and growth of travelling endometrial cells. Both these explanations could account for the fact that endometriosis can occur in tissues very distant from the uterus: in the brain, lung and eye, for instance. There may be an association with reduced immunity, but the link is not understood. Other risk factors include early menarche, short menstrual cycles (less than 27 days), heavy menstrual bleeding and increased maternal age at first pregnancy.

Pathophysiology

Ectopic patches of functional endometrial tissue appear on the surfaces of other body organs or ligaments, usually in the lower pelvis or abdomen, but occasionally in more distant organs including the lung or brain. Because the displaced tissue behaves like normal endometrial tissue, it proliferates when oestrogen levels are high in the proliferative phase of the menstrual cycle, and degenerates when oestrogen levels fall in the menstrual phase. The regular bleeding causes local inflammation, with release of inflammatory cytokines, which in turn causes pain, swelling, fibrosis and adhesions. There is evidence in some women of abnormal T- and B-cell function and complement activation, underpinning the possibility that there is at least some immune contribution to the disorder.

Signs and symptoms

There is pain, especially with menstruation. Adhesions affect the function of affected organs: for example, endometriosis-related inflammation of the intestines, usually affecting the rectum and sigmoid colon, can cause tissues to become fibrotic and adhere to one another (Fig. 14.20). If adhesions affect the intestines, they can impair peristalsis, cause pain on defaecation, and sometimes cause constipation. The uterus can be displaced, and the endometrial lesions can be so large that they are palpable as a pelvic mass. Inflammation, fibrosis, and stricture of the uterine tubes are important contributors to infertility.

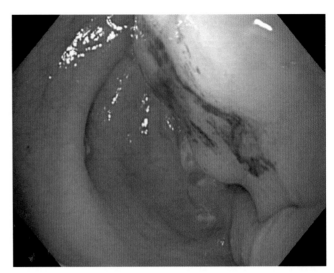

Fig. 14.20 Endometriosis. Colonoscopy photograph of endometrial tissue in the sigmoid colon. (Courtesy Thomas C. Smyrk, MD, Department of Anatomic Pathology, Mayo Clinic, Rochester, MN.)

Management and prognosis

The condition usually resolves at the menopause, when the ovaries fail and oestrogen secretion declines. Suppressing the woman's normal cyclical release of oestrogen with a range of hormonal therapies, including progesterone and oestrogen/progesterone contraceptive preparations keeps the ectopic tissue quiescent and relieves pain. Surgical removal of particularly troublesome areas of tissue is also sometimes an option.

UTERINE PROLAPSE

A prolapse refers to an organ that has slipped forwards and/or downwards out of position relative to adjacent structures. The uterus is secured in its anteverted, anteflexed position superior to the urinary bladder by pelvic ligaments and the musculature of the pelvic floor, particularly the levator ani group, which forms a sling-like structure supporting all the organs lying in the pelvis above it. Gravity pulling on the pelvic organs, and the weight of the abdominal contents pushing from above, especially in overweight or obese women, can progressively stretch and weaken the pelvic floor, and organs may begin to slip relative to one another. The urinary bladder may prolapse backwards and push into the anterior vaginal wall, and the rectum may slip forward and push into the posterior vaginal wall (Fig. 14.21). Frequently, the uterus descends into the vagina, and the prolapse may be so severe that the cervix appears at the vaginal opening. Risk factors include a familial tendency, childbearing, conditions that cause a chronic cough, chronic constipation that causes the woman to strain to pass faeces, and regular lifting of heavy loads. A mechanical support, called a *pessary*, can be inserted below the cervix to hold the uterus in place; surgical repair is also an option.

INFLAMMATORY CONDITIONS

Inflammation of any of the reproductive organs is often secondary to infection, which may be sexually transmitted, or spread via the bloodstream. The inflammatory response may heal with fibrotic changes, causing adhesions that obstruct the movement of sperm and ova through the tract.

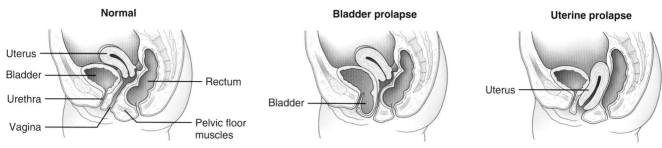

Fig. 14.21   Bladder and uterine prolapse.

PELVIC INFLAMMATORY DISEASE

Pelvic inflammatory disease (PID) is a syndrome of inflammatory changes secondary to infection affecting one or more of the pelvic organs. Most cases are caused by ascending sexually transmitted infections, including gonorrhoea and chlamydia, although infection may also be introduced by insertion of intrauterine contraceptive devices or other procedures. It follows therefore that PID is more frequently seen in younger, sexually active women with multiple partners and a history of known STI. Accurate global statistics on incidence and prevalence are not available. However, even without reliable statistical evidence, the prevalence of PID worldwide is likely to be much higher than current estimates because of the rise in STI, dismissal of minor or embarrassing symptoms by patients, and underdiagnosis by medical professionals.

Pathophysiology

Initial infection is probably more likely at certain times of the menstrual cycle when the cervical mucus barrier is breached: at ovulation, when the thick and crumbly mucus becomes thin and runny to allow the entry of sperm, and during menstruation, when the cervix opens to permit menstrual flow. The use of broad-spectrum antibiotics (e.g., penicillin) to treat infections, including STIs, kills some of the normal vaginal flora and allows other microbes to flourish and ascend, where they may establish infection. Inflammation of the pelvic structures—salpingitis, endometritis, and peritonitis—almost always arise from ascending infection from the vagina and cervix. In serious cases, inflammation spreads into the abdominal cavity and may involve the liver or intestines. A major complication of PID is the development of adhesions between inflamed organs as inflammatory fluids, rich in fibrin, cause adjacent structures to stick together; in addition, healing with scar tissue attaches organs firmly to one another. Uterine tube and ovarian adhesions can significantly reduce fertility because the mechanical processes essential to waft an ovum into the tubal infundibulum, and the muscular contractions of the uterine tubes that propel the ovum towards the uterus, are impeded.

Signs and symptoms

A significant proportion of women have no symptoms, or those they do have (vague occasional grumbling abdominal discomfort, occasional vaginal discharge) are considered too minor to consult a doctor about. However, in more serious cases, acute, constant, aching abdominal pain is usually the presenting symptom. The pain often appears shortly after a menstrual period starts, and usually settles within a week. There may be fever, nausea and vomiting. A vaginal discharge occurs in about 75% of patients.

Management and prognosis

Treating the underlying infection as early as possible is key to reducing the long-term complications of PID and is particularly important in preserving fertility. Prompt and appropriate antibiotic treatment of the patient and identified partners is the main approach. However, even after the infection has resolved, women may still experience persistent pelvic pain. There is evidence that there are even longer-term consequences: increased risk of stroke and myocardial infarction in middle-aged women who experienced PID at a younger age has been reported.

BARTHOLINITIS

Bartholin's glands (see Fig. 14.1), located on either side of the vaginal opening secrete lubricating mucus to facilitate penetration during sexual activity. Blockage of the tiny ducts that carry their secretions to the surface is common, and usually caused by infection, either an STI or contamination from the perineum. Common organisms are *Staphylococcus aureus* and streptococcal species, both common skin commensals. Inflammation distends the duct and involves the gland, as the infection ascends. The resultant swelling is called a Bartholin cyst, which may be painful but is usually asymptomatic. If treatment is indicated (e.g., for a concurrent STI), it is with antibiotics. Warm compresses and warm baths may give comfort and help open up a blocked duct and drain the cyst.

CERVICITIS, VAGINITIS AND VULVITIS

Inflammation of the cervix is usually STI-related, and associated with purulent discharge, although introduction of chemicals (douches, perfumes) or the physical insertion of other items may damage and irritate it. Temporary irritation and inflammation of the vagina and vulva are common; most women experience irritation of the external genitalia and/or the vagina at some point in their lives. This is secondary to a wide range of causes, including irritant soaps, harsh toiletries, sanitary products, tight underwear or clothing, or age-related reduction in vaginal secretions, allowing the membranes to dry out. Skin disorders, for instance psoriasis, sometimes involve the vulva.

GROWTHS AND TUMOURS

The female reproductive organs are subjected to repeated cycles of hormonally mediated proliferation and regression over the decades of a normal reproductively active lifespan.

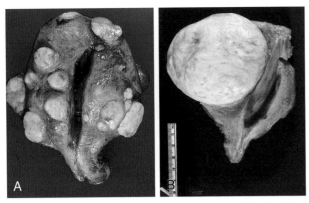

Fig. 14.22 Uterine fibroids. (A) Multiple fibroids within the uterine wall. (B) One large fibroid present. (Modified [by Esther Baranov] from 2 images Elsevier Clinical Key: Figures 19.167 and 19.168. Female reproductive system. *Rosai J: Rosai & Ackerman's surgical pathology*, 19, pp 1399–1657.)

This underpins the high rates of neoplastic disease, much of it malignant, seen in these tissues.

UTERINE TUMOURS

Benign uterine growths include fibroids, uterine polyps and adenomyosis. Malignant change in the uterine cervix is the fourth commonest cancer in women, after breast, lung, and bowel.

Uterine fibroids

Uterine fibroids are benign tumours of the myometrium and are derived from the myometrial smooth muscle. They are sometimes referred to as *leiomyomas*, which means a smooth muscle tumour. They are the commonest benign tumour in women, can reach considerable size and are found in up to 70% of females by the age of 50. Multiple tumours are common. They are up to three times commoner in black women than white women. There is a hereditable factor, so risk increases if close female relatives have also had fibroids. Risk increases significantly with age, but because oestrogen exposure increases risk, most fibroids are found in women of reproductive age.

Pathophysiology

A uterine fibroid is composed of proliferating smooth muscle cells with a significant quantity of fibrous connective tissue. They are very variable in size and location within the uterus (Fig. 14.22), and although considered a benign tumour, some may display indications of malignancy. They are generally firm and well-defined tumours and exhibit varying growth rates: some develop very quickly into large tumours, whereas others grow much more slowly. They are oestrogen-dependent, so women with increased lifetime oestrogen exposure are at increased risk: early menarche, obesity and few or no pregnancies are associated with a higher incidence. A number of genetic abnormalities have been identified, but although the risk factors described previously are well documented, the underlying cause of fibroid development is not known.

Signs and symptoms

Small fibroids often cause no symptoms. When symptomatic, the commonest complaint is heavy menstrual bleeding, and menstrual periods may be painful and last over a week.

Large fibroids may outgrow their blood supply, become ischaemic, and cause pain as they become progressively necrotic. They may also interfere with emptying the urinary bladder and may reduce fertility or contribute to pregnancy loss if they interfere with the attachment or development of the placenta or are large enough to restrict the growth of the baby.

Management and prognosis

Fibroids generally regress after the menopause, so if they are causing few or mild signs and symptoms, they may need no treatment. Heavy, painful periods may be managed with hormonal treatment, and troublesome fibroids may be surgically removed.

Adenomyosis

In this condition, the myometrium is invaded by endometrial tissue. Nests of endometrial glands and their supporting stromal tissue migrate into the uterine smooth muscle and establish there, triggering an inflammatory, hyperplastic response in the myometrium that causes uterine enlargement and cramping pain. Other common symptoms are painful, heavy periods and painful intercourse. The cause is not known, but risk increases with multiple pregnancies, uterine injury or surgery and increased age. The condition cannot be accurately diagnosed until the uterus is removed and examined, and is common in hysterectomy specimens generally, indicating that it is likely to be a frequent change in the ageing uterus, even in the absence of symptoms.

Uterine polyps

These growths arise from the endometrium. They are formed of endometrial glands and stroma with some associated blood vessels and grow on a stalk that extends from the uterine wall into the uterine cavity. They are probably common, but because most are asymptomatic, it is likely that many are never identified. They cause cramping pains and heavy and irregular bleeding. The incidence increases with age, and a small proportion of polyps are pre-malignant.

Cervical cancer

The Global Burden of Disease study showed that cancer of the cervix represented 6.5% of all female cancers in 2020, with over 600,000 new cases. Over 90% of deaths occur in low and middle-income countries, where screening programmes are not routinely implemented. This cancer is strongly associated with human papilloma virus (HPV) infection. At least 15 subtypes of HPV are associated with cancer, but between them, subtypes HPV 16 and 18 are responsible for 70% of pre-malignant cervical lesions and cervical cancer cases. However, because only a small proportion of women with proven HPV infection develop cervical cancer, there must be other factors involved. It is known, for example, that the risk of infected women developing cancer is increased by smoking and poor immunological status, including HIV infection, which increases the risk of cervical cancer five-fold. The risk of acquiring the infection, and therefore any cancer that develops from it, increases with the frequency of sexual activity, the number of sexual partners, and embarking on sexual activity at a young age.

Pathophysiology

In 80% of cases, the cell of origin is a cervical epithelial cell, and most of the remaining 20% are cancers of glandular tissue. The most common site of malignant change is the transformation zone (see Fig. 14.3) where the cells have already undergone metaplastic change. The Pap test, named for its developer, George Papanicolaou, and also called the smear test, has been the cornerstone of cervical screening since the Greek doctor introduced it in the 1930s. A sample of cervical cells is taken on a swab and examined under the microscope. Abnormal cells are usually easily identified, and even early cancers can be accurately detected. Cytological examination of cells from the smear test allows the degree of abnormality to be assessed, using histological features such as the size and shape of the nucleus, the presence of multiple nuclei and irregularities in the size and shape of the epithelial cells themselves. Mild dysplasia, referred to as low-grade cervical intraepithelial neoplasia or CIN I, is not cancer, and may actually regress. Moderate dysplasia, CIN II, is considered pre-cancerous; severe dysplasia, CIN III, is also pre-cancerous or may be diagnosed as carcinoma in situ (carcinoma that has not breached its underlying basement membrane so has not yet spread).

The degree to which an established cervical carcinoma has spread must be accurately assessed (staging of the cancer; Fig. 14.23) to ensure the best possible treatment options are offered. Staging is determined according to the International Federation of Gynecology and Obstetrics (FIGO) system. Stage 1 is confined to the cervix. Stage 2 has spread locally, involving the upper third of the vagina, but not to the pelvic wall. Stage 3 cancers have invaded the lower third of the vagina and/or the pelvic wall. Stage 4 cancers have spread the furthest, involving the bladder and/or the rectum, and/or extending outside of the pelvis. Early-stage cancers carry a 5-year survival rate of over 90%, whereas metastatic disease is associated with 5-year survival rates of only 17%.

Nearly all cases are associated with HPV infection. HPV is a DNA virus that enters the cervical cell and releases its viral DNA, which is then incorporated into the cervical cell's own DNA. This induces the host cell to produce a range of viral proteins. The two viral proteins key to the development of cancer, E6 and E7, inactivate important tumour suppressor genes, including *p53* (p. 75), triggering cell proliferation and inhibiting apoptosis. The tumour tends to grow locally, and can involve the vagina, the bladder, and the rectum, and invade the pelvic wall. It spreads readily through the lymphatic system, and the commonest sites of distant metastasis are the liver, lung, and bone.

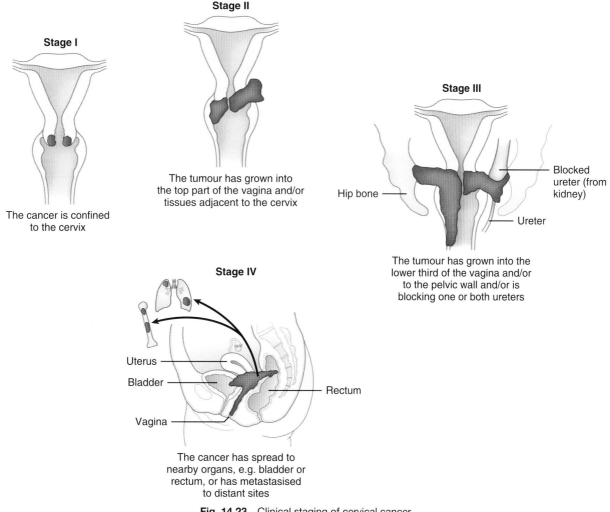

Fig. 14.23 Clinical staging of cervical cancer.

Signs and symptoms

Most countries have routine cervical screening programmes, allowing the disease to be detected on an abnormal Pap test before any signs or symptoms have appeared. If the disease is symptomatic, the usual first indication is abnormal vaginal bleeding. If the disease is advanced, there may be symptoms from metastatic growths, for example pain from involved bone tissue.

Management and prognosis

The earlier the cancer is detected, the better the prognosis. Cancers that have spread extensively carry a poorer outcome than those that have invaded only locally or not at all. Surgery in early cases is often curative; in more advanced disease, a combination of radiotherapy and chemotherapy is used. The introduction of screening, which instantly increased the proportion of tumours caught early enough for cure, greatly reduced death rates, and vaccination against HPV has proved immensely effective in reducing HPV infection and therefore the rates of HPV-related pre-malignant and malignant lesions.

Endometrial cancer

International Agency for Research on Cancer statistics show that, worldwide in 2020, this form of cancer was the fourth commonest in women, and its incidence is increasing worldwide. Globally, the disease is not evenly distributed: incidence in developing countries is much lower than in developed countries. Most cases arise in middle age.

Pathophysiology

Most endometrial cancers (95%) arise in the glandular tissue of the endometrium because, under the influence of oestrogen and progesterone, this tissue undergoes dramatic cyclical proliferative changes during a woman's reproductive life, and tissues with high levels of cellular proliferation are at higher risk of neoplastic change. Endometrial hyperplasia, proliferation of the glandular tissue within the endometrium, is caused by oestrogen exposure, such as in polycystic ovary syndrome, ovarian tumours, obesity (because adipose tissue produces oestrogens) and is associated with hypertension, an early menarche and late menopause, having no children, hormone replacement therapy, diabetes, and a sedentary lifestyle. Endometrial hyperplasia shares some characteristic genetic changes with endometrial cancer and can precede it.

Most endometrial cancers are associated with genetic mutations that increase the responsiveness of the endometrium to oestrogen, deactivate tumour suppressor genes such as *p53* (p. 75) or activate oncogenes such as *RAS* (p. 76). The neoplastic tissue proliferates and invades the myometrium. From there, it can spread to adjacent structures such as the vagina, and in the lymphatic system and bloodstream to distant sites.

Identifying the receptor population on the surface of the tumour cells is important in prognosis and informing treatment. For example, tumours that express oestrogen receptors (ER) are likely to respond well to hormone therapy. Some endometrial cancers express HER2 receptors (p. 76), and these tumours respond less well to chemotherapy and are less likely to give a good outcome.

Signs and symptoms

Unusual vaginal bleeding or discharge is usually the first indication and should never be ignored. Nearly all women with endometrial carcinoma experience bleeding between menstrual periods, or post-menopausal bleeding. There may be pain and unintentional weight loss, and, in the later stages, a pelvic mass.

Prognosis and management

It is important to identify the precise cell type from which the cancer has arisen, as this informs the prognosis and the treatment options. Prognosis depends on this histological identification and on the degree of de-differentiation of the cell of origin. Highly de-differentiated tumours carry a poorer prognosis than tumours that still resemble the parent tissue. In addition, tumour staging is important to identify the anatomical extent of tumour spread. Endometrial cancer is usually staged using the TNM system (p. 81), and prognosis becomes bleaker with more extensive local invasion, lymph node involvement and metastatic spread. Early detection, however, can give a highly optimistic prognosis, with 5-year survival rates in excess of 90% in women whose disease is diagnosed while still localised to the uterus. Treatment may be surgical, but radiotherapy, chemotherapy, and hormone therapy may all be appropriate.

BREAST TUMOURS

Over 80% of breast lumps are benign.

Benign proliferative breast disease

The incidence of breast lumps, caused by some sort of proliferative change in breast tissue, increases with age after puberty until the menopause, after which the incidence declines as oestrogen levels progressively fall. Benign breast proliferative changes may affect any of the tissue types in the breast, including glandular tissue, adipose tissue, smooth muscle tissue and the epithelial lining of the ducts and glands, so there is a wide range of presentations and morphological changes. Some of the more abnormal changes are associated with increased risk of malignant change. Cysts can form if the lobules or their terminal ducts become distended, and can be large and painful, and may rupture. Fibrosis of the proliferating tissue may also occur.

Breast cancer

Worldwide, breast cancer is the commonest cancer in women. It is discussed on p. 84.

OVARIAN CYSTS AND TUMOURS

Most ovarian cysts are benign and arise from the follicles in the cortex of the ovary. These fluid-filled sacs can grow to considerable size and cause compression pain and a palpable mass in the pelvis. They are common in premenopausal women, whose ovaries contain actively developing follicles with each reproductive cycle. Most resolve spontaneously and cause no symptoms. They are much rarer in post-menopausal women, in whom ovulation has stopped. Most ovarian neoplasms (80%) are likewise benign.

Ovarian cancer

Malignant change may occur in any of several cell types present in the ovary, and identifying the cell of origin is important for prognosis and choosing optimal treatment. This is the eighth commonest female cancer but causes a disproportionate number of deaths because it is usually advanced at diagnosis. Increasing age is an important risk factor; most cases occur between 45 and 65 years. Other risk factors include hormone therapy, an early menarche, late menopause and never having had children. Multiple pregnancies confer protection, as does the use of the oral contraceptive. There is a hereditable component, as a woman is up to three times likelier to develop the disease if a first-degree relative is affected, although only a small proportion of affected women (5%–10%) have a family history. Globally, all populations are affected, but not equally; Japan has an incidence of 3 per 100,000 women, but Sweden's incidence is seven times higher.

Pathophysiology

Most ovarian tumours arise from the epithelial cells covering the ovarian surface. Others arise from germ cells or sex cord stromal cells. Some are secondary tumours from primary malignancies elsewhere, including local spread from e.g., cervical cancer, but also after distant spread from e.g., the breast or stomach. There is significant variation in malignant potential of the different types of ovarian cancer. Some forms are slow growing and less invasive and others are much more aggressive with a more rapid clinical progression, so molecular profiling of a tumour is important to predict how it is likely to behave.

The cause of ovarian cancer is not known, although the risk factors listed previously suggest a direct relationship between a high number of ovulatory cycles experienced and increased risk, presumably because the proliferation of follicular tissue driven by oestrogen increases the risk of genetic mutation, which may later progress to malignant change. Factors that decrease the number of ovulatory cycles (e.g., spending a significant portion of the childbearing years pregnant, lactating or taking the contraceptive pill) therefore confer protection, and factors that increase the number of cycles (an extended reproductive period because of an early menarche and late menopause, and never being pregnant) increase risk.

Most cases are caused by random mutation of the cancerous cell, frequently involving key tumour suppressor genes, including *p53* (p. 75), but a wide range of additional mutations have also been identified. *BRCA1* and *BRCA2* mutations (p. 84) are also found in some cases and are associated with familial ovarian cancer.

Signs and symptoms

These are often diffuse and non-specific, and so may be ignored for some time before the woman seeks help. They include lower abdominal discomfort and distension, weight loss, tiredness, constipation, and a feeling of satiety after even small meals.

Management and prognosis

Because presentation is usually late, the disease is often advanced at diagnosis and prognosis may be bleak. Overall 5-year survival rate is around 46%, but it varies hugely depending on the histological type of tumour and the stage at presentation. Diabetic women have poorer survival rates, although the reason for this is not known. Surgery to remove the ovary plus all adjacent structures, followed by chemotherapy, can be curative if the disease is caught at an early enough stage. Surgery to debulk a locally invasive tumour, followed by chemotherapy, can be used in more advanced cases.

DISORDERS OF MALE REPRODUCTION

Healthy men may remain fertile until fairly advanced old age because sperm production is constant rather than cyclical, and there is no real equivalent of the female menopause, when female reproductive capacity ceases.

DEVELOPMENTAL AND STRUCTURAL ABNORMALITIES

CRYPTORCHIDISM (UNDESCENDED TESTES)

The testes develop in the abdominal cavity and begin their descent through the inguinal canal into the scrotum at about the beginning of the seventh month of gestation. At birth, the testes should be fully descended and occupy the scrotal pouch. In up to 3% of newborn boys, one or both testes are not fully in place. Sometimes the testis is still in the abdomen, or it may have travelled only part of the way down through the inguinal canal. It is more common for only one testis to be affected (usually the right), but sometimes both testes are undescended.

The main risk factor is low birth weight, although there is a familial tendency. Exposure to certain chemicals (e.g., pesticides and oestrogen) may increase risk because they interfere with normal hypothalamic-pituitary function, essential for normal testicular development. Prematurity and maternal obesity, smoking, and alcohol consumption are also implicated. Although it may occur as a lone abnormality, it is associated with other congenital defects, including abnormalities of the vas deferens and the epididymis, and is a risk factor for testicular cancer in later life. It is also associated with reduced fertility.

In about two thirds of affected boys, the testes descend normally within 3 months of birth. Surgery brings the testes into their normal position if they do not descend naturally.

PHIMOSIS AND PARAPHIMOSIS

This is a tight foreskin that cannot be retracted over the glans penis (Fig. 14.24A). It is normal in boys under the age of three, but the foreskin generally loosens naturally with erections before the age of six. It is usually secondary to inflammatory skin conditions such as eczema and psoriasis, causing fibrosis and constriction of the foreskin, but it can also arise for no apparent reason. In paraphimosis, a retracted foreskin is too tight to be brought forward over the glans, constricts the penis and may obstruct blood flow (Fig. 14.24B). Both conditions can cause pain and infection and may interfere with sexual function.

TESTICULAR TORSION

The testis is suspended in the scrotum by the spermatic cord, in which the testicular artery and vein provide and drain the organ's blood supply. Rotation of the testis twists the cord, compresses the artery, and cuts off blood flow (Fig. 14.25). If not treated immediately, the testis becomes ischaemic and eventually necrotic. The window of opportunity to salvage

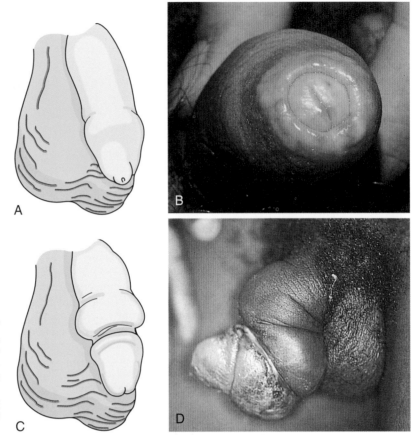

Fig. 14.24 (A) Phimosis. The foreskin cannot be retracted over the glans penis. (B) Paraphimosis. The retracted foreskin is too tight to be pulled forward over the glans, causing constriction and swelling. (From (A and C) Monahan FD, Sands J, Neighbors M, et al. (2007) *Phipps' medical-surgical nursing: health and illness perspectives*, 8th ed. St. Louis; Mosby; (B) Taylor PK (1995) *Diagnostic picture tests in sexually transmitted diseases*, St. Louis, Mosby; (D) Morse SA, Holmes KK, and Ballard RC (2011) *Atlas of sexually transmitted diseases and AIDS*, 4th ed. London; Saunders.)

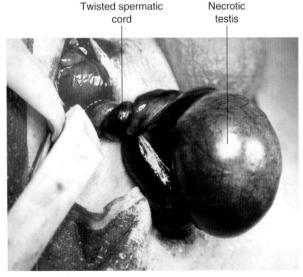

Fig. 14.25 Testicular torsion. The testis is necrotic and the twisted spermatic cord is clearly visible. (From Kliegman R, Stanton B, St. Geme J, et al. (2011) *Nelson's textbook of pediatrics*, 19th ed. Philadelphia; Saunders.)

the testis is small: restoration of blood flow within 4 to 6 hours usually leads to resolution and the testis recovers fully, but by 24 hours post-torsion, necrosis has usually developed. The condition is commonest in young males, including neonates, in whom the immature testis is more mobile in the scrotum than in older men. They experience significant, often sudden, scrotal pain and swelling, the swelling being the result of obstruction of venous outflow. The pain can be severe enough to elicit nausea and vomiting. The cause is not known, but torsion can develop after exercise or after testicular injury and is more common if there is a family history or previous torsion.

INFLAMMATORY CONDITIONS

Inflammation of male reproductive structures is a frequent consequence of sexually transmitted infections, but a range of other conditions and infections may cause inflammatory changes. Conditions may be chronic or acute.

Balanitis

Inflammation of the penis (balanitis) usually involves the glans and foreskin. There is a wide range of causes: infections, trauma, phimosis, chemical irritants (toiletries, latex, laundry products or other chemicals) or some skin conditions (e.g., psoriasis).

PROSTATITIS

This is a common feature of many genitourinary conditions but may be caused by systemic conditions such as sarcoidosis. Up to 10% of men will suffer from prostatitis at some point in their lives.

Pathophysiology

Over 90% of cases of inflammatory prostatitis are not associated with infection, and the underlying cause may not be identified. It is characterised by infiltration of the gland with inflammatory cells, which enlarges and may cause a similar raft of symptoms to benign prostatic hyperplasia. Infective causes include STI, blood-borne or lymphatic infection spread from other body organs, or from direct contamination from local infection in a neighbouring structure. Reflux of urine from the urethra up the prostatic ducts or an indwelling catheter may cause infection. Disseminated tuberculosis may cause mycobacterial prostatitis. Irrespective of the origin, most infections are bacterial, but viral infection may also occur, for example cytomegalovirus infection in HIV-positive men, and fungal infections have also been reported.

Signs, symptoms, and management

Depending on the cause of the condition, the disorder may be acute or chronic. Many cases of prostatitis will cause pain, but many cases are asymptomatic. There may be systemic indications of infection: fever, chills, malaise or joint pains; there may be lower urinary tract symptoms if the swollen prostate compresses the urethra, penile discharge and pain on ejaculation. Management depends on identifying the cause, treating any infection, and controlling any underlying condition.

ORCHITIS AND EPIDIDYMITIS

Orchitis is acute inflammation of the testis. The commonest cause of viral orchitis is mumps, once a common childhood illness but now uncommon in countries with vaccination programmes. The affected testis is swollen, red and painful, and infiltrated with large numbers of inflammatory cells. Mumps orchitis may reduce male fertility because a high proportion of boys who develop orchitis as part of the clinical course of their mumps suffer testicular atrophy, which may not resolve.

Sometimes orchitis develops as a consequence of epididymitis (epididymoorchitis). Epididymitis usually originates as a urinary tract or sexually transmitted infection, so has usually ascended through the urethra, the ejaculatory duct, and the vas deferens, from where it spreads through the epididymis to the testis. Sometimes it is appropriate to allow the condition to resolve without treatment, but antimicrobial therapy may be required.

GROWTHS AND TUMOURS

These may be caused by inflammatory, infective, or neoplastic conditions.

THE PENIS

Benign tumours include condyloma acuminatum (genital warts), caused by human papilloma virus.

Carcinoma of the penis

The incidence of this disorder varies significantly worldwide. High risk is conferred by HPV infection, particularly HPV subtypes 16 and 18, the two subtypes most implicated in HPV-mediated cervical cancer. Up to 50% of penile cancers involve HPV infection. In cultures where circumcision is routinely practised when the child is very young, the disease is very rare. This is thought to relate to another major risk factor, poor genital hygiene, believed to increase the chance of acquiring the disease because of the build-up of smegma below the foreskin. Circumcision as an adult does not give protection. Cigarette smoking is another risk factor.

Pathophysiology

The cell of origin is usually (90% of cases) the squamous epithelial cell of the skin covering the penis. Almost 70% of tumours occur on the glans penis or the foreskin. The internal compartments of the penis present some barrier to spread of the tumour as it invades the deeper tissues, but without treatment it spreads to the femoral and inguinal lymph nodes, where it may cause death from sepsis or haemorrhage. Preferred sites of distant metastasis are liver, brain, and bone.

Signs and symptoms

Lesions appear as painless thickened grey areas of skin, ulcers that do not heal or cauliflower-like masses. Secondary infection may be present.

Management and prognosis

In the initial stages, the tumour is usually slow growing, and men are often reluctant to seek help, perhaps because of embarrassment, ignorance, fear, or self-neglect. As a result, the disease may be well advanced with local lymph node involvement and even metastatic spread at presentation. Five-year survival rates are mainly dependent on whether the inguinal lymph nodes are involved: if they are clear at treatment, they are between 65% and 90%, but can be as low as 20% if local lymph nodes are involved. Treatment options must balance the need to save life, but also to preserve, if possible, a cosmetically and functionally acceptable result. Penis-preserving surgery can walk a thin line between clearing the tumour and providing an acceptable result because surgery that does not take adequate margins has high recurrence rates. Squamous cell carcinomas usually respond poorly to radiotherapy, but there is a range of effective cytotoxic drugs available.

THE SCROTUM AND TESTES

These conditions may involve the testicular tissue itself, or one or more of the membranes that enclose it within the scrotum.

Hydrocele

Hydrocele is a collection of fluid within the tunica vaginalis, the closed sac around the testis that is the remains of the peritoneal pouch in which the testis descends during embryonic life (Fig. 14.26A). Congenital hydrocele is common in newborn babies because the peritoneal pouch has not yet closed off, but usually seals naturally before the baby is 18 months old (Fig. 14.26B). If the channel fails to fully close in early childhood, or if the testis is inflamed or damaged by infection, a tumour, or trauma, hydrocele may develop (Fig. 14.26C) and can cause significant swelling. Swelling may obstruct blood flow and cause ischaemia.

Varicocele

This is dilation of the veins in the spermatic cord, which drain blood from the testis, the epididymis, and the vas deferens, and empty it into the testicular veins. If the valves in the testicular veins are faulty, backflow of blood into the spermatic cord veins leads to their becoming swollen and tortuous, much like faulty valves in leg veins cause varicose veins of the leg. Sometimes obstruction of venous drainage

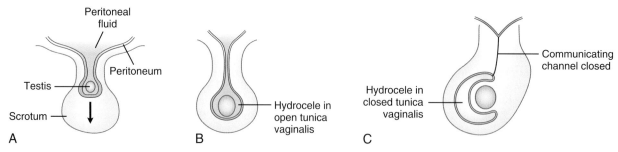

Fig. 14.26   Formation of the tunica vaginalis and hydrocele. (A) In late fetal development, the testis descends into the scrotum from the abdominal cavity, taking its wrappings of peritoneal membrane with it. (B) Congenital hydrocele: the channel between the peritoneum and the tunica vaginalis does not close properly. (C) Closed hydrocele.

from the area is caused by congenital malformation of the veins, or by, for example, a nearby tumour, such as a renal tumour, growing into the vein. The scrotum becomes warm and congested, and the varicose veins may be clearly visible through the scrotal skin, looking like a bag of worms. It may be painful, but many varicoceles give no significant trouble and are diagnosed only when the man seeks help for infertility. The increased temperature associated with venous engorgement impairs spermatogenesis, and varicocele is therefore associated with lower semen quality and reduced fertility.

Testicular cancer

Although this disease is overall relatively uncommon, with an incidence of only 5 per 100,000 men, it is the commonest malignancy in young adult males between the ages of 15 to 40, and globally its incidence is increasing, although geographical distribution is not equal. Caucasian men are at much higher risk than African and Asian men, and risk is higher in developed than in developing countries. Despite this, mortality is much higher in less wealthy countries: about 80% of recorded deaths from testicular cancer occur here. Other risk factors include undescended testes, high oestrogen exposure in the womb and a positive family history (an affected brother increases risk up to tenfold).

Pathophysiology

Malignancy usually occurs in the germ cells lining the seminiferous tubules and responsible for sperm cell production: 90% of testicular cancers are of this origin. With their high rate of division, the risk of producing a mutated cell line is significantly higher than in other, more stable, cell populations. The early stage of tumour development, in which the tumour has not yet invaded the basement membrane of the wall of the seminiferous tubule, is called germ cell neoplasia in situ (GCIS), analogous to DCIS seen in breast cancer. GCIS can give rise to a range of testicular tumours, the commonest of which (40%) is called a **seminoma**. Seminomas are usually slow growing, and occur in older men. Because the germ cells are at such an early stage of development, they have the capacity to produce a wide range of body tissues and when they proliferate in a malignant growth, can produce tumours containing a range of cell types and tissue architecture: for example, there may be cartilage or nerve tissue, or primitive tubular or cystic structures, lined with epithelium, resembling sections of the gastrointestinal tract or the airways. This type of tumour is called a **teratoma** and is also sometimes seen in ovarian malignancies because the

ovary also contains large numbers of germ cells for ovum development. Other types of testicular tumour arising from the germ cells include **carcinomas** and **yolk sac tumours**. Very often, the non-seminoma germ cell tumours present as a combination of the different types, and the resultant tumour has a varied and diverse range of malignant cells.

Not all testicular neoplasms originate from the germ cells. A small proportion arise from other cell types, for example Leydig cells or Sertoli cells. Leydig cell tumours can cause early sexual development because these are the cells that secrete testosterone. However, tumours from either of these cell types are usually benign.

Each of these different types of tumour cells express different surface molecules and receptors and release different markers, so for optimal management it is important to identify the specific composition of the tumour. Identifying benign tumours is obviously essential to allay worries and avoid non-essential treatment. Important serum markers in testicular cancer include alpha-fetoprotein (AFP) and human chorionic gonadotrophin (hCG), which are characteristic of non-seminomas. Plasma concentrations of these markers correlate well with tumour size. No comparable marker for seminomas has been found. Key genetic mutations in testicular cancer include a mutation in the short arm of chromosome 12, which appears to be very common in germ cell tumours and in specific genes on chromosomes 5 and 6. Studies have shown that possessing these key mutations significantly increases the risk of developing the cancer and could be used to identify high-risk individuals.

Signs and symptom

These tumours usually present as a painless testicular mass.

Prognosis and management

Generally, these tumours have an excellent outcome, unless they have already metastasised at presentation. Surgical removal, radiotherapy and chemotherapy may all be options, depending on the stage and type of tumour. Sometimes a 'watch and wait' approach is appropriate in a slow growing, non-aggressive tumour, and regular measurement of serum tumour markers is then important to monitor tumour development. Serum tumour markers can also be used to evaluate response to treatment, and to identify recurrence early.

THE PROSTATE GLAND

Disorders of the prostate gland are common, especially in older men. Swelling, inflammation or tumours of the prostate compress the urethra and obstruct urine flow.

Benign prostatic hyperplasia

The incidence of benign prostatic hyperplasia (also called benign prostatic enlargement or benign prostatic hypertrophy) rises with age, particularly after 50 years. Up to three quarters of men aged 70 to 80 years have symptoms of the disorder. Other risk factors include diabetes and obesity, and there may be a familial tendency.

Pathophysiology

This is not a malignant condition, although it is caused by cellular proliferation within the gland. The main prostatic androgen is dihydrotestosterone (DHT), produced from testosterone by 5α-reductase (Fig. 14.17). In addition to hormone levels within the gland, circulating DHT also affects it. This hormone stimulates cell proliferation and inhibits apoptosis (p. 65), contributing to the steady increase in size of the gland with age. Androgens play an important role in the development of this condition, and castrated males and men with hypogonadism, in whom testosterone levels are very low, do not develop it. However, other factors must also play a part because testosterone levels decrease naturally with age. For example, there is increasing evidence that hyperinsulinaemia plays a part. Insulin stimulates tissue growth and cell division. In insulin resistance, associated with type 2 diabetes, insulin levels may be very high, and diabetes is a known risk factor for prostatic hyperplasia.

The gland enlarges, with growth of proliferative nodules especially within glandular tissue immediately enclosing the urethra (Fig. 14.27A). Affected glands may weigh as much as 100 g (normal weight in the young adult is about 20 g). The main consequence of this is urethral compression. There is also evidence that the smooth muscle in the gland expresses an increased number of α₁-adrenergic receptors and becomes increasingly sensitive

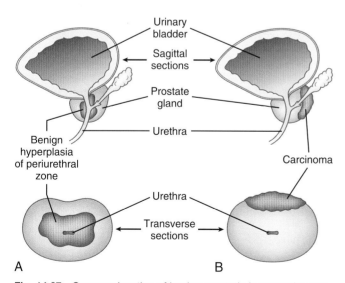

Fig. 14.27 Common location of benign prostatic hypertrophy compared with prostate carcinoma. (A) Benign prostatic hypertrophy usually involves glandular tissue immediately encircling the urethra, so quickly restricts urine flow. (B) Prostatic carcinoma usually arises from glandular tissue in the periphery of the organ. (Modified from Cross S (2019) *Underwood's pathology: a clinical approach*, 7th ed, Fig. 20.9. Oxford; Elsevier Ltd.)

to adrenaline and noradrenaline. This increases the muscle tone of the gland, further compressing the urethra. As the disorder progresses, the detrusor muscle of the bladder thickens and becomes irritable because it is required to generate more force to void urine against the developing obstruction.

Signs and symptoms

The main symptoms at presentation relate both to voiding of urine and storage of urine. Urine flow is slow, weak, and spurting. The increased sensitivity of the detrusor muscle causes frequency and urgency of urination. Normally, awareness of a filling bladder develops when it contains about 150 mL of urine, but as little as 30 mL of urine may trigger the need to pass urine in an irritable bladder. As the prostate gets progressively bigger, urination takes so much time that the bladder may not be completely emptied, causing urinary retention, which may back up into the ureters and kidneys. Infections and kidney stones may follow.

Management and prognosis

Acute urinary retention requires emergency catheterisation to relieve the pressure in the bladder. α₁-adrenergic blockers relax the detrusor and prostatic smooth muscle, relieving the obstruction, and 5α-reductase inhibitors reduce the size of the prostate by blocking the production of DHT. Surgical removal or laser ablation of a portion of the prostate gland may also help.

Prostate cancer

The main risk factor for prostate cancer is increasing age, with the average age at diagnosis being about 66 years. Other risk factors include obesity, family history, and ethnicity, with men of African origin at higher risk than non-Africans. Mutations in the *BRCA1* and *BRCA2* genes (p. 84), implicated in several cancers including breast and cervical cancer, also increase risk. Globally, it is the second commonest male cancer, although incidence is not evenly distributed from country to country. Incidence is significantly higher in Europe, Australia, and North America than in Asia, Africa, and Central and South America, for reasons that are not clear.

Pathophysiology

Most prostate cancers arise from glandular tissue (i.e., they are adenocarcinomas) and usually arise in the peripheral zone of the organ (Fig. 4.27B). A range of genetic mutations may be present, including in the key tumour suppressor gene *p53* (p. 75). There is a wide variation in the clinical course of this disorder. Most tumours are relatively slow growing in the early stages, but they tend to grow faster as they get bigger because the more aggressive malignant cells in the tumour begin to predominate. Some prostate cancers are much more aggressive from the outset and metastasise early.

Prostate epithelial cells secrete the enzyme **prostate specific antigen (PSA)** into semen. PSA may be detected in the bloodstream in healthy men, but its levels are low. In prostate inflammation, infection or cancer, however, PSA escapes through the capillary walls into the bloodstream in much higher quantities and is an accurate and reliable indicator of prostate disease. PSA levels have been used as a

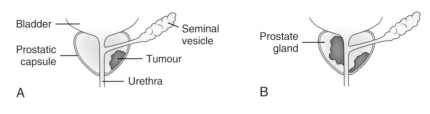

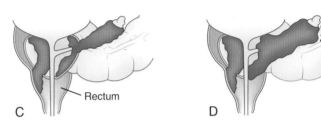

Fig. 14.28 Clinical staging of prostate cancer. (A) Stage I: The tumour occupies less than one half of one side of the gland. (B) Stage II: The tumour is larger than stage I but is contained within the prostatic capsule. (C) Stage III: The tumour has breached the prostatic capsule and invaded locally (e.g., the rectum, bladder, or seminal vesicles). (D) Stage IV: There is local lymph node involvement and/or distant metastases.

standard screening and diagnostic test for prostate cancer since the early 1990s.

The cancer spreads locally, invading nearby structures including the bladder and also to distant sites, usually via the lymphatic system. Bone is a common site for secondary growth.

Signs and symptoms

Screening programmes are in place in some countries, including the United States, where many cases are now identified early while the man is still asymptomatic. There is currently no screening programme in the UK because the test does not pick up all cancers, generates a number of false positives, and current evidence suggests that although screening programmes pick up more cases at an early stage, they do not improve the mortality rate. Symptoms include urinary retention, haematuria and low back pain. If the disease is more advanced, there may be cachexia and indications of metastatic disease, such as bone pain from bone secondaries.

Management and prognosis

Prognosis depends on the aggressiveness of the particular cancer subtype and the stage at diagnosis and more general factors such as the age and health of the patient. Stage 1 prostate cancer is a small tumour, occupying less than half of one side of the prostate gland, and completely contained within the prostatic capsule. Stage 2 is also completely contained within the capsule, but is larger, occupying more than one half of one side of the gland. Stage 3 tumours have breached the capsule and may have grown into immediately neighbouring structures, such as the seminal vesicles. In stage 4, there is lymph node involvement, and/or invasion of nearby structures such as the rectum, and/or distant metastases (Fig. 14.28). In stage 1 and stage 2 disease, 5-year survival rates are nearly 100%. In stage 4, the 5-year survival rate is only 30%. Treatment options include surgery, which offers the best possibility of cure if the cancer is localised, radiotherapy and chemotherapy. Hormone therapy is also used because the prostate gland and its tumours are androgen-sensitive. Suppression of androgen activity with anti-androgenic drugs, or removal of the testes (orchidectomy) to deplete natural androgen production are therefore also options.

BIBLIOGRAPHY AND REFERENCES

Abraham, S., Juel, H. B., Bang, P., et al. (2019). Safety and immunogenicity of the chlamydia vaccine candidate CTH522 adjuvanted with CAF01 liposomes or aluminium hydroxide: A first-in-huan, randomised, double-blind, placebo-controlled phase 1 trial. *The Lancet Infectious Diseases, 19*(10), 1091–1100.

Bhatla, N., Berek, J. S., Cuello, F. M., et al. (2019). Revised FIGO staging for carcinoma of the cervix uteri, Int. *Journal of Gynaecology and Obstetrics, 145*(1), 129–135.

De Martel, C., Plummer, M., Vignat, J., & Franceschi, S. (2017). Worldwide burden of cancer attributable to HPV by site, country and HPV type. *International Journal of Cancer, 141*, 664–670.

Laghzaoui, O. (2016). Congenital imperforate hymen. *BMJ Case Reports.* https://doi.org/10.1136/bcr-2016-215124.

Leslie, S. W., Sajjad, H., & Villanueva, C. A. (2019). Cryptorchidism 2019. *StatPearls.* https://www.ncbi.nlm.nih.gov/books/NBK470270/.

Park, J. S., Kim, J., Elghiaty, A., & Ham, W. S. (2018). Recent global trends in testicular cancer incidence and mortality. *Medicine, 97*(37), e12390. https://www.ncbi.nlm.nih.gov/pmc/articles/PMC6155960/.

Report on globally sexually transmitted infection surveillance 2018. (2018). *WHO.* https://www.who.int/news-room/fact-sheets/detail/sexually-transmitted-infections-(stis).

Styer, A. K., & Rueda, B. R. (2016). The epidemiology and genetics of uterine leiomyoma. *Best Practice & Research Clinical Obstetrics & Gynaecology, 3*, 3–12.

Tampa, M., Sarbu, I., Matei, C., et al. (2014). Brief history of syphilis. *Journal Medicine Life, 7*(1), 4–10.

Taylor, M., Loo, V., & Wi, T. (2018). *WHO Report on globally sexually transmitted infection surveillance.* https://www.researchgate.net/publication/329877512_Report_on_global_sexually_transmitted_infection_surveillance_2018.

Zhang, Y., Zhao, D., Gong, C., et al. (2015). Prognostic role of hormone receptors in endometrial cancer: A systematic review and meta-analysis. *World Journal of Surgical Oncology, 13*, 208–320.

Useful Websites

WCRF data on endometrial cancer 2018: https://www.wcrf.org/dietandcancer/cancer-trends/endometrial-cancer-statistics.

WHO 2019 data on STI: https://www.who.int/news-room/detail/06-06-2019-more-than-1-million-new-curable-sexually-transmitted-infections-every-day.

CHAPTER OUTLINE

INTRODUCTION
 The structure of skin
 The skin microbiome
INFLAMMATORY AND INFECTIVE
CONDITIONS
 Eczema (dermatitis)
 Acne
 Rosacea
 Dermatophyte (tinea) infections
 Infestations
 Bacterial infections

Viral infections
AUTOIMMUNITY AND THE SKIN
 Psoriasis
 Immune mediated skin blistering disorders
TUMOURS OF THE SKIN
Malignant tumours
 Basal cell carcinoma
 Malignant melanoma
 Actinic keratosis and squamous cell
 carcinoma

INTRODUCTION

The skin is the body's heaviest organ, contributing on average about 15% of body weight. It is subject to damage from a range of external insults: trauma, extremes of temperature, chemical or irradiation injuries, and infection, so skin disease and damage is common. Its self-renewal capacity is impressive, and it possesses specialised defensive proteins and immune cells to protect itself and, by extension, the body that it covers. In addition, it is frequently involved in systemic disease, and because cell turnover is high as the skin constantly renews itself, it is vulnerable to drug side effects and malignancy. Skin changes, whether associated with disease or not, manifest in a wide range of ways and the definitions of some common terms are given in Table 15.1.

THE STRUCTURE OF SKIN

Healthy skin varies in thickness depending on its body location but possesses the same basic structure everywhere: a vascular dermis lying beneath and firmly attached to the superficial epidermis by a basement membrane (Fig. 15.1).

The dermis

This collagen-rich connective tissue contains elastic fibres, blood vessels, nerves, free nerve endings, hair follicles, sweat glands, and specialised sensory receptors (which are modified nerve endings). It nourishes and supports the epidermis and gives the skin strength and elasticity.

The epidermis

The epidermis consists of multiple layers of epithelial cells, called **keratinocytes**, because they contain the tough fibrous protein keratin and other specialised cell types including defensive **Langerhans cells** and pigmented **melanocytes**. It has no blood supply and relies on the dermal blood vessels for nourishment. The layers of the epidermis are shown in Fig. 15.2. Its basal layer, anchored to the basement membrane that separates it from the dermis, is made of cuboidal epithelial cells that constantly divide, producing new keratinocytes that are pushed upwards as the basal layer continues to generate new cells below. As keratinocytes move further and further away from the basal layer, and further away from the blood supply provided by the dermis, they die; they lose their nucleus and other internal organelles and become tough, flattened, keratin-rich cells called **squames**. This stratified arrangement allows the upper layers of dead squames to be constantly rubbed off and lost without breaching the skin barrier. Epidermal thickness varies significantly depending on the degree of mechanical stress to which it is subjected: the skin of the soles of the feet, for example, is much thicker than that on the palm of the hand.

The skin is an excellent barrier provided it is intact. With abrasion or injury, microbes can access the tissues below. Keratinocytes are equipped with collections of cell-surface receptors to detect the presence of pathogenic organisms or their products, including lipopolysaccharide (p. 17); they constantly monitor their local environment for unfamiliar and potentially dangerous microbes, and immediately activate immune cells when they find them. The Langerhans cells of the epidermis are macrophages, which ingest microbes or foreign particles that have penetrated the upper epidermal layers. They act as antigen presenting cells (p. 90) and stimulate an inflammatory and immune response in response to skin infection. The basal keratinocytes also produce a range of antimicrobial lipids, which permeate the lower layers of the epidermis and reinforce its barrier properties. Sebum is a lipid-rich material with antimicrobial properties produced by dermal sebaceous glands, which is excreted onto the skin surface for waterproofing and protection.

Table 15.1 Definitions of common skin lesions in dermatological disorders

Term	Definition	Example
Acanthosis	Skin thickening caused by epidermal hyperplasia	Viral wart
Comedones	Dilated and blocked hair follicle. A closed comedo (whitehead) is blocked deep in the duct with sebum and skin debris with no visible opening on the skin; an open comedo (blackhead) is blocked at the skin surface with keratin, which appears black.	Acne
Macule	A flat area of skin with clear boundary different in colour to surrounding skin	Freckle
Papule	Small, raised area of skin but containing no fluid; there may be no sign of inflammation or discolouration	Viral wart
Papulopustule	A raised lesion with features of both papule and pustule	Acne
Plaque	A raised area of skin greater than 2 cm in diameter	Psoriasis
Pustule	A blister-like elevation of the skin containing pus	Acne
Vesicle	A raised blister-like lesion containing fluid	Herpes zoster

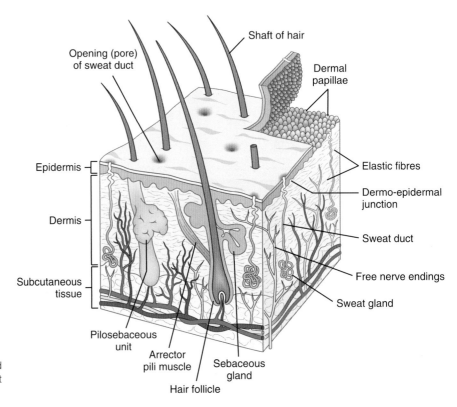

Fig. 15.1 The structure of the skin. (Modified from Standring S (2016) *Gray's anatomy*, 41st ed, Fig. 7.1. Oxford: Elsevier Ltd.)

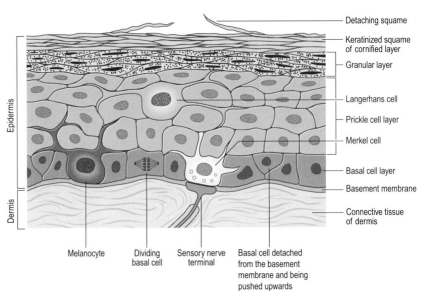

Fig. 15.2 The layers of the epidermis. (Modified from Standring S (2016) *Gray's anatomy*, 41st ed, Fig. 7.3. Oxford: Elsevier Ltd.)

Melanocytes are derived from nervous tissue and produce the pigment melanin. They are found in various tissues of the body; for instance, they give colour to the iris of the eye and to the retinal pigmented epithelium on which the rods and cones of the retina rest. One form of melanin, called neuromelanin, is responsible for the dark colour of the substantia nigra in the brain (see Parkinson disease; Ch. 8). Melanin absorbs harmful ultraviolet (UV) radiation in sunlight and is important in protecting the skin against solar radiation injury. Skin melanocytes produce two types of melanin: **eumelanin**, which is dark and is the predominant form in dark-haired and dark-skinned people, and **pheomelanin**, which is the main form in fair-skinned people with blonde or red hair. Pheomelanin is less effective than eumelanin at absorbing UV radiation, so light-haired, fair-skinned people burn more easily than those with dark skin and hair. Sun exposure increases melanin production in the skin, causing tanning.

The pilosebaceous unit

Hair follicles in the skin, embedded deep in the dermis, are enclosed in a sheath of epidermis (Fig. 15.1). Sebaceous glands open into the hair follicle, secreting **sebum**, a lipid-rich waxy material that waterproofs the hair and the skin and a key contributor to the barrier function of the skin. In addition, it has antimicrobial properties and discourages microbial growth in the hair follicle and skin surface.

The dermo-epidermal junction

The interface between the dermis and epidermis, called the *dermo-epidermal junction*, is irregular and convoluted, helping to hold the two layers firmly together. The basement membrane on which the epidermis sits is manufactured by the keratinocytes themselves and is made mainly of type IV collagen and a protein called laminin. The cell membrane of keratinocytes in immediate contact with the basement membrane features hemidesmosomes (p. 10), responsible for attaching the two firmly together.

THE SKIN MICROBIOME

The skin is colonised by a diverse collection of commensal microbes and mites that live harmlessly on and in the skin and its appendages. One key benefit they give their human host is prevention of pathogenic organisms from establishing themselves and causing infection. They are also involved in educating the immune system to distinguish between pathogenic and non-pathogenic organisms in the skin, essential for appropriate immunological responses. The microbial population varies depending on the region of skin considered: the warm, moist environment within skin folds, for example, supports a different range of organisms to exposed, drier skin, and a different set of microbes is found on hairy skin compared with hairless skin. A wide range of bacteria, including *Staphylococcus*, *Cutibacteria*, and *Corynebacteria* species, are normal skin commensals; fungal species include *Malassezia;* and *Demodex* mites, tiny insects, live in the pilosebaceous unit. The skin microbiome usually lives in balanced harmony with its host, and disturbance of this balance is associated with a range of dermatological conditions.

INFLAMMATORY AND INFECTIVE CONDITIONS

Intact skin is highly resistant to infection. The upper layers are constantly shedding, carrying with them any microbes that may have established themselves on the skin surface. Sebum, the epidermal lipid content and Langerhans cells are all protective. However, inflammatory and infective skin conditions are common.

ECZEMA (DERMATITIS)

Eczema can be caused by a range of irritants, allergens, and injuries. Irrespective of the cause, the skin becomes red, inflamed, swollen, itchy, and sometimes blistered. In chronic eczema, in response to its prolonged inflammatory state and the scratching and rubbing this causes, the skin thickens and becomes leathery (lichenification).

Seborrhoeic dermatitis

This condition is found on areas of skin rich in sebaceous glands, especially the scalp, face, and trunk. It appears as dandruff on the scalp (cradle cap in babies). It is associated with skin colonisation by the yeast *Malassezia*, a very common human commensal that feeds on the lipids in sebum and normally lives peacefully on the skin and mucosal surfaces. However, in susceptible individuals, it triggers an abnormal and excessive immune response in affected skin, although the precise mechanism is not understood. It is very common, affecting up to 5% of people, occurs in all racial groups and is most troublesome in young adults; after the age of 40 it tends to subside. Affected skin is crusty, red, flaky, itchy, and greasy. There may be secondary infection, especially if the person scratches. Antifungal drugs can help, but *Malassezia* is robust and generally rebounds when treatment stops. *Malassezia* is associated with other skin conditions, including atopic dermatitis and psoriasis. It is also associated with some systemic disorders: for example, the incidence of seborrhoeic dermatitis is very high in people with Parkinson disease, and it sometimes causes systemic fungal infections.

Contact dermatitis

Contact dermatitis is an umbrella term referring to skin inflammation in response either to an irritant or abrasive material (irritant contact dermatitis) or to an allergen that triggers a type IV hypersensitivity reaction (p. 101; allergic contact dermatitis). Susceptible people coming into direct contact with an irritant or a particular antigen develop a localised red, often intensely itchy rash, sometimes with blisters, at and around the site of contact. Contact dermatitis may be caused by a failure in the barrier function of the skin, allowing substances to penetrate the upper protective layers and reach the basal epidermal layers, where they trigger an inflammatory and/or immune response from the damaged keratinocytes.

Irritant contact dermatitis

Non-specific barrier failure may be caused by, for example, excessive handwashing or exposure to detergents that strip the skin of its upper layers and waterproofing lipids, leading to irritant contact dermatitis. This is very common and is often occupation-related, in jobs that involve regular exposure to irritant chemicals (e.g., hairdressing, cleaning) or frequent handwashing (e.g., healthcare and food preparation professions). Its prevalence is significantly higher in women than men because women predominate in high-risk occupations. Avoiding the irritant or reducing handwashing resolves the condition.

Allergic contact dermatitis

Allergic dermatitis has an immunological basis. Barrier failure allows an allergen to penetrate to the basal epidermis, where it is phagocytosed by Langerhans cells. Activated Langerhans cells in turn activate innate immune mechanisms, including T cells, and induce a type IV hypersensitivity reaction (p. 101) to the intruding substance. Unlike irritant contact dermatitis, allergic contact dermatitis has a strong genetic predisposition, and multiple genes are involved. One such gene codes for a protein called **filaggrin**, produced by keratinocytes. It is essential for stabilising keratin within keratinocytes and maintaining the intracellular scaffolding that directs keratinocyte maturation as the cell moves from the basal epidermal layer to the cornified outer layer. If the filaggrin gene is mutated, the skin is deficient in filaggrin, keratinocyte maturation is inhibited, the squames lose their flattened, waterproof structure, and the skin's barrier function is reduced. This increases water loss through the skin, allowing allergen entry, and the skin becomes dry and cracked. Filaggrin deficiency is thought to be a major factor both in allergic contact dermatitis and in atopic dermatitis. Many substances can act as allergens and trigger allergic contact dermatitis; they include nickel (often found in jewellery and metal watch straps), some plants (e.g., poison ivy), chemicals (e.g., laundry detergents), and latex (in rubber gloves). Management centres around identifying, and then avoiding, the antigen responsible.

Atopic dermatitis

This is an example of a type I hypersensitivity reaction (p. 99) and is mediated by histamine release in response to antigen exposure. It is the commonest form of eczema, runs in families and is strongly associated with other type I hypersensitivity disorders, including food allergy and asthma. Globally, incidence is rising sharply, indicating the importance of environmental influences. Like allergic contact dermatitis, it is immunological in origin, but it is important to understand that the two conditions are very different. The aetiology is multifactorial, complicated, and not fully understood. Genetic predisposition is very important. Filaggrin gene mutations significantly increase the risk of atopic dermatitis, indicating that impairment of barrier function, allowing the skin to dry out and facilitating antigen entry, contributes to the condition. Environmental factors also play a part. Antenatal factors (e.g., maternal smoking, alcohol consumption, and stress) predispose to atopic dermatitis in the child. Incidence is higher in people exposed to pollutants (e.g., in urban environments) and in those eating diets high in processed and high-fat foods. It is lower in breastfed children and those eating diets high in fish, fruit, and vegetables.

Atopic dermatitis can occur at any age, but it is commonest in babies and children and often improves with age and may disappear by adulthood. The skin is dry, red,

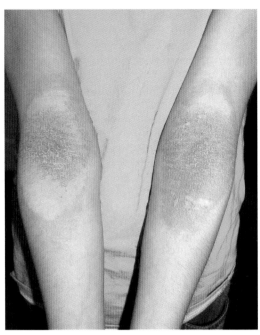

Fig. 15.3 Atopic dermatitis. Scaly, itchy rash in the elbow flexures and extending down the forearms. (From Lebwohl MG, Heymann WR, Coulson IH, et al. (2022) *Treatment of skin disease*, 6th ed, Fig. 17.1. Oxford: Elsevier Ltd.)

and flaky, and often relentlessly itchy (Fig. 15.3). When the child scratches, the risk of infection is high. A range of sites may be affected: on the face, skin creases at joints, and on the feet, ankles, and neck. The condition can have significant and long-lasting consequences in terms of lost sleep, interrupted schooling and impaired normal childhood development. Avoiding extended contact with water and using moisturisers and emollients help reduce skin dryness. Anti-inflammatory corticosteroids and antihistamines are also useful. Severe cases can be offered phototherapy and systemic treatment with potent immunosuppressants and anti-inflammatories.

ACNE

Acne is inflammation and infection of the pilosebaceous unit. The commonest form—acne vulgaris—is found globally and is most common in adolescence, when the sex hormone testosterone levels are rising in both boys and girls. Testosterone increases sebum production and predisposes to blockage of the pilosebaceous duct with consequent inflammation and infection. The face and trunk are most commonly affected. The Global Burden of Disease study estimates that acne vulgaris affects about 85% of young adults between the ages of 12 and 25. However, acne can occur at any age and up to 5% of adults over the age of 40 have acne, and globally, the incidence of acne is rising. There is a genetic component and a familial tendency. The disease can cause great distress, to the extent that young people can withdraw from social interaction including schooling, develop severe depression and experience long-term effects on self-esteem and the capacity to form normal relationships.

Pathophysiology

The condition is associated with increased sebum production, which blocks the sebaceous duct (Fig. 15.4). In addition, there is epidermal proliferation, which blocks the opening of the pilosebaceous duct at the skin surface. The dilated, inflamed ducts produce the characteristic comedones of acne. The blocked duct becomes inflamed and infected, producing inflamed pustules. The principal organism responsible is *Cutibacterium acnes* (formerly *Propionibacterium acnes*). This anaerobic bacterium is a normally harmless skin commensal, but when it accesses the deeper, lipid-rich low-oxygen environment of the hair follicle, it proliferates and triggers inflammation. The dilated and hyperactive sebaceous gland, unable to secrete its products through the blocked pilosebaceous duct, may rupture, triggering dermal inflammation.

Signs and symptoms

The skin is greasy, with varying degrees of inflammation. Mild acne is characterised by comedones, principally whiteheads, with the occasional papule or pustule. Moderate acne has a greater number of comedones, with a greater proportion of blackheads, papulopustules, and a larger degree of inflammation. Severe acne has multiple comedones, papulopustules, extensive inflammation, and a greater incidence of scarring. The most aggressive forms of acne may feature

large inflammatory nodules and cysts (nodulocystic acne). Fig. 15.5 gives examples.

Management and prognosis

Generally, the condition improves with age. Mild to moderate disease is managed with topical antiseptic and anti-comedogenic agents such as benzoyl peroxide, topical anti-proliferative agents (isotretinoin), and topical or oral antibiotics (typically oral tetracyclines, although microbial resistance is an increasing problem). With more severe disease, oral isotretinoin is used, and large, troublesome nodules and cysts can be surgically removed or drained. Residual scarring is common.

ROSACEA

Rosacea is a chronic inflammatory skin disorder affecting the face, which can resemble acne. Its aetiology is unclear, however, and unlike acne, sebum production is normal. It is most common in fair-skinned people of Celtic and northern European extraction, and there is a genetic contribution; half of rosacea sufferers report a family history. It tends to follow a relapsing/remitting course, with periods of exacerbation interspersed with remissions.

Pathophysiology

The underlying cause is not understood, although a variety of factors seem to contribute. Skin blood vessel numbers and reactivity are higher than normal, and vasodilation in response to triggers causes the characteristic flushing, although it is not understood why (Fig. 15.6). There is a range of triggers, which vary from person to person, including alcohol, irritant cosmetics or other products, extremes of temperature, some drugs (e.g., topical steroids), and sunlight. Links have been made to infection with a mite, *Demodex*, that may live in hair follicles, but the evidence is not conclusive: many people with *Demodex* infestation do not develop rosacea. There are degenerative changes in the dermal matrix, but it is not known if these changes are the cause or the result of the inflammation in rosacea.

Signs and symptoms

There are different forms of rosacea, each characterised by a particular collection of signs and symptoms, so not all of the following may be present in an individual patient. There may be facial flushing, thickening, and reddening of the skin and a papulopustular rash that resembles acne. A dense network of dilated blood vessels may be visible under the

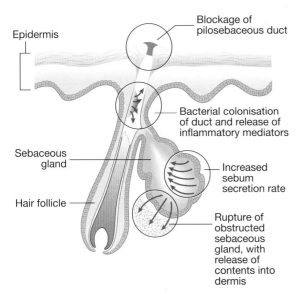

Fig. 15.4 The pilosebaceous unit in acne. (Modified from Ralston S, Penman I, Strachan M, et al. (2018) *Davidson's principles and practice of medicine*, 23rd ed, Fig. 29.28. Edinburgh: Elsevier Ltd.)

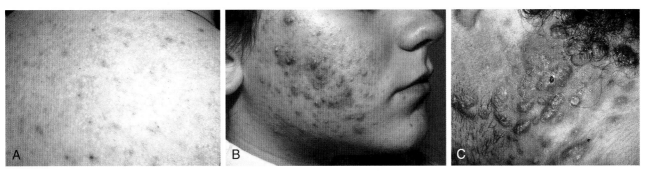

Fig. 15.5 Acne vulgaris. (A) Mild. (B) Moderate. (C) Severe. (From (A) Klatt E (2020) *Robbins and Cotran atlas of pathology*, 4th ed, Fig. 16.77. Philadelphia: Elsevier Inc; (B) courtesy Kalman Watsky, MD; and (C) courtesy Andrew Zaenglein, MD, and Diane Thiboutot, MD.)

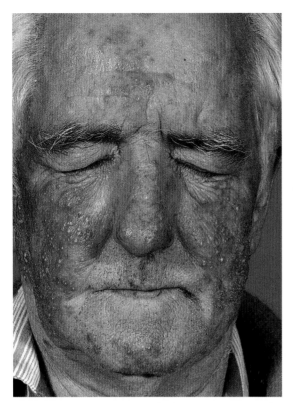

Fig. 15.6 Rosacea. There is typical flushing and erythema, with papulopustules. (From Innes JA (2020) *Davidson's essentials of medicine*, 3rd ed, Fig. 18.8. Edinburgh: Elsevier Ltd.)

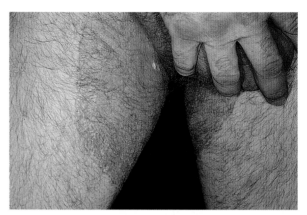

Fig. 15.7 Tinea cruris. (From Callen JP, Greer KE, Paller AS, et al. (2000) *Color atlas of dermatology*, 2nd ed, Fig. 13. Philadelphia: WB Saunders.)

skin (**telangiectasia**, sometimes called 'spider veins'). The nose may thicken and become disfigured (**rhinophyma**), a feature more common in men. There may be conjunctivitis and swelling around the eyes.

Management and prognosis

The disease is chronic, but most people can achieve a relatively stable state, although the most severe forms are disfiguring and respond poorly to treatment. Sunscreens are recommended. Pustular forms of the disease are treated with antibiotics, and some people respond to corticosteroids or isotretinoin. Laser therapy to ablate abnormal blood vessels is also useful if facial flushing and telangiectasia are predominant features.

DERMATOPHYTE (TINEA) INFECTIONS

Fungal species that thrive in the skin, hair, and nails because they feed on keratin are called *dermatophytes* or *tinea* and cause a range of superficial infections. There is evidence that dermatophytes dampen the host immune response and inhibit keratinocyte division, reducing epidermal shedding and therefore reducing clearance of the fungus from the upper skin layers.

Tinea infections are spread via direct contact and are commonest in people with chronic disease (e.g., diabetes), the immunocompromised and in damaged or poorly perfused skin. Other predisposing factors are tropical climates, and increased urbanisation and increasing population densities, making spread easier. Treatment with antifungals generally gives complete resolution although the spread of drug resistance is of concern. Three main genera of dermatophytes

are responsible for human infection: *Trichophyton*, *Microsporum*, and *Epidermophyton*, but tinea infections are usually considered according to the region infected rather than their fungal classification.

Tinea pedis (athlete's foot)

This is the most common tineal infection and is usually caused by *Trichophyton* and *Epidermophyton*. It usually affects the soles of the feet and the spaces between the toes. Warm, moist conditions inside occlusive shoes (e.g., trainers) provide an ideal environment for the fungus to proliferate, and going barefoot in communal showers and swimming pools increases the risk of infection. There does appear to be a heritable component because there is a familial tendency, but the basis of this is not known.

Tinea capitis

This is dermatophyte infection of the hair follicles of the scalp, caused by *Trichophyton* and *Microsporum* infections and is commonest in children. The skin of the scalp becomes inflamed, crusted, and scaly. There may be pustules and hair loss.

Tinea cruris (jock itch)

This dermatophyte infection of the groin is usually caused by *Trichophyton* or *Epidermophyton*. It is three times more common in men than women and is found worldwide, although it is commoner in tropical climates. Well-demarcated areas of red, itchy skin extend from the groin down the thigh (Fig. 15.7). The spreading edge of the infection is often redder and raised compared with the inner part of the lesion. It is spread by direct contamination (e.g., from infected hands or feet) and also by contaminated linens (towels, sheets, clothing).

Tinea versicolour

This is caused by infection with *Malassezia* (see also seborrhoeic dermatitis) and causes variations in skin pigmentation, which usually manifest as macules on the trunk. The macules may be either hyperpigmented or hypopigmented.

Tinea corporis (ringworm)

This is usually caused by *Trichophyton* and begins as a red, scaly plaque that progressively enlarges. The centre may clear, giving a ring-shaped border that gives the infection its common name (although the 'worm' reference is inaccurate).

INFESTATIONS

When the organism colonising the skin is not a microbe but an insect, the condition is referred to as an **infestation** rather than an infection. Treatment is with a topical insecticide, but drug resistance is becoming increasingly problematic.

Scabies

This infestation is caused by the mite *Sarcoptes scabiei* (Fig. 15.8). The global burden of scabies, borne largely by impoverished populations in tropical climates and developing countries, is substantial. The WHO (2015) estimates that 200 million people, mainly children and elderly people, are affected worldwide at any one time. Scabies is included in the WHO 2021 to 2030 roadmap for neglected tropical diseases, which introduces policies and programmes aimed at achieving global control of a range of common, preventable tropical diseases.

The mite is transmitted mainly by direct contact, so the infestation spreads most rapidly in overcrowded living conditions. The mites tunnel into the skin and take up residence in the upper layers of the epidermis. Their burrows are

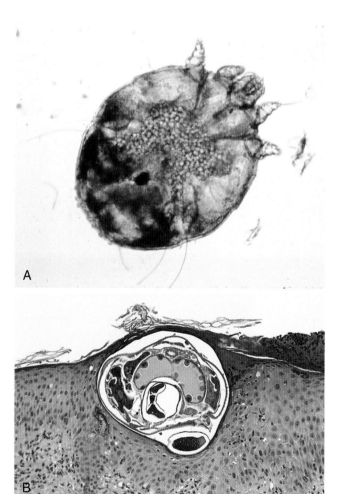

Fig. 15.8 The scabies mite. (A) Magnified x400. (B) Biopsy specimen, showing a mite in its burrow. (From (A) Marks J, and Miller J (2014) *Lookingbill and Marks' principles of dermatology*, 5th ed, Fig. 11.22. London: Saunders; and (B) courtesy James E. Fitzpatrick, MD.)

clearly visible as tracklike marks on the skin surface. Once she has made her burrow, the female mite lays 10 to 25 eggs within, which take 3 to 4 days to hatch. The main symptoms are inflammation and intense, relentless itch, but there is an initial asymptomatic phase after first infestation. This is because the immunological response to the infestation is a type IV (delayed) hypersensitivity reaction, mediated by T cells, which takes time to develop (p. 101). The main areas infested are between the fingers, the soles of the feet, the elbows, waist, genitalia, and the front of the wrists. Scratching leads to secondary bacterial infections, which in turn can invade deeper tissues and lead to serious systemic infection, including post-streptococcal kidney disease. Sepsis is a significant cause of death in this situation.

Lice

Lice infestations (pediculosis) affect the head (the louse *Pediculus capitis*), the body (the closely related *Pediculus corporis*), and the pubic area (the louse *Pthirus pubis*). The insects do not fly or jump, and they or their eggs are transferred by direct person to person contact or on contaminated objects (e.g., combs, clothing, or bedding). Eggs can remain viable for several weeks on contaminated objects, although the live insects do not survive very long when not in contact with their human host. Head and pubic lice live at the base of hair shafts and in her 6-week lifespan each female louse lays about 200 eggs, which she glues to the hair shaft as close to the warm skin as she can. Head lice preferentially glue their eggs to the hairline at the back of the head or behind the ears, the warmest places on the scalp. The eggs hatch in about 9 days, leaving the empty egg case (seen as white dots on the hair—these are called nits). Body lice do not live on the skin; they live in clothing or in bedding, lay their eggs on the fibres of the fabric, and only crawl on to the skin to feed. Female lice take several blood meals a day from their host. The insect's saliva usually triggers an allergic reaction, initiating itch and scratching, but not everyone reacts and so not every infested person scratches.

Head lice are found in all communities worldwide, but infestation is commonest in school age children. It is not related to economic class or level of personal hygiene. Body louse infestation is associated with poverty, poor personal hygiene, and homelessness. Pubic louse infestation is commonest in young sexually active adults.

BACTERIAL INFECTIONS

Streptococcal and staphylococcal species are normal skin residents but can become pathogenic if host immunity is impaired in the presence of chronic disease (e.g., diabetes) if the barrier function of the skin is reduced or the organisms access areas other than their usual habitat.

Erysipelas

This streptococcal infection affects the dermis and may extend into the local lymphatics. Affected skin is well demarcated, tender, and swollen; when it extends into the dermis and subcutaneous tissues, it is called *cellulitis*. it is seen mainly on the legs and face (Fig. 15.9). The organism enters deeper tissues through a traumatic injury of some sort, often minor. Predisposing factors include poor circulation or locally blocked lymphatic flow, which reduces local defence mechanisms. It is treated with antibiotics.

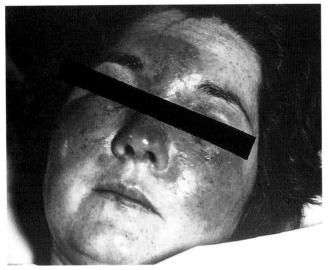

Fig. 15.9 Erysipelas. (From Kumar V, Singh M, Abbas A, and Aster J (2020) *Robbins & Cotran pathologic basis of disease: South Asia edition*, 10th ed, Fig. 8.16. India: Elsevier India.)

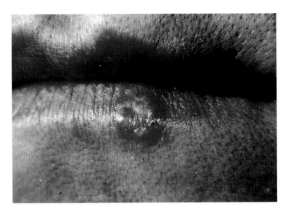

Fig. 15.11 Oral herpes. (From Grimes DE (1991) *Infectious diseases*. St Louis: Mosby.)

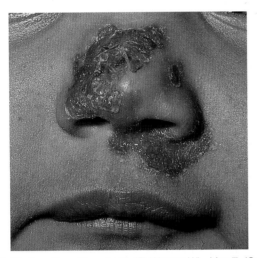

Fig. 15.10 Impetigo. (From Lane AT, Weston WL, Morelli JG (2007) *Color textbook of pediatric dermatology*, 4th ed, Fig. 5.2. Edinburgh: Mosby.)

Impetigo and staphylococcal scalded skin syndrome

Impetigo, usually seen in children, is caused by *Streptococcus pyogenes* or *Staphylococcus aureus* and is highly contagious. Outbreaks are usually associated with institutions, immunocompromise, poverty, and overcrowded living conditions. The condition affects the upper epidermal layers, usually around the mouth and nose and produces vesicles or pustules that rupture and crust (Fig. 15.10). It is not usually painful or itchy. Bullous impetigo, a form of the infection associated with blister formation, is caused by toxins produced by *S. aureus*. The toxin is epidermolytic, that is, it disrupts connections between layers of the epidermis, which separate, forming blisters (compare with the more serious toxic epidermal necrolysis, where the dermis and epidermis separate along the dermo-epidermal junction). The same toxin causes a serious disorder seen mainly in newborn babies and children: staphylococcal scalded skin syndrome. The toxin, released by bacteria at the site of infection, enters the bloodstream and the blistering and epidermal sloughing can therefore be widespread. Most children recover completely unless there is an underlying health condition. Adults fare less well, usually because most cases of adult staphylococcal scalded skin syndrome occur in those with pre-existing conditions (e.g., immunosuppression), and mortality approaches 50%.

VIRAL INFECTIONS

Several clinically important viruses infect the skin, including herpes simplex. Additionally, skin rashes are a common manifestation of systemic viral infection (e.g., measles, German measles, and chickenpox).

Herpes simplex virus (HSV)

Herpes simplex (HS) types 1 and 2 (p. 21) infect skin and mucous membranes. HS-1 is mainly associated with oral herpes, and HS-2 with genital herpes, but this is not exclusive. HS-1 infection is very common in most populations and is usually acquired in childhood. It is usually asymptomatic, but in susceptible people it causes painful blistering and ulceration at the site of infection, flaring up as cold sores in and around the lips and mouth that may burst and crust (Fig. 15.11). The virus is usually transmitted by direct mouth-to-mouth contact, penetrates the skin or mucous membrane and enters local autonomic nerve fibres, where it is protected from immunological attack. It travels up the nerve to the dorsal root ganglion where it takes up permanent residence, alternating periods of latency with recurring episodes of reactivation for the remainder of the individual's life.

Viral warts

Viral warts are caused by human papilloma virus (HPV) infection of basal keratinocytes, which triggers keratinocyte proliferation. Infection with HPV 16 and 18 is a major risk factor for cervical cancer and some oropharyngeal, vaginal, and penile cancers, all associated with sexual transmission. Viral warts are rough, raised, dry papules or plaques caused by hyperkeratosis and acanthosis. There are over 100 types of HPV, which can cause warts on any part of the body. Verruca vulgaris, the common wart (Fig. 15.12), is usually caused by HPV types 2 and 7. Most viral warts clear up themselves within a couple of years, but some may have malignant potential: for example, HPV infection is associated with some forms of squamous cell carcinoma (SCC).

Molluscum contagiosum

This viral infection causes multiple small, pearly, dome-shaped papules (Fig. 15.13) with a tiny central indentation (umbilication). The causative virus belongs to the poxvirus family and is most likely to cause infection in people with additional conditions, including atopic dermatitis and any degree of immunocompromise. It enters epithelial cells and triggers cellular proliferation. It is spread by direct contact and can be spread by the patient themselves from one part of the body to another. Children can acquire the infection by sharing baths, towels, gym equipment, or by close skin-to-skin contact. Adults can spread the infection by sexual contact. It is usually self-limiting and clears up without treatment within about eighteen months in otherwise healthy people, although larger lesions may leave scars.

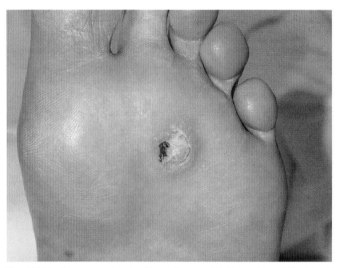

Fig. 15.12 **Verruca vulgaris.** (From Burrow JG, Rome K and Padhiar N (2020) *Neale's disorders of the foot and ankle,* 9th ed, Fig. 18.19. Oxford: Elsevier Ltd.)

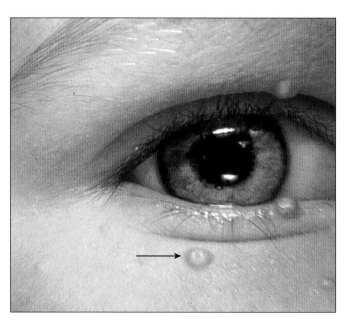

AUTOIMMUNITY AND THE SKIN

Autoantigens present in the skin may activate an autoimmune reaction against that skin component. This may be one facet of a systemic autoimmune disorder that involves tissues elsewhere (e.g., systemic scleroderma and systemic lupus erythematosus), or the skin may be the primary target.

PSORIASIS

This inflammatory disorder of the epidermis, characterised by the presence of raised, reddened scaly skin plaques, is very common in Caucasian and Scandinavian populations, with a prevalence of 11%, and is much less common in people of Asian and African extraction. The aetiology of psoriasis is complex and not well understood. There is a very strong familial tendency; the concordance rate between identical twins is 60% and 70%. Immunological factors also play a part, and there is strong evidence for autoimmune involvement, although the autoantigen has not been identified. Males and females are equally affected.

Pathophysiology

In psoriasis, keratinocyte turnover is significantly increased, and the epidermis thickens, forming raised, dry rough, reddened plaques on the skin, with a silvery white superficial layer of dead squames. Plaques may be painful or itchy, and they may crack and bleed. Affected skin displays a marked inflammatory cell presence, including macrophages and large numbers of T cells, and there may be growth of networks of new blood vessels (neovascularisation). The cytokines produced by the inflammatory cells activate keratinocyte proliferation and promote the ongoing inflammatory response. Identification of the specific agents and pathways directs research into potentially useful drugs; for example, blocking the activity of interleukins and tumour necrosis factor alpha (TNFα), released by T cells in psoriatic plaques, has proved to be an effective treatment.

Fig. 15.13 Molluscum contagiosum. Arrowed papule shows central umbilication. (Modified from Mannis M and Holland E (2022) *Cornea,* 5th ed, Fig. 30.3. Philadelphia: Elsevier Inc.)

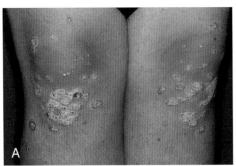
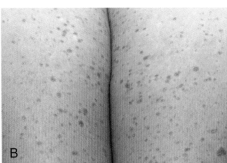
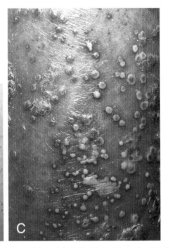

Fig. 15.14 Psoriasis. (A) Plaque psoriasis. (B) Guttate psoriasis. (C) Pustular psoriasis. (From (A) Paller A and Mancini A (2021) *Hurwitz Clinical pediatric dermatology*, 6th ed, Fig. 4.6. St Louis: Elsevier Inc; (B) courtesy Kalman Watsky, MD; and (C) Wilkinson J, Shaw S, and Orton D (2004) *Dermatology in focus*. Edinburgh: Churchill Livingstone.)

Many genes have been implicated in the pathogenesis of psoriasis, many of which belong to the HLA (MHC) complex of genes on chromosome 6 (p. 91). This group of genes is involved in immunological self-recognition, programming immune cells to distinguish between self and non self, and mutations in these genes are implicated in practically all autoimmune disorders yet studied. There is therefore strong support for an autoimmune component in psoriasis. However, at least 70 mutations in other genes have also been associated with increased susceptibility to the disorder. Some of these genes produce proteins important in the barrier function of the skin, and others upregulate the production of inflammatory mediators such as interleukins, and key immune cells including T cells. Clearly, the underlying aetiology of psoriasis is complex and multifactorial.

There are several distinct forms of the disease, which differ significantly in the distribution of skin lesions. The commonest form is **plaque psoriasis**, which presents mainly on the extensor surfaces of the elbows and knees, on the scalp, and may involve the nails (Fig. 15.14A). The second commonest form is **guttate psoriasis** (Fig. 15.14B), which usually appears suddenly, often after a streptococcal throat infection. Numerous small red plaques erupt, scattered over the trunk, and although it usually clears up with treatment, it increases the risk of developing plaque psoriasis in later life. **Pustular psoriasis** is characterised by small blisters filled with pus (Fig. 15.14C). The pus is sterile, that is, it contains no bacteria and is composed of white blood cells. The pustules usually appear on the hands or feet, but the eruption can be widespread, in which case the patient is generally febrile and ill and requires immediate medical treatment. Up to 30% of patients develop psoriatic arthritis. The nails are also commonly involved.

A wide range of trigger factors may cause flare-ups, including cold or dry weather, alcohol, skin trauma (this is called *Koebner phenomenon*), stress, and some drugs (e.g., lithium and some beta blockers).

Prognosis and management

Psoriasis is linked to other conditions including renal and inflammatory gastrointestinal disease, which can impact quality of life; in addition, there may be psychological problems including depression, which can be severe. Standard treatments include retinoids and vitamin D analogues (which are anti-proliferative), emollients, anti-inflammatory glucocorticoids, and phototherapy. An increasing range of biologics are available for serious and resistant disease, for example infliximab, which blocks TNFα.

IMMUNE MEDIATED SKIN BLISTERING DISORDERS

There are several blistering disorders of the skin caused by autoimmune mechanisms that disrupt the normal attachment mechanisms anchoring the layers of the skin together. Autoantibodies are produced against key proteins involved in cell-cell adhesion, leading to separation. Disorders can be primary (i.e., arise with no identifiable trigger) or secondary, in which the trigger is known.

Bullous pemphigoid

This primary blistering disorder is one of a number of blistering disorders (called collectively the *pemphigoid disorders*) characterised by loss of adhesion between the epidermis and the dermis caused by autoantibody production to adhesion proteins. Bullous pemphigoid is the commonest of this group. It is usually seen in middle aged and elderly people, is found in all races and affects men and women equally. Although statistics reporting incidence of this disorder are patchy, it is believed to be low (fewer than 5 in 100,000 people) but is on the increase.

Pathophysiology

In bullous pemphigoid, autoantibodies are produced to two target proteins: BPAg1 and BPAg2. Both proteins are part of the hemidesmosomes attaching the basal keratinocytes to the basement membrane between the dermis and epidermis. Antibody-antigen binding activates complement, inflammatory cell recruitment and inflammation at the dermo-epidermal junction, destroying hemidesmosomes and allowing the epidermis to separate from the dermis (Fig. 15.15A). One well-established risk factor for bullous pemphigoid is pre-existing neurological disease, including multiple sclerosis, possibly because autoantibodies

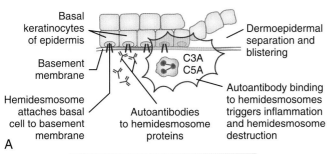

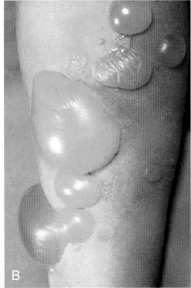

Fig. 15.15 Bullous pemphigoid. (A) Pathogenesis. (B) Blistering. (B, From Innes JA (2020) *Davidson's essentials of medicine*, 3rd ed, Fig. 18.1. Edinburgh: Elsevier Ltd.)

associated with this condition attack both skin and nerve proteins.

Signs and symptoms

The disease follows a chronic path, and initially manifests with an itchy, red rash that develops into large, swollen blisters (Fig. 15.15B).

Management and prognosis

Anti-inflammatory steroids and immunosuppressants are the mainstay of treatment. The disorder generally improves and resolves over a period of years.

Pemphigus vulgaris

This uncommon condition affects people from all racial populations but is most common in people of Jewish and Mediterranean extraction (the prevalence in Jerusalem is 1.6 per 100,000 people, while in Finland, the prevalence is only 0.076 per 100,000 people). In most populations, the male:female ratio is equal. Onset is usually in middle age.

Pathophysiology

The epidermis splits above the level of the dermo-epidermal junction (compare with bullous pemphigoid, where the blistering occurs at the dermo-epidermal junction), causing blistering of the skin and mucous membranes. Keratinocytes in the epidermis lose cell-cell adhesion because of a circulating IgG antibody to **desmoglein**, an adhesion protein that

is part of the desmosomes (p. 10) holding keratinocytes together. With this loss of cell-cell adhesion, blisters develop within the epidermis. The disorder may arise spontaneously, but may be induced by a range of drugs, including captopril and non-steroidal anti-inflammatory agents, which seem to trigger production of the autoantibodies. Pemphigus vulgaris may also follow herpes virus infections.

Signs and symptoms

Recurrent blisters in the mouth are very common and may be the presenting symptom. Most people go on to develop blistering of the skin. The blisters are often painful, are filled with clear fluid and are usually soft rather than tight. They usually appear on skin that looks otherwise healthy, and are fragile, so burst readily leaving a raw and painful surface below. Even slight traction on the skin can produce blistering, which can be widespread and leave large areas of the skin denuded of epidermis.

Management and prognosis

Steroid therapy is the standard treatment, which is anti-inflammatory and immunosuppressive. Without treatment, most people die because of infection or fluid and electrolyte disturbances. Even with treatment, mortality sits between 5% and 15%, and the prognosis is worse in older people and those with more extensive blistering.

Toxic epidermal necrolysis

Along with Stevens–Johnson syndrome, this serious condition is thought to be caused by a type IV delayed hypersensitivity reaction (p. 101), usually to certain drugs or their metabolites. A range of drugs can trigger this abnormal immune response, including a range of antibiotics and anti-convulsants, and some non-steroidal anti-inflammatory agents. There may be a genetic predisposition in some people and the female: male incidence ratio is 1.5:1. Globally, the incidence is between 0.4 and 1.3 per million population, so it is fortunately uncommon, as the mortality rate is up to 70%.

Pathophysiology

The exact mechanism is not clear and likely to be complex. Skin keratinocytes are prime targets, but other epithelial cells of mucous membranes are also affected. However, it is known that in response to drug exposure (occasionally the precipitating event is an infection, usually in children) a population of activated cytotoxic CD8 T-cells (p. 91) is produced. The CD8 T cells react to epithelial proteins, causing massive cell damage, and the damaged cells undergo apoptosis. Septicaemia is a leading cause of death because of the massive failure of the barrier function of the skin, allowing potentially overwhelming infection. There can be bleeding (e.g., in the gastrointestinal tract) as epithelial layers slough off. Fluid loss from denuded skin surfaces can be significant enough to cause hypovolaemia, shock, and renal failure.

Signs and symptoms

Two or three weeks after beginning drug treatment, the patient begins to feel unwell, with a flu-like syndrome including fever, cough, joint pain, anorexia, and headache. Initial skin changes usually involve the appearance of macules over large areas of the body, which coalesce into large blisters that burst;

large sheets of skin may then slough off (Fig. 15.16). The condition is very painful, and if the upper gastrointestinal tract lining is affected, which is common, swallowing is painful, and people do not tolerate oral intake. The lining of the genitourinary tract is also frequently affected. Corneal involvement is also common, with painful corneal ulcers and conjunctivitis.

Management and prognosis

Prognosis depends on a range of factors, including increasing age and the severity of the clinical response. Surviving patients may be left with permanent skin scarring, including an inability to sweat caused by destruction of sweat glands, alopecia, oesophageal stricture, changes in skin pigmentation, loss of hair and nails and corneal scarring. It is essential to identify and discontinue the offending drug.

TUMOURS OF THE SKIN

Skin growths are very common. The skin is constantly exposed to UV light, a potent carcinogen, and cellular

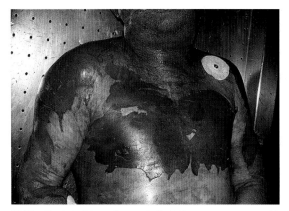

Fig. 15.16   Toxic epidermal necrolysis. This case was caused by the drug captopril. (Courtesy James E. Fitzpatrick, MD.)

proliferation rates in the epidermis are very high, another risk factor for the development of neoplasms. Certain chemicals (e.g., arsenic and tars are known skin carcinogens). The skin may also be the site of metastatic growth of a primary cancer elsewhere.

MALIGNANT TUMOURS

Conventionally, these are considered under two headings: malignant melanoma and non-melanoma skin cancer (NMSC). NMSC includes squamous cell carcinoma (SCC), basal cell carcinoma (BCC), and Bowen disease, among others. World Cancer Research Fund statistics (2020) show that NMSC ranks 5th in global cancer incidence, and the WHO calculates an incidence of 10.1 per 100,000 population. The incidence of malignant melanoma is 3.1 per 100,000 population, and it ranked 17th in the world cancer tables in 2020. Worldwide, skin cancer rates are rising, in both males and females, and especially in older age groups. Exposure to natural ultraviolet (UV) light (i.e., in sunlight) and artificial UV light (e.g., sunbeds) is a key risk factor in all types of skin cancer. Other risk factors include fair, freckled skin, and light-coloured eyes. People who burn in the sun rather than tan or who have a family history of skin cancer are also at increased risk. As with many cancers, the rates of skin cancer increase with age.

UV radiation and skin cancer risk

UV radiation in natural sunlight is responsible for sunburn caused by excessive sun exposure. Sunburned skin is red, hot, and painful, and may blister. UV radiation is at the high energy, short wavelength end of the electromagnetic spectrum (Fig. 15.17). Sunlight reaching the surface of the Earth has two forms of UV rays: UVA and UVB. Both are linked to skin cancer because both damage DNA in proliferating keratinocytes. DNA is damaged directly because it absorbs the energy in UV radiation, which disrupts its molecular structure. In addition, UV rays ionise other cellular macromolecules, producing damaging free radicals that also

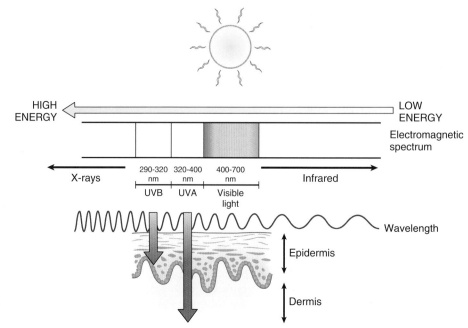

Fig. 15.17   The electromagnetic spectrum. UVA light penetrates to the dermis. UVB light penetrates to the deeper layers of the epidermis.

damage DNA and predispose to mutagenesis and the generation of potentially carcinogenic cells. UVA has less energy than UVB, but it has a longer wavelength (320–400 nm) and penetrates more deeply into the skin. It damages proteins in the dermis and is linked to the ageing effects of sunlight on the skin, including sagging and wrinkling. UVB penetrates less deeply into the skin but has more energy and is particularly damaging to cells in the lower epidermis, significantly increasing the risk of producing a cancerous cell line in keratinocytes or melanocytes. Sun-induced ageing and the incidence of skin cancer are closely correlated.

Field cancerisation

Developing a malignant skin tumour increases the chances of developing others, not necessarily of the same type. This is considered because of the concept of **field cancerisation**, that is, exposing an area of skin to UV light induces pre-cancerous mutations in multiple skin cells, predisposing large numbers to malignant change. This phenomenon explains why people who develop skin cancer frequently develop more than one tumour and are at increased risk of other types of skin cancer as well.

BASAL CELL CARCINOMA

The incidence of this cancer is rising worldwide; globally, it is currently the most common cancer. Risk factors include UV radiation exposure, fair skin, and geographical latitude, and 85% of tumours develop on the face, head, or neck. Australia has the highest rates, where over half the population will have developed the disease by the age of 70 years. In younger age groups, more women than men are diagnosed (perhaps related to the popularity of sunbeds), but this is reversed in older age groups. Intermittent intense periods of exposure increase risk, especially with episodes of sunburn when young. Fair skin, a personal or family history of skin cancer, increasing age, and immunosuppression all increase risk. Although this cancer is common, it is usually slow growing and rarely metastasises, and mortality rates are very low.

Pathophysiology

The cell of origin is a keratinocyte stem cell, often associated with hair follicles, and most tumours arise on hair-bearing skin. Multiple genetic mutations have been demonstrated in BCC; in fact, neoplastic cells from BCCs display more genetic mutations than any other human cancer. It may be that this is the reason why this cancer is generally slow growing and rarely metastasises; its cells carry so many genetic abnormalities that they are rapidly identified and destroyed by the immune system.

Hedgehog signalling and BCC. The Hedgehog signalling pathway is a fundamental biochemical control mechanism in embryonic development and in growth and repair of adult tissues after injury. This pathway activates key genes involved in cell division, blood vessel growth, and cell differentiation, resulting in cell and tissue proliferation. It drives regeneration in multiple body tissue types, including the keratinocytes of the skin, and establishes an environment favourable to tumour growth, including promoting an inflammatory environment, inhibition of apoptosis, destabilising the cell's genetic material and increasing the risk of mutation and conferring resistance to the body's immune defences. Abnormal activation of this pathway has been associated with a range of cancers including breast, lung, prostate, and ovarian cancers, but BCC is the most strongly linked; nearly all BCCs express overactivity of this pathway. Identifying inhibitors of this pathway to treat BCC and other cancers has become an important area of research in the hunt for new cancer therapies.

The commonest form, accounting for 50% to 80% of all BCCs, is called **nodular BCC** and appears as a smooth, pearly papule or nodule that often has a characteristic rolled edge and telangiectases (Fig. 15.18A). The second commonest form, **superficial BCC**, appears as a well-defined, red plaque with the same characteristic rolled borders as nodular BCC (Fig. 15.18B). It accounts for 10% to 30% of all cases. The central area may show clearing because although the tumour is expanding, its central region may become atrophic because of insufficient blood supply, and this area loses the characteristic appearance of the rest of the growth. Additionally, there are a number of rarer subtypes that may resemble scar tissue or polyps. These may have varying degrees of pigmentation and may present either as a raised or indented lesion of the skin. The variable presentation can confuse or delay diagnosis.

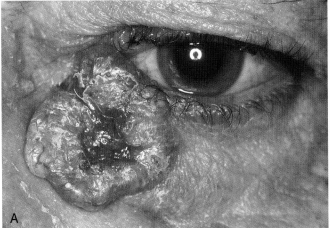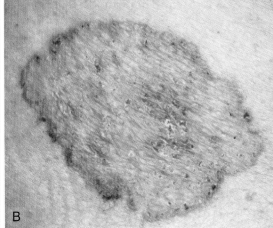

Fig. 15.18 Basal cell carcinoma (BCC). (A) Nodular BCC. Note the raised, rolled pearly edges. (B) Superficial BCC. (From (A) Mannis M and Holland E (2022) *Cornea*, 5th ed, Fig. 28.1. Philadelphia: Elsevier Inc; and (B) courtesy James E. Fitzpatrick, MD.)

Signs and symptoms

The cancer usually appears as an enlarging skin lesion that may ulcerate, bleed, and/or itch, but that consistently fails to heal.

Management and prognosis

Developing one BCC increases the chances that further BCCs (and other skin cancers) will develop (see field cancerisation above). BCC rarely metastasises, but it can cause extensive local destruction, and the enlarging, ulcerating lesion is sometimes called a rodent ulcer. Management is usually surgical, which is curative if the tumour is removed at an early enough stage. For recurrent resistant disease, Hedgehog pathway inhibitors such as vismodegib are available.

MALIGNANT MELANOMA

The incidence of malignant melanoma correlates with the risk factors described previously. However, unlike SCC (described under Squamous cell cancer below), intermittent intense episodes of sun exposure, including sunbed use and beach holidays, especially when the skin is allowed to burn, seem to be more important than the lifetime degree of cumulative exposure. Having large numbers of moles also increases risk. The rates are highest in Queensland, Australia, with a reported rate of 57 cases per 100,000 people, and worldwide the disease is 20 times more common in white-skinned people than dark-skinned people. Although the average age of diagnosis is 55 years, it is frequently found in much younger people (probably related to the increasing use of sunbeds) and is the most lethal form of skin cancer, accounting for most skin-cancer related mortality. Most cases are sporadic, although about 10% occur in family clusters with a clear hereditable component.

Pathophysiology

The cell of origin is the melanocyte, which produces melanin as a fundamental protective mechanism when skin is exposed to the sun. Melanomas may arise in pre-existing moles or other skin growths or may appear spontaneously on a previously normal area of skin. Damage to a wide range of genes can cause this disease, most notably the oncogene (p. 76) called *BRAF* and a tumour suppressor gene (p. 75) called *CDKN2A*. The *MC1R* (melanocortin-1 receptor) gene is also implicated in this cancer. This gene codes for a protein that directs melanin production. *MC1R* mutations can reduce the skin's ability to produce eumelanin, the dark form of melanin, which impairs its ability to tan and absorb UV rays.

There is also a link between malignant melanoma and Parkinson disease. Having one disease significantly increases the risk of the other. The reason for this is not known, but it is not a coincidence that the neurones of the nigrostriatal pathway, which degenerate in Parkinson disease, originate in the substantia nigra, which is rich in a form of melanin called neuromelanin. It may be that an underlying abnormality or deficiency in melanin chemistry increases the risk of both melanoma and Parkinson disease, explaining the correlation.

Signs and symptoms

Of all malignant melanomas, 95% arise on the skin, although some appear on the iris of the eye or the mucous membranes of the mouth. Typical lesions are irregularly shaped, asymmetrical macules or nodules, often with variable pigmentation, that are changing, often getting bigger (Fig. 15.19). There are different forms of the disease, with different growth patterns. **Superficial spreading melanoma** presents as a pigmented macule that steadily enlarges over the skin surface. Eventually, however, it enters a vertical growth phase and invades the dermis, after which metastasis is often rapid. **Nodular melanoma** enters the vertical growth phase very quickly and appear as a raised and rapidly enlarging nodule, often heavily pigmented, bleeding, and ulcerating. It can metastasise at a very early stage. **Lentigo maligna melanoma** is a slow growing, superficial form usually seen in older people. It presents as a slowly enlarging macule that can spend years in this superficial spreading stage before developing vertical growth.

Management and prognosis

Prognosis depends how quickly the tumour is identified and treated. If surgically removed while it is superficial and localised, the cure rate is almost 100%. The most frequent sites of distant metastasis are brain, lungs, and liver. Once metastasis has occurred, 5-year survival rate is only in the order of about 20%. A poorer prognosis is associated with older people, male sex, larger, thicker, and ulcerated lesions, a previous history of malignant melanoma, and lymphatic or distant tissue involvement. Surgery is the treatment of choice wherever possible, although there is an increasing number of options using biologics to manage the disease in patients whose cancer is too widespread to be removed surgically.

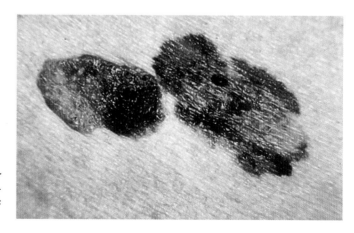

Fig. 15.19 Superficial spreading malignant melanoma. The tumour has an irregular boundary, variable pigmentation, and central clearing. (From Burrow JG, Rome K, and Padhiar N (2020) *Neale's disorders of the foot and ankle*, 9th ed, Fig. 4.32. Oxford: Elsevier Ltd.)

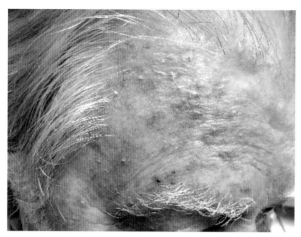

Fig. 15.20 Actinic keratosis. (Courtesy Dr Robert Norman.)

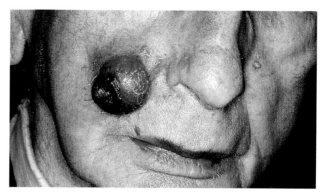

Fig. 15.21 Squamous cell carcinoma. These tumours develop most frequently on sun-exposed skin. (From Underwood J and Cross S (2009) *General and systematic pathology*, 5th ed, Fig. 24.15. Edinburgh: Churchill Livingstone.)

Identifying the specific genetic abnormalities in a particular tumour is important, to best match tumour-specific immunotherapies and biologics in treatment plans.

ACTINIC KERATOSIS AND SQUAMOUS CELL CARCINOMA

Actinic keratosis is a dry, red, scaly lesion on sun-exposed skin, usually seen in older people (Fig. 15.20). It is caused by cumulative sunlight damage, so is usually seen on the face, scalp, ears, and the backs of the hands and forearms. Its incidence varies significantly between countries, but it is common in most populations, especially in sunny countries. It has been estimated, for example, that half of all Australians have actinic keratosis lesions by the age of 40 years. Initially, the lesions are small, but they are often multiple and as they enlarge, they can merge into larger plaque-like patches.

Pathophysiology of actinic keratosis

Basal keratinocytes in actinic keratosis are generally large and clearly abnormal under the microscope; they vary in size and shape and have abnormal nuclei. Examination of their DNA shows a range of characteristic gene mutations in associated with UV irradiation damage, including inactivation of the tumour suppressor gene *p53* (p. 75). The epidermis is abnormal, with nucleated keratinocytes present much higher in the epidermis than usual, and with keratin production abnormally high in the deeper layers of the epidermis.

Prognosis

Individual lesions can be removed with cryotherapy or surgery or treated topically with cytotoxic drugs such as 5-fluorouracil. Although for most people actinic keratosis progresses very slowly and may even spontaneously regress, it warrants careful examination and treatment because a small number of lesions may progress to SCC.

Squamous cell carcinoma

About 60% of cases of SCC of the skin arise in pre-existing actinic keratosis lesions, although the great majority of these lesions remain benign. SCC risk factors include fair skin, living in equatorial or subequatorial countries, cumulative sun exposure (most occur on chronically sun-exposed skin, e.g. the face), increasing age, male gender, smoking and immunosuppression. Australia has the highest incidence, at 1.17 per 100 people. Its incidence is currently rising worldwide, despite vigorous health education initiatives, possibly because of an ageing population and the increased use of sunbeds. Most cases arise in the elderly, but the disease appears at a younger age in higher risk groups (e.g., those living in sunny climates).

Pathophysiology

UV radiation induced genetic mutations in basal keratinocytes are very similar to those seen in actinic keratosis, including *p53* mutations and mutations in the *RAS* oncogene. As these damaged keratinocytes divide, they accumulate further mutations and may become malignant and transform into SCC. As long as the cancerous growth remains in the epidermis and does not break into the dermis, it is referred to as carcinoma in situ (CIS). At this stage, it is called *Bowen disease*.

Signs and symptoms

Initial presentation can be quite diverse. The cancer can appear as an inflamed ulcer that fails to heal, as a raised plaque or a firm, pink nodule, either of which may be dry, crusty, and scaly or inflamed and ulcerated (Fig. 15.21). Occasionally they bleed, and they may be painful. The most common metastatic sites are lung, bone, thyroid, and liver.

Management and prognosis

If caught early enough, surgery is almost always curative. Some body sites (e.g., lips and eyelids) are associated with more aggressive tumours and a poorer prognosis. Also, if the tumour invades local nerves, the prognosis is poorer. Recurrence is likelier in these cases. Five-year survival rates are over 90% if the cancer is diagnosed at stage 1 (small, thin lesions with no lymphatic involvement or distant spread), but advanced stage disease with metastatic growths have survival rates as low as 25%.

BIBLIOGRAPHY AND REFERENCES

Achterman, R. R., & White, T. C. (2013). Dermatophytes. *Current Biology*, *23*(13), PR551–552.

Cameron, M. C., Lee, E., Hibler, B. P., et al. (2019). Basal cell carcinoma. Epidemiology; pathophysiology; clinical and histological subtypes; and disease associations. *Journal of the American Academy of Dermatology*, *80*(2), 303–317.

Grice, E. A., & Segre, J. A. (2011). The skin microbiome. *Nature Reviews Microbiology, 9*(4), 244–253.

Hanna, A., & Shevde, L. A. (2016). Hedgehog signaling: Modulation of cancer properties and tumour microenvironment. *Molecular Cancer, 15*, 24.

Kantor, R., & Silverberg, J. I. (2017). Environmental risk factors and their role in the management of atopic dermatitis. *Expert Review Clinical Immunol, 13*(1), 15–26.

Lynn, D. D., Umari, T., Dunnick, C. A., & Dellavalle, R. P. (2016). The epidemiology of acne vulgaris in late adolescence. *Adolesc Health Medicine Theraphy, 7*, 13–25.

Platsidaki, E., & Dessinioti, C. (2018). Recent advances in understanding Propionibacterium acnes (Cutibacterium acnes) in acne. *F1000Res.* https://doi.org/10.12688/f1000research.15659.1.

Rainer, B. M., Kang, S., & Chien, A. L. (2017). Rosacea: Epidemiology, pathogenesis and treatment. *Dermatoendocrinol, 9*(1), e1361574.

Rendon, A., & Schakel, K. (2019). Psoriasis pathogenesis and treatment. *International Journal of Molecular Sciences, 20*(6), 1475–1500.

Theelen, B., Cafarchia, C., Gaitanis, G., et al. (2018). Malassezia ecology, pathophysiology and treatment. *Medical Mycology, 56*, S10–S25.

Verkouteren, J. A. C., Ramdas, K. H. R., Wakkee, M., & Nijsten, T. (2017). Epidemiology of basal cell carcinoma: Scholarly review. *British Journal of Dermatology, 177*, 359–372.

Useful websites

WCRF skin cancer statistics. (2018): https://www.wcrf.org/dietandcancer/cancer-trends/skin-cancer-statistics.

WHO skin cancer information and statistics: https://www.who.int/uv/faq/skincancer/en/index1.html.

Index

Note: Page numbers followed by *f* indicate figures and *t* indicate tables.

A

A-type antigens, in ABO system, 107
ABCC11 gene, 28
Abdominal aorta, 159–160
Abdominal cavity, 369
Abnormal cells, 63
Abnormal immune cells, 1–2
Abnormalities, 53–54
    deletions, 53–54
    insertions, 53–54
    inversions, 54
    translocations, 54
ABO system, 107–108
Abscess formation, 15, 17f
Absence seizures, 221
    abnormal EEG activity during, 221f
Absorption, 112
Accessory muscles of respiration, 168, 169f
Accessory organs, 272
Accommodation, 239
Acetylcholine (ACh), 199b, 328
    receptors, 323–324
Acetylcholinesterase (AChE), 323–324
Achilles tendon, 341
Acidification, 315
Acidosis, 130
Acne, 378–379
    management and prognosis, 379
    pathophysiology, 378–379
    signs and symptoms, 379
    vulgaris, 378
Acoustic meatus, external, 247f
Acoustic neuromas, 223, 224f
Acquired aplastic anaemia, 126b
Acquired coagulation deficiencies, 130–131
    management and prognosis, 130
    pathophysiology, 130
Acquired diseases, 3
Acquired haemolytic anaemia, 121–123
Acquired hypopituitarism, causes of, 255
Acquired immunity, 88, 90–92
Acquired myopathies, 331
Acquired platelet deficiencies, 131
Acromegaly, 255
Acromion process, 345f
Actin, 9
Actinic keratosis, 389
    pathophysiology of, 389
    prognosis, 389
Action potentials, 197–198
Acute appendicitis, 292
Acute coronary syndrome, 139–141
Acute gastritis, 288
Acute glomerulonephritis, 306–308
    management and prognosis, 308
    pathophysiology, 306–308
        Berger disease, 307
        membranous GN, 307
        post-streptococcal GN, 307
    signs and symptoms, 308

Acute heart failure, 161
Acute inflammation
    consequences of, 15–16
    main events of acute inflammatory
        response, 11–16
Acute kidney injury (AKI), 316–318
    categories of, 317f
    management and prognosis, 318
    pathophysiology, 316–318
        post-renal AKI, 317–318
        pre-renal AKI, 317
        renal AKI, 317
Acute leukaemias, 114–115
Acute lymphoblastic leukaemia (ALL), 117.
    See also Chronic lymphocytic leukaemia
    (CLL)
    management and prognosis, 117
    pathophysiology, 117
    signs and symptoms, 117
Acute myeloid leukaemia (AML), 115,
    115f. *See also* Myeloid (myelogenous)
    leukaemia (CML)
    management and prognosis, 115
    multiple fungal brain abscesses in, 116f
    pathophysiology, 115
    signs and symptoms, 115
Acute myeloid leukaemia, 114–115
Acute otitis externa, 249
Acute otitis media, 250
Acute pain, 235
Acute pancreatitis, 296–297
    management and prognosis, 297
    pathophysiology, 296
    signs and symptoms, 296
Acute phase reactants, 16–17
Acute pyelonephritis, 311
    management and prognosis, 311
    pathophysiology, 311
    signs and symptoms, 311
Acute renal failure (ARF), 316
Acute respiratory distress syndrome (ARDS),
    178
Acute respiratory distress syndrome, 187–189
    aetiological agents in, 188f
    management and prognosis, 188–189
    pathophysiology, 188
Acute trauma, coagulopathy of, 130
Acute tubular necrosis (ATN), 317
Addison disease, 270–271
Addisonian crisis, 270–271
Adenine (A), 25
Adenocarcinomas, 83
    oesophageal, 279–280
Adenoma, 66
Adenomyosis, 366
Adenosine deaminase (ADA), 96
Adenosine triphosphate (ATP), 6, 139
Adherens junctions, 10
Adhesions, 291
Adipocytes, 5–6

Adipose tissue, 6, 363
Adrenal cortex, 268–271
    adrenocortical insufficiency, 270–271
    glucocorticoids and excessive
        glucocorticoid secretion, 269–270
    mineralocorticoids and disorders of
        mineralocorticoid secretion, 268–269
Adrenal gland
    adrenal cortex, 268–271
    adrenal medulla, 267–271
        phaeochromocytoma, 267–268
    and disorders, 267–271
Adrenaline, 373
Adrenocortical insufficiency, 270–271
    management and prognosis, 271
    signs and symptoms, 271
Adrenocorticotrophic hormone (ACTH),
    255
    oversecretion and Cushing disease, 255
Adult-onsetasthma, 184
Advanced glycation end products (AGEs),
    261, 308–309
Aetiology of illness, 2–3, 183
Afatinib, 83–84
Afferent arteriole, renal, 301
Afferent pain pathways, 235
African trypanosomiasis, 22
Afterload, 136–137
Age, 78–79, 127
Age-related eye disease, 246
Age-related macular degeneration (AMD),
    244–246
    dry AMD, 244–246
    management and prognosis, 246
    signs and symptoms, 246
    wet AMD, 245
Ageing process, 238, 314
Air, alveolar, 173
Airways, 175
Albumins, 110
Alcohol intake, 264
Alcoholic liver disease, 285–288
    management and prognosis, 288
    pathophysiology, 285–288
    signs and symptoms, 287–288
Aldosterone, 334
    functions of, 268
Alkaline ammonia, 288
Alleles, 27–28
Allergen, 99–101
Allergic contact dermatitis, 378
Allergic dermatitis, 378
Allergic rhinitis, 102
Allergy, 101–103
Allodynia, 236–237
Alpha-fetoprotein (AFP), 294–295, 372
Alpha-thalassaemia, 51, 51f
Alveolar stability, surface tension and role of
        surfactant in, 171f
Alveolar wall, 170f

Alveoli, 168
Alzheimer disease (AD), 212–213, 213f, 245
  management and prognosis, 213
  pathophysiology, 213
  signs and symptoms, 213
Amacrine cells, 238–239
Amenorrhoea, 361–362
  pathophysiology, 361–362
    failure of ovary to secrete oestrogen, 362
    failure of pituitary gland to secrete FSH and LH, 361–362
    hypothalamic failure to secrete gonadotrophin releasing hormone, 361
Amino acids, 30
Ammonia, 311
Amoebiasis, 283
Amoebic dysentery, 283
Amygdala, 203
Amylase, 275–276
Amyloid precursor protein (APP), 213
Amyotrophic Lateral Sclerosis (ALS), 214–215
  management and prognosis, 214–215
  pathophysiology, 214
  signs and symptoms, 214
Anabolic hormone, 258
Anaemia, 121–126, 312–313, 320
  aplastic, 126
  haemolytic, 121–124
  pernicious, 124
  secondary to reduced erythrocyte production, 124–126
  sickle cell, 124
  vitamin B_{12}/folic acid deficiency, 124
Anaerobic metabolism, shift from aerobic to, 163
Anaphase, 54–55
Anaphylactic shock, 161–162
Anaphylaxis, 101–102, 102f
Anaplasia, 71
Anaplasia-loss of differentiation, 69–70, 70f
Anatomical dead space, 175–176
Anatomy
  of brain, 203f
  of lung tissue, 169–171
  of respiratory passageways, 168–169
  of respiratory system, 168–176
Anchoring fibrils, 4
Androgen, 362
Anencephaly, 229, 230f
Aneuploidy, 53
Aneurysm, 159–160, 159f
Angina, 138–139
Angina pectoris, 138
Angioedema, 94
Angiogenesis, 69
Angiogenic factors, 69
  production of, 69
Angiogenic switch, 69
Angiotensin, 309
  angiotensin I, 165
  angiotensin II, 143, 165, 168, 178
Angiotensin converting enzyme (ACE), 145, 165, 178
  ACE2, 178
Angiotensinogen, 165
Ankylosing spondylitis, 340
  management and prognosis, 340
  signs and symptoms, 340
Anorexia, 79–80
Anteflexion, 350
Anterior cerebral artery, 199–200

Anterior eye, disorders of, 242–244
  cataract, 244
  infection and inflammatory conditions, 242–244
Anterior pituitary hormones, disorders of, 252–257
  ACTH oversecretion and Cushing disease, 255
  causes of acquired hypopituitarism, 255
  causes of congenital hypopituitarism, 255
  growth hormone disorders, 255–256
  hyperprolactinaemia, 256–257
Anterior root, 205
Anti-diuretic hormone (ADH), 252, 302
Anti-HPV vaccination, 360–361
Anti-inflammatory drugs, 290–291, 340
Anti-neutrophil cytoplasmic antibody (ANCA), 311
Antibiotic treatment, 311, 358, 365
Antibiotics, 244, 335
Antibody deficiencies, 97–98
Antibody production, 89
Antibody subtypes, 92, 93f
Antibody-mediated rejection, 109
Antibody-type hypersensitivity, 101
Anticipation, 43
Anticholinesterase drugs, 329–330
Anticoagulant mechanisms, activation of, 130
Antiemetics, 232–233
Antifungal drugs, 377
Antigen presenting cells (APCs), 85–86, 90–91, 298
Antigens, 107
  presentation, 90–91, 91f
Antiinflammatory corticosteroids, 378
Antiinflammatory steroids, 212
Antimicrobial substances, 276
Antiretroviral treatment (ART), 99
α1-Antitrypsin deficiency and emphysema, 186–187
Anuria, 308
Anxiety, 216–217
  management and prognosis, 217
  pathophysiology, 216–217
  signs and symptoms, 217
Aorta
  arch of, 134
  coarctation of, 153–154, 154f
Aortic aneurysm, 159–160
Aortic dilation, 44–45
Aortic valve disease, 151. *See also* Mitral valve disease
  management and prognosis, 151
  pathophysiology, 151
  signs and symptoms, 151
Aplastic anaemia, 126
  pathophysiology, 126
Apoptosis, 62, 64–65, 66f
Appendicitis, 292
Appendix, 291–292
Aqueous humour, 239–240
Arachidonic acid products, 12–13
Arachnoid mater, 200
Arachnoid villi, 201–202
Areolar tissue, 6
Arms, 54
Arrhythmias, 140, 145
Arterial blood gases, 23
Arterial blood pressure, 142
Arterial blood supply to brain, 227f
Arterial thrombosis, 127
Arteries, 74
  blood flow in, 127
  carotid, 137
  coronary, 137

Arteries *(Continued)*
  lenticulostriate, 200
  pulmonary, 151–152
  transposition of great arteries, 153
Arterioles, 308–309
Arteriosclerosis, 157–160
Arthritis, 336
Asbestos, 189t
Ascending colon, 86
Ascites, 287
Asperger syndrome, 219
Aspergillus, 22, 95–96
Aspirin, 304
Asthma, 183–187
  atopic and non-atopic asthma, 183
  chronic obstructive pulmonary disease, 184–185
  genetics of, 183–187
  management and prognosis, 184
  pathophysiology, 183–184
  signs and symptoms, 184
Asthmatic airway, pathological changes in, 184f
Astrocytes, 198
Astrocytoma, 222
Atelectasis, 193–195, 193f
Atheroma, 137–138
Atherosclerosis, 137–138, 157–160
  pathophysiology, 158
  risk factors for, 159b
Athlete's foot, 380
Atoms, 264
Atopic asthma, 184
Atopic dermatitis, 102, 378
Atopic eczema, 102
Atopic-atopic asthma, 183
Atrial arrhythmias, 146–147
Atrial fibrillation (AF), 145–146, 147f
  management and prognosis, 146
  pathophysiology, 146
  signs and symptoms, 146
Atrial flutter, 146–147, 147f
  management and prognosis, 147
  pathophysiology, 147
  signs and symptoms, 147
Atrial septal defect, 152–153, 153f
Atrioventricular block (AV block), 149
Atrioventricular node (AV node), 134–135
Atrioventricular valves, 133–135
Auditory nerve, 208
Auditory ossicles, 248–249
Aura, 219–222
Auricle, 247
Autism, 219
  management and prognosis, 219
  pathophysiology, 219
  signs and symptoms, 219
Autoantibodies, 384
Autoimmune Addison disease, 271
Autoimmune anti-basement membrane disease, 307
  glomerular capillary vasculitis, 307–308
Autoimmune disease, 284
Autoimmune disorders, 103, 328–330
  myasthenia gravis, 328–330
Autoimmune thrombocytopenic purpura, 131
Autoimmunity, 103–106, 383–386
  immune mediated skin blistering disorders, 384–386
  psoriasis, 383–386
Automatisms, 219–220
Autonomic nervous system (ANS), 206, 206f
Autoregulation, 303
Autorhythmicity, 134

Autosomal abnormalities, 57–58
Autosomal dominant inheritance, 33–35, 34f
Autosomal dominant polycystic kidney disease, 314
Autosomal inheritance, 33–35
Autosomal recessive inheritance, 35, 35f
Autosomes, 25
Axial skeleton, 332
Axon, 197–198
Axon terminal, 197–198
Axons, 197–198
Azithromycin, 358
Azotemia, 319–320
Aδ fibres, 235

B

B cells and immunity, 92
B-cell Lymphomas, 65
B-lymphocyte deficiencies, 96–99
B-type antigens, in ABO system, 107
Babesia, 121
Bacillary dysentery, 283
Bacillus, 19
    B. cereus, 281–282
Bacteraemia, 281
Bacteria, 19, 243–244
Bacterial endocarditis, 281
Bacterial infections, 311, 381–382
    erysipelas, 381–382
    impetigo and staphylococcal scalded skin syndrome, 382
Bacterial labyrinthitis, 250
Bacterial meningitis, 208f
Bacterial pathogenicity, mechanisms of, 19–20
Bacterial sexually transmitted infections, 357–360
    chlamydia, 357–358
    gonorrhoea, 358
    syphilis, 358
Balance, 281
Balanitis, 370
    orchitis and epididymitis, 371
    prostatitis, 370–371
Baroreceptor reflex, 137
Baroreceptors, 137
Barrett oesophagus, 280, 279–280, 293
Barrier function of enterocytes, 276
Bartholin's glands, 350
Bartholinitis, 365
Bartonella, 121
Basal cell carcinoma (BCC), 387–388
    management and prognosis, 388
    pathophysiology, 387–388
        Hedgehog signalling and BCC, 387
    signs and symptoms, 388
Basal ganglia, 203, 224–225
Basal keratinocytes, 389
Basal metabolic rate, 264
Basal secretion, 259
Base, 169
Basement membrane, 5, 306–307, 375
Basic calcium phosphate deposition disease, 342
Basilar artery, 199
Basilar membrane, 248
Basophils, 114
Bcl-2 proteins, 65
Bcr-abl gene, 116
Becker muscular dystrophy, 41
Beethoven's deafness, 332
Bell palsy, 234

Benign neoplasms, differences between malignant and, 70–74, 71f
    degree of de-differentiation, 71
    growth rates, 70–72
    histological appearance, 72
    local invasiveness, 70
    metastasis, 72
    presence of capsule, 70–71
Benign prostatic enlargement. *See* Benign prostatic hyperplasia
Benign prostatic hyperplasia, 373
Benign prostatic hyperplasia, 373
    management and prognosis, 373
    pathophysiology, 373
    signs and symptoms, 373
Benign prostatic hypertrophy. *See* Benign prostatic hyperplasia
Benign tumours, 335
    chondrosarcoma, 336
    osteosarcoma, 335–336
Berger disease, 307
Berry aneurysm, 160
Beta lactam ring, 102–103
Beta-amyloid protein, 213
Beta-thalassaemia, 52
Bicarbonate, 273
Bile, 275
    acids, 275
Biliary tract, 275
    bile, 275
    jaundice, 275
Bilirubin, 275
Biologics, 12
Bipolar cells, 238–239
Bipolar disorder, 216
    management and prognosis, 216
    pathophysiology, 216
    signs and symptoms, 216
Birth, 277
Bladder cancer, 313–314
    endoscopic of urothelial bladder tumour, 313f
    management and prognosis, 314
    pathophysiology, 313–314
    signs and symptoms, 314
Blastic metastases, 335
Blastomas, 66
Bleeding, 79
Blindness, 357
Blisters, 377
β-blocker treatment, 334
Blood, 6
    biochemical markers in, 139–140
    disorders, 110, 127
    increased coagulability of, 163
    plasma protein, 303
    spread, 74
    transfusion reactions, 107–108
    typing, 123
    viscosity, 191
Blood cells, 301
    developmental tree of, 110–114, 111f
    formation, 110
Blood clotting, 112–113, 113t, 126
    standard tests of, 126t
Blood flow, 11–12
Blood pressure, 142–143, 165
    disorders of, 165–167
    hypertension, 165–167
    pulmonary hypertension, 167
    regulation of blood pressure, 165
Blood smear, 49
Blood supply
    to brain, 199–202
    left ventricular failure and systemic, 143

Blood vessels, 157–160
    arteriosclerosis and atherosclerosis, 157–160
    peripheral venous disease, 160
    PVD, 158–160
    response in inflammation, 11–12
    structure of, 157f
    thromboembolism, 160
Blood-borne organisms, 340
Blood-borne spread, 340
Blood-Brain Barrier (BBB), 207, 207f
Body mass index, 277–278
Body tissues, 173, 315
Bone, 6, 324–327
    bone cells, 325, 325f
    classification of bones, 324
        structure of Long Bone, 324
    compact and spongy bone, 325–326
    disorders of bone, 331–336
    embryonic development of bone, 326–327
    injury, 344–347
    osteomyelitis, 334–335
    spinal deformity, 336
    structural and degenerative disorders, 331–334
        endocrine-related bone conditions, 333–334
        osteogenesis imperfect, 331
        osteomalacia and rickets, 333
        osteoporosis, 331–332
        paget disease, 332
    tissue, 335
    tumours of bone and cartilage, 335–336
Bone cells, 325, 325f
Bone fracture and healing, 345–347
    delayed union or non-union, 347
    factors interfere with fracture healing, 346–347
Bone health, 320
    effect of chronic kidney disease on, 320f
Bone marrow, 284
Borrelia burgdorferi, 340
Botulism, 282–283
Bouchard nodules, 338
Bowen's disease, 386, 389
Bowman capsule, 300–301
Bradycardia, 135
Bradykinin, 14
Brain
    anatomy of, 203f
    arterial blood supply to, 227f
    blood supply to, 199–202
    changes in brain associated with migraine, 232f
    functional anatomy of, 202–203
    main regions of, 202f
    venous drainage of, 200
    volume, 217–218
Brainstem, 202
*BRCA*1 genes, 84, 369
*BRCA*2 genes, 84, 369
Breast, 354
Breast cancer, 74–75, 84–85, 368
    management and prognosis, 85
    manifestations of, 85
    risk factors for, 84
    types of, 84–85
Breast tumours, 368
    benign proliferative breast disease, 368
    breast cancer, 368
Breathing, 41
Breathlessness, 115
Brittle bone disease, 46, 331
Bronchi, 168
    left, 168
    right, 168

Bronchiectasis, 97
Bronchioles, 168
Bronchitis, 183
Bronchoconstriction, 183
Bronchodilation, 168–169
Bronchopneumonia, 180–181
Bronchospasm, 267
Bruch's membrane, 244–245
Bruton's agammaglobulinaemia, 97–98
Bulbar ALS, 215
Bulbar involvement, 211
Bullae, 185–186
Bullous pemphigoid, 384–385
    management and prognosis, 385
    pathophysiology, 384–385
    signs and symptoms, 385
Bundle branch blocks, 149
Burkitt's lymphoma, 21, 119
Burns, 16, 161

C

C-peptide, 258–259
C-reactive protein (CRP), 16–17, 339
C1 inhibitor (C1INH), 89, 94
Cachexia, 80
Cadherins, 69
Caecum, 276
Café au lait spots, 45–46
Caffeine, 289
Calcitonin, 327
Calcitonin gene-related peptide (CGRP), 232
Calcium, 113, 266–267
    absorption, 315
    stones, 315
Calcium pyrophosphate, 341
Calculi, renal, 309
Calf muscles, 41
Callus, 345–346
Campylobacter, 281
Campylobacter jejuni, 233
Canal of Schlemm, 239–240
Canaliculi, 6, 325
Cancer antigen 125 (CA125), 80
Cancers, 31, 70, 74, 82–86, 368
    assessment, 80–81
        and treatment of, 79–82
    cells, 64–65, 69, 72
    development of, 74–79
    epidemiology, 62
        global trends in cancer incidence and
            survival, 62
    genetics of, 74–77
    metastasises, 313
    risk factors for, 77–79, 78f
Candida albicans, 22
Capillaries, 252
    glomerular, 261
Capsule, presence of, 70–71
Carbohydrates, 38, 263
Carbon dioxide (CO$_2$), 120, 173
Carcinogenesis, 74–79
    process of, 77, 78t
Carcinoma in situ (CIS), 69, 389
Carcinomas, 66, 372
    of penis, 371
        management and prognosis, 371
        pathophysiology, 371
        signs and symptoms, 371
Cardiac arrhythmias, 268
Cardiac cycle, 135, 136f
Cardiac implants, 155
Cardiac muscle, 10, 41
Cardiac output (CO), 135–137
Cardiac tamponade, 156

Cardiac troponins, 140
Cardiogenic shock, 161, 163
Cardiovascular centre (CVC), 137
Cardiovascular disease (CVD), 132
Cardiovascular function, control of, 137
Cardiovascular system, 132, 268
Caries, dental, 105
Carotid bodies, 143
Carpal tunnel syndrome, 233, 233f
Carrier, 33–34
Cartilage, 6
    cartilage-rich skeleton, 333
    model, 326–327
Caseation tissue, 181–182
Cataracts, 244
    management and prognosis, 244
    pathophysiology, 244
    signs and symptoms, 244
β-catenin gene, 294
Caudate nucleus, 224–225
Cavity seeding, 74
*CD*20, 82
CD8 cells, 91–92
*CDH*1, 294
CDKN2A, 388
Cell body, 197–198
Cell cycle, 62
    and control, 63, 64f
Cell division, 62–66
Cell membrane, 6–8
    structure of, 9f
Cell nucleus, 6
Cell numbers, 62
Cell senescence, 29
Cell structure, 6–11
    cell–cell and cell–matrix adhesion, 9–11
    intracellular organelles, 6–9
Cell-ECM adhesion, 10–11
Cell-mediated hypersensitivity, 101
Cell–cell adhesion, 9–11
Cell–cell junctions, 10
    adherens junctions, 10
    desmosomes, 10
    gap junctions, 10
    tight junctions, 10
Cell–matrix adhesion, 9–11
Cells, 4–6, 63, 89
    age, 62
    of nervous system, 197–199
α-Cells, 258
β-cells, 258–259
Cellular phase, 110
Cellular proliferation, 306–307
Cellular response to injury and infection,
    11–23
Cellulitis, 381
Central canal, 275
Central chemoreceptors, 137
Central nervous system (CNS), 99, 197,
    199–205, 199b
    immunological defence in, 207
    infections, 207–211
    inflammatory and immune mediated CNS
        disorders, 211–212
    pathophysiology, 207–233
    tumours, 222–223
        consequences of, 222
Central sensitisation, 236–237
Centromere, 25
Cerebellum, 202–203
Cerebral artery, middle, 200
Cerebral cortex, 202–203
Cerebral cortex, 203
Cerebral haemorrhage, sites of, 228f
Cerebral hemispheres, 202–203

Cerebral palsy (CP), 229
    causes of, 231b
Cerebral ventricles, 201–202
Cerebrospinal fluid (CSF), 199, 201–202
    production, circulation, and reabsorption
        of, 201f–202f
Cerebrovascular accident (CVA), 226
Cerebrovascular disease, risk factors
        for, 226
Cerebrovascular disorders, 226–228
Cerebrum, 203
Cerumen, 247
Cervical cancer, 21, 317–318, 366–368
    management and prognosis, 368
    pathophysiology, 367
    signs and symptoms, 368
Cervical carcinoma, 350
Cervical erosion, 350
Cervical intraepithelial neoplasia, 367
Cervicitis, 365
Cervix, 367
CFTR gene, 37, 40
Chaperone therapy, 51
Chemical digestion, 272
Chemoreceptors, 304
Chemotaxins, 12
Chemotaxis, 12
Chemotherapy, 83–84, 86, 294
Chenodeoxycholic acid, 275
Childbirth, 18
Chlamydia, 19–20, 340–341, 357–358
    management and prognosis, 358
    pathophysiology, 357–358
    signs and symptoms, 358
Chlamydia trachomatis, 242–243
Cholangiocarcinoma, 294–296
Cholecystitis, 298
Cholecystokinin, 235
Cholelithiasis, 297–298
    cholecystitis, 298
Cholera, 283–284
    management and prognosis, 284
    pathophysiology, 284
Cholestasis, 297–298
    gallstones, 297–298
Cholesterol stones, 298
Chondrocytes, 5–6, 338
Chondromas, 335
Chondrosarcoma, 336
Chordae tendineae, 133–134
Choroid, 238
Choroid plexuses, 201–202
Christmas disease, 42
Chromaffin cells, 267
Chromatids, 54–55
Chromatin, 25
Chromosomal abnormalities, 57–58
Chromosomal mosaicism, 56–57
Chromosome 22, 116
Chromosome 22q11.2 deletion syndrome,
    96–97
Chromosomes, 6, 24–32, 53–54
    deletions, 53–54
    insertions, 53–54
    inversions, 54
    translocations, 54
Chronic anaemia, physiological adaptations
        to, 121
Chronic blood loss, 125
Chronic bronchitis, 187
    pathophysiology of, 185, 185f
Chronic disease, 131
Chronic disorders, 190
Chronic exposure to irritant, 16
Chronic glaucoma, 242

Chronic glomerulonephritis, 308–309
  diabetic nephropathy, 308–309
Chronic granulomatous disease (CGD), 95–96
  management and prognosis, 96
Chronic ILD, 190
Chronic inflammation, 16
  consequences of, 16
Chronic kidney disease (CKD), 318–321
  causes of, 318b
  management and prognosis, 321
  national kidney foundation stages of, 319t
  pathophysiology, 319–321
    CKD and anaemia, 320
    CKD and bone health, 320
    CKD and fluid and electrolyte balance, 320
  signs and symptoms, 321
  systemic manifestations of, 319f
Chronic leukaemias, 114–115
Chronic lymphocytic leukaemia (CLL), 117–118. See also Acute lymphoblastic leukaemia (ALL)
  management and prognosis, 116–118
  pathophysiology, 116–118
  signs and symptoms, 117, 116
Chronic obstructive pulmonary disease (COPD), 183–185
Chronic pain, 235
Chronic pancreatitis, 297
  management and prognosis, 297
  signs and symptoms, 297
Chronic pyelonephritis, 311–312
  management and prognosis, 312
  pathophysiology, 311–312
  signs and symptoms, 312
Chronic renal failure. See Chronic kidney disease (CKD)
Circulus arteriosus, 199, 200f
Circumflex artery (CX), 134
Cirrhosis, 285
  hepatic encephalopathy, 285
  increased tendency to bleed, 285
  portal hypertension, 285
Classical pathway, 89
Classification systems, 1
Claudins, 10
Clonal expansion, 91
Closed pneumothorax, 194–195, 194f
Closed spina bifida, 229
Clostridium, 19, 121, 281
Clostridium botulinum, 282–283
Clostridium difficile, 283
Clostridium perfringens, 281–282
Clotting, 113
  control, 113
  deficiencies of clotting inhibitors, 127
  disorders, 126–131
  measurement of clotting parameters, 126
  reduced levels of clotting factors, 130
Cluster headache, 230
Coagulation stage, 113
Coagulative necrosis, 139
Coal dust, 189t
Cochlea, 248
Cochlear duct, 248
Codons, 30
Coeliac disease, 297–298
  management and prognosis, 299
  pathophysiology, 298–299
  signs and symptoms, 298–299
Cognitive symptoms, 218
COL1A1 gene, 46
Colchicine, 341
Collagen, 4, 46

Collecting duct, 300, 302
Colon cancer, 2–3
Colonisation, 277, 340
Colorectal cancer, 85–86
  management and prognosis, 86
  manifestations of, 86
  risk factors for, 85–86
  types of, 86
Commensals, 17–18
Common cold, 176–177
Compact bone, 325–326
Compensated shock, 165
Complement, 15, 89
Complement activation, control of, 89
Complement deficiencies, 93–95
Complement pathways, 89, 89f
Complement proteins, 89
Complete carcinogens, 77
Compliance, 170–171
Complication, 3
Compression, 80
Compression collapse, 193
Computed tomography (CT), 48, 80
Conduction abnormalities, 145–150
  atrial arrhythmias, 146–147
  heart block, 148–149
  ventricular arrhythmias, 147–148
  Wolff-Parkinson-white syndrome, 149–150
Conductive deafness, 248–249
  otosclerosis, 248–249
Cones, 238–239
Congenital diseases, 3
Congenital disorders, 228–229, 314
  horseshoe kidney, 314
  polycystic kidney disease, 314
  renal agenesis, 314
Congenital heart defects, 145
Congenital heart disease, 151–154
Congenital hypopituitarism, causes of, 255
Congenital kyphosis, 336
Coning, 202
Conjunctivitis, 242
Connective tissue, 5–6
  disorders of, 342
  Ehlers-Danlos syndrome, 342
  mucopolysaccharidoses, 342
Consanguinity, 33–36
Constipation, 278–279
  common causes of, 279b
  gastro-oesophageal reflux disorder, 279–280
  intestinal pseudo-obstruction, 280
  management and prognosis, 279
  pathophysiology, 278–279
Consumption, 181–182
Contact dermatitis, 103, 377–378
  allergic contact dermatitis, 378
  irritant contact dermatitis, 377–378
Contact inhibition, 68–69
Conus medullaris, 203–204
Convulsion, 219
Cornea, 238
Coronary artery atherosclerosis, 137–138
Coronary artery blood flow, 137
Coronary artery bypass graft (CABG), 141, 142f
Coronary artery disease (CAD), 137
Coronary circulation, 134–137, 134f
Coronaviruses, 177–178
  infections, 177–179
Corpora cavernosa, 356
Corpulmonale, 182
Corpus callosum, 203
Corpus luteum, 352
Corpus spongiosum, 356

Corpuscles, 300–301
Cortical spreading depolarisation, 231
Cortical spreading depression, 231
Corticotrophs, 254–255
Cortisol, 269
  functions of, 269
Corynebacteria species, 377
COVID-19, 178
  possible manifestations in, 179f
Cranial nerve syndromes, 234
Cranial nerves, 205, 206t
Creatinine kinase MB, 139–140
Crepitus, 338
Cri-du-chat syndrome, 58
  genetics, 58
  management and prognosis, 58
  pathophysiology, 58
Crohn disease, 290–291
  management and prognosis, 291
  pathophysiology, 291
  signs and symptoms, 291
Crossing over, 56
Cryptococcus, 208
Cryptorchidism, 369
Cryptosporidium, 281–282
Crypts of Lieberkuhn, 276
Crystal-induced arthritis, 341–342
  crystal-related arthritides, 342
  gout, 341
  pseudogout, 341–342
Crystal-related arthritides, 342
Crystallins, 239
Crystals, 341
Cupula, 248
Current of injury, 140
Cushing disease, 255, 269–270
Cushing syndrome, 269–270
Cutibacteria, 377
Cutibacterium acnes, 378–379
Cyclins, 63
Cyclo-oxygenase (COX-2), 86
CYP2E1, 285–286
Cystic fibrosis (CF), 38–40, 187
  in airways, 40f
  genetics, 39–40
  management and prognosis, 40
  pathophysiology, 40
Cystic fibrosis transmembrane conductance regulator (CFTR), 39–40
Cystine stones, 316
Cystinuria, 316
Cystitis, 309–312
  management and prognosis, 310
  non–infection-related cystitis, 310
  pathophysiology, 310
  signs and symptoms, 310
Cysts, 314, 368
Cytokines, 12, 278, 334–335
Cytomegalovirus (CMV), 21, 250
Cytoplasm, 6
Cytoplasmic enzymes, 307–308
Cytosine (C), 25
Cytoskeleton, 9
Cytosol, 6
Cytotoxic drugs, 389
Cytotoxic T cells (Tc cells), 91–92
Cytotoxic therapy, 81–82

D

De-differentiation, degree of, 71
Deep venous thrombosis (DVT), 128
Delayed union, 347
Delayed-type hypersensitivity, 101
Deletion, 37

Deletions, 53
Delusions, 215
Dementia, 212
Demodex, 377
Dendrites, 197–198
Dental disease, systemic consequences of, 281
Deoxyribonucleic acid (DNA), 24–32, 293, 315, 389
  and chromosomes, 25
    from DNA to proteins, 25–30
    functional unit of DNA, 25–28
    methylation, 31
    mitochondrial DNA, 32
    mutations, 36–37
    virus, 367
Depolarisation, 135
Depolarising, nerve, 198
Depressive illness, 215–216
  pathophysiology, 215
  prognosis and management, 216
  signs and symptoms, 215–216
Dermatitis, 377–383
  atopic, 378
  contact, 377–378
  seborrhoeic, 377
Dermatophyte infections, 380
Dermis, 375
Dermo-epidermal junction, 377
Descending inhibition, 236
Desmoglein, 10, 385
Desmosomes, 9–10
Detoxifying processes, 274
Detrusor muscle, 305
Developmental disorders, 228–229, 314
  polycystic kidney disease, 314
Dexamethasone, 179
Diabetes insipidus, 257
Diabetes mellitus (DM), 166, 257–264, 308
  complications of, 260–262
    diabetic foot, 262
    features of, 259–260
      glycosuria, 260
      hyperglycaemia, 259
      polyuria, 260
    ketoacidosis, 262
    macrovascular complications, 262
    microvascular complications, 261–262
      diabetic nephropathy, 261
      diabetic neuropathy, 261
      diabetic retinopathy, 261
    types of, 262–264
      diabetes of specific types, 264
      hyperglycaemia of pregnancy, 264
      type 1 diabetes mellitus, 262–263
      type 2 diabetes mellitus, 263–264
Diabetic foot, 262
  infections, 334
Diabetic ketoacidosis (DKA), 262
Diabetic nephropathy, 261, 308–309
  management and prognosis, 309
  pathophysiology, 308–309
  renovascular disease in, 308f
  signs and symptoms, 309
  time course of, 309f
Diabetic neuropathy, 261
Diabetic retinopathy, 261
Diarrhoea, 278–280, 291
  management and prognosis, 278
  pathophysiology, 278
Diastolic pressures, 165
Diencephalon, 202–203
Diet, 290–291
Diffuse tumours, 294

Digeorge syndrome, 96–97, 97f
  management and prognosis, 97
Dihydrotestosterone (DHT), 355–356, 373
Diploid, 53
Disease, 1
  cellular basis of disease, 4–11
    cell structure, 6–11
    cells and tissues, 4–6
  chromosomes and abnormalities, 53–54
  course, 50
  DNA, genes, and chromosomes, 24–32
  gene disorders, 36–53
  key concepts and definitions of, 1–3
    aetiology, 2–3
    complication, 3
    congenital and acquired diseases, 3
    iatrogenic and idiopathic disease, 3
    morbidity and mortality, 3
    pathology, pathophysiology, and pathogenesis, 1–3
    prognosis, 3
    remission and relapse, 3
    signsand symptoms, 3
    syndromes, 3
  in migrant populations, 53
  patterns of inheritance, 32–36
Disease-modifying antirheumatic drugs (DMARDs), 339
Disseminated intravascular coagulation (DIC), 129
  management and prognosis, 129
  pathophysiology, 129
  signs and symptoms, 129
Disseminated TB, 182
Distal convoluted tubule (DCT), 300–302
Distributive shock, 161–164
Diuretic therapy, 341
Diverticular disease, 292
  pathophysiology, 292
  signs and symptoms, 292
Diverticulosis, 292
Dominant allele, 33–34
Domperidone, 280
Dopamine, 199b, 215, 217, 257
Down syndrome, 58
  features of, 58f
  genetics, 58
  management and prognosis, 58
  pathophysiology, 58
Doxycycline, 358
Driver mutations, 77
Drugs, 246, 268, 385
  associated with interstitial lung disease, 190b
  resistance, 381
  treatment, 232–233
Dry cough, 83
Duchenne muscular dystrophy (DMD), 41
  genetics, 41
  management and prognosis, 41
  pathophysiology, 41
Ductal carcinoma in situ (DCIS), 84
Duodenum, 276
Dura mater, 200
Dural venous sinuses, 200
*DUX*4, 330
Dwarfism, 334
Dysaesthesias, 234
Dysentery, 283
  amoebic, 283
  bacillary, 283
Dysplasia, 66, 67f
Dystrophin, 41

E

Early phase response, 184
Ears, 238, 246–250
  deafness, 248–249
    conductive deafness, 248–249
    sensorineural deafness, 249
  ear infections, 249–250
    otitis externa, 249
    otitis media, 249–250
  inner ear disorders, 250
  normal ear, 247–248
    inner ear, 247–248
    interior of eyeball, 239f
    middle ear, 247–248
Economic price, 1
Ectocervix, 350
Ectoderm, 228
Ectopialentis, 44–45
Eczema, 377–383
Eggs, 381
Ehlers-Danlos syndrome, 342
  management and prognosis, 342
  pathophysiology, 342
  signs and symptoms, 342
Elastase, 186–187
Elastic cartilage, 6
Elastic connective tissue, 44–45
Elasticity, 170–171
Electrocardiogram (ECG), 135
Electroencephalograph (EEG), 221–222
Electrolyte, 327
  balance, 320
Elongation, 30, 30f
Embolism, 191
Embryonic cells, 313
Embryonic development of bone, 326–327
  maintenance of mature bone tissue, 327
Emmetropia, 242
Emphysema, 184–185, 186f, 187
  loss of radial traction in airways in, 186f
  management and prognosis, 187
  pathophysiology of, 185–187
  pleural bullae in, 187f
  signs and symptoms, 187
Empyema, 193
Encephalitis, 209
  management and prognosis, 209
  pathophysiology, 209
  signs and symptoms, 209
Encephalocele, 229
End-diastolic volume (EDV), 135
Endocardium, 133, 154–155
Endocervix, 350
Endocrine disorders, 251
Endocrine function
  adrenal gland and disorders, 267–271
  endocrine pancreas and diabetes mellitus, 257–264
  parathyroid glands, 266–267
  pituitary gland and disorders, 251–257
  principles of endocrine control, 251
  thyroid gland and disorders, 264–266
Endocrine glands, 251
Endocrine pancreas, 257–264
  glucose and energy metabolism, 259
  insulin and glucagon, 258–259
Endocrine pancreas, tumours of, 296
Endocrine system, 197
Endocrine-related bone conditions, 333–334
  aldosterone, 334
  growth hormone, 334
  parathormone, 333–334
  steroid hormones, 333–334
  sympathetic hormones, 334
Endoderm, 228

Endogenous pyrogenic factor, 14
Endolymph, 247
Endometrial cancer, 368
    pathophysiology, 368
    prognosis and management, 368
    signs and symptoms, 368
Endometrial glands, 366
Endometrial tissue, 364
Endometriosis, 364
    management and prognosis, 364
    pathophysiology, 364
    signs and symptoms, 364
Endometrium, 350
Endomysium, 323
Endoplasmic reticulum (ER), 8
Endorphins, 199b
Endosteum, 324
Endothelial cells, 113
Energy metabolism, 259
Entamoeba histolytica, 22, 281, 283
Enteric nervous system, 276
Enterobacter, 180
Enterocytes, 276
    barrier function of, 276
Enterotoxin secretion, 281
Enthesitis, 340
Environmental carcinogens, exposure to,
        78–79
Enzymes, 272–273
Eosinophil accumulation, 183–184
Ependymal cells, 198
Epidemiology, importance of, 3–4, 3b
Epidermal growth factor (EGF), 76–77, 222
Epidermal growth factor receptor (EGFR),
        76–77, 83–84
Epidermis, 375–377
    pilosebaceous unit, 377
Epidermophyton, 380
Epididymis, 354–355
Epididymitis, 371
Epididymoorchitis, 371
Epidural space, 200
Epigenetic control, 31
Epilepsy, 219–222
    causes and triggers of, 221
Epileptogenic focus, 219
Epiphyseal plates, 327
Epithelial tissue, 5
    characteristics and function of, 5t
Epithelium, 272–273, 354
Epstein-Barr virus (EBV), 21, 77, 293
ER-negative, 85
ER-positive, 84–85
Erysipelas, 381–382
Erythrocyte sedimentation rate (ESR), 17
Erythrocytes, 6, 111–112, 121b, 125–126
    control of erythrocyte production, 112,
        112f
    count, 121b
    sedimentation, 338
    structure, 121b
    transport oxygen, 120
Erythropoietin, 112, 320
Escherichia coli, 20, 281–282, 309–310
Essential hypertension, 165
Eumelanin, 377
Eustachian tubes, 249
Exogenous steroids, 269–270
Exons, 28
Expansion collapse, 193
Expiratory reserve volume (ERV), 174–175
Expressivity, 33
Extracellular matrix (ECM), 4–6, 4f
Extraglandular symptoms, 105
Extrapulmonary TB, 182

Extrapyramidal pathways, 205
Extrapyramidal tracts, 205
Extrasystoles, 147
Extrinsic asthma, 183
Extrinsic pathway, 113
Exudative AMD. *See* Wet AMD
Eyes, 238–246
    accommodation, 241f
    disorders of anterior eye, 242–244
    glaucoma, 241–242
    normal eye, 238–240
        floaters, 240
        intraocular pressure, 239–240
        lens, 239
        retina, 238–240
    refractive errors, 242
    retinal disorders, 244–246

F

F8 gene, 43
F9 gene, 43
Fabry disease, 41
    genetics, 41
    management and prognosis, 41
    pathophysiology, 41
Facioscapulohumeral dystrophy, 330
Facioscapulohumeral muscular dystrophy,
        330–331
Familial adenomatous polyposis (FAP), 85
Family and personal history, 128
Family studies, 52–53
Fanconi anaemia, 126
Fascicles, 323
FBN1, 44
FBN2, 44
Feedback inhibition and regulation of HPA,
        252–254
Female menopause, 309
Female reproduction, disorders of, 361–369
    developmental and structural
        abnormalities, 361–363
        endometriosis, 364
        uterine prolapse, 364
    disorders of hormonal function, 361–363
    growths and tumours, 365–369
    inflammatory conditions, 364–365
        bartholinitis, 365
        cervicitis, vaginitis and vulvitis, 365
        pelvic inflammatory disease, 365
Female reproductive organs, 348
Female reproductive system, 348–354
    breast, 354
    female reproductive anatomy, 348–350
        ovary, 350
        uterus and uterine cervix, 350
        vagina, 350
        vulva, 350
    female reproductive cycle, 350–354
        hormones and regulation of female
            reproductive cycle, 352–354
Female reproductive tract, 361
Fertilisation, 348
Fetal circulation, 151–152
Fever, 17
Fibres. *See* Muscle cells
Fibrillin, 44
Fibrinogen, 17, 110
Fibrinolysis, 113
Fibroblast growth factor, 345–346
Fibroblasts, 5–6
Fibrocartilage, 6
Fibroids, 366
Fibromuscular tube, 350
Fibrotic tissue, 170–171

Fibrous skeleton, 133
Fibula, 347
Filaggrin, 378
Filtration, 301
Fimbriae, 19
Final common pathway, 113
First order neurones, 235
First-degree AV block, 149, 149f
Fit, 219
Flexorretinaculum, 233
Fluid, 320
    balance, 318
Fluorodeoxyglucose (FDG), 80
FMR1 gene, 41–42
Focal aware seizure, 219–220
Focal impaired awareness seizure, 219–220
Focal seizures, 219–220
Focal to bilateral tonic-clonic seizure,
        220–221
Folic acid, 124
    deficiency, 124
        anaemia, 124
        pathophysiology, 124
Follicle stimulating hormone (FSH), 352
    failure of pituitary gland to secrete,
        361–362
Food allergy, 102
Food poisoning, 282–283
    botulism, 282–283
    microbes cause food poisoning, 282b
Foodstuffs, 272
Foramen ovale, 151–152
Forced expiratory volume in one second
        (FEV_1), 175
Forced vital capacity (FVC), 175, 176f
Fracture healing, factors interfere with,
        346–347, 346f
    displaced, separated, or mobile bone ends,
        347
    infection, 347
    nutritional and lifestyle factors, 347
    poor blood supply, 347
    poor bone health, 347
Fractures, 342–347
    bone fracture and healing, 345–347
    types of fracture, 344–345
        fractures involving an active growth
            plate, 344–345
        pathological fractures, 344
        stress fractures, 344–345
Fragile X mental retardation protein
        (FMRP), 41–42
Fragile X syndrome, 41–42, 42f
    genetics, 41–42
    management and prognosis, 42
    pathophysiology, 42
Frameshift errors, 30
Frontotemporal dementia, 214
    pathophysiology, 214
Fulminant MS, 212
Fungal cells, 21–22
Fungal pathogenicity, mechanisms of, 22
Fungal spores, 189t
Fungi, 21–22

G

G_0 phase, 63
G_1 phase, 63
G_2 phase, 63
Gallbladder, 297–298
Gallstones, 297–298
    cholecystitis, 298
Gamete formation, meiosis and, 56
Gametes, meiosis and production of, 54–59

Gamma aminobutyric acid (GABA), 199b, 215, 217, 221–222, 235
Ganglion cells, 238–239, 242
Gangliosides, 50
Gap junctions, 10
Gas exchange, 172–173
  in lungs and tissues, 173–174, 174f
Gastric cancer, 293–294
  management and prognosis, 294
  pathophysiology, 293–294
    diffuse tumours, 294
    intestinal tumours, 293–294
  signs and symptoms, 294
Gastric epithelial protection, 273–274
Gastric mucosal lining, 273
Gastrin, 273
Gastrinomas, 296
Gastritis, 288
  acute gastritis, 288
  Helicobacter pylori gastritis, 288
Gastro-oesophageal reflux disorder (GORD), 279–280
  Barrett oesophagus, 280
  management and prognosis, 280
  pathophysiology, 279–280
  signs and symptoms, 280
Gastroenteritis, 281–283
  dysentery, 283
  enterotoxin secretion, 281
  food poisoning, 282–283
  invasive organisms, 281–283
Gastrointestinal function
  control of GI motility, 276–277
  GI defences, 278
  GI microbiome, 277–278
  infections and inflammatory conditions of GI tract, 280–292
    appendicitis, 292
    cholera, 283–284
    diverticular disease, 292
    gastritis, 288
    gastroenteritis, 281–283
    hepatitis, 284–288
    inflammatory conditions of small and large intestines, 289–292
    oral infections, 281
    peptic ulcer disease, 288–289
    typhoid fever, 284
  motility disorders, 278–280
    constipation, 278–279
    diarrhoea, 278–280
  neoplasms of GI tract, 292–296
  nutritional and malabsorptive disorders, 296–299
  organs of GI system, 272–278
Gastrointestinal tract (GI tract), 96, 272, 292
Generalised convulsion, 220
Generalised onset tonic-clonic seizure, 220–221
Generalised seizures, 220–221
Genes, 24–32, 312
  disorders, 36–53
  expression, 29–30, 33
  mapping, 26–27
  pairs, 27–28
  profiling, 81
  therapy, 96
  transcription process, 29
Genetics, 24
  chromosomes and abnormalities, 53–54
  DNA, genes, and chromosomes, 24–32
  gene disorders, 36–53
  instability, 70
  mutation, 342
  patterns of inheritance, 32–36

Genital herpes simplex, 360
  pathophysiology, 360
    management and prognosis, 360
Genitourinary tumours, 330
Genome, 24–25
Genotype, 24–25
Genus, 19
Geographical atrophy, 244–245
Germ cell neoplasia in situ (GCIS), 372
Germ layers, 228
Gestational diabetes, 264
Ghent criteria, 45
Ghon foci in TB, 181–182
Gigantism, 255
Gigantism in children and acromegaly in adults, 255–256
  management and prognosis, 256
  pathophysiology, 256
Gingivitis, 281
GLA gene, 41
Glandular cells, 252
Glandular tissue, 251–252
Glaucoma, 241–242
  closed-angle glaucoma, 241–242
    circulation of aqueous humour, 241f
  glaucoma of normal IOP, 242
  management and prognosis, 242
  open-angle glaucoma, 242
  pathophysiology, 242
  signs and symptoms, 242
Gliadin, 298
Glial cells, 6, 198
Glioblastoma, 222, 223f
Gliomas, 222
Global Burden of Disease (GBD), 3–4
β-globin, 52
Globotriaosylceramide, 41
Globulins, 110
Glomerular capillary vasculitis, 307–308
Glomerular disorders, 305–309
  glomerulonephritis, 306–309
Glomerular filtration membrane, 302–303
Glomerular filtration rate (GFR), 303
  autoregulation and GFR, 303–304
    juxtaglomerular apparatus and macula densa, 304
    renal autoregulation, 304
  regulation of, 302–304
Glomerular function, 305–306
Glomerulonephritis (GN), 306–309, 317
  acute glomerulonephritis, 306–308
  chronic glomerulonephritis, 308–309
Glomerulonephropathy, 306
Glomerulus, 301–302, 317
Glucagon, 258–259, 275–276
Glucocorticoids, 331, 334
  and excessive glucocorticoid secretion, 269–270
    functions of cortisol, 269
    hypersecretion of glucocorticoids, 269–270
  therapy, 334, 340
Gluconeogenesis, 259
Glucose, 259
Glucose-6-phospate dehydrogenase (G6PD), 123–124, 124f
Glue cells, 198
Glue ear, 249–250
GLUT-4 transporters, 258
Glutamate, 199b, 215, 217
Gluten, 298
Gluten-containing grains, 299
Glycine, 199b
Glycogen, 352–354
Glycogenesis, 258
Glycolysis, 259

Glycosaminoglycans (GAGs), 4–5, 342
Glycosuria, 260
Golgi apparatus, 8
Gonadotrophin releasing hormone (GnRH), 352
  hypothalamic failure to secrete, 361
Gonorrhoea, 358
  management and prognosis, 358
  pathophysiology, 358
  signs and symptoms, 358
Good nutrition, 321
Goodpasture syndrome, 307
Gout, 341
  management and prognosis, 341
  pathophysiology, 341
  signs and symptoms, 341
Graft, 106
Graft rejection, 108–109
  management and prognosis, 109
  pathophysiology, 108–109
  signs and symptoms, 109
Granulation tissue, 15–16
Granulomas, 96, 181–182
  formation, 16
Graves disease, 265–266
  management and prognosis, 266
  pathophysiology, 265
  signs and symptoms, 265–266
Great arteries, transposition of, 153, 154f
Ground substance, 4
Growth hormone (GH), 334
  deficiency in
    adults, 255
    children, 255
  disorders, 255–256
  excess, 255–256
Growth hormone, 334
GSTM1, 314
Guanine (G), 25
Guardian of genome, 75
Guillain-Barré syndrome, 190, 233
  pathophysiology, 233
  prognosis and management, 234
  signs and symptoms, 234
Gummas, 359
Gut microbiome, 280–281
Gut-associated lymphoid tissue (GALT), 278
Guttate psoriasis, 384
Gyri, 203

H

Haemagglutinin, 180
Haematogenous spread, 74, 340
Haematoma, 345–346
Haematometrocolpos, 361
Haematuria, 314, 316
Haemoglobin (Hb), 49, 111, 112f, 121b
  production, 111–112
Haemoglobin S (HbS), 49
Haemolytic anaemias, 121–124
  pathophysiology, 121
Haemolytic disease of newborn, 108, 109f
Haemolytic transfusion reactions, 107
Haemophilia, 42–43
  genetics, 42–43
  management and prognosis, 43
  pathophysiology, 43
Haemophilia A, 36
Haemopoiesis, 110, 322
Haemorrhage, 227
Haemorrhagic disease of newborn, 130
Haemorrhagic injury, 226
Haemothorax, 193
Hallucinations, 215, 218

Haploid, 53
Hashimoto disease, 266
Hashimoto thyroiditis, 266
  management and prognosis, 266
  pathophysiology, 266
  signs and symptoms, 266
HBB gene, 49
Headache syndromes, 230–233
Healing process, 306–307, 347
Healthcare systems, 1
Healthy bone, 46
Healthy lung tissue, 170f
Heart, 133–157
  cardiac cycle, 135
  cardiac output and stroke volume, 135–137
  conduction abnormalities, 145–150
  congenital heart disease, 151–154
  control of cardiovascular function, 137
  coronary circulation, 134–137
  heart failure, 141–145
  IHD, 137–141
  infective and inflammatory conditions of,
    154–157
  interior of, 133f
  myocardium and conducting system,
    134–135
  valve disorders, 150–151
Heart block, 145, 148–149
Heart failure, 141–145
  causes of, 144–145
  compensatory mechanisms in increased
    cardiac workload, 141–142
  management and prognosis, 145
  pathophysiology, 142–144
Heart rate (HR), 135
Heberden nodules, 338
Hedgehog signalling, 387
Helicobacter pylori, 10, 19–20, 77, 119, 281,
    288–289, 293
Helper T cells (Th cells), 91
Hemidesmosome, 10–11
Henoch-Schönlein purpura, 307
Henrietta Lacks, 68
Hepatic encephalopathy, 285
Hepatitis, 284–288
  alcoholic liver disease, 285–288
  cirrhosis, 285
  viral hepatitis, 285
Hepatitis A virus (HAV), 285
Hepatitis B virus (HBV), 285, 294
Hepatitis C virus (HCV), 285, 294
Hepatitis D virus (HDV), 285
Hepatitis E virus (HEV), 285
Hepatocellular carcinoma (HCC), 294–295
  management and prognosis, 295
  pathophysiology, 294
  signs and symptoms, 294–295
Hepatocytes, 275, 285–286
HER2 receptor, 76–77
HER2-negative, 84–85
HER2-positive, 76–77, 84–85
Hereditable kidney cancer, 312
Hereditary angioneurotic oedema (HAE),
    93–94, 94f
  management and prognosis, 94
  pathophysiology, 94
  signs and symptoms, 94
Hereditary haemolytic anaemias, 123–124
Hereditary spherocytosis, 123
Heredity, 79
Herpes simplex (HS), 382
Herpes Simplex Virus (HSV), 360, 382–383
Herpes zoster virus (HZV), 21
Herpesviruses, 21
Heteroplasmy, 32

Heterozygous, 28
HEXA gene, 50
Hexagons, 275
Hiatus hernia, 279
High-fat diets, 78
Hilum, 300
Hippocampus, 203
Histamine, 13–14, 99–101, 199b
Histones, 25
  modification, 31
Hodgkin lymphoma (HL), 118–119, 118b.
    See also Non-hodgkin lymphoma (NHL)
  cervical lymph node swelling in, 119f
  histology of, 118f
  management and prognosis, 118–119
  pathophysiology, 118–119
  signs and symptoms, 118–119
  staging of, 119b
Homo sapiens, 335
Homocystinuria, 43
  genetics, 43
  management and prognosis, 43
  pathophysiology, 43
Homoplasmy, 32
Homozygous, 28
Hormonal function
  disorders of, 361–363
  menstrual disorders, 361–362
  polycystic ovarian syndrome, 362–363
Hormonal imbalances, 167
Hormonal therapies, 364
Hormone replacement therapy, 332
Hormone therapy, 82
Hormones, 251, 272–273, 305
  menstrual cycle, 352–354
  ovarian cycle, 352
  and regulation of female reproductive
    cycle, 352–354
Horseshoe kidney, 314
Host immune response, avoidance of, 69
Human cells, 6, 11
Human chorionic gonadotrophin (hCG), 372
Human cost, 1
Human Genome Project, 25–26
Human immunodeficiency virus (HIV), 18
  infection, 98–99, 98f, 366
  management and prognosis, 99
  pathophysiology, 98
  signs and symptoms, 98–99
Human leukocyte antigen (HLA), 91
  genes, 53
  proteins, 91–92
Human papilloma virus (HPV), 21, 77,
    356–357, 360–361, 366, 382
  HPV-mediated cervical cancer, 371
  management and prognosis, 360–361
  pathophysiology, 360–361
Hunter syndrome, 342
Huntingtin (HTT), 33–34, 33f, 43–44
Huntington disease, 43–44
  genetics, 43
  management and prognosis, 44
  pathophysiology, 44
Hurler syndrome, 342
Hyaline cartilage, 6, 328
Hyaline membrane, 188–190
Hydrocele, 371
Hydrocortisone, 269
Hydronephrosis, 316
5-hydroxytryptophan (5-HT), 14
1,25-hydroxyvitamin D, 333
Hyperaldosteronism, 268–269
  management and prognosis, 269
  primary, 268–269
  secondary, 269

Hyperalgesia, 236–237
Hyperglycaemia, 259, 262, 306
  consequences of, 264
  pathophysiology, 264
  of pregnancy, 264
Hyperinsulinaemia, 363
Hyperkalaemia, 320
Hyperopia, 242
Hyperparathyroidism, 266–267, 333
  primary hyperparathyroidism, 267
  secondary hyperparathyroidism, 267
Hyperperfusion, 319–320
Hyperphosphataemia, 320
Hyperplasia, 65–66, 67f, 79
Hyperprolactinaemia, 256–257
  management and prognosis, 257
  pathophysiology, 256–257
  signs and symptoms, 257
Hypersecretion of glucocorticoids, 269–270
Hypersensitivity, 99–109
  mechanisms of, 100f
  types of, 99–101
Hypertension, 48, 165–167, 305, 308
  classification of, 165–167
    pathophysiology, 166
  and DM, 166
  and inflammation, 166
  management and prognosis, 167
Hypertension-induced atherosclerosis, 308–309
Hyperthyroidism, 265–266
  graves disease, 265–266
Hypertrophy, 65, 67f
Hyperuricaemia, 341
Hypoparathyroidism, 267
Hypopituitarism, 255
Hypothalamic-pituitary axis (HPA), 251–255
  feedback inhibition and regulation of
    HPA, 252–254
  neural connection, 252
  vascular connection, 252
Hypothalamus, 202–203, 352
Hypothyroidism, 266
  Hashimoto thyroiditis, 266
Hypovolaemic shock, 161–165
Hypoxia, 69, 191, 226

I

Iatrogenic disease, 3
Ibuprofen, 304
Idiopathic AF, 146
Idiopathic disease, 3
Idiopathic pulmonary fibrosis, 189–190
Imaging, 80
Immobility, 127
Immortality, 68–70
Immune cells, 211–212
Immune complex, 92
  mediated hypersensitivity, 101
Immune mediated skin blistering disorders,
    384–386
  bullous pemphigoid, 384–385
  pemphigus vulgaris, 385
  toxic epidermal necrolysis, 385–386
Immune mediators, release of, 163
Immune system, 277
Immunity
  B cells and, 92
  disorders of
    hypersensitivity, 99–109
    immunodeficiency, 92–99
  T cells and, 91–92
Immunodeficiency, 79, 92–99
Immunoglobulin (Ig), 91
  function of five classes of, 94t

Immunological defence in CNS, 207
Immunological surveillance, 90
Immunologically mediated haemolysis, 123
Immunosuppression, 80
Immunotherapy, 82
Impetigo, 382
Inborn errors of metabolism (IEMs), 38
Incomplete penetrance, 33
Increased pulmonary blood flow, 191
Incretins, 259
Incus, 247
Indigestible inflammatory agents, presence
    of, 16
Infant respiratory distress syndrome,
    188–189
Infarcted muscle, 141
Infections, 77, 79, 249, 347
    cellular and tissue response to, 11–23
    and inflammatory conditions, 242–244
        conjunctivitis, 242
        trachoma, 242–244
    and inflammatory conditions, 309–312
        pyelonephritis, 311–312
        risk factors for urinary tract infection,
            310f
        urethritis and cystitis, 309–312
    pathogenicity and, 17–23
Infective arthritis, 340
    haematogenous spread, 340
    pathophysiology, 340
    traumatic infection, 340
Infective endocarditis, 154–155
    management and prognosis, 155
    pathophysiology, 155
    signs and symptoms, 155
Infective labyrinthitis, 250
Inferior endocardial cushions, 152
Infestations, 381
    lice, 381
    scabies, 381
Inflammation, 79
Inflammatory bowel disease, 289–292
    Crohn disease, 290–291
    ulcerative colitis, 291–292
Inflammatory effusion, 195
Inflammatory myopathy, 331
Inflammatory response, 11–17, 12f, 307
    chronic inflammation, 16
    indications of systemic inflammation,
        16–17
    main events of acute inflammatory
        response, 11–16
Influenza, 179–180
    management and prognosis, 180
    pathophysiology, 180
    signs and symptoms, 180
Infraspinatus, 344
Inheritance
    autosomal inheritance, 33–35
    patterns of, 32–36, 32f
    sex-linked inheritance, 35–36
Inherited coagulation deficiencies, 129–130
Inherited disorders, 33, 314
    polycystic kidney disease, 314
Inhibiting hormones, 252
Initiating mutation, 77
Initiation, 30, 30f
Initiators, 77
Injury, cellular and tissue response to, 11–23
Innate immunity, 88–91
Inner ear, 247–248
    disorders, 250
        labyrinthitis, 250
        Ménière's disease, 250
    vestibular apparatus, 247–248

Insertions, 37–38, 53
Inspiratory reserve volume (IRV), 174–175
Insulin, 166, 258–259
    receptors, 258
    release, 258–259
    resistance, 263–264, 363
Insulin growth factor-1 (IGF-1), 78
Insulin growth factors (IGFs), 255
Integrins, 10–11
Interleukin-1 (IL-1), 14, 79
Interleukin-10 (IL-10), 80
Interleukin-2 (IL-2), 14
Interleukin-8, 14
Interleukins (ILs), 14
Intermediate filaments, 9
Intermittent claudication, 159
International Agency for Research on Cancer
    (IARC), 62
International Federation of Gynecology
    and Obstetrics system (FIGO system),
    367
Interstitial cystitis, 310
Interstitial lung disease (ILD), 189–190
    connective tissue disorders associated with,
        189t
    drugs associated with, 190b
    inhaled irritants associated with, 189t
    management and prognosis, 190
    pathophysiology, 190
    signs and symptoms, 190
Intestinal bacteria, 292
Intestinal pseudo-obstruction, 280
    management and prognosis, 280
    pathophysiology, 280
    signs and symptoms, 280
Intestinal tumours, 293–294
Intracellular organelles, 6–9
Intracellular pathogens, 19–20
Intracranial haemorrhage, 227–228
Intracranial pressure (ICP), 201–202
Intraocular pressure (IOP), 239–241
Intrinsic asthma, 183
Intrinsic factor (IF), 124
Intrinsic pathway, 113
Introns, 28
Invasive breast cancers, classification of,
    84–85
Invasive organisms, 281–283
Inversions, 53
Iris-corneal angle, 242
Iron
    absorption and metabolism, 112
    deficiency anaemia, 125–126
        chronic blood loss, 125
        impaired absorption, 125
        insufficient intake, 125
        management and prognosis, 126
        pathophysiology, 125–126
    in haemoglobin, 111
    supplements, 321
Irritable bowel syndrome (IBS), 289
    pathophysiology, 289
    prognosis and management, 289
    signs and symptoms, 289
Irritant contact dermatitis, 377–378
Ischaemic heart disease (IHD), 137–141,
    144
    acute coronary syndrome, 139–141
    angina, 138–139
    management and prognosis, 141
    pathophysiology, 137–138
    riskfactors, 138, 138b
Ischaemic injury, 226
Ischaemic stroke, 226–227
Isograft, 106–107

J
JAK2 gene, 120
Jaundice, 275
Joint injury, 347
    sprained ankle, 347
Joints, 327–328
    cartilage, 328
    disorders of joints, 336–342
        crystal-induced arthritis, 341–342
        infective arthritis, 340
        juvenile idiopathic arthritis, 339–340
        osteoarthritis, 336–342
        rheumatoid arthritis, 338–339
        spondyloarthritis, 340–341
    mice, 337–338
    structure of synovial joints, 328
Junk DNA, 28–29
Juvenile idiopathic arthritis (JIA), 339–340
Juxtaglomerular apparatus (JGA), 165, 304

K
Karyotyping, 25
Keloid scars, 15
Keratin, 380
Keratinocytes, 375
    stem cell, 387
Kernicterus, 275
Ketoacidosis, 262
Ketogenesis, 262
Kidneys, 300, 305
    pressure, 165
Kininogen, 14
Kinins, 14
Klebsiella, 180, 309, 334
Klinefelter syndrome, 59, 59f
    genetics, 59
    management and prognosis, 59
    pathophysiology, 59
Koebner phenomenon, 384
Kupffer cells, 274, 286
Kyphosis, 336

L
Labia majora, 350
Labia minora, 350
Labyrinth, 247
Labyrinthitis, 250
    infective, 250
Lactase, 276
Lactotrophs, 254–255
Lacunae, 6, 325
Lamellae, 6, 325
Laminin, 4, 377
Langerhans cells, 375
Large intestine, 276
Large neurofibromas, 46
Laser therapy, 380
Latephase response, 184
Lateral epicondylitis, 343
Lectin pathway, 89
Left anterior descending (LAD), 134
Left primary bronchi, 168
Left ventricle, 133
Left ventricle hypertrophies, 143
Left ventricular failure, 142–144
    and lungs, 142–143
    signs and symptoms of, 144, 144f
    and systemic blood supply, 143
Left-sided heart failure, 191
Leigh syndrome, 44
    genetics, 44
    management and prognosis, 44
    pathophysiology, 44

Leiomyomas, 366
Lens, 239
    replacement, 244
Lenticulostriate arteries, 226–227
Lentigo maligna melanoma, 388
Leukaemias, 114–118
Leukocyte adhesion deficiency (LAD), 95
Leukocytes, 6, 114
    emigration, 12
Leukotrienes (LTs), 12–13
Leydig cell tumours, 372
Lice, 381
Lifestyle choices, 78
Limbic system, 203
Lipopolysaccharide (LPS), 17, 162
Liposomes, 40
Lipoxins, 12–13
Liver, 274–275
    biliary tract, 275
    enzyme, 287–288
    liver lobules, 275
    metastases, 73f
Liver cancer, 294–296
    cholangiocarcinoma, 295–296
    colorectal neoplasms, 296
    hepatocellular carcinoma, 294–295
    pancreatic cancers, 296
Lobar pneumonia, 180–181
Lobes, 169
Lobstein's disease, 46
Lobules, 169, 275
Local invasion, 69
LOH genes, 222
Lone AF, 146
Long bone, structure of, 324
Long COVID, 179
Loop of Henle, 300–301
Loose connective tissue, 6
Lordosis, 336
Lordotic curves, 336
Low back pain, 342–343
    management and prognosis, 343
    pathophysiology, 343
Low-density lipoproteins (LDLs), 158
Lower limb arterial disease, 158–159
    management and prognosis, 159
    signs and symptoms, 159
Lower motor neurones (LMN), 205, 214
Lower urinary tract, 305, 311
    ureters, 305
    urinary bladder, 305
Lung cancer, 82–84
    management and prognosis, 83–84
    manifestations of, 83
    risk factors for, 82
    types of, 82–83
Lung tissue, 171
    anatomy of, 169–171
Lungs, 142–143
    collapse, 193–195
    elasticity, 171
    function tests, 190
    gas exchange in, 173–174, 174f
    tumours, 83
    volumes and capacities, 174–175, 175f
Luteinising hormone (LH), 352
    failure of pituitary gland to secrete,
        361–362
Lymph nodes, 313, 371
Lymphatic spread, 73–74
Lymphocytes, 5–6, 91, 311–312, 345–346
Lymphoid follicles, 276
Lymphoid malignancies, 114
Lymphomas, 114, 118–119
Lyonisation, 31

Lysosomes, 8
Lysozyme, 88, 242
Lytic metastases, 335

M

M phase, 63
Macrophages, 5–6, 90–91
Macrovascular complications of diabetes
        mellitus, 262
Macula densa, 304
    chemoreceptors, 304
Magnetic resonance imaging (MRI), 48, 80
Major histocompatibility complex (MHC), 91
    proteins, 91–92
Malabsorptive disorders, 296–299
    cholestasis, 297–298
    coeliac disease, 297–298
    pancreatitis, 296–299
Malar rash, 105
Malaria, 121–123
Malassezia, 377
Male reproduction
    developmental and structural
        abnormalities, 369–370
        cryptorchidism, 369
        phimosis and paraphimosis, 369
        testicular torsion, 369–370
    disorders of, 369–374
    growths and tumours, 371–374
    inflammatory conditions, 370–371
        balanitis, 370
Male reproductive organs, 348
Male reproductive system, 354–356
    male reproductive anatomy, 354–356
        prostate gland, 356
        testes, 355–356
    penis, 356
    regulation of sperm production, 356
Males, 307
Malformations, 1
Malfunctions, 62
Malignant cells, 72
Malignant disease, 127
Malignant melanoma, 66, 388–389
    management and prognosis, 388–389
    pathophysiology, 388–389
    signs and symptoms, 388
Malignant pituitary neoplasms, 255
Malignant pituitary tumours, 255
Malignant skin tumour, 387
Malignant tumours, 66, 70–71, 81, 386–389
    degree of de-differentiation, 71
    differences between benign neoplasms
        and, 70–74, 71f
    growth rates, 70–72
    histological appearance, 72
    local invasiveness, 70
    metastasis, 72
    presence of capsule, 70–71
    UV radiation and skin cancer risk, 386–387
Malleus, 247
Maltase, 276
Man-made carcinogens, 78–79
Marfan syndrome, 44–45, 45f, 336
    genetics, 44
    management and prognosis, 45
    pathophysiology, 44–45
Mast cells, 5–6, 13–14
Mature bone tissue, maintenance of, 327
Mature plaques, 158
Mean cell haemoglobin (MCH), 121b
Mean cell volume (MCV), 121b
Measles, 250
Mechanical injury, 342–347

Mediastinum, 169
Medically important pathogenic
        bacteria, 20
Medically important pathogenic
        viruses, 21
Medulla oblongata, 202
Medullary pyramids, 300
Medulloblastoma, 223
Meiosis, 55–57
    and gamete formation, 56
    meiosis I, 55–56
    meiosis II, 55–56
Melanin, 246, 377
Melanocortin-1 receptor (MC1R), 388
Melanocytes, 246, 375, 377
Membrane attack complex (MAC), 89
Membranous GN, 307
    autoimmune anti-basement membrane
        disease, 307
Membranous nephropathy, 307
Memory T cells, 92
Ménière's disease, 250
    management and prognosis, 250
    pathophysiology, 250
    signs and symptoms, 250
Meninges, 200–202, 200f
Meningioma, 223
Meningitis, 207–208
    causative organisms in, 208b
    pathophysiology, 208
    prognosis and management, 208
    signs and symptoms, 208
Meningocele, 229
Menstrual cycle, 352–354
Menstrual disorders, 361–362
    amenorrhoea, 361–362
Mental health disorders, 215–219
Merlin, 223
MERS-CoV, 179
Mesocortical pathway, 217
Mesoderm, 228
Mesolimbic pathway, 217
Mesothelial cells, 196
Mesothelioma, 195
    management and prognosis, 196
    pathophysiology, 196
    signs and symptoms, 196
Messenger RNA (mRNA), 29
Metabolic adaptability, 69
Metabolism, inborn errors of,
        38, 39t
Metalloproteinases, 338
Metaphase, 54–55
Metaplasia, 65–66, 67f, 185
Metastasis, 69, 72
    routes of, 73–74
    stages of, 72–73
Metastatic lung cancer, 183
Metastatic spread, 72–74
Metatarsophalangeal joints, 343
Metformin, 363
Methotrexate, 340
Microbes, 17–18, 242, 278, 309–310
Microbial colonisation, 309
Microbiome, 277–278
Microglia, 198
Microscopic organisms, 17–18
Microsporum, 380
Microtubules, 9
Microvascular damage, 22–23
Midbrain, 202
Middle cerebral artery, 226
Middle ear, 247–248
Middle East Respiratory Syndrome (MERS),
        179

Migraine, 230–233
  changes in brain associated with migraine, 232f
  management and prognosis, 232–233
  pathophysiology, 231–232
  signs and symptoms, 230–233
  stages of migraine episode, 232f
Migraineur, 230
Migrant populations, disease in, 53
Miliary TB, 182
Mineralocorticoid secretion, disorders of, 268–269
  functions of aldosterone, 268
  hyperaldosteronism, 268–269
Mineralocorticoids, 267–269, 334
  functions of aldosterone, 268
  hyperaldosteronism, 268–269
Mitochondria, 6
Mitochondrial DNA (mtDNA), 32, 44
Mitosis, 54–55
Mitotic spindle, 54–55
Mitral valve disease, 150. *See also* Aortic valve disease
  management and prognosis, 150
  pathophysiology, 150
  signs and symptoms, 150
Mixed nerves, 205
Mobile bone ends, 347
Molecular mimicry, 233
Molluscum contagiosum, 383
Monoamine hypothesis, 216f
Monogenic disorders, principal, 38–52
Mononeuropathy, 233
Monosomy, 53
Morbidity, 3
Mortality, 3
Mosaicism, 56–57
Motor control, 205, 205f, 224–226
  disorders of, 223–226
Motor neurone disease (MND), 214–215, 214f
Moulds, 21–22
mRNA translation, 30
Mucopolysaccharides, 342
Mucopolysaccharidoses, 342
Mucous cells, 272–273
Mucus, 273
Multiple myeloma, 119–120
  management and prognosis, 120
  pathophysiology, 119–120, 120f
  signs and symptoms, 120
Multiple sclerosis (MS), 211–212
  management and prognosis, 212
  pathophysiology, 211–212
  signs and symptoms, 212
Muscle cells, 323
  death, 41
Muscle injury, 344
  muscle strain, 344
  rotator cuff injury, 344
Muscle strain, 344
Muscle tissue, 6, 344
  types of, 8t
Muscle tumours, 330
  rhabdomyosarcoma, 330
Muscular dystrophies, 330–331
  facioscapulohumeral dystrophy, 330
  myotonic dystrophy, 330–331
Muscular pump of calf, 160
Musculoskeletal function
  disorders of bone, 331–336
  disorders of connective tissue, 342
  disorders of joints, 336–342
  skeletal muscle, 322–324, 323f
  sprains, fractures, and mechanical injury, 342–347

Musculoskeletal function (*Continued*)
  bone injury, 344–347
  joint injury, 347
  low back pain, 342–343
  muscle injury, 344
  plantar fasciitis, 343
  tennis elbow, 343
Musculoskeletal system, 322
Musculoskeletal tissues, 342
Myasthenia gravis (MG), 234, 328–330
  management and prognosis, 329–330
  pathophysiology, 328–330
  signs and symptoms, 328–329
MYC gene, 119
Mycelium, 21–22
Mycobacter, 181
Mycobacteria, 19–20, 182
Mycobacterium africanum, 181
Mycobacterium bovis, 181
Mycobacterium tuberculosis, 181
Mycoplasma pneumonia, 233
Myeloma, 119–120
Myelomeningocele, 229
Myeloperoxidase (MPO), 95
Myenteric plexus, 276
Myocardial infarction (MI), 139
  pathophysiology of, 139–140, 140f
  spreading from zone of infarction, 140f
Myocardium, 133
  and conducting system, 134–135
Myoglobin, 112
Myomas, 330
Myometrium, 350
Myopathies, 330–331
  acquired, 331
  muscular dystrophies, 330–331
Myopia, 242
Myotonic dystrophy, 330–331
Myxoedema, 265–266

N

Naming microorganisms, 18–22
*NAT*2, 314
Natural carcinogens, 78–79
Natural killer cells (NK cells), 90, 110–111
Negative symptoms, 218
Neisseria gonorrhoeae, 340, 356–358
Neonatal HSV infection, 360
Neoplasia, 61–62
  assessment and treatment of cancer, 79–82
  cancer epidemiology, 62
  carcinogenesis, 74–79
  cell division and tissue growth, 62–66
  characteristics of, 66–74
    tumour nomenclature, 66–68
    tumour structure, 66–68
  major cancers, 82–86
Neoplasms, 254–255
  gastric cancer, 293–294
  of GI tract, 292–296
  liver cancer, 294–296
  oesophageal cancer, 293
  tumours of salivary glands, 292–296
Neoplastic cells, 70
  properties and behaviours of, 68–70, 68f
Neovascular AMD. *See* Wet AMD
Nephrectomy, 312
Nephroblastoma, 313
  management and prognosis, 313
  pathophysiology, 313
  signs and symptoms, 313
Nephrocalcin, 315

Nephrons, 318
  distal convoluted tubule and collecting duct, 302
  loop of nephron, 302
  parts of, 300–302
  proximal convoluted tubule, 301–302
  renal corpuscles, 301
Nerve cells, 198
Nerve tissue, 251–252
Nerve–nerve communication, 198–199
Nervous system
  cells of, 197–199
  disease, 278–279
Nervous tissue, 6
Neural connection, 252
Neural plate, 228
Neural retina, 238–239
Neural tube, 228
Neural tube defect (NTD), 228–229
  development of, 229f
  risk factors for, 228–229
Neuraminidase, 180
Neurodegenerative disorders, 212–215
Neurofibrillary tangles, 213
Neurofibroma, 45
Neurofibromata of skin, 46
Neurofibromatosis, 45–46, 46f
  genetics, 45
  management and prognosis, 46
  pathophysiology, 45–46
Neurofibromatosis type 2 (NF2), 223
Neurofibromatosis types 1 and 2 (NF1 and NF2), 45
Neurofibromin, 45
Neuromelanin, 377
Neuromuscular disorders, 336
Neuromuscular junction, 207, 323–324
Neuronal pruning, 219
Neuronal support cells, 198
Neurone, general structure of, 198f
Neurones, 6
Neuropathic pain, 234
Neurotransmitters, 198–199
Neurulation, 228
Neutrophils, 12, 90, 123
  rolling, adhesion, and emigration, 13f
Newborns, 40, 108
Nicotinic muscarinic receptors, 323–324
Nigrostriatal pathway, 202, 217, 224–226
Nitrogenous waste products, 320
Nociceptive pain, 234–235
Nodular BCC, 387
Nodular melanoma, 388
Non disjunction, 49
Non-atopic asthma, 183
Non-Hodgkin lymphoma (NHL), 119. *See also* Hodgkin lymphoma (HL)
  management and prognosis, 119
  pathophysiology, 119
  signs and symptoms, 119
Non-pulmonary causes of restrictive lung disease, 190
Non-specific immunity, 88
Non-STEM, 140
Non-steroidal anti-inflammatory drugs (NSAIDs), 86, 288–289, 347
Noninfective meningitis, 208
Nonmelanoma skin cancer (NMSC), 386
Noradrenaline, 199b, 215
Normal growth inhibition signals, failure to respond to, 68–69
Nucleotide, 25
Nucleus, 367
Nutrient-rich foods, 257
Nutritional and lifestyle factors, 347

Nutritional disorders, 296–299
    cholestasis, 297–298
    coeliac disease, 297–298
    pancreatitis, 296–299

O

Obesity, 78, 128, 277, 336–337
Obstruction, 80
Obstruction collapse, 193
Obstructive airways disease, 183–187
Obstructive lung disease, 183–190
Obstructive shock, 162, 164
*OCA*2 gene, 28
Ocular malignant melanoma, 246
    management and prognosis, 246
    pathophysiology, 246
    signs and symptoms, 246
Ocular melanoma, 246
Oesophageal cancer, 293
    management and prognosis, 293
    pathophysiology, 293
    signs and symptoms, 293
Oesophageal sphincter, 272
Oestrogen, 78, 331, 354
    failure of ovary to secrete, 362
    receptors, 368
Oligodendrocytes, 198
Oligodendroglioma, 222
Oncogenes, 64, 76
Opacification, 244
Open pneumothorax, 193–194, 194f
Opsonisation process, 89
Oral infections, 281
    systemic consequences of dental disease, 281
Orchitis, 371
Organ-specific metastasis, 73
Organelles, 6
Organic dusts, 189t
Organisation of granulation tissue, 15
Organrejection, 108–109
Organs of GI system, 272–278
    large intestine and rectum, 276
    liver, 274–275
    pancreas, 275–276
    small intestine, 276
    stomach, 272–274
Orolaryngeal squamous cell cancer, 360
Osmotic pressure, 302–303
Ossification, 326–327
Osteitis deformans, 332
Osteoarthritis (OA), 336–342
    management and prognosis, 338
    pathophysiology, 337–338
    signs and symptoms, 338
Osteoarthrosis, 336–342
Osteoblasts, 325
Osteoclasts, 325, 332
Osteocytes, 5–6
Osteogenesis, 342
Osteogenesis imperfecta (OI), 46, 331
    genetics, 46
    management and prognosis, 46
    pathophysiology, 46
Osteoid, 325
Osteomalacia, 333
    management and prognosis, 333
    pathophysiology, 333
    signs and symptoms, 333
Osteomyelitis, 334–335
    management and prognosis, 335
    pathophysiology, 334–335
    of radius, caused by *Mycobacterium
        tuberculosis*, 335f
    signs and symptoms, 335
Osteons, 325

Osteopenia, 331
Osteoporosis, 331–332
    management and prognosis, 332
    pathophysiology, 331–332
    signs and symptoms, 331–332
Osteoporotic vertebrae, 331–332
Osteoprogenitor cells, 325, 335–336
Osteosarcoma, 335–336
    management and prognosis, 336
    pathophysiology, 335–336
    of proximal tibia, 336f
    signs and symptoms, 336
Otitis externa, 249
Otitis media, 249–250
    management and prognosis, 250
    pathophysiology, 249–250
    signs and symptoms, 250
Otosclerosis, 248–249
Ovarian cancer, 368–369
    management and prognosis, 369
    pathophysiology, 369
    signs and symptoms, 369
Ovarian cycle, 352
Ovarian cysts, 368
    ovarian cancer, 368–369
    and tumours, 368–369
Ovarian follicles, 362
Ovaries, 350
Ovary to secrete oestrogen, failure of, 362
Oxidative burst, 90
Oxygen (O₂), 173
Oxytocin, 252, 257

P

p arm, 25
*p*53 gene, 65, 75, 82–83, 222
Packed cell volume (PCV), 121b
Paget disease, 332, 332f, 343
    management and prognosis, 332
    pathophysiology, 332
    signs and symptoms, 332
Pain, 79, 234
    classification of, 234
    signals
        inhibition of, 236–237
        modulation of, 236
    transmission, 235
Pancreas, 275–276
Pancreatic adenocarcinoma, 296
Pancreatic cancers, 296
    management and prognosis, 296
    pathophysiology, 296
    signs and symptoms, 296
    tumours of endocrine pancreas, 296
Pancreatitis, 296–299
    acute pancreatitis, 296–297
    chronic pancreatitis, 297
Panic disorders, 216–217
    management and prognosis, 217
    pathophysiology, 216–217
    signs and symptoms, 217
Pannus, 339
Papilla, 300
Papillary tumours, 313
Paraesthesias, 234
Paraneoplastic syndromes, 80
Paraphimosis, 369
Paraprotein, 119–120
Parasitic sexually transmitted infections, 361
Parasympathetic branches, 206
Parathormone, 266–267, 327, 333–334
Parathyroid glands, 266–267
    hyperparathyroidism, 266–267
    hypoparathyroidism, 267
    role of parathormone, 266–267

Parathyroid hormone (PTH), 320
Parenchyma, 66–67
Parietal cells, 272–273
Parietal pleura, 171
Parkinson disease (PD), 212, 223–226, 377
    management and prognosis, 225–226
    pathophysiology, 225
    signs and symptoms, 225
Patent ductus arteriosus, 153
Patent foramen ovale, 152–153
Pathogenesis, 1–3
Pathogenicity
    and infection, 17–23
    pathogenic groups, 18–22
Pathology, 1–3
    in rheumatoid disease, 2f
Pathophysiology, 1–3, 22–23
    cellular and tissue response toinjury and
        infection, 11–23
        inflammatory response, 11–17
        pathogenicity and infection, 17–23
    cellular basis of disease, 4–11
    importance of epidemiology, 3–4
    key concepts and definitions of disease,
        1–3
    in rheumatoid disease, 2f
Patisiran, 31
Peak flow (PF), 175
Peanut exposure, 102
Pediculus capitis, 381
Pediculus corporis, 381
Pelvic inflammatory disease (PID), 365
    management and prognosis, 365
    pathophysiology, 365
    signs and symptoms, 365
Pemphigoid disorders, 384
Pemphigus vulgaris, 385
    management and prognosis, 385
    pathophysiology, 385
    signs and symptoms, 385
Penetrance, 33
Penicillin, 155–156, 358
    allergy, 102–103
Penis, 356, 371
    carcinoma of penis, 371
    internal structure of, 356f
Peptic ulcer disease (PUD), 273–274,
        288–289
    management and prognosis, 289
    pathophysiology, 289
    signs and symptoms, 289
Periaqueductal grey matter (PAG), 203, 236
Pericardial effusion, 156
Pericardial rub, 156
Pericarditis, 156–157
    causes of, 156t
    management and prognosis, 156–157
    pathophysiology, 156–157
    signs and symptoms, 156
Pericardium, structure of, 156f
Perimetrium, 350
Perimysium, 323
Periodontitis, 281
Periosteum, 324
Peripheral arterial disease, 158–159
Peripheral nervous system (PNS), 197,
        205–207, 233, 261
    pathophysiology, 233
Peripheral neuropathy, 233
Peripheral resistance, 136–137
Peripheral sensitisation, 236–237
Peripheral vascular disease (PVD), 158–160
Peripheral venous disease, 160
Pernicious anaemia, 124, 125f
Persistent inflammatory agents, presence
    of, 16

Peyer's patches, 278
Phaeochromocytes, 267
Phaeochromocytoma, 267–268
  management and prognosis, 268
  pathophysiology, 268
  signs and symptoms, 268
Phagocytes, 90–91
  deficiencies, 95–96
Phagocytosis, 90, 90f
Phagosome, 90
Phantom limb pain, 235
Phenotype, 24–25
Phenylketonuria (PKU), 47, 47f
  genetics, 47
  management and prognosis, 47
  pathophysiology, 47
Pheomelanin, 377
Philadelphia chromosome, 54, 116
Phimosis, 369
Phosphate stones, 315
Phospholipase A_2 receptor, 307
Physiotherapy, 211
Pia mater, 200
Pick bodies, 214
Pili, 19
Pituitary adenoma, 254–255
Pituitary dwarfism, 255
  management and prognosis, 255
  pathophysiology, 255
Pituitary gland, 255
  and disorders, 251–257
  disorders of anterior pituitary hormones, 255–257
  disorders of posterior pituitary, 257
  failure of pituitary gland to secrete FSH and LH, 361–362
  hypothalamic-pituitary axis, 251–255
  pituitary tumours, 254–255
    malignant pituitary tumours, 255
    pituitary adenoma, 254–255
Plantar fasciitis, 343
  management and prognosis, 343
  pathophysiology, 343
  signs and symptoms, 343
Plaque psoriasis, 384
Plaques, 158, 211
Plasma, 110
  calcium, 333
  proteins, 158
Plasmin, 113
Plasmodium, 121–123
Plasmodium falciparum, 121–123
Plasmodium malariae, 121–123
Plasmodium ovale, 121–123
Plasmodium vivax, 121–123
Platelet-derived growth factor, 345–346
Platelets, 6, 112–113
  deficiency, 116
  dysfunction, 130
  stage, 113
Pleura space, 171–172
Pleural disorders, 192–196
Pleural effusion, 193, 195
  management and prognosis, 195
  pathophysiology, 195
  signs and symptoms, 195
Pleural fluid, 171
Pleural rub, 193
Pleural space, 171–172
Pleurisy, 193
Plexiform neurofibromas, 46
Plicae, 276
Pneumonia, 180–181, 180b, 181f
  management and prognosis, 181
  pathophysiology, 180–181
  signs and symptoms, 181

Pneumothorax, 193–195
  management and prognosis, 195
  signs and symptoms, 194–195
Poliomyelitis (POLIO), 211
  management and prognosis, 211
  pathophysiology, 211
  signs and symptoms, 211
Polycystic kidney disease (PKD), 47–48, 48f, 314
  autosomal dominant polycystic kidney disease, 314
  genetics, 47–48
  management and prognosis, 48
  pathophysiology, 48
Polycystic ovarian syndrome (PCOS), 362–363
  management and prognosis, 363
  pathophysiology, 362–363
  signs and symptoms, 363
Polycystin-1, 47
Polycystin-2, 47
Polycythaemia, 120
Polycythaemia vera, 120–121
  management and prognosis, 121
  pathophysiology, 120–121
  signs and symptoms, 120
Polygenic disorders, 52–53
  polygenic inheritance, 52–53
Polymorphisms, 28
  association between traits and gene, 53
Polyneuropathy, 233
Polysaccharides, 248
Polyuria, 260
Pons, 202
Portal hypertension, 285
Positive chronotropy, 141–142
Positive inotropy, 141–142
Positive symptoms, 218, 234
Positron emission tomography (PET), 80
Post-MI complications, 140–141
Post-renal AKI, 317–318
Post-streptococcal GN, 307
Posterior cerebral artery, 200
Posterior pituitary, 252
  diabetes insipidus, 257
  disorders of, 257
Posterior root, 205
Prader-Willi syndrome, 31
Pre-renal AKI, 317
  acute tubular necrosis in pre-renal AKI, 317f
  loss of glomerular filtration pressure in, 318f
Pregnancy, 127, 167
Preload, 135–136
Premature beats, 147
Premonitory phase, 230–231
Presbycusis, 249
Presbyopia, 242
Pressure effusion, 195
Primary afferents, 235
Primary amenorrhoea, 361
Primary CNS
  lymphoma, 223
  malignancies, 222
Primary hyperparathyroidism, 267
Primary immunodeficiency, 92–93
Primary lateral sclerosis, 215
Primary oocytes, 56
Primary pneumothorax, 194
Primary Raynaud disease, 160
Primary TB, 181
Primaryhypertension, 165–167
Primordial follicles, 350
Procalcitonin, 17
Prodromal event, 219
Prodromal phase, 230–231
Prodromal signs and symptoms, 227–228

Prognosis, 3, 311, 374
Progressive bulbar palsy, 215
Prokaryotes, 6
Prolactin, 256
Prolactin inhibitory hormone (PIH), 256
Prolactinomas, 257
Proliferative erythrocyte disorders, 120–121
Promoters, 77
Prophase, 54–55
Propionibacterium acnes, 378–379
Prostaglandins (PGs), 12–13
Prostate cancer, 373–374
  management and prognosis, 374
  pathophysiology, 373–374
  signs and symptoms, 374
Prostate gland, 356, 372–374
  benign prostatic hyperplasia, 373
  prostate cancer, 373–374
Prostate specific antigen (PSA), 74, 80, 355–356, 373–374
Prostatitis, 370–371
  pathophysiology, 370–371
  signs, symptoms, and management, 371
Proteases, 90
Proteins, 1–2
  assembly, 30
  from DNA to, 25–30
  from gene to protein, 28–30
  in rheumatoid disease, 2f
Proteoglycans, 4–5, 341–342
Prothrombin, 113
Proto-oncogenes, 75–76
Protozoa, 22
Proximal convoluted tubule (PCT), 300–302
Pseudogout, 341–342
  management and prognosis, 342
  pathophysiology, 341–342
Pseudomonas, 309
Pseudomonas aeruginosa, 40, 340
Pseuodomonas, 180
Psoriasis, 340, 383–386
  pathophysiology, 383–384
  prognosis and management, 384
Psoriatic arthritis, 340
Psychosis, 215–216
Pthirus pubis, 381
Pulmonary blood pressure and flow, control of, 172–173, 173f
Pulmonary blood vessels, destruction or obstruction of, 191
Pulmonary circulation, 172–173
Pulmonary embolism (PE), 176, 191–192, 192f
Pulmonary hypertension, 145, 167, 188, 190–191
  in COPD, 185
Pulmonary oedema, 142–143
  in raised pulmonary capillary pressure, 143f
Pulmonary shunting, 176
Pulmonary thromboembolism, 191–192
  management and prognosis, 192
  pathophysiology, 191–192
  signs and symptoms, 192
Pulmonary vascular disease, 190–192
Pulmonary vascular system, 172–173
Punnett square, 33–34, 34f
Purine-rich foods, 316
Purkinje fibres, 135
Pustular psoriasis, 384
Putamen, 224–225
Pyelonephritis, 311–312
  acute pyelonephritis, 311
  chronic pyelonephritis, 311–312
Pyramidal tract, 205
Pyrexia, 17
Pyrogens, 17

Q

q arm, 25
QRS complex, 135

R

Rabies, 209–210
  management and prognosis, 210
  pathophysiology, 210
  rabies infection, 210f
  signs and symptoms, 210
Radiation, 2, 77
  injury, 310
Radiotherapy, 82, 86, 374
Raised ICP, consequences of, 202
Raised intracranial pressure, 201–202
Raynaud disease, 160
Raynaud phenomenon, 104, 160, 160f
  pathophysiology, 160
RB gene, 75–76, 82–83
Re-entry circuits, 145–146, 146f
Reactive arthritis, 340–341
Reactive cells, 118
Reactive oxygen species (ROS), 90, 285–286
Recessive, 28
Reciprocal translocation, 54
Recombination, 56
Rectum, 276
Red blood cells, 111
  disorders, 120–126
Red bone marrow, 110–111
5α-reductase inhibitors, 373
Reed-Sternberg cell, 118
Referred pain, 235, 235f
Reflux nephropathy, 311–312
  features of, 312f
Refractive errors of eye, 242
  hyperopia, 242
  myopia, 242
  presbyopia, 242
Refractive power, 242
Regulatory T cells (T-regs), 69, 92
Relapse, 3
Relapsing pattern, 212
Remission, 3
Remitting pattern, 212
Renal adenomas, 312
Renal agenesis, 314
Renal AKI, 317
Renal autoregulation, 304
Renal blood flow, regulation of, 302–304
Renal cancer, 312–313
  nephroblastoma, 313
  renal cell carcinoma, 312–313
Renal cell carcinoma, 312–313
  management and prognosis, 313
  pathophysiology, 312
  signs and symptoms, 312–313
Renal corpuscles, 301
  glomerulus within Bowman capsule, 302f
Renal disease, 167
Renal function
  acute kidney injury, 316–318
  chronic kidney disease, 318–321
  congenital, inherited, and developmental disorders, 314
  glomerular disorders, 305–309
  gross structure of kidney, 300
  hypertension and kidney, 305
  infections and inflammatory conditions, 309–312
  lower urinary tract, 305
  renal nephron, 300–304
    composition of urine, 304
    parts of nephron, 300–302

Renal function (*Continued*)
    regulation of renal blood flow and glomerular filtration rate, 302–304
  urinary calculi, 314–316
  urinary tract tumours, 312–314
Renal malignancies, 312
Renal osteodystrophy, 320
Renal pelvis, 300
Renal process, 300
Renal tubule necrosis, 311
Renal tumours, 312–313
  renal cancer, 312–313
Renin, 165
Renin-angiotensin system (RAS), 76, 143, 165, 166f, 168, 269, 305, 312
Renin-angiotensin-aldosterone system (RAAS), 178
Repair, 15
Repolarisation, 135, 198
Residual volume, 174
Resistant strains, 18
Respiratory distress of newborn (RDN), 187
Respiratory infections, 249
Respiratory membrane, 172
Respiratory passageways, anatomy of, 168–169, 170f
Respiratory system, 168
  anatomy of, 168–176
  structures of, 169f
Respiratory tract
  infections of, 176–182
  malignancies of, 183
Rest, 313
Restriction point, 63
Restrictive lung disease, 183–190
  musculoskeletal conditions, 190
  neurological conditions, 190
  non-pulmonary causes of, 190
Reticulocyte, 111
Retina, 238–240
  healthy retina viewed through ophthalmoscope, 239f
  rods and cones, 239
  structure, 240f
Retinal blood vessels, 238
Retinal detachment, 244–246
  management and prognosis, 246
  pathophysiology, 246
  signs and symptoms, 246
Retinal disorders, 244–246
  age-related macular degeneration, 244–246
  ocular malignant melanoma, 246
  retinal detachment, 244–246
  retinoblastoma, 246
Retinal neovascularisation, 261
Retinoblastoma, 48, 49f, 246
  genetics, 48
  management and prognosis, 48
  pathophysiology, 48
Retroflexion, 350
Retrograde conduction, 145
Retroversion, 350
Retroviruses, 20–21
Reverse transcriptase, 20–21
Rhabdomyoma, 330
Rhabdomyosarcoma, 330
  management and prognosis, 330
  pathophysiology, 330
  signs and symptoms, 330
Rhesus antigen, 107–108
Rhesus incompatibility, 107–108
Rheumatic fever, 155
Rheumatic heart disease, 155–156, 338
  management and prognosis, 155–156
  pathophysiology, 155–156
  signs and symptoms, 155

Rheumatoid arthritis (RA), 189t, 338–339
  management and prognosis, 339
  pathophysiology, 338–339
  signs and symptoms, 339
Rheumatoid disease, pathology, pathophysiology, and pathogenesis in, 2f
Rheumatoid factors (RFs), 338–339
Ribosomes, 8
Richter's transformation, 117–118
Rickets, 333
  management and prognosis, 333
  pathophysiology, 333
  signs and symptoms, 333
Right coronary artery (RCA), 134
Right primary bronchi, 168
Right ventricular failure, 144
  signs and symptoms of, 144, 144f
Rituximab, 82
RNA, 315
  interference, 31, 32f
  viruses, 177–178
Robertsonian translocation, 54
Rods, 238–239
Root, 169
Rosacea, 379–380
  management and prognosis, 380
  pathophysiology, 379–380
  signs and symptoms, 379–380
Rotator cuff injury, 344, 345f
Rotator cuff muscles, 344
Rough ER, 8
Rubella infection, 250

S

S phase, 63
Saccule, 247–248
Saddle embolus, 191
Salivary glands, 272
  tumours of, 292–296
Salmonella, 281, 340–341
Salmonella typhi, 284
Sarcoidosis, 105–106, 189t
  management and prognosis, 106
  pathophysiology, 106
  signs and symptoms, 106
Sarcomas, 66
Sarcoptes scabiei, 381
SARS-CoV, 178
SARS-CoV-2, 178–179
  management and prognosis, 179
  pathophysiology, 178
  signs and symptoms, 178–179
  structure of, 177f
Satellites, 28–29
  cells, 323
  satellite DNA, 29
Scabies, 381
Scar formation, 15–16
Scar tissue, development of, 15f
Schistosoma haematoblum, 313
Schizophrenia, 217–219
  management and prognosis, 218–219
  MRI brain scans of identical twins showing enlarged ventricles in, 218f
  pathophysiology, 217–219
  positive and negative symptoms of, 218b
  signs and symptoms, 218
Schwann cells, 198
Schwannoma, 223
Scirrhous, 67–68
Scleroderma, 104–105
  management and prognosis, 104–105
  pathophysiology, 104–105
  signs and symptoms, 104
Scleroderma, 322

Scoliosis, 336
Scotoma, 230–231
Scrotum and testes, 371–372
  hydrocele, 371
  testicular cancer, 372
  varicocele, 371–372
Seborrhoeic dermatitis, 377
Sebum, 88, 375, 377
Second order neurone, 235
Second-degree AV block, 149, 149f
Secondary amenorrhoea, 361
Secondary complement deficiencies, 95
Secondary hyperparathyroidism, 267, 333
Secondary hypertension, 165, 167
Secondary immunodeficiency, 93
Secondary lymphocyte-related deficiencies,
    98–99
Secondary oocyte, 56
Secondary phagocyte deficiencies, 96
Secondary pulmonary hypertension, 190–191
  causes of, 191
  pathophysiology, 191
Secondary tumours of bone, 335
Secretion, 301–302
Seed, 73
Seeding, 74
Segments, 169
Seizures, 219–222
  causes and triggers of, 221
  key terminology associated with, 220t
  management and prognosis, 222
  pathophysiology of, 221–222
Selective IgA deficiency, 97
Self-renewal, 69
Semicircular canals, 248
Seminiferous tubules, 355
Seminoma, 372
Senescence, 64–65
Sensation, 250
Sensitisation, 236
Sensorineural deafness, 248–249
  presbycusis, 249
Sensory pain pathways, 235
Sentinel node, 73–74
Sepsis, 22–23, 381
Septa, 169
Septic arthritis, 340
Septic shock, 161–162
Septicaemia, 385
Septum, 133
Serotonin, 14, 112, 199b, 215, 217
Serotonin selective reuptake inhibitors
    (SSRIs), 214–215
Severe acute respiratory syndrome (SARS), 178
Severe combined immunodeficiency (SCID),
    96
  management and prognosis, 96
Sex chromosomes, 25
Sex chromosome disorders, principal, 58–59
Sex steroids, 256
Sex-linked inheritance, 35–36
Sexual reproduction, 348
Sexually transmitted infection (STI), 356–361
  bacterial sexually transmitted infections,
    357–360
  parasitic sexually transmitted infections, 361
  viral sexually transmitted infections,
    360–361
SGLT transporters, 260
Shigella species, 281, 340–341
Shock, 161–165
  compensatory mechanisms in, 162, 162f
  four types of, 161f
  management and prognosis, 165
  metabolic changes in, 164f
  pathophysiology of, 162–163

Shock (Continued)
    increased sympathetic drive, 162–163
    increasedcoagulability of blood, 163
    release of inflammatory and immune
      mediators, 163
    shift from aerobic to anaerobic
      metabolism, 163
  signs and symptoms, 163–165, 164f
Shunting occurs, 185
Sickle cell anaemia, 48–49, 50f
  genetics, 49
  management and prognosis, 49
  pathophysiology, 49
Sickle cell disease, 124
Signs, 3, 23
Silicates, 189t
Sino-atrial node (SA node), 134
Sinus rhythm, 135
Sinusoid walls, 275
Sjögren disease, 105
  management and prognosis, 105
  pathophysiology, 105
  signs and symptoms, 105
Sjögren syndrome, 339
Skeletal muscle, 322–324, 323f
  bone, 324–327
  disorders of skeletal muscle, 328–331
    autoimmune disorders, 328–330
    muscle tumours, 330
    myopathies, 330–331
  joints, 327–328
  neuromuscular junction, 323–324
  skeletal muscle cell structure, 323
  tissue, 344
Skin, 375
  autoimmunity and skin, 383–386
  blood vessel, 379
  inflammatory and infective conditions,
    377–383
    acne, 378–379
    bacterial infections, 381–382
    dermatophyte infections, 380
    eczema, 377–383
    infestations, 381
    rosacea, 379–380
    viral infections, 382–383
  microbiome, 377
  skin lesions in dermatological disorders, 376t
  structure of skin, 375–377
    dermis, 375
    dermo-epidermal junction, 377
    epidermis, 375–377
  symptoms, 41
  tumours of skin, 386–389
Skin cancer risk, 386–387
  field cancerisation, 387
Skip lesions, 291
Sleeping sickness, 22
Slower-than-normal healing, 347
Small and large intestines
  inflammatory bowel disease, 289–292
  inflammatory conditions of, 289–292
  irritable bowel syndrome, 289
Small cell lung cancer, 82
Small intestine, 276
  barrier function of enterocytes, 276
Smoking, 127
Smooth ER, 8
Soil, 73
Solid tumours, 69
Somatic nervous system, 207
Somatic pain, 235
Somatotrophs, 254–255
Special senses
  ear, 246–250
  eye, 238–246

Sperm production, regulation of, 356
Spermatic cords, 354–355
  veins, 371–372
Spermatids, 356
Spermatocytes, 356
Spermatogenesis, 371–372
Spermatogonia, 355–356
Spermatozoa, 356
Spina bifida, 229
Spina bifida occulta, 229
Spinal cord, 203–205, 204f
  cross-section of, 205f
Spinal defects, 231f
Spinal deformity, 336
  kyphosis, 336
  lordosis, 336
  scoliosis, 336
Spinal muscular atrophy, 215
Spinal nerves, 205
Spinal tracts, 204–205
Spirogram, 174–175
Spirograph, 174–175
Splicing, 29
Spondyloarthritides, 340
Spondyloarthritis, 340–341
  ankylosing spondylitis, 340
  psoriatic arthritis, 340
  reactive arthritis, 340–341
Spongy bone, 325–326
Sprains, 342–347
Squames, 375
Squamocolumnar junction, 350
Squamous cell carcinoma (SCC), 82–83, 293,
    313–314, 389
  management and prognosis, 389
  pathophysiology, 389
  signs and symptoms, 389
SRY gene, 36
ST-elevation MI (STEMI), 140
Stable angina, 138–139
Staghorn calculus, 316
Stapes, 247
Staphylococcal scalded skin syndrome, 382
Staphylococcal species, 381
Staphylococci, 281–282
Staphylococcus, 20, 377
Staphylococcus aureus, 19–20, 40, 95–96, 180,
    334, 347, 365, 382
Staphylococcus epidermidis, 19
Starling's law, 135–136
Status epilepticus, 221
Stem cells, 61–62
Steroids, 291
  hormones, 333–334
  replacement, 271
  therapy, 385
Stevens-Johnson syndrome, 385
Stomach, 272–274
  gastric epithelial protection, 273–274
Streptococcal species, 381
Streptococcus, 20
Streptococcus pneumonia, 181
Streptococcus pyogenes, 19, 382
Stress fracture, 344
Stressors, 11
Striatum, 203
Stroke, 226–227
Stroke volume (SV), 135–137
Stroma, 66–67
Struvite, 316
  stones, 316
Sub classification systems, 1
Subarachnoid haemorrhage, 227–228
Subarachnoid space, 200
Subdural space, 200
Subscapularis muscles, 344

Substitution, 37–38
Sucrase, 276
Sudden cardiac death, 140
Sulci, 203
Superficial BCC, 387
Superficial spreading melanoma, 388
Superficial thrombophlebitis, 128
Superior endocardial cushions, 152
Superoxide dismutase, 214
Suppurative infection, 15
Supraspinatus, 344
Surfactant, 169–170
Surgery, 81–82, 127
Swayback, 336
Sympathetic hormones, 334
Sympathetic nervous system, 280
    overactivity, 166
Sympatheticbranches, 206
Symptoms, 3, 23
Synapse, 198–199
Synaptic pruning, 219
Synaptic transmission, 199f
Syndromes, 3
Synovial cavity, 328
Synovial fluid, 328, 342
Synovial joints, structure of, 328
    joint cartilage, 328
Synovial membrane, 328
Syphilis, 358–360
    immunological changes in, 359
    management and prognosis, 359–360
        congenital syphilis, 359–360
    pathophysiology, 359
        primary syphilis, 359
        secondary syphilis, 359
        tertiary syphilis, 359
Systemic hypertension, 145
Systemic immune disorder, 307
Systemic inflammation, indications of, 16–17
Systemic lupus erythematosus (SLE), 105, 189t
    management and prognosis, 105
    pathophysiology, 105
    signs and symptoms, 105
Systemic sclerosis, 104–105, 189t
Systemic vasculitis disorders, 307–308
Systolic pressures, 165

T
T cells, 285, 340–341
    and immunity, 91–92
    and rejection, 108–109
    subtypes, 91–92
T wave, 135
T-helper cells, 181–182
T-lymphocytes, 90–91
    deficiencies, 96–99
Tachycardia, 135
Tamoxifen, 82
Tau protein, 213
Tay-Sachs disease, 49–51, 51f
    genetics, 50
    management and prognosis, 51
    pathophysiology, 50
TDP-43, 214
Tectorial membrane, 248
Telangiectasia, 379–380
Telomerase, 64–65
Telomere, 25
Telophase, 54–55
Template strand, 29
Tennis elbow, 343
Tension headache, 230
Tension pneumothorax, 194–195, 194f
Teratoma, 372
Teres minor, 344

Terminal bouton, 197–198
Terminally differentiated tissue, 61–62
Termination, 30, 30f
Testicular cancer, 372
    pathophysiology, 372
    prognosis and management, 372
    signs and symptom, 372
Testis, 354–356
    testosterone, 355–356
Testosterone, 355–356, 378
Tetanus, 145
Thalamus, 202–203
Thalassaemia A, 51
Thalassaemia B, 51
Thalassaemias, 51–52, 124
    genetics, 51–52
    management and prognosis, 52
    pathophysiology, 52
Third-degree heart block, 149, 149f
Third-order neurones, 235
Thromboembolism, 141, 160
Thrombophilia, 126
Thrombosis, risk factors for, 127–129
Thrombotic disorders, 126–129
Thromboxane (TX), 13
Thymine (T), 25
Thyroglobulin, 264
Thyroid follicles, 264
Thyroid gland and disorders, 264–266
    actions of thyroid hormones, 264–266
    control of thyroid hormone levels, 264–265
    hyperthyroidism, 265–266
    hypothyroidism, 266
Thyroid stimulating hormone (TSH), 252, 264–265
Thyroid transcription factor-1 (TTF-1), 83
Thyroid-binding protein, 110
Thyrotoxicosis, 265
Thyrotrophin releasing hormone (TRH), 252, 264–265
Thyroxine (T_4), 264
Tibia, 347
Tidal volume, 174
Tight junctions, 10
Tinea capitis, 380
Tinea corporis, 380
Tinea cruris, 380
Tinea infections, 380
    tinea capitis, 380
    tinea corporis, 380
    tinea cruris, 380
    tinea pedis, 380
    tinea versicolour, 380
Tinea pedis, 380
Tinea versicolour, 380
Tissue graft, types of, 107f
Tissue growth, 62–66
Tissue growth patterns, adaptive adjustments in, 65–66
Tissue inflammation, 11
Tissue injury, 11–12
Tissue response toinjury and infection, 11–23
Tissue-specific autoantibodies, 306
Tissues, 2, 4–6
    gas exchange in, 173–174, 174f
    rejection, 106–109
Tonic-clonic seizures, 220–221
Tophi, 341
Torsades de pointes, 148
Total lung capacity (TLC), 174
Toxic epidermal necrolysis, 385–386
    management and prognosis, 386
    pathophysiology, 385
    signs and symptoms, 385–386
Trachea, 168

Trachoma, 242–244
    management and prognosis, 244
    pathophysiology, 243–244
Tracts, 204–205
Transcription, 29, 29f
Transferrin, 110, 112
Transforming-growth factor beta (TGFβ), 158
Transient ischaemic attack (TIA), 227
    management and prognosis, 227
    signs and symptoms, 227
Translation, 29–30, 30f
Translocations, 53
Transmission patterns in X-linked inheritance, 36
Transmural, 139
Trastuzumab, 76–77
Trauma, 127
Traumatic infection, 340
Traumatic injury, 340
Treatment approaches, major, 81–82
Treponema pallidum, 358
Tri-iodothyronine (T_3), 264
Trichomonas vaginalis, 22, 361
Trichophyton, 380
Trigeminal neuralgia, 234
Triploid, 53
Trisomy, 53
Trypanosoma brucei, 22
Tuberculosis (TB), 181–182
    management and prognosis, 182
    pathophysiology, 181–182
    signs and symptoms, 182
    stages of, 182f
Tuberculosis, 255
Tubero infundibular pathway, 217
Tumour, Nodal involvement and Metastases (TNM), 81
Tumour biology, 68t
Tumour cells, 69
Tumour grading, 81
Tumour growth factor alpha (TGFα), 69
Tumour growth factor beta (TGFβ), 80
Tumour markers, 80–81
Tumour necrosis factor alpha (TNFα), 15, 79, 383
Tumour necrosis factor inhibitors, 340
Tumour nomenclature, 66–68
Tumour promoter genes, 75–77
Tumour staging, 81
Tumour structure, 66–68, 68f
Tumour suppressor genes, 75–77
Tumours, growths and, 365–369, 371–374
    breast tumours, 368
    ovarian cysts and tumours, 368–369
    penis, 371
    prostate gland, 372–374
    scrotum and testes, 371–372
    uterine tumours, 366–368
Tumours of bone and cartilage, 335–336
    benign tumours, 335
    secondary tumours of bone, 335
Tumours of skin, 386–389
    actinic keratosis and squamous cell carcinoma, 389
    basal cell carcinoma, 387–388
    malignant melanoma, 388–389
    malignant tumours, 386–389
Tunica albuginea, 355
Tunica vaginalis, 355
Tunica vasculosa, 355
Turner syndrome, 59, 314, 362
    genetics, 59
    management and prognosis, 59
    pathophysiology, 59
Twin studies, 52–53
Tympanic duct, 248

Type 1 diabetes mellitus (T1DM), 262–263
 pathophysiology, 263
 prognosis and management, 263
 signs and symptoms, 263
Type 1 pneumocytes, 169
Type 2 diabetes mellitus (T2DM), 85–86,
 263–264
 pathophysiology, 263–264
 prognosis and management, 264
 signs and symptoms, 264
Type I hypersensitivity, 99–101
Type II hypersensitivity, 101
Type III hypersensitivity, 101
Type IV hypersensitivity, 101
Typhoid fever, 284
 management and prognosis, 284
 pathophysiology, 284
 signs and symptoms, 284

U

Ulcerative colitis (UC), 2–3, 278, 291–292
 management and prognosis, 292
 pathophysiology, 292
 signs and symptoms, 292
Ulcers, 289
Ultrasound, 48
 in pregnancy, 59
Ultraviolet B (UVB), 333
Ultraviolet radiation (UV radiation), 377
Uncompensated shock, 165
United States National Kidney Foundation,
 318–319
Unstable angina, 138–139
Upper motor neurones (UMN), 205, 214
Ureterovesicular junction, 305
Ureters, 305
 ureterovesicular junction, 305
Urethritis, 309–312
 management and prognosis, 310
 non–infection-related cystitis, 310
 pathophysiology, 310
 signs and symptoms, 310
Uric acid, 315
 stones, 315
 urinary stones, 316f
Urinary bladder, 305, 309
Urinary calculi, 314–316
 pathophysiology, 315–316
  calcium/phosphate stones, 315
  cystine stones, 316
  struvite stones, 316
  uric acid stones, 315
 prognosis and management, 316
 signs and symptoms, 316
Urinary stones, 315
Urinary system, 312, 314
Urinary tract infection (UTI), 309, 315
Urinary tract tumours, 312–314
 bladder cancer, 313–314
 renal tumours, 312–313
Urine, 300, 304
 composition of, 304
Urolithiasis, 314
Urothelial cancers, 314
Urothelium, 305
Uterine cervix, 350
 positions of uterus, 350
 squamocolumnar junction and cervical
  erosion, 350
Uterine fibroids, 366
 management and prognosis, 366
 pathophysiology, 366
 signs and symptoms, 366
Uterine polyps, 366
Uterine prolapse, 364

Uterine tumours, 366–368
 adenomyosis, 366
 cervical cancer, 366–368
 endometrial cancer, 368
 uterine fibroids, 366
 uterine polyps, 366
Uterus, 350
 positions of uterus, 350
 squamocolumnar Junction and Cervical
  Erosion, 350
 structure of, 351f
Utricle, 247–248
UV radiation, 386–387, 389
 field cancerisation, 387

V

Vagina, 350
Vaginitis, 365
Valve disorders, 150–151
Variable expressivity, 33
Variable immunodeficiency, 97
Variable segments, 92
Varicocele, 371–372
Varicose veins, 160, 161f
Vasa vasorum, 157
Vascular connection, 252
 anterior pituitary hormones, functions,
  and hypothalamic hormones, 254b
Vascular dementia, 213–214
 pathophysiology, 213–214
Vascular endothelial growth factor (VEGF),
 69, 244–245
Vascular network, 157
Vascular stage, 113
Vasodilation, 304
Venous stasis, 127
Venous thrombosis, 127–129
 of left leg, 128f
 pathophysiology, 128
 risk factors for thrombosis, 127–129
 treatment and prognosis, 129
Ventilation-perfusion matching, 175–176, 176f
Ventilation-perfusion mismatch, 176
Ventilation/perfusion (V/Q), 175–176
Ventral tegmental area (VTA), 202, 217
Ventricular arrhythmias, 147–148
Ventricular ectopic beats, 147
 management and prognosis, 147
 pathophysiology, 147
 signs and symptoms, 147
Ventricular fibrillation (VF), 147–148
Ventricular rupture, 140–141
Ventricular septal defect, 152
Ventricular tachycardia (VT), 147–148
 management and prognosis, 148
 pathophysiology, 147–148
Verruca vulgaris, 382
Vertebral column, 336
Vestibular apparatus, 247–248
 cochlea, 248
 semicircular canals, 248
Vestibular duct, 248
VHL gene, 313
Vibrio cholerae, 283–284
Viral hepatitis, 285
 pathophysiology, 285
  HBC, 285
  HBV, 285
 signs and symptoms, 285
Viral infections, 382–383
 herpes simplex virus, 382–383
 molluscum contagiosum, 383
 viral warts, 382
Viral labyrinthitis, 250
Viral pathogenicity, mechanisms of, 21

Viral respiratory tract infections, 176–180
Viral sexually transmitted infections, 357–358
 genital herpes simplex, 360
 human papilloma virus, 360–361
Viral warts, 382
Virchow's triad, 128
Virulence, 18–19
Viruses, 20–21, 360
Visceral pain, 235
Visceral pleura, 171
Vision, 238
Vital capacity (VC), 174
Vitamin B$_{12}$, 124
 deficiency, 124
Vitamin C, 327
Vitamin D, 266, 320, 327, 333
Vitamin k deficiency, 130–131
 management and prognosis, 131
 pathophysiology, 130–131
 signs and symptoms, 131
Vitreous humour, 239–240
Volkmann's canals, 325
Voluntary nervous system, 207
Von Recklinghausen's disease, 45
Von Willebrand disease (vWD), 129–130
 management and prognosis, 130
 pathophysiology, 130
Von Willebrand factor (vWF), 129–130
Vulva, 348, 350
Vulvitis, 365

W

Water molecules, 169–170
Weight loss, 79–80
Wet AMD, 245
White blood cells
 arrival and activity, 12
 malignancies of, 114–120
Wilms tumour, 313
Wolff-Parkinson-White syndrome (WPW),
 145, 149–150, 150f
 management and prognosis, 150
 pathophysiology, 149–150
World Health Assembly, 244
World Health Organisation (WHO), 1, 125,
 132, 178–179, 211
Worsening hypertension, 309

X

X chromosomes, 25, 31, 35–36
X-linked agammaglobulinaemia,
 97–98
 management and prognosis, 98
X-linked disorder, 36
X-linked dominant pattern, 42
X-linked inheritance, transmission patterns
 in, 36, 37f
X-rays, 80
X-SCID, 96

Y

Y chromosome, 25, 36
Yeasts, 21–22
Yersinia species, 340–341
Yolk sac tumours, 372

Z

Zollinger-Ellison syndrome, 279, 296
Zoonotic infection, 177
Zygote, 27–28